ORAL RADIOLOGY

Principles and Interpretation

ORAL RADIOLOGY

Principles and Interpretation

PAUL W. GOAZ, B.S., D.D.S., S.M.
Professor Emeritus, Department of Diagnostic Sciences
Baylor College of Dentistry
Dallas, Texas

STUART C. WHITE, D.D.S., Ph.D.
Professor, Section of Oral Radiology
University of California School of Dentistry
Center for the Health Sciences
Los Angeles, California

THIRD EDITION
with 1125 illustrations

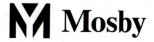

St. Louis Baltimore Boston Chicago London Madrid Philadelphia Sydney Toronto

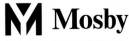

Dedicated to Publishing Excellence

Publisher: George Stamathis
Editor-in-Chief: Don Ladig
Executive Editor: Linda L. Duncan
Developmental Editor: Melba Steube
Project Manager: John Rogers
Production Editor: George B. Stericker, Jr.
Designer: Julie Taugner
Manufacturing Supervisor: John Babrick
Cover Design: Renee Duenow
Production: Graphic World Publishing Services

THIRD EDITION
Copyright © 1994 by Mosby–Year Book, Inc.

Previous editions copyrighted 1982, 1987

Printed in the United States of America
Composition by Graphic World, Inc.
Printing/binding by Maple Vail Book Mfg. Group

Mosby–Year Book, Inc.
11830 Westline Industrial Drive
St. Louis, Missouri 63146

Library of Congress Cataloging in Publication Data

Goaz, Paul W., 1922-
     Oral radiology : principles and interpretation / Paul W. Goaz,
Stuart C. White.—3rd ed.
          p.   cm.
     Includes bibliographical references and index.
     ISBN 0-8016-7295-3
     1. Teeth—Radiography. 2. Jaws—Radiography. 3. Mouth—
Radiography. I. White, Stuart C. II. Title.
     [DNLM: 1. Radiography, Dental.   WN 230 G573o 1994]
     RK309.G63   1994
     617.6'07572—dc20
     DNLM/DLC
     for Library of Congress   93-45306
                                                             CIP

94 95 96 97 98 / 9 8 7 6 5 4 3 2 1

Contributors

KATHRYN A. ATCHISON, D.D.S., M.P.H.

Associate Professor
Section of Public Health Dentistry
University of California School of Dentistry
Center for the Health Sciences
Los Angeles, California

BYRON W. BENSON, D.D.S., M.S.

Associate Professor
Division of Oral and Maxillofacial Radiology
Department of Diagnostic Sciences
Baylor College of Dentistry
Dallas, Texas

DONALD D. BLASCHKE, D.D.S.

Private Practice, Oral and Maxillofacial Surgery
Lompoc, California;
Formerly Assistant Professor and Director of
Maxillofacial Radiology
Section of Oral Radiology
University of California School of Dentistry
Center for the Health Sciences
Los Angeles, California

ALLAN G. FARMAN, B.D.S., Ph.D. (Odont), M.B.A.

Professor of Radiology and Imaging Sciences
University of Louisville
School of Dentistry
Louisville, Kentucky

NEIL L. FREDERIKSEN, D.D.S., Ph.D.

Director, Oral and Maxillofacial Radiology
Department of Diagnostic Sciences
Baylor College of Dentistry
Dallas, Texas

BARTON M. GRATT, D.D.S.

Professor and Chairman
Section of Oral Radiology
University of California School of Dentistry
Center for the Health Sciences
Los Angeles, California

ALAN G. LURIE, D.D.S., Ph.D.

Professor and Head
Division of Oral and Maxillofacial Radiology
University of Connecticut
School of Dental Medicine
Farmington, Connecticut

STEPHEN R. MATTESON, D.D.S.

Professor and Chairman
Department of Dental Diagnostic Science
University of Texas Health Science Center
Dental School
San Antonio, Texas

CHRISTOFFEL J. NORTJÉ, B.Ch.D., Ph.D.

Professor and Head
Department of Maxillofacial Radiology
University of Stellenbosch
Faculty of Dentistry
Tygerberg, Cape, Republic of South Africa

ALBERT G. RICHARDS, B.S.E., M.S.

Emeritus Professor
Department of Oral Diagnosis and Radiology
University of Michigan School of Dentistry
Ann Arbor, Michigan

ABDUL H. SHAWKAT, B.D.S., D.M.D., M.Sc.

Formerly Professor and Coordinator
Section of Oral Radiology
University of Louisville School of Dentistry
Louisville, Kentucky

VIVEK SHETTY, D.D.S., Dr.Med.Dent.

Adjunct Assistant Professor
Section of Oral and Maxillofacial Surgery
University of California School of Dentistry
Center for the Health Sciences
Los Angeles, California

ROBERT E. WOOD, D.D.S., M.Sc.

Assistant Professor
Department of Dentistry
University of Toronto
Faculty of Dentistry;
Ontario Cancer Institute/Princess Margaret
    Hospital
Toronto, Ontario, Canada

To our wives and daughters

VIRGINIA

Mary

Karan

LIZA

Heather

Kelly

"Man erblickt nur, was man schon weiss und versteht."

Johann Wolfgang von Goethe

Gespräche mit F.V. Müller

24.4.1819

One recognizes only what one already knows and understands.

Preface

Of course, the ideas in this book are not ours.

We pinched them from William Morgan and Jean Nolet.

We snatched them from Nikola Tesla.

We appropriated them from Otto von Guerike.

We plagiarized them from Michael Faraday.

We borrowed them from William Conrad Röntgen.

We copied them from Otto Walkoff.

We pillaged them from William J. Morton.

We pirated them from Sir Joseph John Thomson.

We apprehended them from W.D. Coolidge.

We stole them from Howard R. Raper.

We swiped them from William Herbert Rollins.

We scrounged them from C. Edmund Kells.

We pilfered them from Clyde Snook.

We lifted them from Franklin W. McCormack.

We took them from Niels Bohr,

   and many more.

If you don't like these sources, who would you use?

   —with apologies to Dale Carnegie.

Time has a way of slipping by. It is hard to realize that some 15 years have passed since we first seriously contemplated composing a book on oral radiology. We visualized a book that would explain the fundamental physical principles involved in the generation of x rays and the application of radiation physics, as well as a book that would be clinically relevant and practical to use; all this in as comprehensive and comprehendible manner as possible, without sacrificing accuracy for simplicity. This, in spite of the fact that we were aware that some teachers were and still are complaining that there is too much emphasis being placed on the physical basis of radiology, while others believed it was being gracefully neglected for an overemphasis on interpretation. Despite this difference of opinion, we believed there could be no question that the better the dentist's training in physics and photochemistry, the more intelligently he or she can use his or her equipment; and the better the orientation in clinical pathology, the better the interpretation of images. It is now 11 years since the publication of the first edition and the looming of the third, so it seems appropriate to thank the many people who recommended and purchased the first and second editions, making the third possible.

This revised edition includes new material and some changes in emphasis.

Three chapters that appeared in the second edition have been discontinued, two have been rewritten by new authors, and three new chapters have been added. The remaining chapters that appeared in the second edition have been carefully scrutinized, and information that others and we, grudgingly, finally considered less relevant in this setting has been removed, making the book more straightforward for the uninitiated student. These changes were adopted as the result of comments, direct and indirect, mostly from students, and secondarily from teachers and colleagues, as well as the changing emphasis in dentistry.

Three chapters were omitted from the third edition: Origins of Dental Radiology, Quality Assurance, and Endodontic Radiology. The decision to eliminate these resulted from the perpetual prompting by the publisher to reduce the number of pages and the feeling that we could succumb to this bane of all authors and emphasize the principles in these lost chapters at other appropriate points in the text. The exception to this was the material of historical interest that had to give way to the seeming, current, flagging concern for tradition.

The chapters on Radiation Biology and Radiation Safety and Protection have been carefully evaluated and updated since radiobiology is assuming an ever greater significance. This is not only because of the dentist's concern for patients, staff, and himself or herself, but it is increasingly frequent that he or she has to interact with more and more patients concerned about the effects of diagnostic radiation on their well-being as well as with government bureaus with newly found "teeth" that regulate the use of ionizing radiation.

New authors have rewritten the chapters Specialized Radiographic Techniques and Principles of Radiographic Interpretation.

There have been explosive developments in diagnostic radiology with the exploitation of CT, MRI, ultrasound, and nuclear medicine since the advent of the first edition. Fortunately, there has developed a rapid application of these techniques to aid in the diagnosis of oral and head and neck diseases since the second edition. In view of this happenstance, Specialized Radiographic Techniques has been extensively rewritten to include new information, and all appropriate oral and maxillofacial applications are so adequately described that the dentist will have little difficulty in requesting and interpreting the image that is most suitable to a particular circumstance.

Notwithstanding, the increased attention to the application of the more sophisticated imaging techniques, conventional radiography, from "bitewings to lateral jaws," is still emphasized as a necessary and often sufficient method for the diagnosis of most dental problems.

The current chapter Principles of Radiographic Interpretation, in contrast to the more or less theoretical approach used in the first two editions, has a more practical and clinical approach that we anticipate will make the discussions more relevant for the student and practicing dentist.

In this edition, we are introducing discussions of Guidelines for Prescribing Dental Radiographs, Radiographic Infection Control, Salivary Gland Radiology, and Implant Radiology. The inclusion of these topics is a reflection of the changing face of dentistry.

The admonitions and recommendations set forth in the chapter Guidelines for Prescribing Dental Radiographs stresses the fact that dental radiographs are indicated only when there is high probability that they will detect disease and/or demonstrate its extent as suggested by the history, clinical examination, or a specific test. In consequence, this chapter describes the radiographic examinations that are the most likely to provide evidence that will affect the treatment plan.

The infection control procedures described in Radiographic Infection Control were designed to interfere with the development of disease by impeding the spread of the disease agents. In the radiology area, this can be achieved only by reducing contamination, and since efforts to prevent contamination are never completely successful, by subsequently killing or reducing the number of microbes to a safe level (disinfection) after contamination has occurred. An effective and easily executed series of procedures is described.

The absence of a chapter on Salivary Gland Radiology from the first two editions was responsible for our most frequent criticism. Currently, discussion of the uses of the standard sialogram and the new imaging techniques for the diagnosis of congenital, traumatic, neoplastic and inflammatory salivary gland diseases are included in this edition.

The success of a dental implant is dependent upon the amount and quality of the bone and the location of significant anatomical landmarks in the jaws. Radiographic techniques that will usually provide this information are described in the last chapter, Implant Radiology.

Clearly this is a collaborative effort and is a testament to the dedication of all the collaborators. We are especially grateful for their unselfish commitment to teaching and their generosity of spirit. Significant credit must also be given to the many people at Mosby who eased the mechanics of publication.

I (PWG) wish to recognize the contribution of my chairman, William H. Binnie, who quietly provides encouragement and support for all reasonable academic pursuits. I am likewise indebted to my associates, Neil Frederiksen, who wrote two chapters for this edition, and Byron "Pete" Benson, who took the responsibility for another. It is also important to emphasize my appreciation for their continuous, constructive critique of the book. And I (SCW) wish to especially recognize the contributions of my colleague, Barton Gratt, who over the years has provided innumerable valuable suggestions regarding this book and has also contributed three chapters. Finally, we both thank our students and fellow teachers for their support and constructive criticisms that have helped to make writing this book a thoroughly happy adventure.

PAUL W. GOAZ
STUART C. WHITE

Contents

SECTION FIVE ▪ RADIOGRAPHIC INTERPRETATION OF PATHOLOGY

ORAL RADIOLOGY

Principles and Interpretation

1

in collaboration with ALBERT G. RICHARDS

Radiation Physics

COMPOSITION OF MATTER

Matter is the substance of which all physical things are composed. It is anything that occupies space and has inertia. It has mass and can exert force or be acted on by a force. It occurs in three states—solid, liquid, or gas—and may be divided into elements or compounds. *Elements* are accumulations of a single species of atom. *Compounds* are recurring units of atoms in a definite arrangement, with at least two of the atoms different. *Atoms,* which are the fundamental unit of any particular element, cannot be subdivided by ordinary chemical methods but may be broken down into smaller (subatomic) particles by special high-energy techniques. Although more than 100 *subatomic particles* have been described, it is only the so-called "fundamental" particles (electrons, protons, and neutrons) that are of greatest interest in radiology.

Atomic structure

The importance of an understanding of atomic structure relates to the fact that generation, emission, and absorption of radiation occur at the subatomic level. An appreciation of atomic physics is essential for comprehending the uses, operation, and interpretation of the images produced by such diagnostic systems as nuclear medicine, positron emission tomography, magnetic resonance imaging, and diagnostic ultrasound. (See Chapter 13.)

To describe the structure of an atom and its components, it has been customary since the time of the ancient Greeks (500 BC) to use models. The model used to depict the atom depends to some extent on the event to be described. The phenomena associated with radiology employ one of the simplest: that proposed by Niels Bohr in 1913. This is the quantum mechanical model. It quantizes or separates the atom into its finite parts. Bohr conceived the atom to be like a miniature solar system, at the center of which is the nucleus, analogous to our sun. Revolving around this nucleus at high speeds, analogous to the planets orbiting about the sun, are one or more particles. For most purposes, in all atoms except hydrogen, the nucleus can be considered to consist of two kinds of (subatomic) particles, protons and neutrons, collectively called *nucleons.* A single proton constitutes the nucleus of the hydrogen atom. The particles that orbit the nucleus are electrons. All electrons are alike, as are all protons and all neutrons, regardless of the atoms with which they are associated.

Subatomic particles

The primary subatomic particles of interest to diagnostic radiology are electrons, protons, and neutrons. Each of these has unique characteristics. The electron carries an electrical *charge* designated as -1, the proton a charge of $+1$, and the neutron no charge at all. The *mass* of an electron at rest is about 9.1×10^{-28} gram. In contrast, the mass of a proton is 1.67×10^{-24} gram, which is 1838 times that of an electron. The mass of a neutron is 1.68×10^{-24} gram, 1841 times heavier than an electron and thus slightly heavier than a proton. Most of an atom's mass consists of protons and neutrons concentrated in the nucleus. The nucleus contributes only a small fraction of the atom's total size (about $1/100,000$), most of which is contributed by the cloud of electrons orbiting it (and this cloud is mostly empty space).

The nucleus has a positive charge equal to the number of protons in its nucleus. Because any atom in its ground state is electrically neutral, the total number of protons and electrons it carries must be equal. The number of protons in the nucleus, and similarly the number and arrangement of the orbital electrons, determines the identity of an element—

1

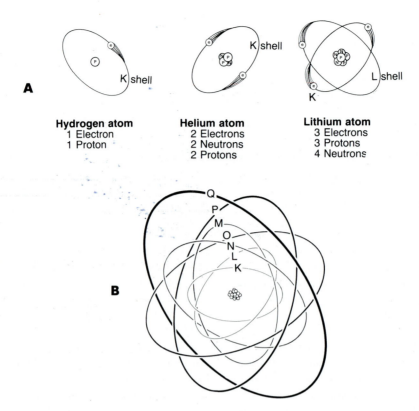

FIG. 1-1. A, Atomic structure of hydrogen, helium, and lithium showing orbiting electrons surrounding neutrons and protons in the nucleus. **B,** Atom showing the structure and identification of electron shells around the nucleus.

makes it distinctly different from all other atoms. The distinguishing number of protons (positive charges) in the nucleus of an atom is its *atomic number* which is designated by the symbol Z. Consequently, each species of atom has a definitive atomic number, a corresponding number of orbital electrons, and as a result its own unique chemical and physical properties. As indicated above, nearly the entire mass of the atom consists of the protons and neutrons in the nucleus. The total number of protons and neutrons in an atom's nucleus is its *atomic mass*, designated by the symbol A.

Figure 1-1, *A,* illustrates Bohr's concept, with the stylized structure of three atoms. The paths of the electrons are drawn as sharply defined orbits to facilitate graphic representation of the generation of x rays and their interaction with matter. This is an oversimplification, since in reality the orbit should be represented by broad parameters defining a space in which there is a significant probability that the electron will be found. The orbits, or shells, lie at defined distances from the nucleus and are identified by letter (Fig. 1-1, *B*). The innermost shell is the K shell, and the next in order are the

L, M, N, O, P, and Q shells. The shells also have numbers for identification: 1 for the K shell, 2 for the L shell, and so on. These are the *principal quantum numbers,* represented by the letter *n*. No known atom has more than seven shells. Only two electrons may occupy the K shell, with increasingly larger numbers in the outer shells. The maximum number of electrons in a given shell is $(2n)^2$, the principal quantum number.

The electrostatic attraction between a positively charged nucleus and its negatively charged electrons balances the centrifugal force of the rapidly revolving electrons and maintains them in their orbits about the nucleus. Consequently, the amount of energy required to remove an electron from a given shell must exceed the electrostatic force of attraction between it and the nucleus. This is called the *binding energy* of the electron and is specific for each shell of each atom. Electrons in the K shell of a given atom have the greatest binding energy, because they are closest to the nucleus. The binding energy of the electrons in each successive shell decreases as the shells are located progressively farther from the nucleus. To move an electron from a specific orbit to another orbit farther from the nucleus, energy must be supplied in an amount equal to the difference in binding energies between the two orbits. The displaced electron in the orbit further from the nucleus has absorbed energy and is now considered to be at a higher energy level, as are all the electrons in this orbit and all orbits that are located progressively further from the nucleus. The magnitude of the energy level at each successive orbit is defined as the difference between the binding energy of the orbit and the binding energy of the atom's K orbit. In contrast, when an electron is moved from an orbit at a higher energy level to one at a lower energy level, closer to the nucleus, energy must be lost and is given up in the form of electromagnetic radiation. (See "Characteristic Radiation," p. 14.)

The coulomb force of attraction pulling electrons toward the nucleus decreases with the square of the distance between the electron and the nucleus. (This inverse square law applies to all electromagnetic radiation, magnetic fields, and gravity.) Also, the opposing or balancing centripetal force that keeps electrons in orbit decreases inversely with the radius of the orbit. The K-shell electrons, as well as the electrons in any shell, of large (high-Z) atoms have greater binding energies than those in a comparable shell of smaller (low-Z) atoms. This is because large atoms have higher atomic numbers and therefore more positive charges in their nuclei. These nuclei pull the orbital electrons deep within the atomic structure, forming tight clusters of particles that are more difficult to penetrate with an x ray.

Ionization

When the number of orbiting electrons in an atom is equal to the number of protons in its nucleus, the atom is electrically neutral. When an electrically neutral atom loses an electron, it becomes a *positive* ion, and the free electron a *negative ion*. The process of converting atoms to ions is termed "ionization." Ionization also occurs by the addition of an electron to an electrically neutral atom, resulting in a *negative ion*. Note that protons do not participate in this process; their role is entirely passive. Heating or interactions (collisions) with high-energy x rays or particles such as protons can remove electrons from an atom. To cause such ionization, by whatever means, requires sufficient energy to overcome the electrostatic force binding the electrons to the nucleus.

The electrons in the inner shells—K, L, and M—are so tightly bound to the nucleus that only x rays, gamma rays, and high-energy particles can remove them. In contrast, the electrons in the outer shells have such low binding energies that they can be easily displaced by photons of lower energy (e.g., ultraviolet or visible light).

NATURE OF RADIATION

Radiation is the transmission of *energy* through space and matter. There are two types: particulate and electromagnetic.

Particulate radiation

Particulate radiation consists of atomic nuclei or subatomic particles moving at high velocity. Alpha rays, beta rays, and cathode rays are examples of particulate radiation. *Alpha rays* are high-speed doubly ionized helium nuclei. They consist of two protons and two neutrons with an atomic number of 2 and an atomic mass of 4. On acquisition of two electrons, they become neutral helium atoms. Because of their double charge and heavy mass, they densely ionize the atoms of matter through which they pass. Accordingly, they quickly give up their energy and penetrate only a few microns of body tissue. (An ordinary sheet of paper absorbs them.) Alpha particles result from the decay of many radioactive elements. Beta and cathode rays are both high-speed electrons that if emitted by radioactive nuclei are *beta* rays and if originating in some manufactured device (e.g., an x-ray tube) are *cathode rays*. Beta particles ejected from the radioactive nuclei travel at speeds approaching that of light. Those that constitute the current in an x-ray tube travel at about half the speed of light. The very high-speed beta particles from radionuclides are able to penetrate matter to a greater depth than the alpha particles, up to a maximum of 1.5 cm in tissue. This deeper penetration occurs because beta particles are smaller and lighter and carry a single negative charge; therefore, they have a much lower probability of interacting with matter than alpha particles have. They ionize matter through which they penetrate much less readily than alpha particles do.

The capacity of particulate radiation to ionize atoms depends on its kinetic energy (mass × velocity) and its charge. The rate of loss of energy from a particle as it moves along its track through matter (tissue) is its *linear energy transfer* (LET). A particle loses kinetic energy at each ionization; the greater its physical size and charge and the lower its velocity, the greater will be its LET. For example, alpha particles (with their large charge and low velocity) are densely ionizing and, as a consequence, lose kinetic energy rapidly and have short paths. Beta particles (that are much less densely ionizing because of their lighter mass and lower charge) have a lower LET than alpha particles and are thus more penetrating of tissue.

These differences in properties of alpha and beta particles will result in different patterns of ionization caused by the particles. Beta particles will ionize atoms relatively sparsely, up to a depth of a few centimeters. Alpha particles, however, ionize atoms very densely, but only in the most superficial layer. Accordingly, alpha particles transfer more energy in a given path length and are more damaging per unit dose. Beta particles are used in radiation therapy for treatment of skin lesions.

Electromagnetic radiation

Electromagnetic radiation is the movement of energy through space as a combination of electric and magnetic fields. It is generated when the velocity of an electrically charged particle is altered (Fig. 1-2). Gamma rays, x rays, ultraviolet rays, visible light, infrared radiation (heat), television, radar, microwaves, and radio waves are all examples of electromagnetic radiation (Fig. 1-3). Gamma rays are photons in the same energy range as x rays but they originate in the nucleus of radioactive atoms. X rays, however, originate from the interaction of electrons and atoms. The types

of radiation in this spectrum are also ionizing or nonionizing depending on their energy. If there is sufficient energy associated with the radiation to remove orbital electrons from the atoms in the irradiated matter, the radiation is ionizing.

An explanation of the characteristics of electromagnetic radiation requires a dualistic theory. Some of the properties of electromagnetic radiation

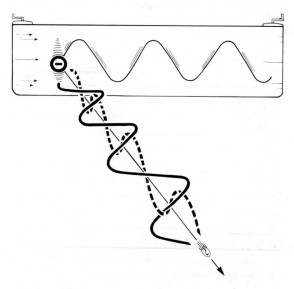

FIG. 1-2. A vibrating negatively charged particle generates electromagnetic radiation. Oscillations of the particle are being traced on a strip recorder and can be seen to be of equal frequency with the frequency of electromagnetic waves produced.

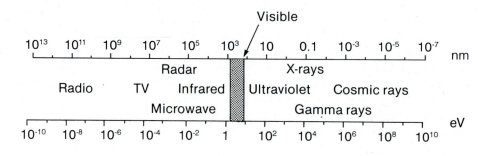

FIG. 1-3. Electromagnetic spectrum showing the relationship between wavelength, photon energy, and physical properties of various portions of the spectrum. Note that the photons with shorter wavelengths have higher energy. Photons used in dental radiography have a wavelength of 0.1 to 0.001 nm.

are best expressed in terms of *wave theory;* others are more successfully described on the basis of *quantum theory,* which depicts electromagnetic radiation as small bundles of energy called *quanta* or photons. Wave theory is more useful for considering radiation in bulk when millions of quanta are being examined, as in diffraction experiments. Quantum theory is more convenient when individual particles are being considered. Consequently, radiation is assumed to be either a wave or a beam of quanta depending on which assumption is more appropriate for the problem at hand.

The *wave theory* of electromagnetic radiation maintains that radiation is propagated in the form of waves, not unlike the waves resulting from a disturbance in water. Such waves consist of electrical and magnetic energy (Fig. 1-4). The electrical and magnetic fields are in planes at right angles to one another and are oscillating perpendicular to the direction of motion. They move forward in much the same way as a ripple moves over the surface of water. All electromagnetic waves travel at the velocity of light, 3.0×10^8 meters per second in a vacuum. Waves of all kinds exhibit the properties of wavelength (λ) and frequency (ν). For electromagnetic radiation, wavelength and frequency are related by the formula:

$$\lambda \times \nu = c = 3 \times 10^8 \text{ meters/second}$$

where λ is in meters and ν is in cycles per second (Hertz). Wave theory best accounts for the results of experiments dealing with refraction, reflection, diffraction, interference, and polarization.

In contrast, the *quantum theory* assumes that the transfer of energy by electromagnetic radiation occurs not as waves but as a flux of *quanta* or *photons* (finite bundles of energy). Each photon travels at the speed of light and contains a specific amount of energy. The unit of photon energy is the *electron volt* (eV) (Fig. 1-5). The relationship between wavelength and photon energy is

$$E = hc/\lambda$$

where E is energy in kiloelectron volts (keV), h is Planck's constant (6.25×10^{34} joule-seconds*), c is the velocity of light, and λ is wavelength in nanometers. This expression may be simplified to

$$E = 1.24/\lambda$$

---

*The joule is the fundamental unit of work. Work is measured as the product of a force exerted and the distance through which it acts. The fundamental unit of force is the newton (1 newton = 0.225 lb), and the unit of distance is the meter, so the unit of work is the newton-meter. (This unit is called a joule.) Another useful unit is the erg (1 erg = 10^{-7} joule).

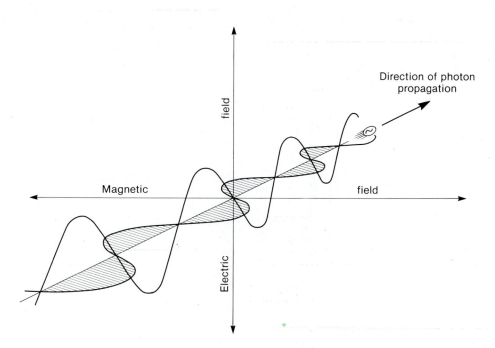

Direction of photon propagation

Magnetic   field

field

Electric

FIG. 1-4. Electromagnetic radiation illustrating the electric and magnetic fields associated with a photon.

The quantum theory of radiation has been more successful in correlating experimental data on the interaction of radiation with atoms, the photoelectric effect, and the production of line spectra and x rays.

THE X-RAY MACHINE

An x-ray machine consists of an x-ray tube, its power supply, and the tube head, support arm, and control panel. The x-ray tube is positioned within the tube head along with some components of the power supply (Fig. 1-6). Often the tube is recessed

to improve the quality of the radiographic image. (See Chapter 6.)

The basic apparatus for generating x rays, the x-ray tube, is composed of a *cathode*, consisting of a focusing cup and filament that serve as a source of electrons, and an *anode*, consisting of a copper stem and target at which the beam of high-speed electrons is directed (Fig. 1-7). The cathode and target lie within an evacuated glass envelope or tube. Electrons from the filament strike the target and produce x rays. For the x-ray tube to function, an electrical power supply is necessary to establish high potentials across the tube and accelerate the electrons to very high speeds. Various circuits control the flow of electrons and tube performance (Fig. 1-8).

Cathode

The cathode (Fig. 1-7) of an x-ray tube consists of the filament and the focusing cup.

The *filament* is the source of electrons within the x-ray tube. It is a coil of tungsten wire about 0.2 cm in diameter and 1 cm or less in length. It is mounted on two stiff wires that support it and carry the electric current. These two mounting wires lead through the glass envelope to serve as a connection to both the high- and the low-voltage electrical sources. The filament is heated to incandescence through a range of temperatures by varying the voltage (around 10 volts) across the filament from a step-down transformer (*A* in Fig. 1-8) in a low-

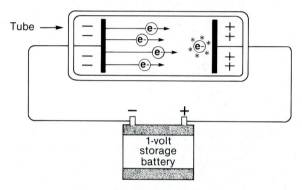

FIG. 1-5. An electron volt is the amount of energy acquired by one electron accelerating through a potential difference of 1 volt (1.602×10^{-19} joule).

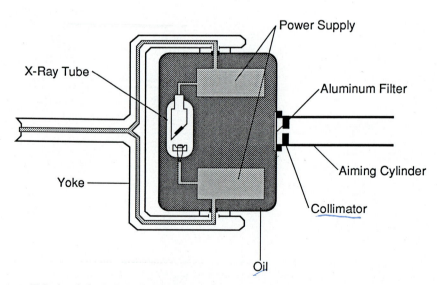

FIG. 1-6. Tube head (including the recessed x-ray tube), components of the power supply, and the oil that conducts heat away from the x-ray tube.

voltage circuit. The hot filament emits electrons that are separated from the outer orbits of the tungsten atoms at a rate proportional to the temperature of the filament by a process called *thermionic emission*. The electrons lost by the filament form a cloud or space charge about the filament and are replaced in the tungsten atoms from the negative side of the high-voltage circuit, which is connected to one of the filament mounting wires. A *milliampere* (mA) control (*B* in Fig. 1-8) provides for fine adjustment of the voltage across the filament and, in turn, the flow of heating current through it. The milliampere control thereby modulates the quantity of electrons

that the filament emits, which in effect controls the *tube current* (flow of electrons through the tube, measured by the milliammeter, *H* in Fig. 1-8). Thus the tube current and, hence, the number of x-ray photons subsequently produced are a function of the filament temperature.

The filament lies in a *focusing cup* (Figs. 1-7 and 1-9, *A*), a negatively charged concave reflector of molybdenum. The focusing cup electrostatically focuses the electrons emitted by the incandescent filament into a narrow beam directed at a small rectangular area on the anode called the *focal spot* (Figs. 1-7 and 1-9, *B*). The electrons move in this

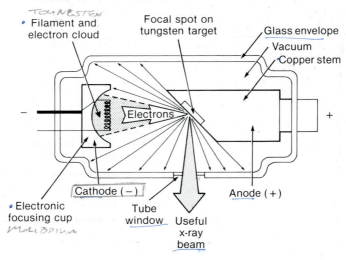

FIG. 1-7. X-ray tube with the major components labeled.

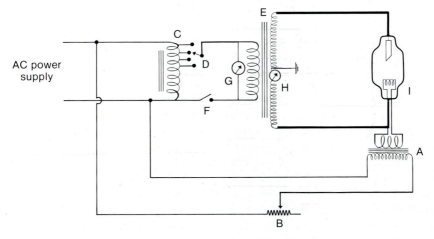

FIG. 1-8. Dental x-ray machine circuitry with the major components labeled. *A*, Filament step-down transformer; *B*, filament current control (mA switch); *C*, autotransformer; *D*, kVp selector dial (switch); *E*, high-voltage transformer; *F*, x-ray timer (switch); *G*, tube voltage indicator (voltmeter); *H*, tube current indicator (ammeter); *I*, x-ray tube.

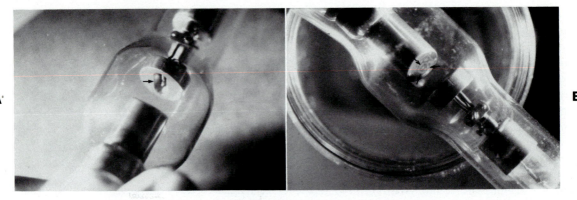

FIG. 1-9. A, Focusing cup *(arrow)* containing a filament in the cathode of the tube from a dental x-ray machine. **B,** Focal spot (area) *(arrows)* on the target of the tube. Note how the size and shape of the focal area approximate those of the focusing cup.

direction because of the strong electrical field between the negatively charged cathode and the positively charged anode. The negatively charged cathode repels electrons while the positively charged anode attracts them. The x-ray tube is evacuated as completely as possible to facilitate the movement of these high-speed electrons. The vacuum prevents collision of the moving electrons with gas molecules, which would significantly reduce their speed. It also prevents oxidation and "burnout" of the filament.

Anode

The anode consists of a tungsten target and copper stem (Fig. 1-7). The purpose of the *target* in an x-ray tube is to convert the kinetic energy of the electrons generated from the filament into x-ray photons. The target is made of tungsten, because tungsten represents an effective compromise between the many features of an ideal target material. It has a high atomic number, high melting point, and low vapor pressure at the working temperatures of an x-ray tube. A target material with a *high atomic number* is best because it is more efficient for the production of x rays. A *high melting point* is also important for the target material. In practice, only a very small amount of the kinetic energy of electrons coming from the filament generates x-ray photons when the electrons impact at the focal spot of the target. Since the production of x rays is a rather inefficient process, with more than 99% of the electron kinetic energy converted to heat, the requirement for a high melting point is clear. Although the atomic number of tungsten (74) is lower than that of several other metals (e.g.,

platinum [78] and lead [82]), its melting point (3370° C) is much higher. The *low vapor pressure* of tungsten at high temperatures also precludes compromising the vacuum in the tube at the high operating temperatures.

Since the thermal conductivity of tungsten is relatively low, the tungsten target (usually a button of metal) is frequently embedded in a large block of copper. Copper, a good *thermal conductor,* dissipates heat from the tungsten and copper anode, thus reducing the risk of target melting. In addition, an insulating oil may circulate between the glass envelope and the protective tube housing. This type of anode is a *stationary anode*.

Radiographic image quality is dependent in part on the size of the target. The sharpness of the radiographic image increases as the size of the radiation source, the *focal spot,* decreases. (See Chapter 6.) The focal spot is the area on the target to which the focusing cup directs the electrons from the filament. The heat generated per unit target area, however, becomes greater as the focal spot decreases in size. To take advantage of the smaller focal spot and yet distribute the electrons over the surface of a larger target, the target is placed at an angle with respect to the electron beam (Fig. 1-10). The projection of the focal spot perpendicular to the electron beam (the *effective focal spot*) will be smaller than the actual size of the focal spot. In practice, the target is inclined about 20 degrees with respect to the central ray of the x-ray beam. This provides the geometry to cause the effective focal spot to be almost 1 × 1 mm as opposed to the actual focal spot, which is about 1 × 3 mm. The effect is a small apparent source of x rays and

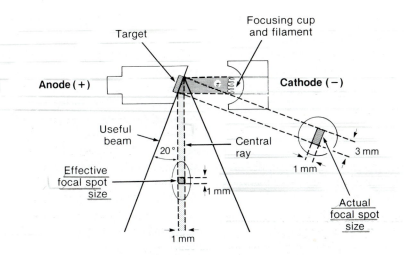

FIG. 1-10. Line focus principle showing that because of the oblique angle of the target to the central ray, the effective focal spot size is much smaller than the actual focal spot size.

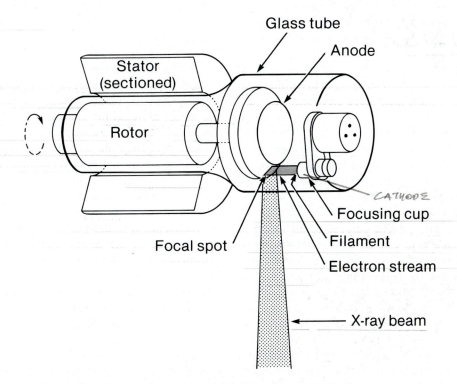

FIG. 1-11. X-ray tube with a rotating anode, which allows heat at the focal spot to spread out over a large surface area.

an increase in sharpness of the image (Fig. 6-2) with a larger actual focal spot for heat dissipation.

Another method of dissipating the heat from a small focal spot is to use a *rotating anode*. In this case the tungsten target is in the form of a beveled disk that rotates when the tube is in operation (Fig. 1-11). As a result of this arrangement the electrons strike successive areas of the target as it rotates, which effectively widens the focal spot by an amount corresponding to the circumference of the beveled disk and distributes the heat over this expanded area. As a consequence small focal spots can be used with currents of 100 to 500 mA, 10 to 50 times that possible with the stationary target.

The target and the rotor (armature) of the motor lie within the x-ray tube, and the stator coils (which drive the rotor at about 3000 rpm) lie outside the tube. Such rotating anodes are not used in conventional dental x-ray machines but may be used in cephalometric units and in medical x-ray machines.

Power supply

The primary functions of the power supply are (1) to provide current to heat the x-ray tube filament by use of a step-down transformer and (2) to generate a potential difference between the anode and the cathode by use of a high-voltage transformer. These transformers and the x-ray tube lie within an electrically grounded metal housing called the *head* of the x-ray machine. An electrical insulating material, usually oil, surrounds the transformers.

The *filament step-down transformer* (A in Fig. 1-8) reduces the voltage of the incoming alternating current (AC) to about 10 volts. Its operation is regulated by the filament current control (mA switch) (B in Fig. 1-8), which adjusts the current flow through the low-voltage circuit and thus the filament. This, in turn, regulates the heating of the filament and thus the quantity of electrons emitted. The electrons emitted by the filament travel to the anode and constitute the *tube current*. The mA setting on the filament current control refers to the intensity of the tube current, which is measured by the ammeter (H in Fig. 1-8).

The output of the *autotransformer* (C in Fig. 1-8) is regulated by the kVp (kilovolts peak) selector dial (D in Fig. 1-8). The kVp dial selects varying voltages from different levels on the autotransformer and applies them across the primary of the high-voltage transformer. It therefore controls the voltage between the anode and cathode of the x-ray tube. The *high-voltage transformer* (E in Fig. 1-8) provides the high voltage required by the x-ray tube to accelerate the electrons and generate x rays. It accomplishes this by boosting the voltage of the incoming line current to 60 to 100 kV and the energy of the electrons passing through the tube to 60 to 100 keV.

Because the line current is AC (60 cycles per second), the polarity of the x-ray tube will alternate at the same frequency. When the polarity of the alternating high voltage applied across the tube is such that the target anode is positive and the filament is negative, the electrons around the filament accelerate toward the positive target and current flows through the tube. As the tube voltage is increased, the speed of the electrons toward the anode increases. Because the line voltage is variable, the voltage potential between the anode and cathode will also vary. The kVp selector dial setting (D in Fig. 1-8) controls the peak kilovoltage across the tube (I in Fig. 1-8) during one cycle. When the electrons strike the focal spot of the target, some of their energy converts to x-ray photons. X rays are produced at the target with greatest efficiency when the voltage applied across the tube is high. Thus the intensity of x-ray pulses will tend to be sharply peaked at the center of each cycle (Fig. 1-12, C). During the following half (or negative half) of the cycle, the polarity of the AC reverses and the filament becomes positive and the target negative (Fig. 1-12, B). At these times the electrons stay in the vicinity of the filament and do not flow across the gap between the two elements of the tube. This reverse voltage is called *inverse voltage* or *reverse bias* (Fig. 1-12, B). No x rays are generated during this half of the voltage cycle (Fig. 1-12, C). Thus, when an x-ray tube is powered with 60-cycle alternating current, 60 pulses of x-rays are generated each second, each having a duration of $1/120$ second. This type of power supply circuitry, in which the alternating high voltage is applied directly across the x-ray tube, limits x ray production to half the AC cycle. It is called *self-* or *half-wave rectified*. Almost all conventional dental x-ray machines are self-rectified.

A tube energized with a self-rectifying power supply must not be operated for extended periods or the temperature of the target may reach the point of electronic emission. If the target gets that hot, there is the possibility that during the negative half-cycle the inverse voltage will drive electrons to the filament, causing it to overheat and melt. The glass envelope may also be damaged if the electrons are driven in the wrong direction by the reverse bias on the tube.

Recently some dental x-ray equipment manufacturers have replaced the conventional 60-cycle AC high-voltage current to the x-ray tube with a direct-current high-voltage supply. This is achieved with a step-up transformer amplifying the current from a generator that produces an AC current with a frequency of 800 or more cycles per second instead of the customary 60 cycles. The minor ripples in the high-voltage current from the transformer are then electronically smoothed to provide essentially a direct current to the x-ray tube. The effect is that the energy of the x-ray beam produced by the direct current x-ray machine is higher than that

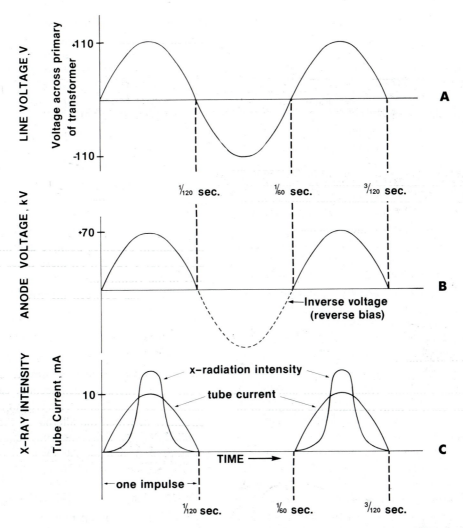

FIG. 1-12. A, Sixty-cycle AC line voltage at a primary transformer. **B,** Voltage at the anode varies up to the kVp setting (70 in this case). **C,** The intensity of radiation produced at the anode increases as the anode voltage increases. (Modified from Johns HE, Cunningham JR: *The physics of radiology,* ed 3, Springfield Ill, 1969, Charles C Thomas.)

from a conventional half-wave rectified machine operated at the same high voltage. This is because the lower-energy (nondiagnostic) x rays, which are produced as the voltage across the x-ray tube increases to a maximum and then decreases during the voltage cycle in the half-wave rectified machine, are eliminated. (See "Production of X Rays," on p. 12.)

Timer

A device to control the x-ray exposure time (*F* in Fig. 1-8) is in the primary circuit of the high-voltage supply. The timer completes the circuit with the high-voltage transformer. This controls the time that the high voltage is applied to the tube and thus the time during which tube current flows

and x rays are produced. Before the high voltage is applied across the tube, however, the filament must be at the proper operating temperature to assure an adequate rate of electron emission. It is not practical to subject the filament to prolonged heating at normal operating current. As in an ordinary light bulb, the filament will remain intact for only a certain number of hours. The higher the temperature is maintained, the shorter the life of the filament will be. Most x-ray tube failures result from filament burnout. To minimize filament burnout, the timing circuit first sends a current through the filament for about half a second to bring it to the proper operating temperature; once the filament is heated, a time delay switch applies power to the high-voltage circuit. In some circuit designs there is a continuous low-level current passing through the filament that maintains it at a safe low temperature. In this case the delay to preheat the filament before each exposure is even shorter.

Some x-ray machine timers are calibrated in fractions of seconds and in whole numbers of seconds. The time intervals on other timers are expressed as numbers of impulses per exposure (1, 2, 3, 4). The number of impulses divided by 60 (the frequency of the power source) gives the exposure time in fractions of a second. Thus 30 impulses is equivalent to a half-second exposure.

Tube rating and duty cycle

Although few x-ray tubes fail as a result of damage to the target from overheating, the operating parameters recommended for tubes are based on the capacity of their anodes to accumulate heat without melting the target. Each x-ray tube comes with rating specifications that describe the operating limits of the tube. These specifications are on *tube rating charts*. They describe in a graphlike presentation the maximum safe intervals (seconds) that the tube can be energized for a range of voltages (kVp) and filament current (mA) values. These tube ratings generally do not impose any restrictions on tube use for dental periapical radiography. If a dental x-ray unit is to be used for both intraoral and extraoral exposures, however, it is recommended that the tube rating chart be mounted by the machine. This will remind the technician that the tube's operation has limits.

The *duty cycle* relates to how frequently successive exposures can be made. The heat buildup at the anode is measured in heat units defined by the equation: Heat units* (HU) = kVp × mA × seconds (watt-sec), an actual measure of energy. The heat storage capacity for the anodes of various diagnostic tubes ranges from 100,000 to perhaps 250,000 HU. Because of this heat generated at the anode, the interval between successive exposures must be long enough for its dissipation. This characteristic is a function of the size of the anode and the method used to cool it. The cooling characteristics of anodes are described by the maximum number of heat units it can store without damage and the heat dissipation rate, which can be determined from the cooling curves provided by the manufacturer for each tube.

Careful attention not to exceed the tube rating

---

*One heat unit equals about 0.24 calorie.

and duty cycle of a particular x-ray machine will maximize tube life and performance. In general, an increase in kVp has less wearing effect on the anode than does an increase in mA or time for the production of the same film density.

PRODUCTION OF X RAYS

The kinetic energy of electrons in the tube current converts to x-ray photons at the focal spot of an x-ray tube by the formation of bremsstrahlung and characteristic radiation.

Bremsstrahlung radiation

Bremsstrahlung interactions, the primary source of x-ray photons from an x-ray tube, is produced by the sudden stopping or braking of high-speed electrons at the target. This process occurs, first, through the acceleration of electrons to a high velocity by a high voltage applied across the gap between the filament and the target of the x-ray tube. When the electrons interact with the electrostatic field of target nuclei or collide with nuclei, their direction of travel is altered. This process of rapidly decelerating the high-speed electron is called *inelastic collision* and gives rise to bremsstrahlung, or braking radiation. Although its mass is small, an electron accelerates to a very high velocity by the high voltage across the tube. This increases its mass, so it acquires appreciable kinetic energy. If a high-speed electron hits the nucleus of a target atom, all its kinetic energy will transform into a single x-ray photon (Fig. 1-13, *A*). The energy of the resultant photon (in units of kiloelectron volts) is numerically equal to the energy of the electron. This, in turn, is equal to the kilovoltage applied across the x-ray tube at the instant (time) of its passage.

Most high-speed electrons, however, have encounters with the atomic nuclei ranging from near to wide misses (Fig. 1-13, *B*). In these interactions the negatively charged high-speed electrons are attracted toward the positively charged nuclei, being deflected from their original paths and losing some of their velocity. This deceleration causes them to lose some kinetic energy, which is given off in the form of photons of electromagnetic radiation with an energy equal to that lost by the deflected electrons. The closer the high-speed electrons come to the nuclei, the greater will be the electrostatic attraction on the electrons. This, in turn, will increase the braking effect and the energy of the resulting photons of bremsstrahlung radiation.

Bremsstrahlung interactions generate photons

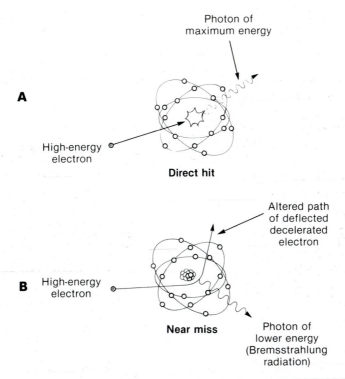

Photon of
maximum energy

A

High-energy
electron

Direct hit

Altered path
of deflected
decelerated
electron

B High-energy
electron

Near miss

Photon of
lower energy
(Bremsstrahlung
radiation)

FIG. 1-13. **A,** Bremsstrahlung radiation is produced by the direct hit of electrons on the nucleus in the target, or **B,** by the passage of electrons near the nucleus, which results in electrons' being deflected and decelerated,

having a *continuous spectrum* of energy. The energy of an x-ray beam may be described by identifying the peak operating voltage, designated kVp (kilovolt peak). A dental x-ray machine operating at a peak voltage of 70,000 volts (70 kVp), for example, applies a fluctuating voltage of up to 70 kVp across the tube. This tube thus produces x-ray photons with energies ranging up to a maximum of almost 70,000 eV (70 keV). The spectrum of the beam can be represented by graphing the relative number of photons in the beam at each energy level. Figure 1-14 demonstrates the continuous spectrum of photon energies produced from an x-ray machine operating at 100 kVp. The reasons for this continuous spectrum are as follows:

1. The continuously varying voltage difference between the target and filament, which is characteristic of half-wave rectification, cause the electrons striking the target to have varying levels of kinetic energy.
2. Most electrons participate in many interactions before all their kinetic energy is expended. As a consequence, an electron will carry differing amounts of energy at the time

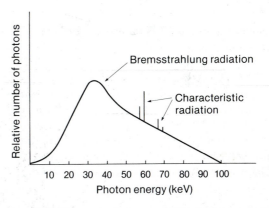

Relative number of photons

Bremsstrahlung radiation

Characteristic
radiation

10 20 30 40 50 60 70 80 90 100
Photon energy (keV)

FIG. 1-14. Spectrum of photons emitted from an x-ray beam generated at 100 kVp. Note the vast preponderance of bremsstrahlung, but with a minor addition of characteristic radiation.

of each interaction with a tungsten atom that results in the generation of an x-ray photon.
3. The bombarding electrons pass at varying distances around tungsten nuclei and are thus deflected to varying extents. As a result, they give up varying amounts of energy in the form of bremsstrahlung photons.

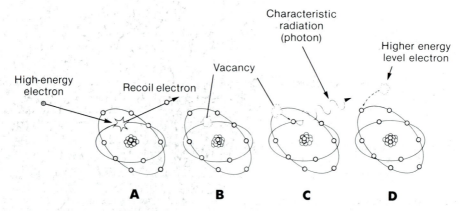

FIG. 1-15. Characteristic radiation. **A,** An incident electron in an inner orbit ejects a photoelectron, creating a vacancy. **B,** This vacancy is filled by an electron from an outer orbit. **C,** A photon is emitted with energy equal to the difference in energy levels between the two orbits. **D,** Electrons from various orbits may be involved, giving rise to other photons. The energies of the photons thus created are characteristic of the target atom.

Characteristic radiation

Characteristic radiation occurs as the result of electronic transition when a bombarding electron of the tube current displaces an electron from a shell of a target (tungsten) atom, thereby ionizing the atom. Another electron in an outer shell of the tungsten atom and at a higher energy level is quickly attracted to the void in the deficient inner shell (Fig. 1-15). When the displaced electron is replaced, a photon is emitted with an energy equivalent to the difference in the two orbital binding energies. Characteristic radiation from the K shell occurs only above 70 kVp with a tungsten target and occurs as discrete increments to the bremsstrahlung radiation (Fig. 1-14). The energies of characteristic photons are a function of the energy levels of various electron orbital levels and hence are characteristic of the target atomic composition. Characteristic radiation is only a minor source of radiation from an x-ray tube.

FACTORS CONTROLLING THE X-RAY BEAM

The x-ray beam emitted from an x-ray tube may be modified to suit the requirements of the application by altering the conditions of tube operation (exposure time, mA, kVp), manipulating the beam produced by the tube (filtration, collimation, target-patient distance), and controlling the results of the interactions between the beam and the patient. (See "Grids," p. 94.)

Exposure time

Figure 1-16 portrays the changes in the x-ray spectrum that result when the exposure time is increased while the tube current (mA) and voltage (kVp) remain constant. When the exposure time is doubled, the number of photons generated is doubled but the range of photon energies is unchanged. Thus the effect of changing time is simply to control the "quantity" of the exposure (the number of photons generated).

Tube current   (mA)

Figure 1-17 illustrates the changes in the spectrum of photons that result from increasing tube current (mA) while maintaining tube voltage (kVp) and exposure time. Theoretically there is a linear relationship between mA and tube output. Thus the quantity of radiation produced by an x-ray tube (i.e., the number of photons that reach the patient and film) is directly related to the tube current and the time the tube is operated. The quantity of radiation produced is expressed as the product of time and tube current (mAs). The quantity of radiation will remain constant regardless of how mA and time are changed if their product remains constant. A machine operating at 10 mA for 1 second (10 mAs) would produce the same quantity of radiation when operated at 20 mA for 0.5 second (10 mAs). Although this is generally true, in practice some dental x-ray machines fall slightly short of this ideal (Fig. 1-17).

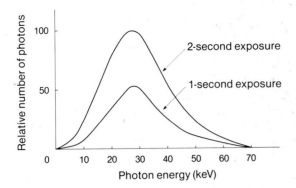

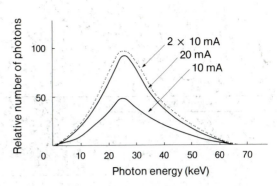

FIG. 1-16. Spectrum of photon energies showing that as exposure time is increased the total number of photons increases but the mean energy and maximum energy of the beams are unchanged.

FIG. 1-17. Spectrum of photon energies showing that two 10 mA exposures result in slightly more radiation than one 20 mA exposure. The difference, however, is slight.

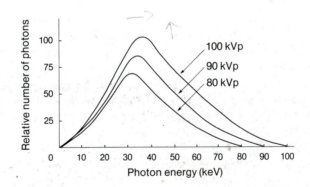

FIG. 1-18. Spectrum of photon energies showing that as the kVp is increased (with mA held constant) there is a corresponding increase in the mean energy of the beam, the total number of photons emitted, and the maximum energy of the photons.

Tube voltage   (KVP)

Figure 1-18 represents how the range of photon energies in the beam increases with the tube voltage (kVp). When kVp is increased the spectrum or energy range, as well as, the number of photons produced at each energy value, and the average energy of the beam of photons will be increased. The number of photons present at each energy value and the average energy of the beam increase as the kVp increases. Thus, as the kVp is increased there is an increase in the energy of each electron when it strikes the target. This results in an increased efficiency of conversion of electron energy into x-ray photons, and thus in an increase in the (1) number of photons generated, (2) mean energy of the photons, and (3) maximum energy of the photons.

The increased number of high-energy photons

produced per unit time by use of higher kVp results from the greater efficiency in production of bremsstrahlung photons when increased numbers of higher-energy electrons interact with the target.

The ability of x-ray photons to penetrate matter is dependent on their energy.

High-energy x-ray photons have a greater probability of penetrating matter whereas relatively low-energy photons have a greater probability of being absorbed. Thus, the higher the kVp, and hence the higher the mean energy of the x-ray beam, the greater will be the penetrability of the beam through matter. A useful way to designate the penetrating quality of an x-ray beam is by its *half-value layer* (HVL). The HVL is the thickness of an absorber, such as aluminum, required to reduce the number of x-ray photons passing through it by one half. As the average energy of an x-ray beam increases, so does its HVL. The term "quality" refers to the mean energy of an x-ray beam.

Filtration

An x-ray beam consists of a spectrum of x-ray photons of different energies, but only photons with sufficient energy to penetrate anatomic structures are useful for diagnostic radiology. Those that are of low penetrating power (long wavelength) contribute to patient exposure but not to the information on the film. Consequently, in the interest of patient safety, it is necessary to increase the mean energy of the x-ray beam by removing the less penetrating photons. This can be accomplished by placing an aluminum filter in the path of the beam.

Figure 1-19 illustrates how the addition of an aluminum filter alters the energy distribution of the unfiltered beam. The aluminum removes many of the lower energy photons with little affect on those that are able to penetrate the patient and reach the film.

When determining the amount of filtration that may be required for a particular x-ray machine, it is necessary to consider kVp and inherent filtration of the tube and its housing. The *inherent filtration* consists of the materials that x-ray photons encounter as they travel from the focal spot on the target to form the usable beam outside the tube enclosure. These materials include the glass wall of the x-ray tube, the insulating oil that surrounds many dental tubes, and the barrier material that prevents the oil from escaping through the x-ray port. The inherent filtration of most x-ray machines ranges from the equivalent of 0.5 to 2 mm of aluminum.

Total filtration is the sum of the inherent filtration plus any added external filtration supplied in the form of aluminum disks placed over the port in the head of the x-ray machine. Governmental regulations require the total filtration in the path of a dental x-ray beam be equal to the equivalent of 1.5 mm of aluminum up to 70 kVp, and 2.5 mm of aluminum for all higher voltages. (See Chapter 3.)

Collimation

When an x-ray beam is directed at a patient, about 90% of the x-ray photons are absorbed by the tissues. Ten percent of the photons pass through the patient and are available to form an image on a film. Many of the absorbed photons generate scattered radiation within the exposed tissues through a process called *Compton scattering*. These scattered photons travel in all directions (Fig. 1-20). The scattered photons that travel in the same direction as the original beam can carry some useful information to the film. The vast majority, however, travel in other directions. Many reach the film but contribute no useful information. They only add fog to the film and degrade the image by uniformly exposing the film.

The detrimental effect of scattered radiation on the formation of images can be minimized by reducing the amount of scattered radiation formed and by preventing the scattered radiation from reaching the film.

Collimation means to shape an x-ray beam, usu-

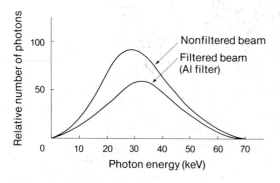

FIG. 1-19. Filtration of an x-ray beam with aluminum results in the preferential removal of low-energy photons, reducing the intensity of the beam but increasing its mean energy.

ally by the use of a metallic barrier with an aperture in the middle. Collimation reduces the size of the x-ray beam and thus the volume of irradiated tissue within the patient from which the scattered photons originate. Collimation thereby *reduces patient exposure and increases film quality.*

Diaphragm, tubular, and rectangular collimators are useful in dentistry. The *diaphragm collimator* (Fig. 1-21, *B*) is a thick plate of radiopaque material (usually lead) with an aperture or opening in it that is usually placed over the port in the x-ray head through which the x-ray beam emerges. The size and shape of the aperture determine the size and shape of the useful beam. The *tubular colli-*

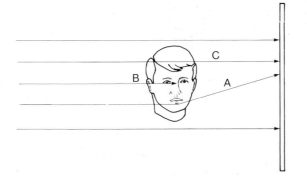

FIG. 1-20. Scattered radiation resulting from Compton interaction *(A)* may strike the film and degrade the radiographic image by causing film fog. Photons may also be absorbed *(B)* or pass through the object without interacting *(C)*.

mator (Fig. 1-21, *C*) is simply a tube lined with or constructed of a radiopaque material. One end of the tube, in conjunction with a diaphragm collimator, covers the x-ray port. *Rectangular collimators* (Fig. 1-21, *D*) further limit the beam to a size just larger than that of the x-ray film. Some types of film-holding instruments also provide rectangular collimation of the x-ray beam. (See Chapters 3 and 9.)

Inverse square law

The intensity of an x-ray beam at a given point (number of photons per cross-sectional area per unit exposure time) is dependent on the distance of the measuring device from the focal spot. For a given beam, the intensity is inversely proportional to the square of the distance from the source (Fig. 1-22). The reason for this decrease in intensity is that the x-ray beam spreads out as it moves from the source. The "spread out" beam is less intense. Thus, if a dose of 1 Gray (Gy)* is measured at a distance of 2 meters, then a dose of 4 Gy will be found at 1 meter, and 0.25 Gy at 4 meters. The relationship is

$$I_1/I_2 = (D_2)^2/(D_1)^2$$

where *I* is intensity and *D* is distance.

_____

*Table 1-2.

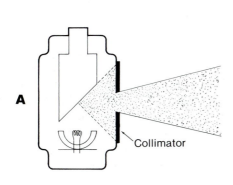

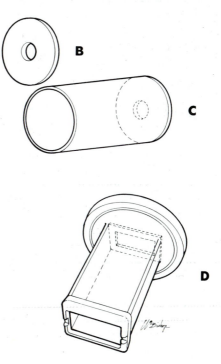

FIG. 1-21. A, Collimation of an x-ray beam (shown as dotted area) is achieved by restricting its useful size. **B,** Diaphragm collimator. **C,** Tubular collimator. **D,** Rectangular collimator.

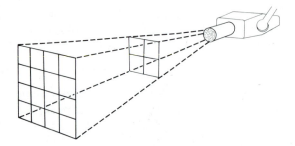

FIG. 1-22. The intensity of an x-ray beam is inversely proportional to the square of the distance between the source and the point of measure.

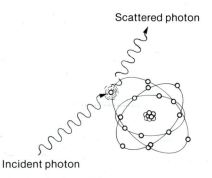

FIG. 1-23. Coherent scattering resulting from the interaction of a low-energy incident photon with an outer electron, causing it to vibrate momentarily. After this a scattered photon of the same energy is emitted at a different angle from the path of the incident photon.

Changing the distance between the x-ray tube and the patient thus has a marked effect on beam intensity. Such a change will require a corresponding modification of the kVp or mAs if the exposure of the film is to be kept constant.

INTERACTIONS OF X RAYS WITH MATTER

The intensity of an x-ray beam is reduced by interaction with the matter it encounters. This *attenuation* results from interactions of individual photons in the beam with atoms in the absorbers. As a result of their interaction with matter, x-ray photons are attenuated by absorption and scattering. In *absorption,* photons convert their energy into kinetic energy of the absorber electrons. In *scattering,* photons are ejected out of the absorber as a result of interactions with the orbital electrons of component atoms. In the case of a diagnostic x-ray beam there are three mechanisms by which these processes take place: (1) coherent scattering, (2) photoelectric absorption, and (3) Compton scattering. In a dental bitewing examination about 9% of the primary photons will pass through the head without interaction (Table 1-1).

Coherent scattering

When a *low-energy photon* passes near an atom's *outer electron* (with a relatively low binding energy of only a few electron volts), it may not be absorbed but *scattered* without a loss of energy (Fig. 1-23). This process is known as coherent scattering (also the Thompson effect or classic scattering). The incident photon interacts with the electron by causing it to vibrate momentarily at the same frequency as the incoming photon. The incident photon then ceases to exist. The vibration causes the electron to radiate energy in the form of another x-ray photon with the same frequency and energy as in the

TABLE 1-1. Fate of 2,000,000 incident photons in bitewing projections

Interaction	Primary photons	Scattered photons*	Total
Coherent scatterings	148,905	156,234	305,139
Photoelectric	536,208	522,082	1,058,290
Compton effect	1,131,878	1,098,720	2,230,598
Exit	183,009	758,701	941,710
	2,000,000	2,535,737	4,535,737

*Scattered photons result from primary, Compton, and coherent interactions.
From Gibbs SJ: Personal communication, 1986.

incident beam. Usually the secondary photon is emitted at an angle to the path of the incident photon. In effect, the direction of the incident x-ray photon is altered. Only low-energy photons (a few keV) may undergo coherent scattering; this interaction accounts for only about 8% of the total number of interactions in a dental examination (Table 1-1). At the energy levels employed in diagnostic radiology the effect of coherent scattering is negligible compared to that of Compton scattering in producing film fog because the total quantity is too small and the energy level of the resulting radiation too low for much of it to scatter out of the patient to the film.

Photoelectric absorption

Photoelectric absorption occurs when an incident photon collides with a bound electron in an atom

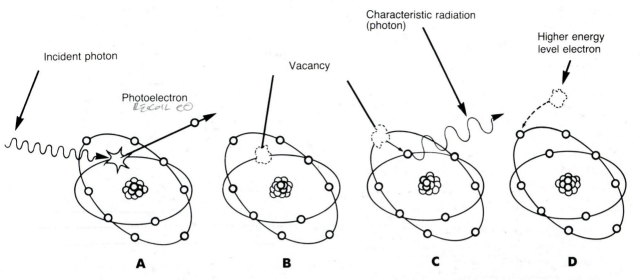

FIG. 1-24. A, Photoelectric absorption occurs when an incident photon gives up all its energy to an inner electron ejected from the atom (a photoelectron). **B,** An electron vacancy in the inner orbit results in ionization of the atom. **C,** An electron from a higher energy level fills the vacancy and emits characteristic radiation. **D,** All orbits are subsequently filled, completing the energy exchange.

of the absorbing medium. At this point the incident photon ceases to exist. The electron is ejected from its shell and becomes a *recoil electron* (photoelectron) (Fig. 1-24). The kinetic energy imparted to the recoil electron is equal to the energy of the incident photon minus that required to overcome the electron's binding energy. The absorbing atom has now lost an electron and is ionized. In the case of atoms with low atomic numbers (e.g., those comprising most biologic molecules) the binding energy is small. As a result the recoil electron acquires most of the energy of the incident photon. A photoelectric interaction with electrons in a given orbit can take place only if the energy of the incident photon exceeds the binding energy of the orbit in question. When the incident photons have sufficient energy, 80% of the photoelectric interactions occur in the K shell (because the density of the electron cloud is greater in this region); thus a higher probability of interaction exists.

An atom that has participated in a photoelectric interaction is ionized. This electron deficiency (usually in the K shell) is instantly filled, usually by an L-shell electron, with the release of characteristic radiation. Whatever the orbit of the replacement electron, the characteristic photons generated are of such low energy that they are absorbed within the patient and will not fog the film.

Photoelectric absorptions are most probable when the energy of the photon slightly exceeds the electron binding energy. The ejected recoil electrons will travel only a short distance in the absorber before they give up their energy. As a consequence, all the energy of incident photons that undergo photoelectric interaction is deposited in the patient. This is beneficial in producing high-quality radiographs, because there is no scattered radiation to fog the film, but bad for the patient because of increased radiation absorption.

About 30% of photons absorbed from a dental x-ray beam are absorbed by the photoelectric process. The frequency of photoelectric interaction varies directly with the third power of the atomic number of the absorber. Accordingly, since the effective atomic number of compact bone (Z = 13.8) is greater than water (Z = 7.4), the probability that a photon will be absorbed by a photoelectric interaction in bone is approximately 6.5 times greater than in an equal distance of water. This difference is readily seen on dental radiographs.

Compton scattering

Compton scattering occurs when a photon interacts with an outer orbital electron having a low binding energy (Fig. 1-25). In this interaction the

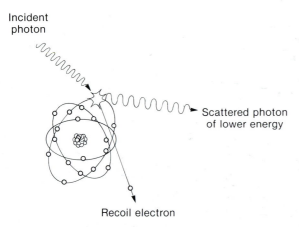

Incident
photon

Scattered photon
of lower energy

Recoil electron

FIG. 1-25. Compton absorption occurs when an incident photon interacts with an outer electron, producing a scattered photon of lower energy than the incident photon and a recoil electron ejected from the target atom.

incident photon collides with an outer electron, which receives kinetic energy and recoils from the point of impact. The incident photon is then deflected by its interaction and is scattered from the site of the collision. The scattered photon loses energy equal to the kinetic energy gained by the recoil electron plus its binding energy. As with photoelectric absorption, Compton scattering results in the loss of an electron and thus ionization of the absorbing atom. Although some characteristic radiation is produced by the return of the ionized atom to the ground state, the binding energies of the involved electrons are so low that the energy of the characteristic radiation is in the optical energy levels and is insignificant. In a dental x-ray beam approximately 62% of the photons undergo Compton scattering.

Scattered photons travel in all directions. The higher the energy of the incident photon, however, the greater the probability that the angle of scatter of the secondary photon will be small and its direction will be forward. Aproximately 30% of the scattered photons formed during a dental x-ray exposure (primarily from Compton scattering) exit the head. This is advantageous to the patient because some of the energy of the incident photons escapes the tissue, but it is disadvantageous to the dentist because it may cause film fog.

A 50 keV photon may transfer up to 17% of its energy to the recoil electron in one interaction. The *recoil electrons* lose energy along their tracks by causing secondary ionizations and consequent biologic damage. If the energy of the incident photon is low, the amount of energy transferred to the electron will be low. By contrast, a high-energy photon generates a high-energy recoil electron. Recoil electrons travel only a short distance before losing all their energy and coming to rest.

The probability of Compton scattering is directly proportional to the electrons per volume *(electron density)*. The number of electrons in bone $(5.55 \times 10^{23}/cc)$ is greater than in water $(3.34 \times 10^{23}/cc)$; thus the probability of Compton scattering is correspondingly greater in bone than in tissue. The importance of photoelectric and Compton absorption in diagnostic radiography relates to the differences in the way photons are absorbed by various anatomic structures. The number of photoelectric and Compton interactions is greater in hard tissues than in soft tissues. As a consequence there are more photons in the beam exiting the patient after passing through soft tissue than through hard tissue and thus a radiograph can readily depict enamel, dentin, bone, and soft tissues.

Secondary electrons

In both photoelectric absorption and Compton scattering, electrons are ejected from their orbits in the absorbing material after interaction with x-ray photons. These secondary electrons give up their energy in the absorber by either of two processes: (1) *collisional interaction* with other electrons, resulting in ionization or excitation of the struck atom and (2) *radiative interactions,* which produce bremsstrahlung radiation resulting in the emission of low-energy x-ray photons. Eventually secondary electrons dissipate all their energy, mostly as heat by collisional interactions, and come to rest.

Beam attenuation

As a dental x-ray beam travels through matter, individual photons are removed, primarily through photoelectric and Compton interactions. The reduction of beam intensity is predictable because it is dependent on physical characteristics of the beam and the absorber. First, consider the case of a *monochromatic beam* of photons, a beam in which all the photons have the same energy. When just the primary (not scattered) photons are considered, a constant fraction of the beam is attenuated as the beam moves through each unit thickness of an absorber. Thus, for example, 1.5 cm of water might reduce a beam intensity by 50%, the next 1.5 cm by another 50% (to 25% of the original intensity), and so on. This is an *exponential* pattern of absorption (Fig. 1-26). The term *half value layer* is a measure of beam energy as it describes the amount of an absorber that reduces the beam intensity by half; 1.5 cm of water in the preceding example. The absorption of the beam is dependent primarily on the thickness and mass of the absorber and the energy of the beam.

For *polychromatic radiation,* generated in an x-ray machine, there is a spectrum of photon energies ranging from very low to quite high (equivalent to the kVp setting). In such a heterogeneous beam the probability of absorption of individual photons depends on their energy. Low-energy photons are much more likely than high-energy photons to be absorbed. As a consequence the superficial layers of an absorber tend to remove the low-energy photons and transmit the higher-energy photons. Thus, as a polychromatic beam passes through matter, each succeeding unit thickness of absorber preferentially removes lower-energy photons and the mean energy of the resultant beam increases. In contrast to the absorption of a monochromatic beam, a polychromatic beam is absorbed less and less by each succeeding unit of absorber thickness. This difference is the result of the increase in mean energy by the polychromatic beam as it passes through the absorber and the low-energy photons are preferentially absorbed. For example, the first 1.5 cm of a water phantom might absorb about 40% of the photons in a polychromatic beam with a mean energy of 50 kVp. The mean energy of the remnant beam might increase 20% as a result of the loss of lower-energy photons. The next 1.5 cm of water would remove only about 30% of the photons as the average energy of the beam increased another 10%. If the water phantom is thick enough mean energy of the remnant beam will reflect the peak voltage applied across the tube and absorption will become similar to that of a monochromatic beam.

The attenuation of a beam depends on both the energy of the incident beam and the composition of the absorber. In general, as the energy of the beam increases, so does the transmission of the beam through the absorber. When the energy of the incident photon is raised to the binding energy of the K-shell electrons of the absorber, however, the probability of photoelectric absorption increases sharply and the number of transmitted photons is greatly decreased. This is called *K-edge*

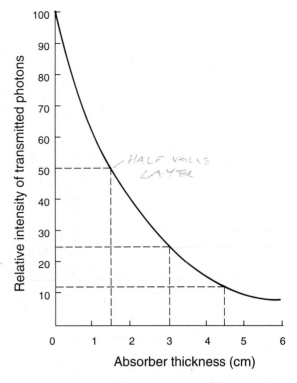

FIG. 1-26. Exponential decay of intensity in a homogeneous photon beam through the absorber, where the half-value layer (HVL) is 1.5 cm of absorber. The curve for a heterogeneous x-ray beam would not drop quite as precipitously because of the preferential removal of low-energy photons and the increased mean energy of the resulting beam.

absorption. (The probability that a photon will interact with an orbital electron is greatest when the energy of the photon equals the binding energy of the electron, and it decreases rapidly as the photon energy increases.) Photons with energy less than the binding energy of K-shell electrons interact photoelectrically only with electrons in the L-shell and in shells even farther from the nucleus, but the energies involved are very low (much below the useful diagnostic energy range) and are of little significance. Rare earth elements are sometimes used as filters because their K edge (50.2 keV for gadolinium) has the effect of greatly increasing the absorption of photons, thereby reducing patient exposure.

DOSIMETRY

Determining the quantity of radiation exposure or dose is termed "dosimetry." *Dose* is used to

TABLE 1-2. Summary of radiation quantities and units

Quantity	SI unit	Traditional unit	Conversion
Exposure	Coulomb per kilogram (C/kg)	Roentgen (R)	1 C/kg = 3876 R 1 R = 2.58×10^{-4} C/kg
Absorbed dose	Gray (Gy)	rad	1 Gy = 100 rad 1 rad = 0.01 Gy (1 cGy)
Effective dose	Sievert (Sv)	rem	1 Sv = 100 rem 1 rem = 0.01 Sv
Radioactivity	Becquerel (Bq)	Curie (Ci)	1 Bq = 2.7×10^{-11} Ci 1 Ci = 3.7×10^{10} Bq

describe the amount of energy absorbed per unit mass at a site of interest. *Exposure* is a measure of radiation based on its ability to produce ionization in air under standard conditions of temperature and pressure (STP). A variety of techniques are available for such measurements that take advantage of specific properties of ionizing radiations.

Units of measurement

Table 1-2 presents some of the more frequently used units for measuring quantities of radiation. In recent years there has been a move to use a modernized version of the metric system called the SI system (Système International d'Unités). This book uses SI units.

Exposure. Exposure is a measure of radiation quantity, the capacity of the radiation to ionize air. The *roentgen* (R) is the traditional unit of radiation exposure measured in air; 1 R is that amount of x- or γ-radiation that will produce in 1 cc of air (STP) 2.08×10^9 ion pairs. It measures the intensity of radiation to which an object is exposed. There is no specific SI unit equivalent to the R, but in terms of other SI units it is equal to coulombs per kilogram (C/kg); 1 R = 2.58×10^4 C/kg, and 1 C/kg equals 3.88×10^3 R. The roentgen applies only for x rays and gamma rays.

Absorbed dose. Absorbed dose is a measure of the energy imparted by any type of ionizing radiation to a mass of any type of matter. The SI unit is the *gray* (Gy), where 1 Gy equals 1 joule/kg. The traditional unit of absorbed dose is the *rad* (radiation absorbed dose), where 1 rad is equivalent to 100 ergs/gm of absorber. One gray equals 100 rads.

Equivalent dose. The equivalent dose (H_T) is used to compare the biologic effects of different types of radiation to a tissue or organ. It is the sum of the products of the absorbed dose (D_T) averaged over a tissue or organ and the radiation weighting factor (W_R).

$$H_T = \Sigma \, W_R \cdot D_T$$

It is expressed as a sum to allow for the possibility that the tissue or organ is exposed to more than one type of radiation. The radiation weighting factor is chosen for the type and energy of the radiation involved. Thus high-LET* radiations (which are more damaging to tissue than low-LET radiations) have a correspondingly higher W_R. For example, the W_R of photons is 1, of 5 keV neutrons and high-energy protons 5, and of alpha particles 20. The unit of equivalent dose is the *sievert* (Sv). For diagnostic x-ray examinations 1 Sv equals 1 Gy. The traditional unit of equivalent dose is the *rem* (roentgen equivalent man). One sievert equals 100 rem.

Effective dose. The effective dose (E) is used to estimate the risk in humans. It is the sum of the products of the effective dose to each organ or tissue (H_T) and the tissue weighting factor (W_T).

$$E = \Sigma \, W_T \cdot H_T$$

The tissue weighting factors include gonads, 0.20; red bone marrow, 0.12; esophagus, 0.05; thyroid, 0.05; skin, 0.01; and bone surface, 0.01. The unit of effective dose is the *sievert* (Sv). The use of this term is described more fully in Chapter 3 (p. 47).

Activity. The measurement of (radio)activity (A) describes the decay rate of a sample of radioactive material. The SI unit is the *becquerel* (Bq), where 1 Bq equals 1 disintegration/second. The traditional unit is the *curie* (Ci), which corresponds to the activity of 1 gm of radium (3.7×10^{10} disintegrations/second). Accordingly, 1 mCi equals 37 megaBq; and 1 Bq equals 2.7×10^{-11} Ci.

---

*Linear energy transfer.

SELECTED REFERENCES

Bushong SC: *Radiologic science for technologists: physics, biology, and protection,* ed 4, St Louis, 1988, Mosby.

Curry TS, Dowdey JE, Murry RC: *Christensen's Physics of diagnostic radiology,* ed 4, Philadelphia, 1990, Lea & Febiger.

International Commission on Radiological Protection: Radiation protection, *ICRP Publ* 60, 1990.

Johns HE, Cunningham JR: *The physics of radiology,* ed 4, Springfield Ill, 1985, Charles C Thomas.

2

Radiation Biology

Radiation biology is the study of the effects of ionizing radiation on living systems. This discipline requires studying many levels of organization within biologic systems spanning broad ranges in size and temporal scale. The initial interaction between ionizing radiation and matter occurs at the level of the electron within the first 10^{-13} second after exposure. These changes result in modification of biologic molecules within the following seconds to hours. In turn, the molecular changes may lead to alterations in cells and organisms that persist for hours, decades, and possibly even generations. They may result in death of the cell or organism.

RADIATION CHEMISTRY

The primary actions of radiation on living systems occur through direct and indirect effects. When the energy of a photon or secondary electron is transferred directly to biologic macromolecules, the effect is *direct*. Alternatively, the photon may be absorbed by water in a biologic system and the water molecules ionized. These ions form free radicals (radiolysis of water) that, in turn, interact with and produce changes in the biologic molecules. This series of events involving water molecules is *indirect*.

Direct effect

Direct alteration of biologic molecules by ionizing radiation involves three steps: absorption of energy by the molecule, transfer of energy between unstable intermediate molecules, and formation of stable damaged molecules. The resultant molecules are rearrangements resulting from dissociation of molecules into free radicals* and subsequently reforming stable configurations by dissociation or cross-linking.

---

*Radicals are atoms or molecules that have an unpaired electron in the valence shell. They are extremely reactive and have a very short life. Free radicals having no charge are designated with a dot following the chemical symbol. When a radical has a charge, it is an ion.

Free radical production

$$R + \text{x-radiation} \rightarrow R^\bullet + H^+ + e^-$$

Free radical fates

Dissociation: $R^\bullet \rightarrow X + Y^\bullet$

Cross-linking: $R^\bullet + S^\bullet \rightarrow RS$

Because the resultant molecules differ structurally and functionally from the original molecules, the consequence is a biologic change in the irradiated organism. *Approximately one third of the biologic effects of x-ray exposure result from direct effects.*

Radiolysis of water

Water plays a major role in the transfer of energy from photons to biologic molecules by the indirect effect. Because water is the predominant molecule in biologic systems (about 70% by weight), it participates in the greatest number of the interactions between x-ray photons and the system's constituent molecules. About two thirds of radiation-induced biologic damage results from such indirect effects. In biologic systems a complex series of chemical changes occurs in water after exposure to ionizing radiation. Collectively these reactions are the radiolysis of water.

The first step in the radiolysis of water is ionization, which may result from the absorption of a photon but generally follows interaction with a photoelectron or Compton electron (see Chapter 1). Displacement of an electron from the water molecule results in an electron pair, a positively charged water molecule (H_2O^+) and the displaced electron.

$$\text{Photon} + H_2O \rightarrow e^- + H_2O^+$$

$$e^- + H_2O \rightarrow 2e^- + H_2O^+$$

The displaced electron will most likely be captured by an un-ionized water molecule to form a hydrated electron (e_{aq}). These negatively charged water molecules (H_2O^-) are not stable and disassociate rapidly to form a hydroxyl ion and a hydrogen free radical.

$$e^- + H_2O \rightarrow H_2O^-$$

$$H_2O^- \rightarrow OH^- + H^\bullet$$

The positively charged water molecule reacts with another water molecule to form a hydroxyl free radical.

$$H_2O^+ + H_2O \rightarrow OH^\bullet + H_3O^+$$

Water may also be excited and dissociate into hydrogen and hydroxyl free radicals.

$$Photon + H_2O \rightarrow H_2O^* \rightarrow OH^\bullet + H^\bullet$$

Whereas the radiolysis of water is extremely complex, water is largely converted to hydrogen and hydroxyl free radicals.

The generation of free radicals occurs in less than 10^{-10} second after the passage of a photon. These radicals play the dominant role producing molecular changes in biologic molecules. The $OH^\bullet$ free radical is believed to be the most destructive.

When dissolved molecular oxygen (O_2) is present in irradiated water, hydroperoxyl free radicals may also be formed:

$$H^\bullet + O_2 \rightarrow HO_2^\bullet$$

Hydroperoxyl free radicals also may contribute to the formation of hydrogen peroxide in tissues:

$$HO_2^\bullet + H^\bullet \rightarrow H_2O_2$$

Both peroxyl radicals and hydrogen peroxide are oxidizing agents that can significantly alter biologic molecules and thus cause cell destruction. They are considered to be major toxins produced in the tissues by ionizing radiation.

Indirect effects

The various free radicals formed in water may change the structure of organic molecules. The interaction of hydrogen and hydroxyl free radicals with organic molecules can result in the formation of organic free radicals. Such reactions may involve the *removal of hydrogen* as follows:

$$RH + OH^\bullet \rightarrow R^\bullet + H_2O$$

$$RH + H^\bullet \rightarrow R^\bullet + H_2$$

Because hydrogen is so prevalent in organic molecules, such breaks occur most often between it and carbon. The $OH^\bullet$ free radical is the more important in causing such damage.

Organic free radicals are unstable and may transform into new molecules by undergoing cross-linking or rearrangement reactions:

Condensation: $R^\bullet + U^\bullet \rightarrow RU$

Rearrangement: $R^\bullet + TH \rightarrow RH + T^\bullet$

Each of these reactions results in the formation of new molecules that have different chemical, and hence biologic, properties from the original molecules. Evidence for the important role of water radiolysis and the indirect action of radiation may be seen by comparing the radiation dose required to inactivate enzymes when dry or in solution. For example, the dose required to inactivate 37% of dry yeast invertase is 110 kGy but only 60 kGy when the enzyme is irradiated in solution.

Changes in biologic molecules

Proteins. Irradiation of proteins in solution usually leads to changes in their secondary and tertiary structure through disruption of side chains or the breakage of hydrogen or disulfide bonds. Such changes lead to denaturation. The primary structure of the protein is usually not significantly altered. Irradiation may also induce inter- and intramolecular cross-linking. When an enzyme is irradiated, the biologic effect of the radiation may become amplified. For example, inactivation of an enzyme molecule will result in its failure to convert many substrate molecules to their products. Thus many molecules become subsequently affected, although only a small number were initially damaged.

In vitro the dose of radiation required to induce significant amounts of protein denaturation (or enzyme inactivation) is much higher than that required to induce gross cellular changes or cell death. Such data suggest that radiation-induced changes in protein structure and function are not the major cause of radiation effects following absorption of moderate doses (2 to 4 Gy) of radiation.

Nucleic acids. During the last few decades there has been a growing appreciation for the critical role of nucleic acids in determining cellular functions. Recent research has tended to focus interest on the effects of radiation on these molecules. It is clear that DNA is the target molecule responsible for cell killing. In general, DNA is more radiosensitive than RNA. Radiation produces a number of different types of alterations in DNA:

1. Change or loss of a base
2. Disruption of hydrogen bonds between DNA strands

3. Breakage of one or both DNA strands
4. Cross-linking of DNA strands within the helix, to other DNA strands, or to proteins

The amount of radiation required to cause disruption of DNA molecules (e.g., one single-strand break per molecule) is much higher than is required to cause cell death. Such evidence suggests that if DNA is the molecular target in a cell, relatively few biochemical lesions of the types listed above may be required to result in cell death. DNA sensitivity to radiation results from its complex replication mechanism in mitotically active cell populations.

RADIATION EFFECTS AT THE CELLULAR LEVEL

Effects on intracellular structures

The effects of radiation on intracellular structures result from radiation-induced changes in their macromolecules. Although the initial molecular changes are produced within a fraction of a second after exposure, cellular changes resulting from moderate exposures usually require hours or longer to become apparent. These changes manifest themselves initially as structural and functional changes in cellular organelles. Later, cell death may occur.

Nucleus. A wide variety of radiobiologic data indicate that the nucleus is more radiosensitive (in terms of lethality) than the cytoplasm, especially in populations of dividing cells. Irradiation of the nucleus also causes inhibition of cell division. *The sensitive site in the nucleus is the DNA within chromosomes.*

Chromosome aberrations. Chromosomes serve as useful markers for radiation injury. They may be easily visualized and quantified, and the extent of their damage is related to cell survival. Chromosome aberrations are observed in irradiated cells at the time of mitosis when the DNA condenses to form chromosomes. The type of damage that may be visualized depends on the stage of the cell in the cell cycle at the time of irradiation.

Figure 2-1 shows the stages of a cell cycle. If radiation exposure occurs after DNA synthesis (i.e., in G_2 or mid- and late S), then only one arm of the affected chromosome will be broken (chromatid aberration) (Fig. 2-2). If the radiation-induced break occurs before the DNA has replicated (i.e., in G_1 or early S), the damage shows as a break in both arms (chromosome aberration) at the next mitosis. The highest frequency of aberrations occurs after irradiation in the G_2 phase, presumably because of the short interval for repair prior to

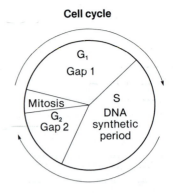

Cell cycle

FIG. 2-1. Cell cycle. A proliferating cell moves in the cycle from mitosis *(M)* to gap 1 *(G₁)* to the period of DNA synthesis *(S)* to gap 2 *(G₂)* to the next mitosis.

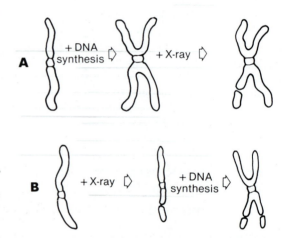

FIG. 2-2. Chromosome aberrations. **A,** Irradiation of the cell after DNA synthesis results in a single-arm chromatid aberration. **B,** Irradiation before DNA synthesis results in a double-arm aberration.

entering mitosis and the greater amounts of chromatin material (which make a larger target). Most simple breaks repair and go unrecognized. If a lesion repairs correctly, it will not be visible. Various forms of misrepair occur, however. Figure 2-3 illustrates several common forms of chromosome aberrations resulting from incorrect repair. Such radiation-induced aberrations may result in unequal distribution of chromatin material to daughter cells or may prevent completion of a subsequent mitosis.

Chromosome aberrations have been detected in peripheral blood lymphocytes of patients exposed to medical diagnostic procedures. Moreover, the survivors of the atom bombings of Hiroshima and

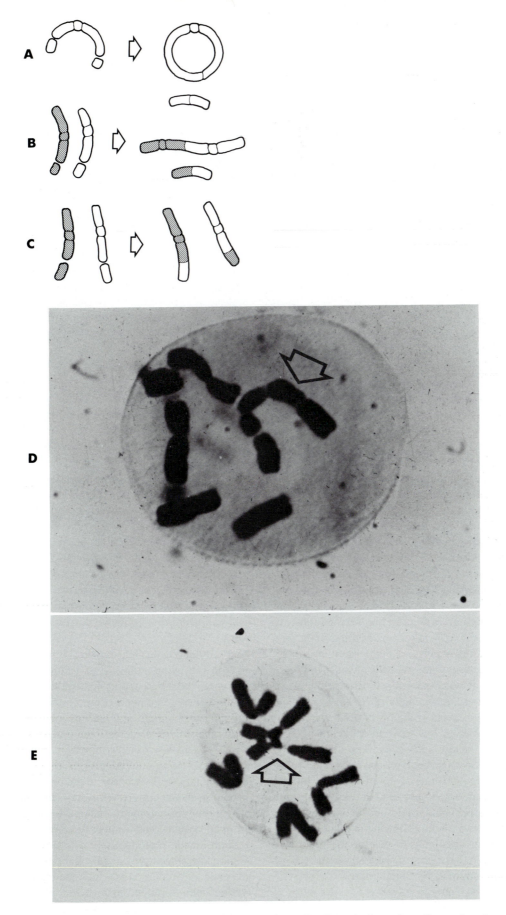

FIG. 2-3. Chromosome aberrations. **A,** Ring formation; **B,** dicentric formation; **C,** translocation. In **D** and **E** the *arrow* points to tetracentric exchange and chromatid exchange taking place in *Tradescantia,* an herb. (**D** and **E** courtesy Dr. M. Miller, Rochester N.Y.)

Nagasaki have demonstrated chromosome aberrations in circulating lymphocytes more than two decades after the radiation exposure. The frequency of aberrations is generally proportional to the radiation dose received. Although the relationship between such aberrations and the health status of the survivors is unknown, accumulation of chromosomal aberrations may be one of the causes of aging.

Cytoplasm. Radiation effects occur in cellular structures other than nuclei and chromosomes. High doses are required to cause visible changes. Numerous experiments have shown that irradiation of plasma membranes causes increased permeability to potassium and sodium ions and changes in active transport mechanisms. Relatively large doses of radiation (30 to 50 Gy) produce marked changes in the membranous structures of the cytoplasm. Mitochondria may demonstrate swelling and disorganization of the internal cristae. Such permeability and structure changes probably play a minor role in the cellular changes seen in rapidly dividing cells after exposure to moderate doses of radiation (2 to 4 Gy).

Effects on cell kinetics

The effects of radiation on the kinetics (turnover rate) of a cell population have been studied in rapidly dividing cell systems such as skin and intestinal mucosa and in cell culture systems. Irradiation of such cell populations will cause a reduction in size of the irradiated tissue as a result of mitotic delay (inhibition of progression of the cells through the cell cycle) and cell death (usually during mitosis).

Mitotic delay. Mitotic delay occurs following irradiation of a population of dividing cells. Although radiation delays cell progression into G_2 by depressing DNA synthesis, cells actually in G_2 are the most affected. Figure 2-4 illustrates the effect of radiation on mitotic activity. In this graph the control mitotic index (fraction of cells in mitosis) is defined as *1*. A low dose of radiation induces mild mitotic delay in G_2 cells. The delayed cells subsequently pass through mitosis with other (nondelayed) cells, giving rise to an elevated mitotic index. A moderate dose results in a longer mitotic delay (G_2 block) and some cell death. The area under the curve of the following supranormal mitotic index is smaller than that of the preceding mitotic delay, indicating some cell death. Larger doses may cause a profound mitotic delay with incomplete recovery.

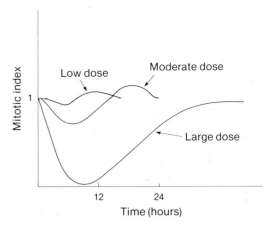

FIG. 2-4. Radiation-induced mitotic delay. The degree of delay in a replicating cell population is dependent on the amount of exposure. Note how a large dose severely depresses mitosis and prolongs recovery.

Cell death. Reproductive death in a cell population is loss of the capacity for unlimited mitotic division. Usually reproductive death results from failure to complete the first few mitoses after irradiation. G_2 and mitosis are the most sensitive stages, and the end of S the least sensitive (when repairing enzymes are at the highest levels). The intimate relationship between chromosomal aberrations and cell death is suggested by three observations: (1) Comparable doses are required to cause cell death and chromosome aberrations, (2) Agents that modify the incidence of chromosome aberrations also modify cell killing in the same manner, and (3) The surviving fraction of an irradiated cell population rarely contains chromosome aberrations.

Reproductive death occurs in a dividing cell population following exposure to a moderate dose of radiation, which accounts for the radiosensitivity of tissues. When a population of nondividing cells is irradiated, much larger doses and longer time intervals are required for induction of interphase death.

Survival curves are used to study the response of replicating cells exposed in culture. Single cells grown in tissue culture are dispersed onto plates, where they form colonies. The plates are irradiated prior to colony growth and the effect of the irradiation on the reproductivity of the cells studied. Figure 2-5 shows typical survival curves for cells exposed to x-radiation in which the fraction of surviving cells is plotted against the absorbed dose.

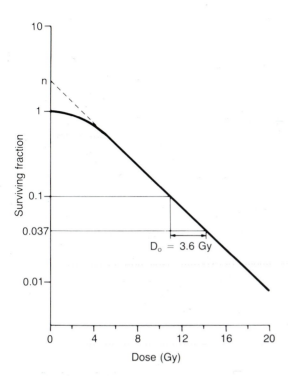

FIG. 2-5. Survival curve for mammalian cells grown in culture following irradiation. In this case the cells have an extrapolation number (n) of about 2 and a D_o of about 3.6 Gy. The n value is a measure of the size of the shoulder; D_o is the amount of radiation required to reduce the surviving population to 37% of its former size.

The shoulder in the survival curve represents either the accumulation of sublethal damage before cells die or a measure of the repair process active early in the period of irradiation. The value *n* is the extrapolation number and measures the size of the shoulder. The value D_0 indicates the slope of the straight portion of the curve. It measures the amount of radiation required to reduce the number of colony-forming cells to 37% and thus is the dose required to deliver an average of one cell killing event per cell. Survival curves have helped to understand the response of cells to irradiation under various conditions.

Recovery. Cell recovery involves enzymatic repair of single-strand breaks of DNA. Because of this repair a higher total dose is required to achieve a given degree of cell killing when multiple fractions are used (e.g., in radiation therapy) than when the same total dose is given in a single brief exposure. Damage to both strands of DNA at the same site (usually caused by particulate radiation) is usually lethal to the cell.

Relationship between radiosensitivity and cell type

Different cells from various organs of the same individual may respond to irradiation quite differently. This variation was recognized as early as 1906 by the French radiobiologists Bergonié and Tribondeau. Their studies on the response of rat testes to irradiation led them to some general conclusions regarding the relationship between sensitivity to radiation and cell type. They observed that the most radiosensitive cells are those that (1) have a high mitotic rate, (2) undergo many future mitoses, and (3) are most primitive in differentiation. These findings are still true except for lymphocytes and oocytes, which are very radiosensitive although they are highly differentiated and nondividing.

Mammalian cells may be divided into the following five categories of radiosensitivity on the basis of histologic observations of early cell death (see Rubin and Casarett, 1968):

1. *Vegetative intermitotic cells* are the most radiosensitive. They divide regularly, have long mitotic futures, and do not undergo differentiation between mitoses. These are stem cells that retain their primitive properties and whose function is to replace themselves. They divide often, so their life span is short and they are frequently in a radiosensitive phase (G_2 or M) of the cell cycle. Examples include early precursor cells, such as those in the spermatogenic or erythroblastic series, and basal cells of the oral mucous membranes.

2. *Differentiating intermitotic cells* are somewhat less radiosensitive than vegetative intermitotic cells because they divide less often. They divide regularly, although they undergo some differentiation between divisions. The more differentiated they become, the less often they divide and the less radiosensitive they are. Examples of this class include intermediate dividing and replicating cells of the inner enamel epithelium of developing teeth, cells of the hematopoietic series that are in the intermediate stages of differentiation, spermatocytes, and oocytes.

3. *Multipotential connective tissue cells* have intermediate radiosensitivity. They divide irregularly, usually in response to a demand for more cells and are also capable of limited differentiation. Examples are vascular endothelial cells, fibroblasts, and mesenchymal cells.

4. *Reverting postmitotic cells* are generally radioresistant because they infrequently divide. They are relatively long lived and usually die without dividing. They divide only under special conditions (e.g., the demand for more cells of their kind) and are generally specialized in function. Examples include acinar and ductal cells of the salivary glands and pancreas as well as parenchymal cells of the liver, kidney, and thyroid.

5. *Fixed postmitotic cells* are most resistant to the direct action of radiation because they do not divide. They are the most highly differentiated cells and, once mature, are incapable of division. Examples of these cells include neurons, striated muscle cells, squamous epithelial cells that have differentiated and are close to the surface of oral mucous membrane, and erythrocytes.

RADIATION EFFECTS AT THE TISSUE AND ORGAN LEVEL

The radiosensitivity of a tissue or organ is measured by its response to irradiation. When the number of lost cells is fairly small, there is no clinical effect. As the number of lost cells increases, there is a clinically evident result that all persons will show. The severity of this change is dependent on the dose and thus the amount of cell loss. Such changes are called *deterministic effects*. The criterion usually employed for deterministic effects is tissue hypoplasia (cell loss), leading to atrophy. The following discussion pertains to the effect of irradiation of tissues and organs when the exposure is restricted to a small area. Moderate doses to a localized area may lead to damage of a tissue that may be repaired. Doses of a comparable size to a whole organism may result in death from damage to the most sensitive systems in the body.

Another type of biologic effect from radiation is called *stochastic effect*. Stochastic changes are those for which the probability of occurrence, rather than the severity, is dose dependent. Radiation-induced cancer is a stochastic effect since greater exposure increases the probability of cancer but not its severity.

Short-term effects

The short-term effects of radiation on a tissue are determined primarily by the sensitivity of its parenchymal cells. When continuously proliferating tissues (e.g., bone marrow) are irradiated with a moderate dose, cells are lost primarily by temporary or permanent inhibition of mitosis and by extensive mitosis-linked death. The extent of cell loss depends on damage to the stem cell pools and the proliferative rate of the cell population. The effects of irradiation of such tissues become apparent relatively quickly as a reduction in the number of final cells in the series. Tissues composed of cells that rarely or never divide (e.g., muscle) demonstrate little or no radiation-induced hypoplasia over the short term. The relative radiosensitivity of various organs is as follows:

High	Intermediate	Low
Lymphoid organs	Fine vasculature	Optic lens
Bone marrow	Growing	Mature
Testes	cartilage	erythrocytes
Intestines	Growing bone	Muscle cells
Mucous	Salivary glands	Neurons
membranes	Lungs	
	Kidneys	
	Liver	

Long-term effects

The long-term deterministic effects of radiation on tissues and organs are dependent primarily on the extent of damage to the fine vasculature. The relative radiosensitivity of the fine vasculature and connective tissue is intermediate between that of differentiating intermitotic cells and reverting postmitotic cells. The effects of radiation on capillaries include swelling, degeneration, and necrosis. These changes, and the subsequent inflammation resulting from irritating products released by degenerating parenchyma, increase the permeability of fine vessels and capillaries. Such changes also initiate a slow progressive fibrosis of the vessels. As a result there is increased deposition of fibrous scar tissue around the vessels, leading to premature narrowing and eventual obliteration of vascular lumens. This impairs the transport of oxygen, nutrients, and waste products. Death of fixed and reverting postmitotic cells following moderate exposure is largely secondary to such vascular changes. The net result is progressive fibroatrophy of the irradiated tissue. This is true for tissues composed of either radiosensitive or radioresistant cells. There will also be reproductive death in the cell pool proportional to the extent that partial cell loss stimulates compensatory hyperplasia. Such progressive atrophic changes lead to a loss of cell function and a reduced resistance of the tissue to infection and trauma. These cellular changes are the basis for long-term radiation-induced atrophy of tissues and organs.

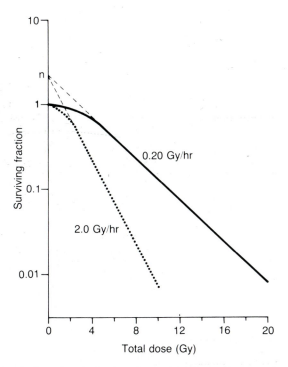

FIG. 2-6. Survival curve for mammalian cells grown in culture following irradiation at low and high dose rates. Note that a high dose kills more cells because there is less time for repair of sublethal damage.

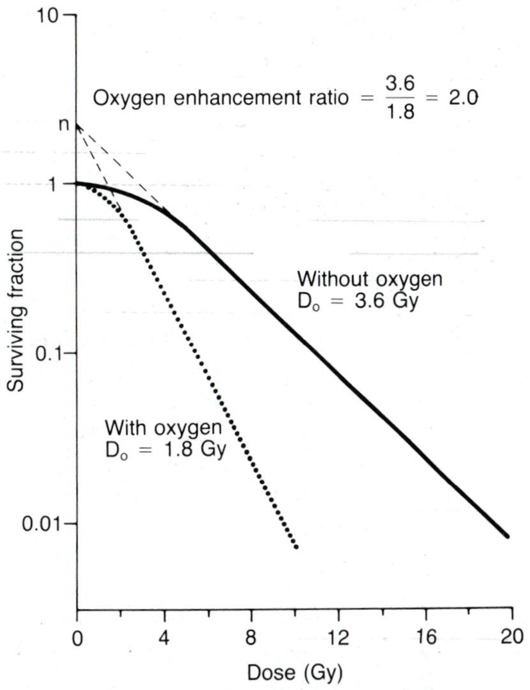

FIG. 2-7. Survival curve for mammalian cells grown in culture following irradiation with and without oxygen. The presence of oxygen increases the cells' sensitivity to radiation: the D_0 value is reduced from 3.6 Gy when irradiated without oxygen to 1.8 Gy with oxygen. The oxygen enhancement ratio measures the influence of O_2.

Modifying factors

The response of cells to irradiation is dependent on variations in exposure parameters and the environment of the cell.

Dose. Generally the severity of deterministic damage seen in an irradiated tissue or organ is dependent on the amount of radiation received. Very often there is a clinical threshold dose below which no adverse effects will be seen. With doses above the threshold level all individuals show damage in proportion to the dose.

Dose rate. The term "dose rate" indicates the rate of exposure. For example, a total dose of 5 Gy may be given at a high dose rate (5 Gy/min) or a low dose rate (5 mGy/min). Exposure of biologic systems to high dose rates causes more damage than exposure to lower dose rates. When organisms are exposed at lower dose rates, there is greater opportunity for repair of damage before termination of the exposure, thereby resulting in less net damage. Figure 2-6 illustrates the effects of dose rate schematically.

Oxygen. The radioresistance of many biologic systems increases by a factor of 2 or 3 when irradiation is conducted under conditions of profound hypoxia. The greater cell damage sustained in the presence of oxygen is related to the increased amounts of hydrogen peroxide and hydroperoxyl free radicals formed. The *oxygen enhancement ratio* measures the extent of this damage. It is the dose required to achieve a given end point (e.g., 50% survival of a cell population) under anoxic conditions divided by the dose required to produce the same end point under fully oxygenated conditions. Figure 2-7 shows the influence of oxygen on cell survival curves.

Normal tissues are nearly saturated with oxygen. Some tumors, however, have a relatively poor vascular supply in their central, necrotic portions and are therefore largely hypoxic. Under such conditions breathing oxygen at several atmospheres pressure may increase the radiosensitivity of tumor cells while not appreciably increasing the radiosensitivity of the surrounding normally saturated tissues. Such oxygen treatment is most effective in patients with quite severe disease and the benefits are limited to short-term palliative improvement.

Linear energy transfer. In general, the dose required to produce a certain biologic effect is reduced as the linear energy transfer (LET) of the radiation is increased (see page 3.) Thus, higher LET radiations (e.g., alpha particles) are more efficient in the induction of damage to biologic systems because their high ionization density is more likely than x rays to induce double-strand breakage in DNA. In addition, high-LET radiations are more efficient at inducing hydrogen peroxide in tissues.

Chemical protectors. A wide variety of chemical compounds are effective in modifying the responses of cells and animals to radiation. Agents enhancing the effects of radiation are radiosensitizers. Chemicals that inhibit radiation effects are radioprotectors. The most effective radioprotectors act as free radical scavengers, thereby reducing the indirect effects of radiation.

RADIATION EFFECTS ON THE ORAL CAVITY
Rationale of radiotherapy

The oral cavity is irradiated during the course of treating radiosensitive oral malignant tumors, usually squamous cell carcinomas. The treatment of choice for a specific lesion will depend on many tumor variables, such as radiosensitivity, histology, size, location, invasion into adjacent structures, and duration of symptomatology.

Radiation therapy for malignant lesions in the oral cavity is usually indicated when the lesion is radiosensitive, advanced, or deeply invasive and cannot be approached surgically. Combined surgical and radiotherapeutic treatment often provides optimum treatment. Increasingly, chemotherapy is being combined with radiation therapy and surgery for treatment.

Fractionation of the total x-ray dose into multiple small doses provides greater tumor destruction than would be possible with a large single dose. Fractionation characteristically also allows increased cellular repair of normal tissues, which are believed to have an inherently greater capacity for recovery than tumor cells. Another value of fractionation is that it increases the mean oxygen tension in an irradiated tumor, rendering the tumor cells more radiosensitive. This results from rapid killing of tumor cells and shrinkage of the tumor mass after

the first few fractions, reducing the distance that oxygen must diffuse through the tumor to reach the remaining viable tumor cells. The fractionation schedules currently in use have been established empirically.

Radiation effect on oral tissues

The following sections describe the deterministic effects of a course of radiotherapy on the normal tissue of the oral cavity. For this discussion it is assumed that 2 Gy is delivered daily, bilaterally through 8 × 10 cm fields over the oropharynx, for a weekly exposure of 10 Gy. This continues until a total of 50 Gy has been administered. (This is a standard procedure.) Cobalt is often the source of radiation; however, on occasion small implants containing radon or iodine-125 are placed directly in a tumor mass. Such implants deliver a high dose of radiation to a relatively small volume of tissue in a short time.

Oral mucous membrane. The oral mucous membrane contains a basal layer composed of radiosensitive vegetative and differentiating intermitotic cells. Near the end of the second week of therapy the mucous membranes begin to show areas of redness and inflammation (mucositis). As the therapy continues, the irradiated mucous membrane begins to break down, with the formation of a white to yellow pseudomembrane. (This membrane is the desquamated epithelial layer.) At the end of therapy the mucositis is usually most severe, discomfort is at a maximum, and food intake is difficult. Good oral hygiene will minimize infection. Topical anesthetics may be required at mealtimes. Secondary infection by *Candida albicans* is a common complication and may require treatment.

After irradiation the mucosa begins to heal rapidly. Healing is usually complete by about 2 months. At later intervals (months to years) the mucous membrane will tend to become atrophic, thin, and relatively avascular. This long-term atrophy results from progressive obliteration of the fine vasculature and fibrosis of the underlying connective tissue. The changes complicate wearing of dentures because they may cause oral ulcerations of the compromised tissue. Ulcers can result from a denture sore, radiation necrosis, or tumor recurrence. A biopsy may be required to make the differentiation.

Taste buds. Taste buds are sensitive to radiation. Doses in the therapeutic range cause extensive degeneration of their normal histologic architecture. Patients often notice a loss of taste acuity during the second or third week of radiotherapy. Bitter and acid flavors are more severely affected when the posterior two thirds of the tongue is irradiated, and salt and sweet when the anterior third of the tongue is irradiated. Taste acuity usually decreases by a factor of 1000 to 10,000 during the course of radiotherapy. Alterations in the saliva may account partly for this reduction, which may proceed to a state of virtual insensitivity, with recovery to near-normal levels some 60 to 120 days after irradiation.

Salivary glands. The major salivary glands are at times unavoidably exposed to 20 to 30 Gy during radiotherapy for cancer in the oral cavity or oropharynx. The parenchymal component of the salivary glands is rather radiosensitive (parotid glands more so than submandibular or sublingual glands); the reason is unknown. Histologically there may be an acute inflammatory response soon after the initiation of therapy, particularly involving the serous acini. In the months following irradiation the inflammatory response becomes more chronic and the glands demonstrate progressive fibrosis, adiposis, loss of the fine vasculature, and concomitant parenchymal degeneration (Fig. 2-8).

During the first few weeks after initiation of radiotherapy there is usually a marked and progressive loss of salivary secretion. The extent of reduced flow is dose dependent and reaches essentially zero at 60 Gy. The scanty saliva that is secreted has an elevated concentration of sodium, chloride, calcium, and magnesium ions and protein. It also loses its normal lubricating properties. The mouth will become dry (xerostomia) and tender, and swallowing will be difficult and painful. Patients with irradiation of both parotid glands are more likely to complain of dry mouth than are those with unilateral irradiation. The small volume of viscous saliva that is secreted usually has a pH value 1 unit below normal (i.e., an average of 5.5 in irradiated patients compared to 6.5 in unexposed individuals). This pH is low enough to initiate decalcification of normal enamel.

As might be expected, salivary changes have a profound influence on the oral microflora and secondarily on the dentition, often leading to radiation caries (see Chapter 15). In saliva and plaque of patients following radiotherapy that includes the major salivary glands there is a pronounced change toward acidogenic microflora. Such patients have increases in *Streptococcus mutans*, *Lactobacillus*, and *Candida*. In addition, the buffering capacity of saliva falls as much as 44% during radiation

therapy. If some portions of the major salivary glands have been spared, dryness of the mouth usually subsides in 6 to 12 months because of compensatory hypertrophy of residual salivary gland tissue. Xerostomia that has persisted beyond a year is less likely to show significant return of function.

Teeth. Irradiation of teeth with therapeutic doses during their development severely retards their growth. Such irradiation may be for local disease (e.g., eosinophilic granuloma) or a generalized condition (leukemia being treated with whole-body irradiation followed by bone-marrow transplantation). If it precedes calcification, it may destroy the tooth bud. Irradiation after calcification has begun may inhibit cellular differentiation, causing malformations and arresting general growth. Children receiving radiation therapy to the jaws may show defects in the permanent dentition such as retarded root development, dwarfed teeth, or failure to form one or more teeth (Fig. 2-9). Teeth irradiated during development may complete calcification and erupt prematurely. In general, the severity of the damage is dose dependent. It is important to note that irradiation of teeth may retard or abort root formation but the eruptive mechanism of teeth is relatively radiation resistant. Irradiated teeth with altered root formation will still erupt.

Adult teeth are very resistant to the direct effects of radiation exposure. Pulpal tissue (which consists primarily of reverting and fixed postmitotic cells) demonstrates long-term fibroatrophy after irradiation. There is no discernible effect of radiation on the crystalline structure of enamel, dentin, or cementum, and radiation does not increase their solubility.

Radiation caries. Radiation caries is a rampant form of dental decay that may occur in individuals who have received a course of radiotherapy that included exposure of the salivary glands. The carious lesions result from changes in the salivary glands and saliva, including reduced flow, decreased pH, reduced buffering capacity, and increased viscosity. Because of the reduced or absent cleansing action of normal saliva, debris accumulates quickly. Irradiation of the teeth per se does not influence the course of radiation caries.

Clinically, there are three types of radiation caries. The most common is widespread superficial lesions attacking buccal, occlusal, incisal, and palatal surfaces. Another type primarily involves the cementum and dentin in the cervical region. These lesions may progress around the teeth circumferentially and result in loss of the crown. A final type

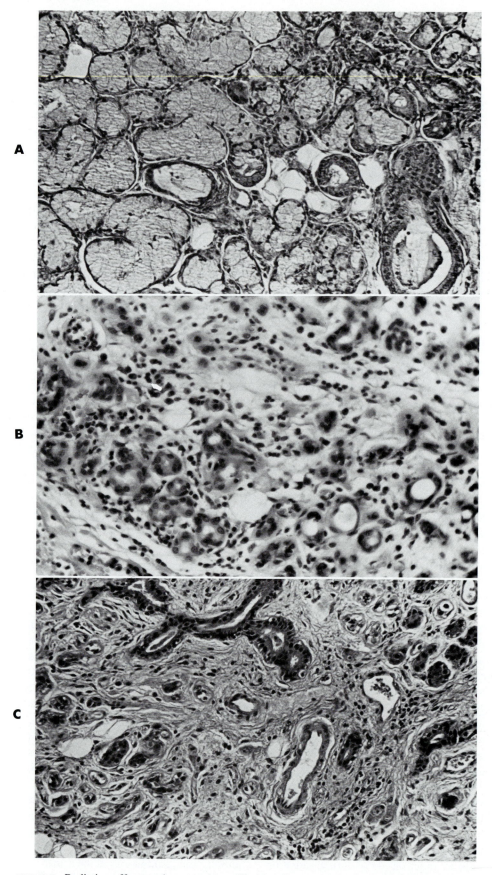

FIG. 2-8. Radiation effects on human submandibular salivary glands. **A,** Normal gland. **B,** A gland 6 months after exposure to radiotherapy. Note the loss of acini and presence of chronic inflammatory cells. **C,** A gland 1 year after exposure to radiotherapy. Note the loss of acini and extensive fibrosis.

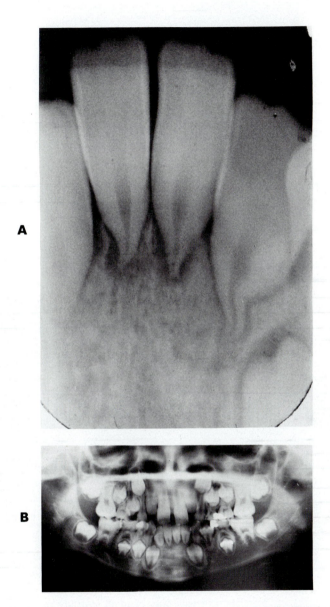

FIG. 2-9. Dental abnormalities following radiotherapy in two patients. The first, **A** and **B,** a 9-year-old girl who received 35 Gy at the age of 4 because of Hodgkin's disease, had severe stunting of the incisor roots with premature closure of the apices at 8 years (**A**) and retarded development of the mandibular second premolar crowns with stunting of the mandibular incisor, canine, and premolar roots at 9 years (**B**).　　　　　　　　　　　　　*Continued.*

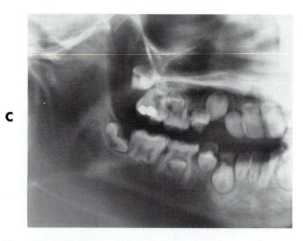

FIG. 2-9, cont'd. The other patient, **C,** a 10-year-old boy who received 41 Gy to the jaws at age 4, had severely stunted root development of all permanent teeth, with a normal primary molar. (**A** and **B** courtesy Mr. P.N. Hirschmann, Leeds England; **C** courtesy Dr. James Eischen, San Diego Calif.)

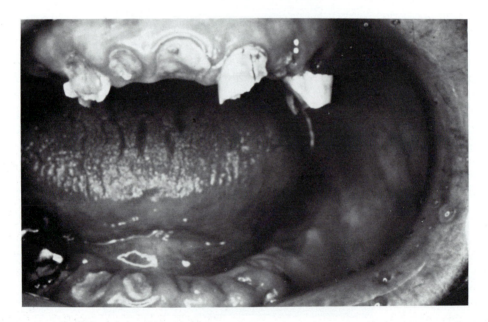

FIG. 2-10. Radiation caries. Note the extensive loss of tooth structure resulting from radiation-induced xerostomia.

appears as a dark pigmentation of the entire crown. The incisal edges may be markedly worn. Some patients will develop combinations of all these lesions (Fig. 2-10). The histologic features of the lesions are similar to those of typical carious lesions. It is the rapid course and widespread attack that distinguish radiation caries.

The best method of reducing radiation caries is daily application of a viscous topical 1% sodium fluoride gel. Use of topical fluoride causes a 6-

month delay in the irradiation-induced elevation of *Streptococcus mutans*. Deletion of dietary sucrose in addition to the use of a topical fluoride further reduces the concentrations of *S. mutans* and *Lactobacillus*. In recent years there has been a tendency to maintain sound teeth with a combination of restorative dental procedures, oral hygiene instruction, and topical applications of sodium fluoride. Patient cooperation in maintaining oral hygiene is extremely important. Teeth with gross caries or periodontal involvement are often extracted before irradiation.

Bone. Treatment for cancers in the oral region often includes irradiation of the mandible. The primary damage to mature bone results from radiation-induced damage to the fine vasculature, which is normally already sparse in a dense bone such as the mandible. The marrow tissue becomes hypovascular, hypoxic, and hypocellular. Subsequent to irradiation there may be a replacement of normal marrow with fatty marrow of fibrous connective tissue. In addition, the endosteum become atrophic, showing a lack of osteoblastic and osteoclastic activity, and some lacunae of the compact bone are empty, an indication of necrosis. Histologic study shows the degree of mineralization to be little altered from that in normal bone.

The clinical complications that occur in bone following irradiation relate to the marked reduction in vascularity and the consequent decreased capacity of the bone to resist infection. There is a strong possibility that infection and necrosis of bone will result in a nonhealing wound if the oral mucous membrane (already compromised by irradiation) breaks down. This may occur spontaneously or following a tooth extraction or denture sore and is known as *osteoradionecrosis* (Fig. 2-11). It is more common in the mandible than in the maxilla, probably because of the richer vascular supply to the maxilla and the fact that the mandible is more frequently irradiated. The role of microorganisms in this process is unclear. They may be only a contaminant rather than etiologic. The most common factors precipitating osteoradionecrosis are pre- and postirradiation extractions and periodontal disease. The higher the radiation dose absorbed by the bone, the greater is the risk of necrosis.

The risks of oral epithelial breakdown and subsequent osteoradionecrosis are significantly reduced by performing any necessary extractions and alveolectomies 2 to 3 weeks before the initiation of radiotherapy. This allows time for the soft tissues to heal before irradiation. Wound healing is compromised in an irradiated region, and posttreatment extraction of teeth should be avoided because of the risk of inducing osteoradionecrosis. This is especially true when 75% or more of the mandible is within the field of irradiation and the bone dose exceeds 65 Gy. Under these conditions endodontic therapy is preferable to extractions. When postirradiation extractions must be performed, it is important that these procedures be accompanied by radical alveolectomy to protect the mucosa against subsequent trauma from a prosthetic appliance. The use of hyperbaric oxygen before oral surgery in irradiated patients is effective for reducing the risk of complications.

It is very important that individuals who have received radiotherapy to the oral cavity be given regular dental care. Often they will require a radiographic examination to supplement the clinical examination. These radiographs are especially important because untreated caries leading to periapical infection can be quite severe with the compromised vascular supply to bone. The amount of added radiation is negligible in comparison to the amount received during therapy and should not serve as a reason to defer radiographs. Whenever possible, however, it is desirable to avoid taking radiographs during the first 6 weeks to 6 months after completion of radiotherapy. This gives the mucosal membrane time to heal and reduces the risk of breaking its integrity.

EFFECTS OF WHOLE-BODY IRRADIATION

When the whole body is exposed to low or moderate doses of radiation, there are characteristic changes (called the *acute radiation syndrome*) that develop. The clinical picture following whole-body exposure is quite different from that seen when a relatively small volume of tissue is exposed.

Acute radiation syndrome

The acute radiation syndrome is a collection of signs and symptoms experienced by persons after acute whole-body exposure to radiation. Information about this syndrome comes from animal experiments and human exposures in the course of medical radiotherapy, atom bomb blasts, and radiation accidents. Individually the clinical symptoms are not unique to radiation exposure; but taken as a whole, the pattern constitutes a distinct entity (Table 2-1). The following discussion pertains to whole-body exposure at a relatively high dose rate.

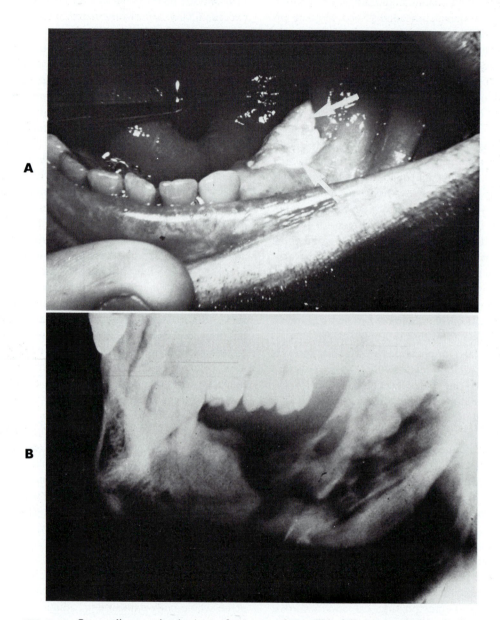

FIG. 2-11. Osteoradionecrosis. **A,** Area of an exposed mandible following radiotherapy. Note the loss of oral mucosa. **B,** Destruction of irradiated bone resu̅ ᶾ from the spread of infection.

Prodromal period. Within the first minutes to hours following exposure to whole-body irradiation of about 1.5 Gy, symptoms characteristic of gastrointestinal tract disturbances may occur. The individual may develop anorexia, nausea, vomiting, diarrhea, weakness, and fatigue. These early symptoms constitute the prodromal period of the acute radiation syndrome. Their cause is not clear but probably involves the autonomic nervous system. The severity and time of onset may be of significant prognostic value because they are dose related: the higher the dose, the more rapid the onset and the greater the severity of symptoms.

Latent period. Following this prodromal reaction there is a latent period of apparent well-being during which no signs or symptoms of radiation sickness occur. The extent of the latent period is also dose related. It extends from hours or days at supralethal exposures (greater than approximately 5 Gy) to a few weeks at sublethal exposures (less than 2 Gy). Symptoms will follow the latent period when individuals are exposed in the lethal range (approximately 2 to 5 Gy) or supralethal range.

Hematopoietic syndrome. Whole-body exposures of 2 to 7 Gy cause injury to the hematopoietic stem cells of the bone marrow and spleen. The high mitotic activity of these cells and the presence of many differentiating cells make the bone marrow a highly radiosensitive tissue. As a consequence, doses in this range cause a rapid and profound fall in the numbers of circulating granulocytes and platelets, and finally erythrocytes. Note that the mature circulating granulocytes, platelets, and erythrocytes themselves are very radioresistant because they are nonreplicating cells. Their paucity in the peripheral blood after irradiation reflects the relative radiosensitivity of their precursors. The differential changes in the blood count do not all appear at the same time (Fig. 2-12). Rather, the rate of fall in the circulating levels of a cell depends on the life span of that cell in the peripheral blood. Granulocytes, with short lives in circulation, fall off in a matter of days whereas red blood cells, with their long lives in circulation, fall off only slowly.

The clinical consequences of the depression of these cellular elements become evident as the circulating levels decline. Hence, in the weeks following such a radiation injury, infection appears first, followed later by anemia. The clinical signs of the hematopoietic syndrome include infection (in part from the lymphopenia and granulocytopenia), hemorrhage (from the thrombocytopenia), and anemia (from the erythrocyte depletion). Individuals may survive exposure in this range if the

TABLE 2-1. Acute radiation syndrome

Dose (Gy)	Manifestation
1 to 2	Prodromal symptoms
2 to 4	Mild hematopoietic symptoms
4 to 7	Severe hematopoietic symptoms
7 to 15	Gastrointestinal symptoms
50 +	Cardiovascular and central nervous system symptoms

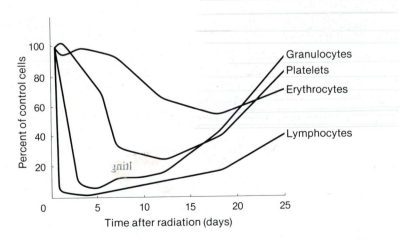

FIG. 2-12. Radiation effects on blood cells. When whole-body exposure inhibits the replacement of circulating cells by stem cell proliferation, the duration of their survival is largely determined by their life span.

bone marrow and spleen recover before the patient dies of one or more clinical complications. The probability of death is low following exposures at the low end of this range but much higher at the high end. When death results from the hematopoietic syndrome, it usually occurs 10 to 30 days after irradiation.

Because chronic inflammatory disease in the mouth is a likely source of entry for microorganisms into the bloodstream, the role of a the dentist is important in preventing death from hematopoietic syndrome. Following moderate injury there is about 7 to 10 days before clinically significant leukopenia develops. During this time the dentist should remove all sites of infection from the mouth. The removal of sources of infection, the vigorous administration of antibiotics, and in some cases the transplantation of bone marrow have saved individuals from the acute radiation syndrome.

Gastrointestinal syndrome. Whole-body exposures in the range of 7 to 15 Gy cause extensive damage to the gastrointestinal system. This damage, in addition to the hematopoietic damage described above, causes signs and symptoms called the gastrointestinal syndrome. Individuals exposed in this range may experience the prodromal stage within a few hours of exposure. Typically from the second through about the fifth day no symptoms are present (latent period) and the patient feels well. Such exposure, however, causes considerable injury to the rapidly proliferating basal epithelial cells of the intestinal villi and leads to a loss of the epithelial layer of the intestinal mucosa. The turnover time for cells lining the small intestine is normally 3 to 5 days. Because of the denuded mucosal surface, there is a loss of plasma and electrolytes; efficient intestinal absorption cannot occur. There is also ulceration with hemorrhaging of the intestines. All these changes are responsible for the diarrhea, dehydration, and loss of weight that are observed. Endogenous intestinal bacteria readily invade the denuded surface, producing septicemia.

The level of radiation required to produce the gastrointestinal syndrome (more than 7 Gy) is much greater than that causing sterilization of the blood-forming tissues, however, death (from destruction of the rapidly self-renewing cells in the intestines) occurs before the full effect of the radiation on hematopoietic systems can be evidenced. At about the time that developing damage to the gastrointestinal system reaches a maximum, the effect of bone marrow depression is just beginning to be manifested. By the end of 24 hours, the number of circulating lymphocytes falls to a very low level and this is followed by decreases in the number of granulocytes and then of platelets (Fig. 2-12). The result is a marked lowering of the body's defense against bacterial infection and a decrease in effectiveness of the clotting mechanism. The combined effects on these stem cell systems cause death within 2 weeks — from a combination of factors that include fluid and electrolyte loss, infection, and possibly nutritional impairment. Several of the fire fighters at Chernobyl, in the former Soviet Socialist Republic, Ukraine, died of the gastrointestinal syndrome.

Cardiovascular and central nervous system syndrome. Exposures in excess of 50 Gy usually cause death in 1 to 2 days. The few humans who have been exposed at this level showed collapse of the circulatory system with a precipitous fall in blood pressure in the hours preceding death. Autopsy revealed necrosis of cardiac muscle. Victims also may show intermittent stupor, incoordination, disorientation, and convulsions suggestive of extensive damage to the nervous system. Although the precise mechanism is not fully understood, these latter symptoms most likely result from radiation-induced damage to neurons and the fine vasculature of the brain. The syndrome is irreversible, and the clinical course may run from only a few minutes to about 48 hours before death occurs. The cardiovascular and central nervous system syndromes have such a rapid course that the irradiated individual dies before the effects of damage to the bone marrow and intestinal systems can develop.

The initial clinical problems govern the management of different forms of the acute radiation syndrome. *Antibiotics* are indicated when infection threatens or the granulocyte count falls. *Fluid and electrolyte replacement* is used as necessary. *Whole blood transfusions* are used to treat anemia, and platelets may be administered to arrest thrombocytopenia. *Bone marrow grafts* are indicated between identical twins, because there is no risk of graft-versus-host disease. Patients also receive such grafts when exposed to 8 to 10 Gy for treatment of leukemia.

Radiation effects on embryos and fetuses

Embryos and fetuses are considerably more radiosensitive than adults because most embryonic cells are relatively undifferentiated and rapidly mitotic, with long mitotic futures. In contrast to adult cells, they represent a relatively larger population in the radiosensitive phases (G_2 and M, Fig. 2-1) per unit tissue volume. Prenatal irradiation may lead to death of the organism or to specific developmental abnormalities depending on the stage of development at the time of irradiation. The description below of abnormalities resulting from embryo or fetal irradiation pertains to exposures far higher than those received during the course of dental radiography. The fetus of a patient exposed to dental radiography receives approximately 0.01 mGy.

The effect of exposure during the preimplantation period (first 10 days after conception in humans) has been studied, mostly in animals. Irradiation of rats with 2 Gy soon after conception usually causes death of the embryo but may have no effect. In the latter instance the surviving offspring show no abnormalities after birth. During the period of implantation (10 to 14 days after conception in humans) the embryo is much less susceptible to death although some malformations may appear.

The effects of radiation on human embryos and fetuses have been studied in women exposed to diagnostic or therapeutic radiation during pregnancy and women exposed to the atom bombs dropped at Hiroshima or Nagasaki. These embryos received exposures of 0.5 to 3 Gy. Exposures during the first few days following conception are thought to cause undetectable death of the conceptus. The most sensitive period for inducing developmental abnormalities is during the period of organogenesis, between 18 and 45 days of gestation. These effects are deterministic in nature. The most common abnormality among the Japanese children exposed early in gestation was reduced growth and reduced head circumference (microcephaly), often associated with mental retardation. Other abnormalities included small birth size, cataracts, genital and skeletal malformations, and microphthalmia. The period of maximum sensitivity of the brain is 8 to 15 weeks postconception. The frequency of severe mental retardation following exposure to 1 Gy during this period is about 43%.

Irradiation during the fetal period (greater than 50 days after conception) does not cause gross malformations. There is, however, general retardation of growth that persists through life. There is also evidence for an increased risk of childhood cancer, both leukemia and solid tumors, following irradiation in utero.

Comparative risks during pregnancy*

Irradiation during gestation

10 mSv	Death from childhood leukemia	1 in 3333
10 mSv	Death from other childhood cancer	1 in 3571

Maternal smoking

1 pack or more/day	Infant death	1 in 3

Maternal alcohol consumption

2 to 4 drinks/day	Signs of fetal alcohol syndrome	1 in 10
	Major malformation at delivery	2.75%

LATE SOMATIC EFFECTS

Somatic effects are those seen in the irradiated individual. The most important are radiation-induced cancers. Such lesions are a stochastic effect of radiation in that the probability of an individual's getting cancer depends on the amount of radiation exposure but the severity of the disease is not related to the dose.

Carcinogenesis

It is important to recognize that in the United States cancer accounts for nearly 20% of all deaths. Accordingly, the estimated number of deaths attributable to low-level radiation exposure is a small fraction of the total number that occur spontaneously. It is estimated that a single brief whole-body exposure of 100 mGy (about 30 times the average annual exposure) to 100,000 people would result in about 500 additional cancer deaths over the lifetime of the exposed individuals. This would be in addition to the 20,000 that would occur spontaneously. By far, the group of individuals most intensively studied for estimating the cancer risk from radiation are the Japanese A-bomb survivors. Over 60,000 individuals have been followed since 1950. An estimated 5936 cases of cancer of all types have been observed in this cohort, most resulting from natural causes. British patients treated with spinal irradiation for ankylosing spondylitis have also demonstrated 36 cases of leukemia and 563 cancers of all other types. Several studies of patients receiving many fluoroscopic examinations in the course of treatment for tuberculosis, as well

---

*Adapted from Mettler and Moseley, 1985.

as women treated with radiation for postpartum mastitis, have helped to understand the risk of inducing breast cancer. The effects of thyroid gland exposure have also been studied in irradiated patients. Some Israeli children were irradiated to the scalp to aid in treatment for ring worm, whereas infants in Rochester N.Y. received radiation treatments to reduce the size of their thymus gland. Many other studies on smaller groups of patients have provided useful information.

The estimation of the number of cancers induced by radiation is very difficult. Most of the individuals in the studies mentioned above received exposure in excess of the diagnostic range. Thus the probability that a cancer will result from a small dose can be estimated only by extrapolation from the rates observed following exposure to larger doses. Furthermore, radiation-induced cancers are not distinguishable from cancers produced by other causes. This means that the number of cancers can only be estimated as the number of excess cases found in exposed groups compared to the number in unexposed groups of people.

Tissues vary in their susceptibility to radiation-induced cancer (Table 2-2). There are some general findings regarding radiation-induced cancers other than leukemia.

1. Most cancers appear approximately 10 years after exposure and the elevated risk remains for as long as most exposed populations are followed, presumably for the lifetime of the exposed individuals.
2. The risk from exposure during childhood is estimated to be about twice as large as the risk during adulthood.
3. The mortality rate from all cancers (other than leukemia) shows no departure in linearity below 4 Sv.
4. The number of excess cancers induced by radiation is considered to be a multiple of the spontaneous rate rather than independent of the spontaneous rate.

The ensuing brief discussion of somatic effects of exposure to radiation will pertain largely to those organs exposed in the course of dental radiography.

Leukemia. The incidence of leukemia (other than chronic lymphocytic leukemia) rises following exposure of the bone marrow to radiation. Atom bomb survivors and patients irradiated for ankylosing spondylitis show a wave of leukemias (appearing within 5 years after exposure and returning to baseline rates within 30 years). The mortality data for leukemia are compatible with a linear-

TABLE 2-2. Susceptibility of different tissues to radiation-induced cancer

High	Moderate	Low
Colon	Breast (women)	Bladder
Stomach	Esophagus	Liver
Lung		Thyroid
Bone marrow		Skin
(leukemia)		Bone surface
		Brain
		Salivary glands

quadratic dose response relationship. Children under 20 are more at risk than adults.

Thyroid cancer. The incidence of thyroid carcinomas (arising from the follicular epithelium) increases in humans following exposure. Only about 10% of individuals with such cancers die from their disease. The best-studied groups are Israeli children irradiated to the scalp for ringworm, children in Rochester, New York, irradiated to the thymus gland, and atom bomb survivors in Japan. Susceptibility to radiation-induced thyroid cancer is greater early in childhood than at any time later in life and children are more susceptible than adults. Females are 2 to 3 times more susceptible than males to radiogenic as well as spontaneous thyroid cancers.

Bone cancer. Irradiation of bone periosteal and endosteal surfaces carries the risk of excess bone malignancies, mostly osteosarcoma. The dosimetry data pertaining to cancers arising from bone surfaces in humans following exposure to low-LET radiation are fairly sparse and not suitable for risk estimation. The Japanese A-bomb survivors showed no elevation in bone tumors following exposures up to 4 Gy.

Esophageal cancer. The data pertaining to esophageal cancer are relatively sparse. Excess cancers are found in the Japanese A-bomb survivors as well as in patients treated with x-ray for ankylosing spondylitis.

Brain and nervous system cancers. Patients exposed to diagnostic x-ray examinations in utero and to therapeutic doses in childhood or as adults (average midbrain dose of about 1 Gy) show excess numbers of malignant and benign brain tumors. Additionally, a case-control study has shown an association between intracranial meningiomas and previous medical or dental radiography. The strongest association was with a history of exposure to full-mouth dental radiographs when less than 20 years of age. Because of their age it is likely that

TABLE 2-3. Estimates of lifetime mortality rates in a population of all ages from specific fatal cancers after exposure to low doses (International Commission on Radiation Protection, 1990)

	Cancers/10^4 people/Sv
Bladder	30
Bone marrow	50
Bone surface	5
Breast	20
Colon	85
Liver	15
Lung	85
Esophagus	30
Ovary	10
Skin	2
Stomach	110
Thyroid	8
Remainder*	50
	500†

* The composition of the remainder is quite different in the two cases. Currently the remainder is composed of the following additional tissues and organs: adrenals, brain, upper large intestine, small intestine, kidney, muscle, pancreas, spleen, thymus, and uterus.
† This figure pertains to the general public. The total fatal cancer risk for a working population is taken to be $400 \times 10^{-4}/Sv^{-1}$.

TABLE 2-4. Risk of fatal cancers per million full-mouth radiographic examinations

Organ	Cancers
Gonads	—
Bone marrow	0.7
Colon	—
Lung	0.1
Stomach	—
Bladder	—
Breast	0.1
Liver	—
Esophagus	0.1
Thyroid	0.8
Skin	—
Bone surface	0.5
Remainder	0.3
	2.5

From White SC: 1992 Assessment of radiation risk from dental radiography, *Dentomaxillofac Radiol* 21:118-126, 1992.

Dental risk implications

The primary risk from dental radiography is radiation-induced cancer. The risk of fatal cancers resulting from a radiographic exposure is the sum of the risks of individual radiosensitive organs. The International Commission on Radiation Protection (ICRP) 1990 report presents the estimated lifetime mortality rates from cancer following low-dose exposure for 12 specific organs (Table 2-3).

The product of these mortality coefficients and the organ doses received during a radiographic examination yields fatality estimates for that examination. The remainder organs are those known to be radiosensitive but whose risk coefficient is too low or not known with sufficient precision to list separately. The risk estimates presented here pertain to the general public in that they are derived on the basis of typical age and sex distributions.

The dental literature contains several studies reporting sufficient dosimetric data for radiosensitive sites in the head and neck to allow estimation of the risk of fatal cancers from intraoral and panoramic radiography. The values from these studies were used to estimate the probability of fatal cancers per million full-mouth examinations shown in Table 2-4. This table assumes the use of typical radiographic technique (D-speed film and round collimation). With optimal technique (E-speed film and rectangular collimation) (described in Chapter 3) the risk can be substantially reduced. The highest estimated risks are for leukemia (bone marrow) and for thyroid and bone surface cancers. The risk of bone cancer following dental exposure is probably

these patients received substantively more exposure than is the case today with contemporary techniques.

Salivary gland cancer. The incidence of salivary gland tumors is increased in patients treated with irradiation for diseases of the head and neck, in Japanese A-bomb survivors, and in persons exposed to diagnostic x irradiation. An association between tumors of the salivary glands and dental radiography has been shown, the risk being highest in persons receiving full-mouth examinations before the age of 20 years. Only individuals who received an estimated cumulative parotid dose of 500 mGy or more showed a significant correlation between dental radiography and salivary gland tumors.

Cancer of other organs. Other organs such as the skin, paranasal sinuses, and bone marrow (with respect to multiple myeloma) also show excess neoplasia following exposure; however, the mortality and morbidity rates expected following head and neck exposure are much lower than for the organs described above.

TABLE 2-5. Risk of fatal cancers per million panoramic radiographic examinations

Organ	Cancers
Gonad	—
Bone marrow	0.06
Colon	—
Lung	0.01
Stomach	—
Bladder	—
Breast	—
Liver	—
Esophagus	0.02
Thyroid	0.06
Skin	—
Bone surface	0.03
Remainder	0.03
	0.21

From White SC: 1992 Assessment of radiation risk from dental radiography, *Dentomaxillofac Radiol* 21:118-126, 1992.

overestimated because of the lack of evidence relating low-LET exposure below 4 Gy to osteosarcoma.

It is possible to estimate the upper extent of the worldwide risk of fatal cancers from dental radiography. The United Nations reports that there were 340 million dental radiographic procedures performed in 1980, with an average of four films per procedure. Given a risk estimate of 2.5 fatalities per million full-mouth examinations, we might project that the risk of one radiographic procedure (four films) would be about 1 fatality per 2 million procedures and, accordingly, the worldwide annual fatality rate would be about 170 cases. This estimate declines to 34 cases with the universal adoption of E-speed film and rectangular collimation.

Published dosimetry data for panoramic radiography allow risk estimation from this source of exposure. Table 2-5 computes the risk of fatal malignancies per million individuals exposed to a panoramic radiograph using rare-earth intensifying screens. As in Table 2-4, the computation was based on original dosimetry and current ICRP risk estimates. In this case leukemia (bone marrow) and thyroid cancer constitute the greatest risk but bone surface cancers are also important. It is noteworthy that panoramic radiography carries about one-tenth the risk of a full-mouth set of radiographs.

The estimates in Tables 2-4 and 2-5 represent extrapolations to the low-dose range beyond the availability of data. As such they cannot be considered as demonstrating that diagnostic exposures cause cancer at the rates estimated. Nor, however,

is there reason to presume that dental radiography is without risk. Although the risk is certainly small in terms of other risks that we readily assume in the course of our daily lives (e.g., from driving, smoking, or eating fatty foods), there is no basis to assume that it is zero. Despite the fact that radiation appears to be but a weak carcinogen, we must have concern because of the large numbers of people exposed to diagnostic radiography. We also must conclude that it is our responsibility to assure that patients avoid receiving even the smallest unnecessary dose of radiation.

Other late somatic effects

A number of late somatic effects other than carcinogenesis are recognized.

Mental retardation. Studies of individuals exposed in utero have shown that the developing human brain is radiosensitive. It is estimated that there is a 4% chance of mental retardation per 100 mSv at 8 to 15 weeks of gestational age, with less risk occurring from exposure at other gestational ages. Again, the exposure to the embryo from dental radiography is in the range of 0.01 mSv.

Cataract. The threshold for induction of cataracts ranges from about 2 Gy when the dose is received in a single exposure to more than 5 Gy when the dose is received in multiple exposures over a period of weeks. These doses are far in excess of those received with contemporary dental radiographic techniques.

RADIATION GENETICS
Gene mutation

Radiation may induce damage in the genetic material of reproductive cells, and the offspring of irradiated parents may reveal the effects of such damage. In his pioneering work in this field (1927) Muller reported radiation-induced mutations in *Drosophila* (fruit flies). Intensive work in this field established a number of basic principles of radiation genetics. He found that radiation induces new mutations rather than simply increases the frequency of spontaneous mutations. Furthermore, the frequency of mutations increases in direct proportion to the dose, even at very low doses, with no evidence of a threshold. The vast majority of mutations are deleterious to the organism.

Mice. The genetic effects of radiation on mammals have been studied most extensively in mice. Unlike *Drosophila,* mice show a mutation rate that is dependent on dose rate. When spermatogonia are irradiated at 900 mGy/min, the number of mutations for a given total dose is about three times

TABLE 2-6. Estimated genetic effects of 10 mSv per generation

Disorder	Current incidence/ 10^6 liveborn offspring	Additional first-generation cases/ 10^6 liveborn offspring/10 mSv
Autosomal dominant		
Severe	2500	5 to 20
Mild	7500	1 to 15
X-linked	400	<1
Recessive	2500	<1
Congenital abnormalities	20,000 to 30,000	10

*Adapted from Committee on the Biological Effects of Ionizing Radiations: *Health effects of exposure to low levels of ionizing radiation, BEIR V,* Washington DC, 1990, National Academy Press, Table 2-1.

higher than when 9 mGy/min is used; and the dose-rate effect is greater when female mice are irradiated. The use of very low dose rates causes no more mutations in oocytes than are seen in controls, which suggests that there may be repair of radiation-induced genetic damage in females. Spermatozoa show no dose-rate dependence below 8 mGy/min, suggesting a lack of such repair mechanisms in males. The mouse studies also revealed that descendents of irradiated individuals had far fewer abnormalities than would have been expected.

Effects on humans. There is little information about the heritable effects of radiation exposure in humans (those effects seen in the progeny of irradiated persons). To date, such effects have not been clearly demonstrated. Nor has there been a statistically significant increase in genetically related disease in the children of atom bomb survivors. Current knowledge of genetic effects following radiation exposure derives largely from work on mice. It is believed that the bulk of genetic damage from low levels of radiation will result from the accumulation of subtle nonvisible changes and lead to a gradual increase in the overall ill health of the irradiated population.

Doubling dose. One way to measure the risk from genetic exposure is by determining the doubling dose. This is the amount of radiation a population requires to produce in the next generation as many additional mutations as arise spontaneously. In humans the genetic doubling dose for mutations resulting in death is approximately 1 Sv. Inasmuch as the average person receives far less gonadal radiation, it is clear that radiation contributes relatively little to the genetic damage in populations. The gonadal dose to patients from a full-mouth radiographic examination is in the range of 2 to 20 μSv. Table 2-6 shows the estimated genetic effects resulting from 10 mSv per generation.

SELECTED REFERENCES
Odontogenesis

Gorlin RJ, Meskin LH: Severe irradiation during odontogenesis, *Oral Surg* 16:35-38,1963.

Kimeldorf DJ: Radiation-induced alterations in odontogenesis and formed teeth. In Berdgis CC (ed): *Pathology of irradiation,* Baltimore, 1971, Williams & Wilkins.

Osteoradionecrosis

Balogh JM, Sutherland SE: Osteoradionecrosis of the mandible: a review, *J Otolaryngol* 18(5):245-250, 1989.

Calhoun KH, Shapiro RD, Stiernberg CM, et al: Osteomyelitis of the mandible, *Arch Otolaryngol Head Neck Surg* 114(10):1157-1162, 1988.

Kluth EV, Jain PR, Stuchell RN, Frich JC Jr: A study of factors contributing to the development of osteoradionecrosis of the jaws, *J Prosthet Dent* 59(2):194-201, 1988.

Larson D, Lindberg R, Lane E, Goepfert H: Major complications of radiotherapy in cancer of the oral cavity and oropharynx: a 10 year retrospective study, *Am J Surg* 146:531-536, 1983.

Makkonen TA, Kiminki A, Makkonen TK, Nordman E: Dental extractions in relation to radiation therapy of 224 patients, *Int J Oral Maxillofac Surg* 16(1):56-64, 1987.

Marciani RD, Ownby HE: Osteoradionecrosis of the jaws, *J Oral Maxillofac Surg* 44(3):218-223, 1986.

Marx RE, Johnson RP: Studies in the radiobiology of osteoradionecrosis and their clinical significance, *Oral Surg* 64:379-390, 1987.

Marx RE, Johnson RP, Kline SN: Prevention of osteoradionecrosis: a randomized prospective clinical trial of hyperbaric oxygen versus penicillin, *J Am Dent Assoc* 111:49-54, 1985.

Maxymiw WG, Wood RE: The role of dentistry in head and neck radiation therapy, *Can Dent Assoc J* 55(3):193-198, 1989.

Rothwell BR: Prevention and treatment of the orofacial complications of radiotherapy, *J Am Dent Assoc* 114(3):316-322, 1987.

Radiation caries

Brown L, Dreizen S, Handler S: Effects of selected caries preventive regimens on microbial changes following irradiation-induced xerostomia in cancer patients, *Microbiol Abstr* 1(suppl):275-290, 1976.

Daly TE, Drane JB: Prevention and management of dental problems in irradiated patients, *J Am Soc Prevent Dent* 6:21-25, 1976.

Dreizen S, Brown L: Xerostomia and dental caries, *Microbiol Abstr* 1(suppl):263-273, 1976.

Frank RM, Herdly J, Philippe E: Acquired dental defects and salivary gland lesions after irradiation for carcinoma, *J Am Dent Assoc* 70:868-883, 1965.

Marciani RD, Plezia R: Management of teeth in the irradiated patient, *J Am Dent Assoc* 88:1021-1024, 1974.

Ripa LW: Review of the anticaries effectiveness of professionally applied and self-applied topical fluoride gels, *J Public Health Dent* 49(5):spec no:297-309, 1989.

Risk estimation

Committee on the Biological Effects of Ionizing Radiations: *Health effects of exposure to low levels of ionizing radiation, BEIR V,* Washington DC, 1990, National Academy Press.

Gibbs SJ: Influence of organs in the ICRP's remainder on effective dose equivalent computed for diagnostic radiation exposures, *Health Phys* 56:515-520, 1989.

Gibbs SJ, Pujol A, Chen TS, et al: Patient risk from intraoral dental radiography, *Dentomaxillofac Radiol* 17:15-23, 1988.

Preston-Martin S, Thomas CC, White SC, Cohen D: Prior exposure to medical and dental x-rays related to tumors of the parotid gland, *J Natl Cancer Inst* 80:943-949, 1988.

Preston-Martin S, White S: Brain and salivary gland tumors related to prior dental radiography: implications for current practice, *J Am Dent Assoc* 120:151-158, 1990.

1990 Recommendations of the International Commission on Radiological Protection, ICRP Publication 60, Annals of the ICRP 21, 1990.

Underhill TE, Chilvarquer I, Kimura K, et al: Radiobiologic risk estimation from dental radiology. I, Absorbed doses to critical organs, *Oral Surg* 66:111-120, 1988; II, Cancer incidence and fatality, *Oral Surg* 66:261-267, 1988.

United Nations Scientific Committee on the Effects of Atomic Radiation: *Sources, effects, and risks of ionizing radiation,* New York, 1988, U.N.

White SC: 1992 Assessment of radiation risk from dental radiography, *Dentomaxillofac Radiol* 21:118-126, 1992.

Saliva and salivary glands

Ben-Aryeh H, Gutman D, Szargel R, Laufer D: Effects of irradiation on saliva in cancer patients, *Int J Oral Surg* 4:205-210, 1975.

Karlsson G: The relative change in saliva secretion in relation to the exposed area of the salivary glands after radiotherapy of head and neck region, *Swed Dent J* 11(5):189-194, 1987.

Kashima HK, Kirkham WR, Andrews JR: Postirradiation sialadenitis: a study of the clinical features, histopathologic changes, and serum enzyme variations following irradiation of human salivary glands, *Am J Roentgenol* 94:271-291, 1965.

Marks J, Davis C, Gottsman V, et al: The effects of radiation on parotid salivary function, *Int J Radiat Oncol Biol Phys* 7:1013-1019, 1981.

Taste

Conger AD: Loss and recovery of taste acuity in patients irradiated to the oral cavity, *Radiat Res* 53:338-347, 1973.

Mossman KL: Gustatory tissue injury in man: radiation dose response relationships and mechanisms of taste loss, *Br J Cancer Suppl* 7:9-11, 1986.

GENERAL REFERENCES

Arena V: *Ionizing radiation and life,* St Louis, 1971, Mosby.

Bergonié J, Tribondeau L: Médicine: interprétation de quelques résultats de la radiothérapie et essai de fixation d'une technique rationnelle, *Comp Rend Acad Sci* 143:983-985, 1906. (English translation by GH Fletcher, *Radiat Res* 11:587, 1959.)

Casarett A: *Radiation biology,* Englewood Cliffs NJ, 1968, Prentice-Hall.

Dalrymple G, Gaulden ME, Kollmorgen G, Vogel H (eds): *Medical radiation biology,* Philadelphia, 1973, WB Saunders.

Hall E: *Radiobiology for the radiologist,* ed 3, Philadelphia, 1988, JB Lippincott.

Mettler F, Kelsey C, Ricks R: *Medical management of radiation accidents,* Boca Raton Fla, 1990, CRC Press.

Mettler F, Moseley R: *Medical effects of ionizing radiation,* Orlando Fla, 1985, Grune & Stratton.

Pizzarello D, Witcofski R: *Medical radiation biology,* ed 2, Philadelphia, 1982, Lea & Febiger.

Prasad K: *CRC handbook of radiobiology,* Boca Raton Fla, 1984, CRC Press.

Rubin P, Casarett G: *Clinical radiation pathology,* Philadelphia, 1968, WB Saunders.

3

Neil L. Frederiksen

Health Physics

FAULTY X-RAY DEVICES, UNTRAINED OPERATORS OVERDOSE U.S. PATIENTS; TESTS SHOW RADIATION'S BAD EFFECTS; RADIATION CLOUD OVER MEDICINE; SINGLE DOSE OF "SAFE" RADIATION FOUND HARMFUL; and DIAGNOSTIC X-RAYS DESERVE THAT NEGATIVE REACTION are headlines that have appeared in newspapers across the United States during the last few years. The night before an appointment with you, your patient may read one of these articles and, understandably, form a negative opinion concerning the use of x rays for diagnostic purposes. Are you prepared to discuss intelligently the benefits and possible hazards involved with their use and to describe the steps you will take to reduce the hazard?

It is essential that practitioners who administer ionizing radiation become familiar with the magnitude of radiation exposure encountered in medicine and dentistry as well as with the possible risk in everyday life that such exposure entails and the methods used to affect exposure and dose reduction. This information will provide the background necessary to discuss intelligently with patients the benefits and possible hazards involved with the use of x rays.

SOURCES OF RADIATION EXPOSURE

A wide variety of conditions and circumstances, some of which we are able to control and others we are not, result in radiation exposure from a multitude of sources. Although the sources of radiation exposure are many and varied, they can be categorized as being derived from two sources: natural and artificial (Table 3-1). The radiation from these sources results in an *average annual effective dose* of 3.60 mSv to a person living in the United States.[71] The *effective dose*, the dosimetric quantity used to relate radiation exposure to risk, is derived as follows: *The equivalent dose (H_T)*, a quantity that expresses all kinds of radiation on a common scale, is defined as the product of the absorbed

TABLE 3-1. Average annual effective dose of ionizing radiations (mSv) to a person in the United States

Source	
Natural	
External	
Cosmic	0.27
Terrestrial	0.28
Internal	
Radon	2.00
Other	0.40
ROUNDED TOTAL	3.00
Artificial	
Medical	
X-ray diagnosis	0.39
Nuclear medicine	0.14
Consumer products	0.10
Other	
Occupational	<0.01
Nuclear fuel cycle	<0.01
Fallout	<0.01
Miscellaneous	<0.01
ROUNDED TOTAL	0.60
Natural plus artificial	3.60

From National Council on Radiation Protection and Measurements, Bethesda, MD: *NCRP Report* 93, 1987; 94, 1987; 95, 1987; 100, 1989.

dose in grays *(D)* and the radiation weighting factor *(w_R)*. The unit of equivalent dose is the *sievert*. The effective dose *(E)* is the sum of the equivalent doses to each tissue *(H_T)* multiplied by each tissue's weighting factor *(w_T)*:

$$E = \Sigma\, H_T \cdot w_T$$

The tissue weighting factors are defined by the International Commission on Radiological Protection.[41] In this manner it is possible to obtain a value for effective dose (estimated to be proportional to the somatic and genetic radiation-induced risks, even though the body was not uniformly exposed).

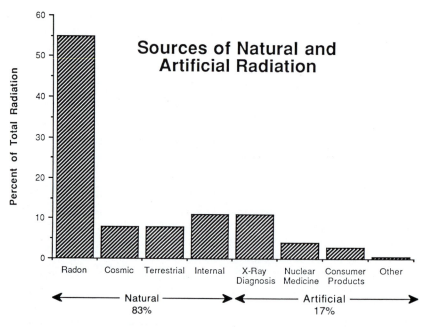

FIG. 3-1. Distribution of natural and artificial background radiation. Note that natural radiation contributes more exposure than artificial radiation and that x-ray diagnosis is the largest component of the artificial radiation.

For each source category in Table 3-1 the *collective effective dose* was obtained by multiplying the *average effective dose to the exposed population by the number of people exposed*. This collective effective dose was then divided by the United States population in 1980 (230 million) to obtain the *average annual effective dose* for a member of that population. It is important to consider that these quantities of dose, listed in Table 3-1, are expressed in millisieverts per year prorated over the total population. Thus the contribution to the radiation exposure of an individual from each component may be expected to vary by one or more orders of magnitude.

Natural radiation

Natural or background radiation is, by far, the largest contributor (83%) to the radiation exposure of people living in the United States today[69,71,74] (Table 3-1 and Fig. 3-1). Background radiation, resulting from external and internal sources, yields an average annual E of about 3 mSv.

External. Exposure in this category is due to cosmic and terrestrial radiation or that originating from the environment. These sources contribute about 15% of the radiation exposure to the population.

Cosmic radiation. Cosmic radiation includes both energetic subatomic particles and photons of extraterrestrial origin that reach the earth (primary cosmic radiation) and, to a lesser extent, the particles and photons (secondary cosmic radiation) generated by the interactions of primary cosmic radiation with atoms and molecules of the earth's atmosphere. In the lower atmosphere the E from cosmic radiation is primarily a function of altitude, almost doubling with each 2000 m increase in elevation. Thus at sea level the exposure from cosmic radiation is about 0.24 mSv per year, at an elevation of 1600 m (approximately 1 mile or the elevation of Denver, Colorado) about 0.50 mSv per year, and at an elevation of 3200 m (approximately 2 miles or Leadville, Colorado) about 1.25 mSv per year. Considering the altitude distribution of the U.S. population and a 20% reduction in exposure because of structural shielding during time spent indoors, it can be calculated that the average cosmic radiation E rate is about 0.26 mSv per year.

Also included in this category is the exposure resulting from airline travel. An airline flight of 5 hours in the middle latitudes at an altitude of 12 km may result in an absorbed dose of about 15 μSv. With 340 million passengers in 1984 undertaking trips with an average duration of 1.5 hours, this would yield an average annual effective dose of approximately 0.01 mSv. Thus, in total, cosmic radiation including that occurring in airline travel contributes an exposure of 0.27 mSv or about 8% of the average annual effective dose to a member of the U.S. population.

Terrestrial radiation. The exposure from terrestrial sources varies with the type of soil and its content of the naturally occurring radionuclide potassium-40 and the radioactive decay products of uranium-238 and thorium-232. Most of the gamma radiation from these sources comes from the top 20 cm of soil, with only a small contribution by airborne radon and its decay products. Indoor exposure from terrestrial radionuclides is very close to that occurring outdoors. This results from a balance between the shielding provided by structural materials and the exposure from radioactive nuclides contained within these shielding materials.

Terrestrial radiation has been measured in air in more than 200 locations over a large portion of the United States. Dose rates vary from about 0.16 mSv per year on the Atlantic and Gulf coastal plains, to 0.63 mSv per year for a region on the eastern slopes of the Rocky Mountains, to about 0.30 mSv for the rest of the country. Combining this information with data on the geographic distribution of the U.S. population, it is estimated that the average terrestrial exposure rate is about 0.28 mSv per year or approximately 8% of the average annual effective dose to a person living in the United States. This quantity of radiation exposure appears minimal compared to that received by individuals living in certain towns and villages of Brazil and India, where the gamma radiation dose levels can be as high as 120 mGy per year. These unusually high terrestrial radiation levels have been recorded because these towns and villages were constructed on soil containing monazite, a mineral with a high content of thorium-232.[3]

Internal. The sources of internal radiation are radionuclides that are taken up from the external environment by inhalation and ingestion. Because an organism cannot discriminate between isotopes of a chemical element, all isotopes, radioactive or not, have an equal chance, modified by frequency of occurrence, of being incorporated into the body. This source, which results in about 67% (2.40 mSv) of the radiation exposure of the population, includes radon and its short-lived decay products.

Radon. Radon is estimated to be responsible for approximately 56% of the radiation exposure of the United States population. As such it is the largest single contributor to natural radiation (2.00 mSv/yr) and one that has only recently been recognized.

Although the ubiquitous noble gas radon is transported in the water and atmosphere that enters our homes and buildings, its short-lived decay products (^{218}Po, ^{214}Po, ^{214}Pb, and ^{214}Bi) are of perhaps more concern. These products are primarily attached to aerosols that can deposit in the respiratory tract, contributing an average annual equivalent dose to the bronchial epithelium in the United States population of 24 mSv. It has recently been estimated[67] that exposure to this quantity of radiation may be causing as many as 10,000 lung cancer deaths per year in the United States.

Other internal sources. Estimates place the average annual E as a result of the presence of uranium and thorium and their decay products (potassium-40, rubidium-87, carbon-14, tritium, and a dozen or more extraterrestrially produced radionuclides) at 0.40 mSv per year. Because some of these radionuclides have always existed in the environment, at least since the origin of mankind, they have always been in the body. Other artificial radionuclides are a product of modern times. Following periods of nuclear weapon testing in the 1950s and early 1960s, the fission products cesium-137 and strontium-90 were discovered in the human body. Released into the environment by nuclear explosions, they reached the body through normal food chains. Of these, strontium-90, a pure beta emitter, is perhaps the most important. Because of its chemical similarity to calcium, it is readily assimilated in the bones and teeth of children and young adults. Once strontium-90 is concentrated in these areas, there is justifiable concern because of its long half-life (28.8 years) and slow turnover rate (the effective half-life in bone is 17.5 years).[3] Currently fallout is no longer a significant source of exposure to the public because of an almost worldwide ban on the atmospheric testing of nuclear weapons.

Artificial radiation

Human beings, with all their technologic advances, have contributed a number of sources of radiation to the environment.[71,74,70] These may be categorized into three major groups—medical diagnosis and treatment, consumer and industrial products and sources, and other minor sources—which contribute an average annual E of about 0.60 mSv or 17% of the annual radiation exposure to the U.S. population (Table 3-1 and Fig. 3-1).

Medical diagnosis and treatment. Studies show that radiation used in the healing arts is the single largest component (0.53 mSv) of artificial radiation to which the U.S. population is exposed and second only to radon as a source. Although sources in this group include radiation therapy and diagnosis, diagnostic x-ray exposure is the larger contributor. It has been estimated that more than 330,000 x-ray units in the United States in 1981 were being used for medical and dental diagnoses, procedures that yield an average annual E of about 0.39 mSv. The contribution made by oral radiography has recently been excluded from this calculated total because dental examinations are estimated[110] to be responsible for an average annual effective dose of less than 0.01 mSv. That dental x-ray examinations are responsible for only 2.5% of the average annual E resulting from x-ray diagnosis and 0.3% of the total average annual E is remarkable when the following facts are considered: in 1981 more than half (204,000) the x-ray units in the United States were used by dentists; in 1982 it was estimated that 105 million x-ray examinations were performed using 380 million films; and in that same year (1982) there were a reported 456 dental x-ray examinations per 1000 population.

Consumer and industrial products and sources. Although only a minor contributor to the average annual effective dose (3%), consumer and industrial products and sources contain some of the more interesting and unsuspected sources. In total this group, which includes the domestic water supply (10 to 60 μSv), combustible fuels (1.0 to 6.0 μSv), dental porcelain (0.1 μSv), television receivers (<10 μSv), pocket watches (1.0 to 5.0 × 10^{-2} μSv), smoke alarms (<1.0 × 10^{-2} μSv), and airport inspection systems (<1.0 × 10^{-2} μSv), contributes about 0.10 mSv to the average annual E.

The contribution resulting from use of tobacco products is also included in this category. With information available, however, it is impossible to estimate the average annual E to the population from this source. Nevertheless, by making several assumptions an estimate of the effective dose for the average smoker can be calculated. The annual average dose to a small area of the bronchial epithelium is estimated[15,56] to be 8.0 mGy as a result of the ^{210}Pb and ^{210}Po contained within tobacco. Applying a radiation quality factor (w_R) of 20 for alpha particles (^{210}Pb and ^{210}Po are alpha emitters) would yield an annual equivalent dose (H_T) to the lungs of 160 mSv. By using a tissue weighting factor (w_T) of 0.08 for the portion of lungs exposed yields an effective dose of approximately 13 mSv for the average smoker.

Other artificial sources. Of the sources in this category (which may contribute in total only about 0.01 mSv to the average annual effective dose), nuclear power is of particular concern to the public. By 1979, 70 nuclear power reactors had been licensed for operation in the United States[17]; and by 1987 this figure had reached almost 100.[71] By the year 2000 it is estimated[17] that the number may reach 250. In spite of this increasing number of nuclear power and support facilities, it is currently estimated that in normal operation these reactors add only about 0.6 μSv to the average annual E, a quantity up to 10 *times less* than that contributed by the combustible fuels, coal, and natural gas, which contain naturally occurring radionuclides that are released to the environment when burned.

History tells us that accidents do happen. Such was the case at the Three Mile Island nuclear plant in 1979. In this case, however, studies showed that the maximum individual dose was less than 1.0 mSv and individuals living within a 16 km radius of the plant received an average dose of only 0.08 mSv, an added exposure equal to some 2.7% of their natural background radiation exposure. A study made 5 years after the Three Mile Island accident[5] reported that residents living near the power plant showed no evidence of increased cancer as a result of the 1979 accident, a finding not unexpected in view of the relatively long latent period for radiation-induced malignancy. It is thought,[18] however, that because of the low exposures that resulted from this accident, if an increase in the number of cancer cases were to occur, it would be negligible and perhaps go undetected.

The nuclear accident at Chernobyl in 1986, in what was then the Ukrainian Soviet Socialist Republic, made clear that the use of nuclear power facilities carries the real potential of causing considerable harm if not properly controlled. In that event, according to the press, 31 persons in the immediate vicinity of the plant died of acute radiation injury (see Chapter 2) in the first months following exposure. In the next 70 years it has been estimated[18] that at least 10,000 excess cancer deaths from leukemia and solid tumors of the thyroid gland and other organs will occur in the Ukrainian people. Risk estimates to the United States population as a result of exposure to airborne debris from Chernobyl are considerably less[11]: three additional lung cancer deaths and an extra four deaths from cancer of the thyroid, breast, or bone marrow may be expected over the next 45 years in the United States because of this accident. (Compare this with the estimated 10,000 annual lung cancer deaths that may be caused by the presence of radon in our environment.)

EXPOSURE AND DOSE IN RADIOGRAPHY

The goal of radiation protection procedures is to minimize the exposure of office personnel and patients during the radiographic examination. To assure that radiographic techniques and procedures are followed that will both achieve this goal and enable the practitioner to comply with federal and state regulations, the radiation exposure of personnel and the radiation dose to patients are continuously monitored and assessed.

Occupational exposure

Recognition of the harmful effects of radiation and of the risk involved with its use has resulted in the establishment of a limitation, termed the *maximum permissible dose equivalent* (MPD), on the amount of radiation received by occupationally exposed individuals. Defined by both the National[72] and the International[41] Council on Radiation Protection and Measurements (NCRP and ICRP), the MPD is "the maximum dose that a person or specified parts thereof shall be allowed to receive in a stated period of time" (Table 3-2). This definition addresses several important radiobiologic facts: the ability of cells to repair radiation damage and the differing radiosensitivities of the organs of the body. The MPD is expressed in sieverts to include both particulate and electromagnetic ionizing radiation. At doses equal to the MPD, the risk is not zero but small and consistent with the risks encountered in other occupations. No "effects" or injuries have been demonstrated as a result of exposure to the MPD.[98]

The MPD is also considered to be the maximum dose of radiation that *in light of present knowledge* would not be expected to produce any significant radiation effects in a lifetime.[66] This expression (of the maximum permissible dose equivalent) assumes significance when it is considered that over the past 60 years the MPD has been revised downward three times and today the whole body MPD stands at 20 mSv per year, only 3% of that established in 1931. These reductions in the value of the MPD are a direct reflection of increased knowledge gained over the years concerning the harmful effects of radiation and the increased ability to use radiation more efficiently.

The current effective dose limit allows occupationally exposed individuals to receive a whole body exposure of 20 mSv per year (Table 3-2). Because of their cellular composition, different or-

TABLE 3-2. Recommendations on annual limits for human exposure to ionizing radiation

	Occupational (mSv)	Public (mSv)
Effective dose	20*	1
Equivalent dose to		
Lens	150	15
Skin	500	50
Hands and feet	500	—

*This value is averaged over 5 years (100 mSv in that length of time).
From International Commission on Radiological Protection: Table 5-4, *ICRP Publ* 60, 1990.

gans or parts of the body have different sensitivities to radiation. Thus, for avoidance of deterministic effects,* an annual equivalent dose limit of 150 mSv for the lens and 500 mSv for all other organs and tissues including the skin and extremities is recommended. The possibility of exposure of the general population and the need to limit this exposure are also recognized by both the NCRP and the ICRP. To this end an annual whole-body effective dose limit of no more than 1 mSv and a tissue and organ dose limit of 50 mSv have been established (Table 3-2).

The MPD described above and in Table 3-2 is based on a linear, nonthreshold, dose-response relationship. Consequently, although 20 mSv of whole body radiation per year may be considered to present minimal risk, every effort should be made to keep the dose to all individuals as low as practical and all unnecessary radiation exposure should be avoided. This is the philosophy of radiation protection currently in practice. It is based on the principles of ALARA (as low as reasonably achievable), which recognizes the possibility that no matter how small the dose there may be some effect.[41] Current data show that workers in radiation industries are acting in accordance with this philosophy, insofar as their average annual individual effective dose in 1980 was approximately 2.3 mSv, 12% of the annual limit. In 1980 the mean annual dose of individuals occupationally exposed in the operation of dental x-ray equipment was even less, 0.20 mSv, 1% of the allowable limit.[55]

---

*Effects for which the severity varies with the dose and for which a threshold usually exists. Examples include cataracts, fibrosis, and certain blood changes.

It is important to realize that the MPD was formulated by the NCRP and ICRP, private nonprofit organizations, and as such have no force of law. It is the responsibility of everyone who administers ionizing radiation to consult with his or her state's bureau of radiation control or safety to obtain information an applicable and current laws. In addition, the MPD is specified as occupational exposure. It should not be confused with the x-ray exposure that patients receive as a result of radiographic procedures. There are *no* state recommended maximum patient exposures.*

Patient exposure and dose

Patient dose from dental radiography is usually reported as the amount of radiation received by a target organ. One of the most common measurements is skin or surface exposure. The surface exposure, obtained by direct measurement, is the simplest way to record a patient's exposure to x rays. Of little significance in itself, it is used in the calculation of doses received by organs that lie at or near the point of measurement. Other target organs commonly reported include the bone marrow, thyroid gland, and gonads. The mean active bone marrow dose is an important measurement because bone marrow is the target organ believed responsible for radiation-induced leukemia. Particular concern has been expressed over exposure of the thyroid because this gland has one of the highest radiation-induced cancer rates.[17] The gonad dose is important because of suspected genetic responses to diagnostic x-ray exposure.

Additionally, patient dose has recently been reported as the effective dose (*E*).[70,113] This method of reporting resulted from an inability to make direct comparisons between radiographic techniques themselves and background radiation exposure in terms of dose because of the limited area of the body exposed during diagnostic radiology. It is only through the *E* that possible adverse effects from irradiation to a limited portion of the body can be compared with possible adverse effects from irradiation of the whole body.

Mean active bone marrow dose. The mean active bone marrow dose was derived as a specific tissue dose relevant to a particular stochastic[†] effect, leukemia. The mean active bone marrow dose is that dose of radiation averaged over the entire active bone marrow.[13] The mean active bone marrow dose resulting from an intraoral full-mouth survey of 21 films exposed with round collimation has been reported to be 0.142 mSv, and one exposed with rectangular collimation only 0.06 mSv.[113] Panoramic radiography was found to contribute a mean active bone marrow dose of about 0.01 mSv per film. For comparison, the mean active bone marrow dose from one chest film is 0.03 mSv.[75]

The risk from exposure to levels of radiation to the bone marrow as described above is discussed in detail in Chapter 2. It can be noted here, however, that studies have found no relationship between the level of background radiation and the incidence of leukemia,[23,24] congenital malformations,[90,91] or neonatal deaths.[37]

Thyroid dose. The proximity of the thyroid gland to the x-ray beam is of critical importance in determining the magnitude of dose received. For example, a radiographic examination of the cervical spine may consist of four separate exposures that in total are responsible for a dose to the thyroid of about 5.5 mGy.[75] During this examination the thyroid gland is almost directly in the center of the radiation field. On the other hand, a radiograph of the chest may result in a thyroid dose of only 0.01 mGy, mainly from scatter radiation.[75]

Studies have reported that the dose to the thyroid from oral radiography is fairly low. A 21-film full-mouth examination results in about 0.94 mGy.[113] This value is but one sixth that resulting from a radiographic examination of the cervical spine. Likewise, the thyroid dose from panoramic tomography has been reported[34] as being about 74 μGy, 1% that from a cervical spinal examination.

Gonad dose. Radiographs that involve the abdomen result in the highest dose to the gonads; and those involving the head, neck, and extremities the lowest. For example, a radiograph of the kidneys, ureters, and bladder (retrograde pyelogram) was reported[75] to deliver a gonad dose of 1.07 mGy to women and 0.08 mGy to men whereas a radiograph of the skull delivered a dose of less than 0.005 mGy to both sexes. Dental x-ray examinations result in a genetically significant dose of only 1.0 mGy.[36][‡] This contribution is only 0.03% of the

---

*With the possible exception of Illinois and Vermont.[40]

†Effect whose probability (rather than severity) is a function of radiation dose without threshold. Examples include cancers and genetic effects.

‡This quantity is close to 1/10,000 of the total beam exposure, an estimate for the gonad dose proposed by Richards.[86] (See "Leaded aprons and collars," p. 59.)

average annual background exposure. The probability that congenital anomalies and childhood malignancies could result from 0.1 Gy (100,000 times the gonad dose resulting from one dental periapical film) in utero is nil.[13]

Effective dose. It is tempting to make a direct comparison of the above values for purposes of risk estimation. However, the statement that a single dental periapical radiograph delivers more than 10 times the radiation of a chest film (in terms of surface exposure, i.e., 300 vs 23 mR is not entirely true because of differences in the exposed area and critical organs. These differences may be compensated for by a calculation of the effective dose, which is an estimate of the uniform whole body exposure carrying the same probability of radiation effect as a partial body exposure. By this method of calculation an optimized full-mouth survey (i.e., E-speed film, rectangular collimation) of 20 films has been found to deliver *one third* the amount of radiation of a single chest film and less than 1% the amount of a barium study of the intestines (Table 3-3).

In addition, the effective dose allows comparison of radiation doses resulting from diagnostic radiography to those received in the course of everyday life. Thus the data in Table 3-3 may be used by the dentist to discuss risk with patients in terms more easily understood. For example, it has been reported that the effective dose resulting from cosmic radiation in Denver is 0.24 mSv higher than the average of the United States. This would mean that a person living in an average location in the United States who had one full-mouth survey and one panoramic film made by optimized techniques every year (total *E* for these examinations = 0.04 mSv, Table 3-3) would incur only *one sixth* the risk of a person living in Denver who was not exposed to dental radiography. The significance of this method of comparison can be made even more dramatic by considering those locations in Brazil and India where the terrestrial gamma radiation levels can be as high as 0.12 Gy per year. This is equivalent to an annual excess exposure of about 40 *years* of average background radiation. Thus, if persons living in an average location in the United States were to receive *at least one* full-mouth survey and one panoramic examination everyday for the rest of their life, they would incur much less risk than individuals in one of these areas of Brazil or India and not exposed to oral radiography. Table 3-4 compares the exposure resulting from dental examinations to that resulting from

TABLE 3-3. Effective dose from diagnostic x-ray examinations (mSv)

Barium enema*	4.06
Upper gastrointestinal tract*	2.44
Computer tomography*	
Head and body	1.11
Abdomen*	0.56
Skull*	0.22
Chest*	0.08
Full-mouth survey†	
20 films, round collimation	0.084
Full-mouth survey†	
20 films, rectangular collimation	0.033
Interproximal survey†	
4 films, round collimation	0.017
Panoramic tomography†	0.007
Interproximal survey	
4 films, rectangular collimation	0.007

*From National Council on Radiation Protection and Measurements: *NCRP Reports* 100, Bethesda, MD, 1989.
†From White SC: *Dentomaxillofac Radiol* 21:118-126, 1992.

TABLE 3-4. Equivalent background exposure from dental radiography

Examination	Film	Collimation	Background equivalent
Full mouth			
	D	Round	10 days
	E	Round	5 days
	D	Rectangular	4 days
	E	Rectangular	2 days
Bitewings (4)			
	D	Round	2 days
	E	Round	1 day
	D	Rectangular	1 day
	E	Rectangular	10 hours
Panoramic			
	Calcium tungstate screens		1 day
	Rare earth screens		10 hours

Modified from White SC: *Dentomaxillofac Radiol* 21:118-126, 1992.

natural background radiation. It can be seen that dental exposures are quite small in terms of the radiation routinely received during the course of everyday life.

METHODS OF EXPOSURE AND DOSE REDUCTION

The decision to use diagnostic radiography rests on professional judgment of its necessity for the benefit of the total health of the patient. This decision having been made, it then becomes the duty of the dental professional to produce a maximum yield of information per unit of x-ray exposure.[19]

Becoming aware of the potential risks associated with the use of ionizing radiation and its contribution to rising health care costs is the first step toward exposure and dose reduction in diagnostic radiography. Once this awareness has been developed, the second step is the utilization of techniques, materials, and equipment that optimize the radiologic process. Optimizing the radiologic process is the best way to ensure maximum patient benefit with a minimum of patient and operator exposure.[12]

In this section methods of exposure and dose reduction are described that can be used in oral radiography. Each subsection begins with a recommendation of the American Dental Association Council on Dental Materials, Instruments, and Equipment based on optimum use of the radiologic process. This is followed by a discussion of how these recommendations can be satisfied. Included in the text are NCRP recommendations and federal regulations concerning the use of ionizing radiation. In addition to federal regulations, many states have their own laws dealing with ionizing radiation. Although most of them closely follow the recommendations of the ADA and the NCRP, it is the responsibility of every practitioner to consult with their state's bureau of radiation control or safety to obtain information on current and applicable state laws.

Patient selection

Professional judgment should be used to determine the type, frequency, and extent of each radiographic examination (patient selection). Diagnostic radiography should be used only after clinical examination and consideration of both the dental and general health needs of the patient.[21]

It has been reported[6] that in 3 out of 4 cases orthodontists were confident in their diagnosis before evaluating any existing radiographic evidence. It has been suggested that in some instances less than 1% of *all* radiographs made have any influence in patient care.[115] These reports may cast some doubt on the reliability of "professional judgment" as the sole criterion for patient selection. Realization of this has prompted two national conferences[77,99] to conclude that there is a need for the development and implementation of more specific radiographic selection criteria to guide the practi-

tioner's "professional judgment." Such criteria could serve as more definitive guidelines for patient selection, which in turn might reduce the number of unproductive radiographic examinations and thus patient exposure to x rays.

Radiographic selection criteria, also known as high-yield or referral criteria, are clinical or historical findings that identify patients for whom there is a high probability that a radiographic examination will provide information that will affect their treatment or prognosis. Selection criteria have been found effective in several medical radiographic examinations.[12,101] The utility of selection criteria for reducing patient exposure has been demonstrated in oral radiography. It is possible to reduce the number of unproductive panoramic radiographs by 73% while missing only a small number of findings (6%) that may influence patient treatment.[114] Similar criteria have been proposed for the bitewing examination[61] and for pediatric[108] and complete intraoral[111] radiography.

The Dental Patient Selection Criteria Panel established by the Center for Devices and Radiological Health of the Food and Drug Administration was assigned the responsibility of formulating selection criteria for oral radiography. It is hoped that the selection criteria recommended by this panel will be accepted by the dental profession as guides for professional judgment. (See Chapter 4.)

Conduct of the examination

When the decision has been made that a radiographic examination is justified (patient selection), the way in which the examination is conducted will greatly influence patient exposure to x radiation. The conduct of the examination may be divided into choice of equipment, choice of technique, operation of equipment, and processing and interpretation of the radiographic image.

Choice of equipment. The choice of equipment includes selection of the image receptor, focal spot–to–film distance, x-ray beam collimation, and filtration and the type of leaded apron and collar.

Receptor selection. The ADA has taken the position that

The basis for selecting films, film-intensifying screen combinations, and other image receptors should be to obtain the maximum sensitivity (speed) consistent with the image quality required for the diagnostic task.[21]

INTRAORAL IMAGE RECEPTORS. In 1920, regular dental x-ray film was introduced by the Eastman

Kodak Company. The images produced by this film were excellent for that time, but the speed was so slow that a radiograph of the maxillary molar area of an adult required 9 seconds of exposure.[87] Since that time, progressively faster films have been developed. Currently, intraoral dental x-ray film is available in two speed groups, D and E. Clinically, film of speed group E is almost twice as fast (sensitive) as film of group D and about 50 times as fast as Regular dental x-ray film[89] (Fig. 3-2). In practice this means that the 9-second exposure required for Regular film in 1920 has been reduced to about 0.2 second with the use of E-speed film.

Faster films are desirable from the standpoint of exposure reduction. However, the possible decrease in image quality associated with increased speed, obtained in part by increasing the size of silver halide crystals in the film's emulsion, must also be considered[27] (Table 3-5). If shorter exposure times are realized at the expense of image quality, there is no benefit in using faster film. Shortly after the introduction of E-speed film in 1981,[93] studies were undertaken to compare film of speed group E with that of speed group D in terms of the diagnostic quality of the image. It was found* that E-speed film had about the same useful density range, a greater latitude with slightly less contrast, and equal image quality as D-speed film if strict

attention was paid to film handling and processing.[26,39,43,104] These and other studies of the comparative diagnostic value of D- and E-speed film*

---

*References 31, 45, 52, 62, 117, 116.

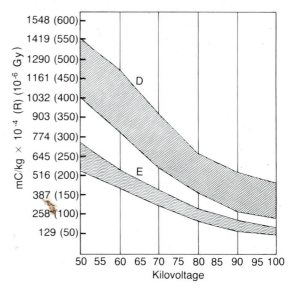

FIG. 3-2. Relationship between surface exposures delivered to a patient by exposure of group D and group E intraoral films and diagnostic density at various kilovoltages. (From HHS Pub [FDA] 85-8245, 1985.)

TABLE 3-5. Factors affecting the radiographic quality of a diagnostic film

	Definition	Image size	Shape distortion	Film density	Radiographic contrast
kVp*	X	X		X	X
mAs*	X	X		X	
Collimation*				X	X
Filtration*				X	X
Focal spot size†	X	X			
Object-to-film distance†	X	X			
Focal spot-to-film distance†	X	X		X	
Motion	X	X			
Alignment‡			X		
Subject density§	X			X	X
Subject shape§	X			X	X
Film speed§	X			X	X
Developing time‖				X	X
Technique‡	X	X	X		
Screen speed§	X	X		X	X

*See Chapter 1.
†See Chapter 6.
‡See Chapter 11.
§See Chapter 5.
‖See Chapter 7.

suggest that the faster E film can be used in routine intraoral radiographic examinations without sacrifice of diagnostic information.

In addition to the use of E-speed film alone several other techniques have been proposed to even further reduce patient exposure. Both double film packets and film that has been folded back on itself and repackaged have been suggested as means of reducing patient exposure by 50%.[16,57] After exposure to half the usual amount of radiation, the processed films are viewed by superimposing one on the other. Although the diagnostic quality of the image obtained by these techniques is reported to be comparable to that of single film packets, it should be kept in mind that the front (tube side) film of a two-film packet has been found[42] to have superior image quality compared to the back film because of parallax unsharpness.

Exposure reductions of up to 90% as compared with D-speed film and 80% as compared with E-speed film have been reported* with rare earth screen–film imaging techniques. Although the feasibility of using these systems intraorally has been demonstrated under laboratory conditions, with one exception[54] their application to clinical radiography has yet to be established.

INTENSIFYING SCREENS. Conventional intensifying screens used in extraoral radiography are made of crystals of calcium tungstate that emit blue light on interaction with x rays. (See Chapter 5.) In recent years, screens using the rare earth elements gadolinium and lanthanum have become commercially available. These phosphors emit green light on interaction with x rays. When combined with green-sensitive films, these screens are up to eight times more sensitive to x rays than conventional intensifying screens using blue-sensitive film, without a significant loss of image quality.[38,53,102] The greater sensitivity or speed of the rare earth screen–film combinations results in a dramatic reduction in patient exposure. Compared with calcium tungstate screens, rare earth screens have been found to decrease patient exposure by up to 55% in panoramic[38,94] and cephalometric[48] radiography.

A further reduction in patient exposure during extraoral radiography may be achieved with the use of T-grain film. Introduced as T-Mat by the Eastman Kodak Company in 1983, this film contains

silver halide grains that are tabular or flat rather than pebblelike in shape. With their flat surface oriented toward the x-ray source, these grains present a greater cross section, which increases their ability to gather light from intensifying screens. T-grain film used with rare earth screens has been found† to be twice as fast as calcium tungstate screen–film combinations and one and a third times as fast as conventional rare earth screen–film combinations with no loss in image quality.

Focal spot–to–film distance. The ADA states that

The combination of proper collimation and extended source-patient distance (focal spot–to–film distance) will reduce the amount of radiation to the patient.[20]

Two standard focal spot–to–film distances (FSFDs) have evolved over the years for use in intraoral radiography, one 20 cm (8 inches) and the other 41 cm (16 inches). When the x-ray tube is operated above 50 kVp, each of these distances satisfies the federal regulation that the x-ray source–skin distance must be not less than 18 cm (7 inches) (assuming a 2.5 cm [1 inch] distance from the skin surface to the film).[14]

Inasmuch as both distances comply with federal law, the decision as to which should be used may then be based on which FSFD results in less patient exposure and the best diagnostic image. One study of patient exposures from intraoral radiographic examinations[33] compared a 40 cm FSFD with a 20 cm FSFD in terms of organ doses. The results showed a 38% decrease in thyroid dose with the longer distance when 90 kVp x rays were used and a 45% decrease with 70 kVp x rays. These results were regardless of film speed used (i.e., D or E) and in spite of the fact that the intraoral examination using the 40 cm FSFD consisted of 21 films and the 20 cm FSFD examination consisted of only 18 films.

In addition to the decrease in thyroid dose obtained with the longer FSFD, use of the longer distance has been estimated to result in a 32% reduction in exposed tissue volume.[29] This is because at the greater distance the x-ray beam is less divergent (Fig. 3-3). The use of a longer FSFD will also result in a smaller apparent focal spot size and thereby increase the resolution of the radiograph. (See Chapter 6.)

The advantage to using a longer FSFD is often not realized because of the complaint that it makes maneuvering the radiographic tube housing difficult. This real or imagined problem has been over-

---

*References 49, 51, 54, 58.
†References 25, 65, 80, 103.

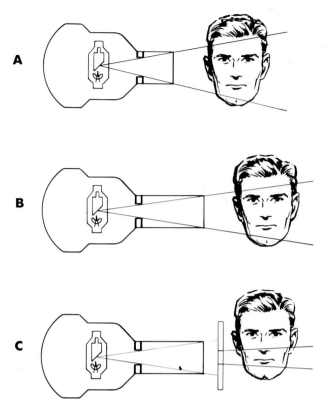

FIG. 3-3. Effect of focal spot–to film distance (FSFD) and collimation on the volume of tissue irradiated. There is a larger volume of irradiated tissue in **A** (with a shorter FSFD) than in **B** (in which the longer FSFD produces a less divergent beam). In **C** the collimator between the round position-indicating device (PID) and the patient produces the effect of a rectangular PID on the tube housing or a rectangular collimating face shield on the film-holding instrument. This rectangular collimator (close to the patient in **C**) results in a smaller, less divergent, beam and a smaller volume of tissue irradiated than in **A** or **B**.

come by the Long Beam tube concept developed by S.S. White Dental Products International, of Philadelphia, and now employed by Keystone X-Ray, Neptune, N.J. In this system the x-ray tube is recessed in the tube housing, which allows a shorter position-indicating device (PID), with increased maneuverability, to be used while maintaining the longer FSFD.

Collimation. The ADA recommendation is that

The tissue area (and volume) exposed to the primary x-ray beam should not exceed the minimum coverage consistent with meeting diagnostic requirements and clinical feasibility. The collimation should comply with federal and state regulations. For periapical and bitewing radiography, restriction of the beam cross section to conform to the size of the image receptor (rectangular collimation) is recommended. Furthermore, shielded open-end position-indicating devices should be used.[21]

The federal government requires[14] that the x-ray beam used in intraoral radiography be collimated so the field of radiation at the patient's skin surface is ". . . containable in a circle having a diameter of no more than 7 cm (2¾ inches) . . ." when the x-ray tube is operated above 50 kVp. In view of the dimensions of no. 2 intraoral film (3.2 × 4.1 cm), a field size of this magnitude is almost three times that necessary to expose the film. Consequently, patient exposure may be significantly reduced by limiting the size of the x-ray beam even more than required by law. This will result in not only decreased patient exposure but also increased image quality (Table 3-5 and Fig. 3-3). Additionally, the amount of radiation scatter generated is proportional to the area exposed. If scatter radiation is decreased, film fog is decreased and image quality is increased.[118] Also the reduction in beam size

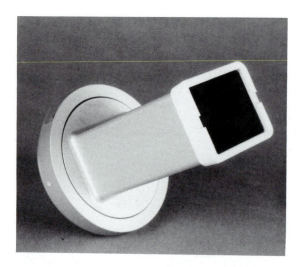

FIG. 3-4. A rectangular position-indicating device, which may be used to reduce the area of patient skin exposed. (Courtesy Rinn Manufacturing Co, Elgin Ill.)

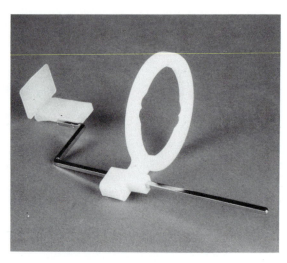

FIG. 3-5. Rinn X-C-P film-holding instrument. (Courtesy Rinn Manufacturing Co, Elgin Ill.)

improves image definition (sharpness) by reducing the geometric phenomenon of penumbra. (See Chapter 6.)

Limiting the size of the x-ray beam can be accomplished by any one or a combination of several methods. *First,* a rectangular position-indicating device (PID) may be attached to the radiographic tube housing (Fig. 3-4). Use of a rectangular PID having an exit orifice of 3.5 × 4.4 cm (1 ⅜ × 1 ¾ inches) will reduce the area of the patient's skin surface exposed by 60% over that of a round (7 cm) PID (Fig. 3-3, *C*). This reduction in beam size, however, may make aiming the beam difficult. To avoid the possibility of unsatisfactory radiographs (cone cutting), a film-holding instrument that centers the beam over the film is recommended (Fig. 3-5).

Second, film holders with rectangular collimators may be used with round PIDs (Fig. 3-6) and will reduce patient exposure the same as rectangular PIDs. In a study reviewing the effective dose delivered during full-mouth examinations made with round and rectangular collimation[113] it was found that rectangular collimation reduced the patient dose from intraoral examinations by about 60% (Table 3-4). Both the Precision instrument (Masel Orthodontics, Bristol, Pa) and the X-C-P instrument (Rinn Manufacturing, Elgin, Ill) with a rectangular collimator clipped to the aiming ring (Fig. 3-7) may be expected to produce similar results.

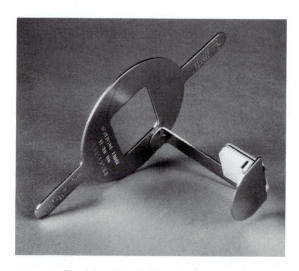

FIG. 3-6. Precision film-holding instrument. The face shield of the instrument absorbs radiation except for that required to expose the film. (Courtesy Masel Orthodontics, Philadelphia.)

Filtration. The ADA recommendation is that

Beam filtration should comply with federal and state regulations. The most judicious use of filtration involves selective filtration of excessively high-energy as well as excessively low-energy radiation.[21]

The x-ray beam, emitted from the radiographic tube, consists of not only high-energy x-ray photons but also many photons with relatively lower energy. (See Chapter 1.) Low-energy photons,

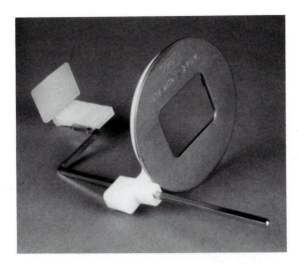

FIG. 3-7. Rinn X-C-P instrument with a rectangular collimator clipped to the aiming ring. As with the Precision instrument (Fig. 3-6), the collimator of this instrument absorbs radiation except for that required to expose the film. (Courtesy Rinn Manufacturing Co, Elgin Ill.)

TABLE 3-6. Minimum total filtration

Operating x-ray tube voltage (kVp)	Minimum total filtration (mm Al Eq*)
<50	0.5
50 to 70	1.5
>70	2.5

*Aluminum equivalent, the thickness of aluminum affording the same attenuation, under specified conditions, as the material in question.
From National Council on Radiation Protection and Measurements: *NCRP Report* 35, Bethesda, MD, 1970.

which have little penetrating power, are mainly absorbed by the patient and contribute nothing to the information on the film. The purpose of conventional filtration is to remove these low-energy x-ray photons selectively from the x-ray beam. This results in decreased patient exposure with no loss of radiologic information (Table 3-5).

The beneficial effect of filtration has been known for many years. When an x-ray beam is filtered with 3 mm of aluminum, the surface exposure is reduced to about 20% of that with no filtration.[105] In light of this and other information, the federal government has designated the specific amount of filtration required for dental x-ray machines operating at various kilovoltages (Table 3-6). Compliance with these regulations by the dental profession was demonstrated in the 1970 national x-ray exposure study,[82] which indicated that more than 90% of all dental x-ray machines in the United States had total filtration equal to or greater than the required minimum amount.

Studies* have suggested that patient exposure may be reduced even further by removing both low- and high-energy x-ray photons from the beam, leaving the mid-range energy photons to expose the film. This suggestion resulted from the finding[88]

---

*References 28, 32, 46, 47, 50, 63, 78, 79, 81, 84, 97, 106, 107.

that the x-ray energies most effective in producing the image are between 35 and 55 keV. Selective filtration of both low- and high-energy photons has been demonstrated with the rare earths samarium, erbium, yttrium, niobium, gadolinium, terbium-activated gadolinium oxysulfide (Lanex, Eastman Kodak), and thulium-activated lanthanum oxybromide (Quanta III, DuPont). The use of these materials in combination with aluminum filtration has reduced patient exposure by 20% to 80% as compared with conventional aluminum filtration alone, which attenuates few high-energy photons.

It should be considered, however, that exposure reduction achieved with rare earth filtration is not without cost. Use of these filters requires a significant increase in exposure time (up to 50%), increasing both x-ray tube loading and the possibility of patient movement during exposure. Additionally, depending on preference, image quality may suffer because of a decrease in contrast.[28]

Leaded aprons and collars. The ADA also states that

Leaded aprons and collars should be used to minimize any unnecessary radiation.[21]

It is generally accepted that the gonad dose resulting from oral radiography is minimal. (See "Gonad dose," p. 52.) The philosophy of radiation protection currently in practice, however, is based on the principles of ALARA (as low as reasonably achievable). This philosophy recognizes the possibility that, no matter how small the dose, there may be some deleterious effect. Consequently, any dose that can be reduced without difficulty, great expense, or inconvenience should be reduced. Current data show that the mean exposure at skin entrance for a single dental periapical film is 300 mR. If it is assumed that the gonad dose is equal to 1/10,000 of the total beam exposure,[86]

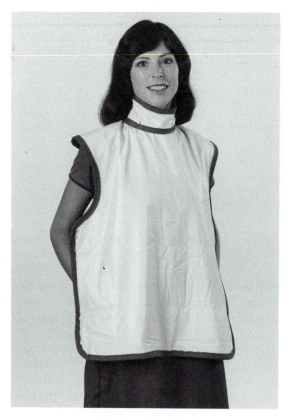

FIG. 3-8. Leaded apron with a thyroid collar attached. (Courtesy Ada Products, Milwaukee.)

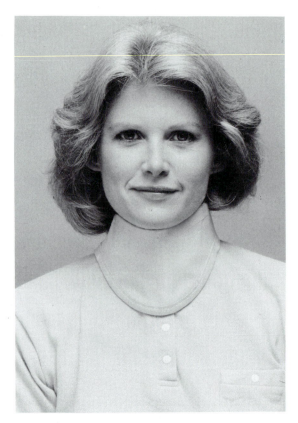

FIG. 3-9. Thyroid collar for use when one is not attached to the leaded apron. (Courtesy Ada Products, Milwaukee.)

the dose from one dental periapical film can be calculated to be 0.03 mR. Put in perspective, this value is 27 times less than the average daily effective dose from natural background radiation and almost 50 times less than the radiation during one airline flight. (See "Sources of Radiation Exposure," p. 47.)

No matter how small, this dose still represents a measurable quantity that, according to ALARA, should be reduced if possible. This can be accomplished with the use of a leaded apron or cervical shield, which may attenuate up to 98% of the scatter radiation to the gonads.[8,44] Thus, with the use of either of these devices, the gonad dose from one dental periapical film can be calculated to be 0.6 μR. This quantity is up to 10 times less than the average annual effective dose to the population resulting from the use of combustible fuels. (See "Sources of Radiation Exposure," p. 47.)

Although these calculations and comparisons demonstrate that the gonad dose is indeed quite small, there is no valid argument for not routinely

using a leaded apron (Fig. 3-8). A similar statement can be made for thyroid shields, which have been found[92] to reduce the exposure of this gland by up to 92% (Fig. 3-9). No difficulty, great expense, or inconvenience is encountered with their use; instead, using them demonstrates a real concern for the welfare of the patient. In 1983 (the most recent year for which figures are available) 12 states were found to mandate the use of leaded aprons in dental radiography.[1] It is unfortunate that these states have found it necessary to dictate good practice to the dental profession.

This and other information regarding the dose to the fetus during oral radiographic procedures, and NCRP recommendations concerning embryo-fetus exposure, resulted in the decision by the Dental Patient Selection Criteria Panel to propose that the oral radiographic examination should not be contraindicated because of pregnancy. Still, however, the decision to use x rays if the patient is pregnant is an individual one. The patient should be made aware of both the need for radiographs and the relative magnitude of exposure before any films are made.

Choice of intraoral technique. Receptor holders that position the (image) receptor to coincide with the collimation should be used. Receptors should not be held in place for the patient.[21] Currently there are no recommendations or regulations dealing specifically with intraoral radiographic techniques. Consequently, the choice of technique—bisection of the angle or paralleling long cone—is left to the practitioner. The decision as to which method is used should be based on the diagnostic quality of the resultant radiographs, the efficiency of using radiation, and the convenience of the technique (Table 3-5). The implication here is that the more efficient the technique the fewer radiograph retakes will be required and the less will be the patient exposure. A study of comparative efficiencies of the bisection and parallel cone techniques[7] found that the number of undiagnostic radiographs was reduced by more than half when intraoral full-mouth examinations were made with the parallel technique. If it is assumed that all undiagnostic radiographs are remade, use of the bisection technique will lead to a significant increase in patient exposure. This study used the Rinn X-C-P instrument for parallel film placement (Fig. 3-5), but similar reports on efficiency have appeared using the Precision instrument[112] (Fig. 3-6). The Precision instrument with rectangular field collimation serves to reduce patient exposure even more, although it would be expected that similar results might be obtained with the Rinn X-C-P instrument and a rectangular PID (Figs. 3-4 and 3-5) or with a rectangular collimator clipped to the aiming ring (Fig. 3-7). (See "Collimation," p. 57.)

Operating the equipment. Operation of the x-ray generating equipment includes selection of the appropriate machine technique factors, kilovoltage, and milliampere-seconds.

Kilovoltage. The recommendation for selection of operating kilovoltage is stated in very general terms.

A kilovoltage best suited to the diagnostic purpose should be used. Exposure should be established for optimal image quality.[21]

This allows the practitioner to select either high (90) or low (70) kilovoltage, whichever is felt more suitable for the diagnostic purpose. Kilovoltage is the exposure factor that controls the energy of the x-ray beam. (See Chapter 1.) As the kilovoltage is decreased, the effective energy of the x-ray beam is decreased and radiographic image contrast increases (Table 3-5). Diagnostically, an image of high contrast is better suited for visualizing large differences in density within an object such as caries or soft tissue calcifications.[95] As the kilovoltage is increased, the effective energy of the x-ray beam is increased and radiographic image contrast decreases. An image of low contrast allows for the visualization of smaller differences in density within an object. This type of image contrast is more useful for periodontal diagnosis where minute changes in bone must be detected.[29] High-kilovoltage techniques, which produce images of low contrast, also reduce the effective dose delivered per intraoral examination. It has been reported[33] that the effective dose resulting from the production of comparable-density radiographs was reduced by up to 23% in one study, with an increase in kilovoltage from 70 to 90.

The introduction of a constant-potential (fully rectified) dental x-ray unit has made possible the production of diagnostic-quality radiographs with lower kilovoltage and at reduced levels of radiation.[96] The Intrex machine (Keystone X-Ray, Neptune, N.J.), which operates at 70 kVp, was compared[64] with a conventional self-rectified x-ray unit also operating at 70 kVp. It was found that the surface exposure required to produce a comparable radiographic density was about 26% less for the constant-voltage Intrex unit. This finding results from the fact that the x-ray beam produced by the fully rectified Intrex machine has an equivalent photon energy approximately equal to that produced by a self-rectified unit operated at about 80 kVp.[30]

Milliampere-seconds. Of the three technical conditions—tube voltage, filtration, and exposure time—exposure time has been shown to be the most critical factor in influencing diagnostic quality.[4] In terms of exposure, optimal image quality means that the radiograph is of diagnostic density, neither overexposed (too dark) nor underexposed (too light). Both overexposed and underexposed radiographs result in needless patient exposure. Image density is controlled by the quantity of x rays produced, which in turn is best controlled by the combination of milliamperage and exposure time, termed *milliampere-seconds* (mAs) (Table 3-5). (See Chapter 1.)

In Table 3-7 are listed average mAs values needed to expose an intraoral film to proper density.

TABLE 3-7. Milliampere-seconds required to expose speed group D and E intraoral radiographic film to diagnostic density at a focal spot–film distance (FSFD) of 16 inches

Operating kilovoltage*	Milliampere-seconds†					
	D			E		
	Low	High	Mean	Low	High	Mean
70	6.7	10.9	8.8	3.6	4.8	4.2
90	3.1	6.0	4.6	1.7	2.6	2.2

*X-ray beam filtered to NCRP recommendations (Table 3-6).
†For an 8-inch FSFD, divide by 4.
Values calculated from DHEW Publ (FDA) 73-8047, 1973; and from information in Figure 3-2.

In general, a radiograph of correct density should demonstrate very faint soft tissue outlines.[29] Such a degree of image density can be obtained by using values within the ranges listed, after consideration has been given to the age and physical stature of the patient. For example, 2.2 mAs is suggested for an average adult when E-speed film and an operating kilovoltage of 90 are used. This value may be arrived at by using a milliamperage of 10 and an exposure time of 0.22 second (13 impulses). If the kilovoltage is increased to reduce image contrast, the mAs must be decreased or the radiograph will be overexposed.

Phototiming is routinely employed in some medical radiographic procedures.[13] This technique uses a phototimer to measure the quantity of radiation reaching the film and automatically terminates the exposure when enough radiation has reached the film to provide the required density. The availability of very small photodiodes has made feasible this type of automatic exposure control in intraoral radiography.[109]

Processing the film. A good darkroom and proper darkroom practices are important parts of performing diagnostic radiography.[22] A major cause of unnecessary exposure of the patient to radiation is the deliberate overexposure of films. Overexposure is compensated for by underdevelopment of the film.[2] Not only does this procedure result in needless overexposure of the patient, however, it also (because of incomplete development) results in films that are of inferior diagnostic quality. On the other hand, a properly exposed radiograph is of no value if all its diagnostic information is lost as a result of poor processing procedures (Table 3-5). A study by one dental insurance carrier[9] reported that some 6% of the dental radiographs it received were not readable because of improper processing. Another study of 500 panoramic radiographs[10] found that the average film contained *at least one* processing error. Time-temperature processing, in an adequately equipped and maintained darkroom, is the best way to assure optimum film quality. (See Chapter 7.)

The use of machines to process dental x-ray film has become widespread. Film processors, however, can actually increase patient exposure if not correctly maintained. One study[35] has shown that 30% of all retakes because of incorrect film density were directly related to processor variability. The introduction of a comprehensive maintenance program was found to reduce this retake rate significantly, resulting in a substantial savings in both *patient exposure* and *operating costs*.

Interpretation of the image. The maximum diagnostic information can be obtained from a radiograph only if it is viewed with even backlighting.

Radiographic images should be viewed under proper conditions with an illuminated viewer or transparent images to obtain maximum available information.[21]

Radiographs are best viewed in a semidarkened room with light transmitted only through the films; all extraneous light should be eliminated. In addition, radiographs should be studied with the aid of a magnifying glass, to detect even the smallest change in image density. A variable intensity light source should also be available. This may compensate for over- or underexposed radiographs or radiographs with processing artifacts. Many radiographs can be "saved" in this way, precluding the necessity of remaking the film and subjecting the patient to additional radiation exposure.

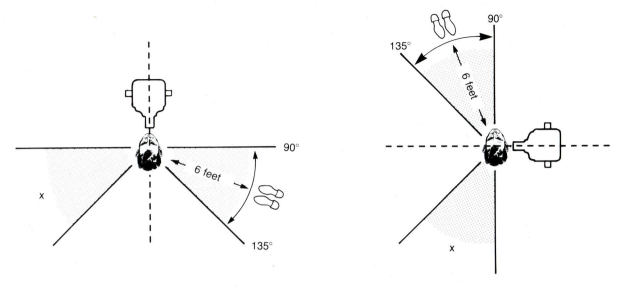

FIG. 3-10. Position-and-distance rule. If no barrier is available, the operator should stand at least 6 feet from the patient, at an angle of 90 to 135 degrees to the central ray of the x-ray beam, when the exposure is made.

Protection of personnel

Unless protective shielding is provided for the operator, the installation should be so arranged so that the operator can stand at least 6 ft from the patient during exposure.[21]

The methods of dose reduction discussed thus far have emphasized their effect on patient exposure. It should be apparent, however, that any procedure or technique that reduces radiation exposure to the patient will also reduce the possibility of operator or office personnel exposure. In addition to those mentioned, several other steps can be taken to ensure against the chance of occupational exposure.

Perhaps the single most effective way of limiting occupational exposure is the establishment of radiation safety procedures that are understood and followed by all personnel. Such written procedures are currently mandated by several states.[76,100] The procedures described below are based on a number of important facts concerning x rays: they travel in straight lines from their source; the intensity of the radiation beam diminishes fairly rapidly as the distance from the source increases (inverse square law); and they can be scattered or deflected in their path of travel.

First, every effort should be made so the operator can leave the room or take a position behind a suitable barrier or wall during exposure of the film. Dental operatories should be designed and con-

structed to meet the minimum shielding requirement of the NCRP.[68] This recommendation states that walls must be of sufficient density or thickness that the exposure to nonoccupationally exposed individuals (e.g., someone occupying an adjacent office) is no greater than 10 mR per week. In most instances it is not necessary to line the walls with lead to meet this requirement. Walls constructed of gypsum wallboard (drywall) have been found to be adequate for the average dental office.[59,85]*

If it is impossible to leave the room or make use of some other barrier, there should be strict adherence to what has been termed the *position-and-distance rule*[83]: that the operator stand at least 6 feet from the patient, at an angle of 90 to 135 degrees to the central ray of the x-ray beam (Fig. 3-10). When applied, this rule not only takes advantage of the inverse square law to reduce x-ray intensity but also considers that in this position most scatter radiation will be absorbed by the pa-

---

*In calculation of specific barrier thicknesses the following factors are considered: (1) workload, an expression of the amount of radiation emitted at a given kilovoltage in milliamperes per week; (2) use, the fraction of time an x-ray beam is directed toward the barrier; (3) occupancy, an estimation of the amount of time the area behind the barrier is occupied; (4) maximum permissible effective dose. Examples of how these parameters are used in the calculation of required barrier thickness can be found in NCRP Report 35 (1970).

R S LANDAUER JR AND CO
SAMPLE REPORT
MAILING ADDRESS

ACCOUNT NO.	SERIES CODE
999999	ABC

PROCESS NO.	REPORT DATE	DOSIMETER RECEIVED	REPORTING TIME IN WORK DAYS	PAGE NO.
	61483	60783	5	1

QUALITY CONTROL RELEASE
JMD

Landauer

R. S. Landauer, Jr. & Co. **Tech/Ops**
Division of Tech/Ops, Inc.
2 Science Road, Glenwood, Illinois 60425-1586
(312) 755-7000

Accredited by the
National Bureau of Standards
through NVLAP

RADIATION DOSIMETRY REPORT

PARTICIPANT ID NUMBER	NAME	SOCIAL SECURITY NUMBER	NOTE	DOSIMETER TYPE	USE	RADIATION QUALITY	EXPOSURE TO BADGE (MILLIREMS) FOR PERIOD(S) INDICATED BELOW		CUMULATIVE TOTALS (MILLIREMS) CALENDAR QUARTER		YEAR TO DATE		PERMANENT		ADJUSTMENTS	UNUSED PART OF PERMISSIBLE ACCUMULATED DOSE (MILLIREMS)	SEX	BIRTH DATE MO DA YR	TO DATE	NUMBER BADGE REPORTS QTR.	INCEPTION DATE OF PERMA- NENT TOTAL MO YR
							DEEP	SHALLOW	DEEP	SHALLOW	DEEP	SHALLOW	DEEP	SHALLOW							
	FOR EXPOSURE PERIOD 05/01/83			TC			05/31/83		SECOND		1983										
00000	CONTROL			G1			M	M	M	M	M	M	30	30						85 2 4 74	
00000	CONTROL			L3				M		M		M		M						6 21 1 75	
00022	SMITH GEORGE	125876499		G1	PM		60	60	60	60	60	60	60	60			M	91 5 49	1	1 5 82	
00022	SMITH GEORGE	125876499		L3				M		M		M		M			M	91 5 49	1	1 5 82	
	FOR EXPOSURE PERIOD 05/01/83			TC			05/31/83		SECOND		1983										
00000	CONTROL			G1			M	M	M	M	M	M	30	30						86 3 4 74	
00000	CONTROL			L3				M		M		M		M						7 31 1 75	
00004	LAND KEN	846432187		G1	CPB		30	100	30	100	30	100	30	1960	A		M	102 350	78	2 6 74	
00004	LAND KEN	846432187		E				70									M	102 350	79	2 6 74	
00005	ROOM 210			G1	CPB		150	330					NO TOTAL								
00005	ROOM 210			E				180													
00006	JAY JONATHAN	567843215		B1	CPN		230	230	230	230	230	230	230	230			M	30 342	9	2 10 75	
00006	ZIM RONALD	567843215		NF			100										M	30 342	9	2 10 75	
00007	SUEZ DERICK	987654335		G1			M		30	30	930	930	3560	3640			M	52 644	71	2 7 74	
00011	SUPERA JACK	878953254		H1	CPN		50	50	50	50	50	50	50	50			M	82 915	10	2 12 75	
00011	SUPERA JACK	878953254		NT			10										M	82 915	10	2 12 75	
00011	SUPERA JACK	878953254		NF			20										M	82 915	10	2 12 75	
00012	ALBERT DON	654687952H		G1			M	M	M	M	M	M				M	22 627	10	2 12 75	
00013	DOE JOSEPH	254336878		G1	CPB		40	110	60	130	190	320	150	320			M	111 547	54	2 12 74	
00013	DOE JOSEPH	254336878		E				70									M	111 547	54	2 12 74	
00015	MARUL JOHN	125468763		G1	P		20	20	20	20	20	20	20	20			M	80 951	10	2 12 75	
00016	MARUL JOHN	125468763		G8	B		M	60	M	60	M	60	M	60			M	80 951	10	2 12 75	
00017	NOLLS JOHN	245635779		G1			M	M	30	30	30	30	30	30			M	122 240	6	2 11 75	
00017	NOLLS JOHN	245635779		U3				1020		1020		1020		36580	C		M	122 240	6	2 11 75	
00017	NOLLS JOHN	245635779		L4				80		80		80		60			M	122 240	6	2 11 75	

USE CODE (COLUMN 6)
1-WHOLE BODY   3-RIGHT FINGER   7-OTHER EXTREMITY
2-LENS OF EYE   4-LEFT FINGER   8-OTHER WHOLE BODY
3-RIGHT WRIST   5-LEFT WRIST   9-MONITOR

AN "H" (HIGH ENERGY) DESIGNATION, WHEN ONLY LOW ENERGY EXPOSURE IS POSSIBLE MAY INDICATE THAT THE FILM PACKET WAS EXPOSED OUT OF THE FILTERED HOLDER.

IMPORTANT: SEE REVERSE SIDE FOR ADDITIONAL EXPLANATIONS

FIG. 3-11. Sample radiation dosimetry report showing that George Smith received an exposure of 0.60 mSv (60 mrem) during the month reported. Note that the report also shows totals for the calendar quarter, year to date, and permanent or lifetime exposure. (Courtesy RS Landauer Jr & Co, Glenwood Ill.)

tient's head. Every practitioner should check their state's regulations for use of ionizing radiation regarding operator position when an x-ray exposure is made. At least one state[76] requires that the operator leave the room during the exposure. Thus, the position and distance rule is in violation of that state's regulations.

Second, films should never be held in place by the operator.[68] Ideally, film-holding instruments should be used. (See "Collimation," p. 57.) If correct film placement and retention are still not possible, a parent or other individual responsible for the patient should be asked to hold the film in place and, or course, be afforded adequate protection with a leaded apron. Under no circumstances should this person be one of the office staff.

Third, the radiographic tube housing should never be stabilized by the operator or patient during the exposure.[68] Suspension arms should be ade-

quately maintained to prevent housing movement and drift.

The best way to ensure that personnel are following office safety rules, such as those described above, is with personnel-monitoring devices. Commonly referred to as "film badges," they provide a useful record of occupational exposure. Their use is not only recommended but also required by law in certain states. Several companies in the United States offer a film badge service. For a reasonable charge they provide the badge, which contains either a piece of sensitive film or a radiosensitive crystal (thermoluminescent dosimeter) and a printed report of accumulated exposure at regular intervals (Fig. 3-11). These reports both indicate any undesirable change in work habits and serve to remove apprehension that office staff may have about the possibility of exposure to x rays.

TABLE 3-8. Guide for establishing maintenance and quality control procedures

Following should be inspected at suitable intervals:
  X-ray unit
    Leakage radiation
    Verification of FSFD
    Stability of radiographic tube housing
    X-ray beam
      Alignment
      Collimation
      Quality
    Timer accuracy
    Integrity of exposure switch
  Darkroom
    Light leaks
    Adequacy of safe lighting
    Cleanliness
  Ancillary equipment
    Leaded aprons and collars
    The brightness and color of view boxes
Procedures should be established for
  Use of a reference film
  Proper handling and storage of film, cassettes,
    screens, grids, and chemicals
  X-ray exposure factors (posted by control console)
  Film processing techniques (posted in darkroom)
  Maintenance of processing systems

From National Council on Radiation Protection and Measurements: *NCRP Report 99*(1990), Washington DC, NCRP Publications.

Quality assurance

A quality assurance program should be established to ensure high-quality radiographic images.[21]

Quality assurance may be defined as "any systematic action to ensure that a dental office will produce consistently high-quality images with minimal exposure to patients and personnel."[60] National studies[60] have indicated that dentists may be needlessly exposing their patients to compensate for improper exposure techniques and film processing and darkroom procedures. It has also been demonstrated that when demands are placed on dentists to improve their techniques there is a significant reduction in the number of unsatisfactory radiographs. In two studies by a dental insurance carrier,[9] it was found that after claims were rejected for unsatisfactory radiographs and the dentist was made aware of the errors and how they could be corrected the number of satisfactory radiographs submitted doubled. This suggests that when the dentist is presented with guidelines for quality assurance, along with proper motivation, patient exposure can be dramatically reduced.

Currently some states require dental offices to establish written guidelines for quality assurance and maintain written records of quality assurance tests.[76,100] Regardless, each dental office should establish maintenance and monitoring procedures as outlined in Table 3-8 according to the NCRP.[73] The frequency of these inspections will vary according to state regulations and manufacturers' directions.

Continuing education

Practitioners should stay informed of new developments in equipment, materials, and techniques and adopt appropriate items to improve radiographic practices.[21]

It is essential that those who administer ionizing radiation become familiar with the magnitude of exposure encountered in medicine and dentistry and everyday life, the possible risks associated with such exposure, and the methods used to effect exposure and dose reduction. This chapter provides some of this information; however, it should be remembered that acquiring knowledge and developing and maintaining skills are a continuous process.

REFERENCES

1. ADA State Legislative Clearing House: *Dental radiography survey results,* Chicago, 1983, American Dental Association.
2. Alcox RW: Biological effects and radiation protection in the dental office, *Dent Clin North Am* 22:517-532, 1978.
3. Arena V: *Ionizing radiation and life,* St Louis, 1971, Mosby.
4. Arnold LV: The radiographic detection of initial carious lesions on the proximal surfaces of teeth. I. The influence of exposure conditions, *Oral Surg* 64:221-231, 1987.
5. Associated Press: Increased cancer not found near TMI, *Dallas Times Herald,* September 6, 1985.
6. Atchison KA, Luke LS, White SC: Contribution of pretreatment radiographs to orthodontist's decision making, *Oral Surg* 71:238-245, 1991.
7. Bean LR: Comparison of bisecting angle and paralleling methods of intraoral radiology, *J Dent Educ* 33:441-445, 1969.
8. Bean LR, Devore WD: The effect of protective aprons in dental roentgenography, *Oral Surg* 28:505-508, 1969.
9. Beideman RW, Pettigrew JC, Green PH: A follow-up study of a third-party radiographic evaluation system, *Oral Surg* 56:103-108, 1983.
10. Brezden NA, Brooks SL: Evaluation of panoramic dental radiographs taken in private practice, *Oral Surg* 63:617-621, 1987.
11. Broadway JA, Smith MJ, Norwood DL, Porter CR: Estimates of radiation dose and health risks to the United States population following the Chernobyl nuclear plant accident, *Health Phys* 55:533-539, 1988.

12. Brown RF, Shaver JW, Lamel DA: The selection of patients for x-ray examinations, *DHEW Publ (FDA)* 80-8104, 1980.

13. Bushong SC: *Radiologic science for technologists: physics, biology, and protection,* ed 4, St Louis, 1988, Mosby.

14. Code of Federal Regulations 21, Subchapter J: *Radiological health,* part 1000, Washington, DC, 1984, Office of the Federal Register, General Services Administration.

15. Cohen BS, Eisenbud M, Harley NH: Measurement of the α-radioactivity on the mucosal surface of the human bronchial tree, *Health Phys* 39:619-632, 1980.

16. Colquitt WN, Richards AG: An old/new idea for reducing exposure to x-rays, *Oral Surg* 54:597-600, 1982.

17. Committee on the Biological Effects of Ionizing Radiations: *The effects on populations of exposure to low levels of ionizing radiation,* Washington DC, 1980, National Academy Press.

18. Committee on the Biological Effects of Ionizing Radiations: *Health effects of exposure to low levels of ionizing radiation. BEIR V,* Washington DC, 1990, National Academy Press.

19. Council on Dental Materials and Devices: Recommendations in radiographic practices: March 1978, *J Am Dent Assoc* 96:485-486, 1978.

20. Council on Dental Materials, Instruments, and Equipment: Recommendations in radiographic practices, 1984, *J Am Dent Assoc* 109:764-765, 1984.

21. Council on Dental Materials, Instruments, and Equipment: Recommendations on radiographic practices: an update, 1988, *J Am Dent Assoc* 118:115-117, 1989.

22. Council on Dental Materials, Instruments, and Equipment: Recommendations for radiographic darkrooms and darkroom practices, *J Am Dent Assoc* 104:886-887, 1982.

23. Court Brown WM, Doll R, Spiers FW et al: Geographical variation in leukaemia mortality in relation to background radiation and other factors, *Br Med J* 5188:1753-1759, 1960.

24. Craig L, Seidman H: Leukemia and lymphoma mortality in relation to cosmic radiation, *Blood* 17:319-327, 1961.

25. D'Ambrosio JA, Schiff TG, McDavid WD, Langland OE: Diagnostic quality versus patient exposure with five panoramic screen-film combinations, *Oral Surg* 61:409-411, 1986.

26. Diehl R, Gratt BM, Gould RG: Radiographic quality control measurements comparing D-speed film, E-speed film, and xeroradiography, *Oral Surg* 61:635-640, 1986.

27. Domon M, Yoshino N: Factors involved in the high radiographic sensitivity of E-speed films, *Oral Surg* 69:113-119, 1990.

28. Farman AG, Perez C, Jacobsen A, Kelley MS: Evaluation of aluminum-yttrium filtration for intraoral radiography, *Oral Surg* 67:244-226, 1989.

29. Frederiksen NL: The radiograph in the diagnosis of periodontal disease: a quality assurance program, Technology Assessment Forum on Dental Radiology, *FDA/BRH* 82:107, 1982.

30. Frederiksen NL, Goaz PW: Parameters affecting radiographic contrast. *Dentomaxillofac Radiol* 19:173-177, 1990.

31. Frommer HH, Jain RK: A comparative clinical study of group D and E dental film, *Oral Surg* 63:738-742, 1987.

32. Gelskey, DE, Baker CG: Energy-selective filtration of dental x-ray beams, *Oral Surg* 52:565-567, 1981.

33. Gibbs SJ, Pujol A, Chen TS, James A: Patient risk from intraoral dental radiography, *Dentomaxillofac Radiol* 17:15-23, 1988.

34. Gibbs SJ, Pujol A, McDavid, WD et al: Patient risk from rotational panoramic radiography, *Dentomaxillofac Radiol* 17:25-32, 1988.

35. Goldman L, Vucich JJ, Beech S, Murphy WL: Automatic processing quality assurance program: impact on a radiology department, *Radiology* 125:591-595, 1977.

36. Gonad doses and genetically significant dose from diagnostic radiology: U.S., 1964 and 1970, DHEW Publ (FDA) 76-8034, 1976.

37. Grahn D, Kratchman J: Variation in neonatal death rate and birth weight in the United States and possible relations to environmental radiation, geology and altitude, *Am J Hum Genet* 15:329-352, 1963.

38. Gratt BM, White SC, Packard FL, Peterson AR: An evaluation of rare-earth imaging systems in panoramic radiography, *Oral Surg* 58:475-482, 1984.

39. Horton PS, Sippy FH, Kohout FJ et al: A clinical comparison of speed groups D and E dental x-ray films, *Oral Surg* 58:104-105, 1984.

40. Hull JB: Faulty x-ray devices, untrained operators overdose U.S. patients, *The Wall Street Journal,* December 11, 1985.

41. International Commission on Radiological Protection: Radiation protection, *ICRP Publ* 60, 1990.

42. Jarvis WD, Pifer RG, Griffin JA, Skidmore AE: Evaluation of image quality in individual films of double film packets, *Oral Surg* 69:764-767, 1990.

43. Kaffe I, Littner MM, Kuspet ME: Densitometric evaluation of introral x-ray films: Ekta speed versus Ultraspeed, *Oral Surg* 57:338-342, 1984.

44. Kaffe I, Littner MM, Shlezinger T, Segal P: Efficiency of the cervical lead shield during intraoral radiography, *Oral Surg* 62:732-736, 1986.

45. Kantor ML, Reisken AB, Lurie AG: A clinical comparison of x-ray films for detection of proximal surface caries, *J Am Dent Assoc* 111:967-969, 1985.

46. Kapa SF, Tyndall DA: A clinical comparison of image quality and patient exposure reduction in panoramic radiography with heavy metal filtration, *Oral Surg* 67:750-759, 1989.

47. Kapa SF, Tyndall DA, Ouellette TE: The application of added beam filtration to intra-oral radiography, *Dentomaxillofac Radiol* 19:67-74, 1990.

48. Kaugars GE, Fatouros P: Clinical comparison of conventional and rare-earth screen-film systems for cephalometric radiographs, *Oral Surg* 53:322-325, 1982.

49. Kircos LT, Staninec M, Chou L: Comparative evaluation of the sensitometric properties of screen-film systems and conventional dental receptors for introral radiography, *Oral Surg* 68:787-792, 1989.

50. Kircos LT, Staninec M, Chou L: Rare earth filters for intraoral radiography: exposure reduction as a function of kV(p) with comparisons of image quality, *J Am Dent Assoc* 118:605-609, 1989.

51. Kircos LT, Vandre RH, Lorton L: Exposure reduction of 96% in intraoral radiography, *J Am Dent Assoc* 113:746-750, 1986.

52. Kleier DJ, Hicks MJ, Flaitz CM: A comparison of Ultraspeed and Ektaspeed dental x-ray film: in vitro study of the radiographic appearance of interproximal lesions, *Oral Surg* 63:381-385, 1987.

53. *Kodak film screen combinations,* Publication M3-138, Rochester NY, 1983, Eastman Kodak.

54. Kogon SL, Stephens RG, Reid JA, Lubus NJ: 1984. A clinical trial of a rare-earth screen/film system in a periapical cassette, *Oral Surg* 57:455-461, 1984.

55. Kumazawa S, Nelson DR, Richardson ACB: *Occupational exposure to ionizing radiation in the United States: a comprehensive review of the year 1980 and a summary of trends of the years 1960-1965,* EPA 520/1-84-005, Washington DC, 1984, Office of Radiation Programs, U.S. Environmental Protection Agency.

56. Little JB, Radford EP, McCombs HL, Hunt VR: Distribution of Polonium[210] in pulmonary tissues of cigarette smokers, *N Engl J Med* 273:1343-1351, 1965.

57. Ludlow JB: Diagnostic imaging assessment of experimental intraoral "folded film", *Oral Surg* 64:123-129, 1987.

58. Lundeen RC, McDavid WD, Barnwell GM, Proximal surface caries detection with direct-exposure and rare earth screen/film imaging, *Oral Surg* 66:734-745, 1988.

59. MacDonald JCF, Reid JA, Berthoty D: Drywall construction as a dental radiation barrier, *Oral Surg* 55:319-326, 1983.

60. Manny EF, Carlson KC, McClean PM et al: *An overview of dental radiology,* Washington DC, 1980, National Center for Health Care Technology (FDA/BRH).

61. Matteson SR, Morrison WS, Stanek EF III, Phillips C: A survey of radiographs obtained at the initial dental examination and patient selection criteria for bitewings at recall, *J Am Dent Assoc* 107:586-590, 1983.

62. Matteson SR, Phillips C, Kantor ML, Leinedecker T: The effect of lesion size, restorative material, and film speed on the detection of recurrent caries, *Oral Surg* 68:232-237, 1989.

63. Mauriello SM, Matteson SR, Tyndall DA, Bader JD: Clinical evaluation of a samarium/aluminum compound filter, *Oral Surg* 68:108-114, 1989.

64. McDavid WD, Welander V, Pillai BK, Morris CR: The Intrex: a constant-potential x-ray unit for periapical dental radiography, *Oral Surg* 53:433-436, 1982.

65. Miles DA, Van Dis ML, Peterson MGE: Information yield: a comparison of Kodak T-Mat G, Ortho L and RP X-Omat films, *Dentomaxillofac Radiol* 18:15-18, 1989.

66. National Council on Radiation Protection and Measurements: Basic radiation protection criteria, *NCRP Report* 39, 1971.

67. National Council on Radiation Protection and Measurements: Control of radon in houses, *NCRP Report* 103, 1989.

68. National Council on Radiation Protection and Measurements: Dental x-ray protection, *NCRP Report* 35, 1970.

69. National Council on Radiation Protection and Measurements: Exposure of the population in the United States and Canada from natural background radiation, *NCRP Report* 94, 1987.

70. National Council on Radiation Protection and Measurements: Exposure of the U.S. population from diagnostic medical radiation, *NCRP Report* 100, 1989.

71. National Council on Radiation Protection and Measurements: Ionizing radiation exposure of the population of the United States, *NCRP Report* 93, 1987.

72. National Council on Radiation Protection and Measurements: Medical x-ray and gamma-ray protection for energies up to 10 MeV: equipment design and use, *NCRP Report* 33, 1963.

73. National Council on Radiation Protection and Measurements: Quality assurance for diagnostic imaging, *NCRP Report* 99, 1990.

74. National Council on Radiation Protection and Measurements: Radiation exposure of the U.S. population from consumer products and miscellaneous sources, *NCRP Report* 95, 1987.

75. Nationwide evaluation of x-ray trends tabulations: representative sample data, January 1, 1983 to December 31, 1983, HHS Publication (FDA), 1984.

76. New Mexico Health and Environment Department, Environmental Improvement Division: *Radiation protection regulations,* Santa Fe, 1989.

77. Nowak AJ, Creedon RL, Musselman RJ, Troutman KC: Summary of the Conference on Radiation Exposure in Pediatric Dentistry, *J Am Dent Assoc* 103:426-428, 1981.

78. Ponce AZ, McDavid WD, Langland OE: The use of added erbium filtration in intraoral radiography, *Oral Surg* 66:513-517, 1988.

79. Ponce AZ, McDavid WD, Lundeen RC, Morris CR: Adaptation of the Panorex II for use with rare earth screen-film combinations, *Oral Surg* 61:645-648, 1986.

80. Ponce AZ, McDavid WD, Lundeen RC, Morris CR: Kodak T-Mat G film in rotational panoramic radiography, *Oral Surg* 61:649-652, 1986.

81. Ponce AZ, McDavid WD, Underhill TE, Morris CR: Use of E-speed film with added filtration, *Oral Surg* 61:297-299, 1986.

82. Population exposure to x-rays: U.S. 1970, DHEW Publ (FDA) 73-8047, 1978.

83. Preece JW, Morris CR: The efficient and effective use of x-radiation in the dental office. III. Office assessment *GP Texas Acad Gen Dent Pub* 6:1-5, 1980.

84. Price C, McDonnell D: Effects of niobium filtration and constant potential on the sensitometric responses of dental radiographic films, *Dentomaxillofac Radiol* 20:11-16, 1991.

85. Reid JA, MacDonald JDF: Use and workload factors in dental radiation: protection design, *Oral Surg* 57:219-224, 1984.

86. Richards AG: Roentgen-ray doses in dental radiography, *J Am Dent Assoc* 56:351-368, 1958.

87. Richards AG: Trends in dental radiography, *Oral Surg* 44:807-810, 1977.

88. Richards AG, Barbor GL, Bader JD, Hale JD: Samarium filters for dental radiography, *Oral Surg* 29:704-715, 1970.

89. Richards AG, Colquitt WN: Reduction in dental x-ray exposures during the past 60 years, *J Am Dent Assoc* 103:713-718, 1981.

90. Schuman LM: Background radiation and Down's syndrome, *Ann NY Acad Sci* 171:441-453, 1970.

91. Segall A, MacMahon B, Hannigan M: Congenital malformations and background radiation in norhtern New England, *J Chron Dis* 17:915-932, 1964.

92. Sikorski PA, Taylor KW: The effectiveness of the thyroid shield in dental radiology, *Oral Surg* 58:225-236, 1984.

93. Silha RE: The new Kodak Ektaspeed dental x-ray film, *Dent Radiogr Photogr* 54:32-35, 1981.

94. Skoczylas LJ, Preece JW, Langlais RP et al: Comparison of x-radiation doses between conventional and rare earth

panoramic radiographic techniques, *Oral Surg* 68:776-781, 1989.

95. Svenson B, Grödahl H, Petersson A, Olving A: Accuracy of radiographic caries diagnosis at different kilovoltages and two film speeds, *Swed Dent J* 9:37-43, 1985.

96. Svenson B, Petersson A: Accuracy of radiographic caries diagnosis using different x-ray generators, *Dentomaxillofac Radiol* 18:68-71, 1989.

97. Tanimoto K, Ogawa M, Tomita S, Wada T: A filter for use in lateral cephalography, *Oral Surg* 68:666-669, 1989.

98. Taylor LS: Let's keep our sense of humor in dealing with radiation hazards, *Perspect Biol Med* 23:325-334, 1980.

99. Technology Assessment Forum on Dental Radiology, *op. cit.* reference 29.

100. Texas Department of Health, Division of Occupational Health and Radiation Control: *Texas regulations for control of radiation,* Austin, 1989.

101. The selection of patients for x-ray examinations: chest x-ray screening examinations, HHS Publ (FDA) S3-8204, 1983.

102. Thunthy KH, Boozer CH, Weinberg R: Sensitometric evaluation of rare earth intensifying screen systems, *Oral Surg* 59:102-106, 1985.

103. Thunthy KH, Weinberg R: Sensitometric and image analysis of T-grain film, *Oral Surg* 62:218-220, 1986.

104. Thunthy KH, Weinberg R: Sensitometric comparison of dental films of groups D and E, *Oral Surg* 54:250-252, 1982.

105. Trout ED, Kelley JP, Cathey GA: The use of filters to control radiation exposure to the patient in diagnostic radiology, *AJR* 67:946-963, 1952.

106. Tyndall DA: Spectroscopic analysis and dosimetry of diagnostic x-ray beams filtered by rare earth materials, *Oral Surg* 62:205-211, 1986.

107. Tyndall DA, Washburn DB: The effect of rare earth filtration on patient exposure, dose reduction, and image quality in oral panoramic radiology, *Health Phys* 52:17-26, 1987.

108. Valachovic RW, Lurie AG: Risk-benefit considerations in pedodontic radiology, *Pediatr Dent* 2:128-146, 1980.

109. van Lujik JA, Sanderink GCH: Application of a photodiode in dental radiology, *Oral Surg* 62:110-116, 1986.

110. Wall BF, Kendall GM: Collective doses and risks from dental radiology in Great Britain, *Br J Radiol* 56:511-516, 1983.

111. Weems RA, Manson-Hing LR, Jamison HC, Greer DF: Diagnostic yield and selection criteria in complete intraoral radiography, *J Am Dent Assoc* 110:333-338, 1985.

112. Weissman DD, Longhurst GE: Clinical evaluation of a rectangular field collimating device for periapical radiography, *J Am Dent Assoc* 82:580-682, 1971.

113. White SC: 1992 Assessment of radiation risks from dental radiography, *Dentomaxillofac Radiol* 21:118-126, 1992.

114. White SC, Forsythe AB: High-yield criteria for panoramic radiography, HHS Publication (FDA) 82-8186, 1982.

115. White SC, Forsythe AB, Joseph LP: Patient-selection criteria for panoramic radiography, *Oral Surg* 57:681-690, 1984.

116. White SC, Hollender L, Gratt BM: Comparison of xeroradiographs and film for detection of calculus, *Dentomaxillofac Radiol* 13:39-43, 1984.

117. White SC, Hollender L, Gratt BM: Comparison of xeroradiographs and film for detection of proximal surface caries, *J Am Dent Assoc* 108(5):755-759, 1984.

118. Winkler KG: Influence of rectangular collimation on intraoral shielding on radiation dose in dental radiography, *J Am Dent Assoc* 77:95-101, 1968.

4

KATHRYN A. ATCHISON

Guidelines for Prescribing Dental Radiographs

The decision to conduct a radiographic examination is based on the individual characteristics of the patient—age, general health, clinical findings, dental history. At the first patient visit it is necessary to obtain the patient's medical and dental history. Following the recording of the medical and dental history, it is important that the patient be clinically examined. This examination may disclose dental problems that will prove critical to decisions relevant to the radiographic examination. It is necessary to make a radiographic examination when the history and clinical examination have not provided enough information to evaluate completely a patient's condition and to formulate an appropriate treatment plan. Exposures should be made only when there is reason to expect that the patient will benefit by finding clinically useful information on the radiograph.

DISEASE DETECTION

The goal of dental care is to preserve and improve the patient's oral health while minimizing other health-related risks. Although the diagnostic information provided by radiographs may be of definite benefit to the patient, the radiographic examination does carry the potential for harm from ionizing radiation. One of the most effective means of reducing possible harm is to avoid making radiographs that will not contribute information pertinent to the patient's care. The judgment that underlies the decision to make a radiographic examination centers on several factors:

1. Prevalence of the disease(s) that may be detected radiographically in the oral cavity
2. Ability of the clinician to detect these diseases clinically and radiographically
3. Consequences of undetected and untreated disease

As a general principle, radiographs are indicated when there is a high probability that they will provide valuable information about a disease that is not evident clinically. Conversely, radiographs are not indicated when they are unlikely to yield information that will contribute to patient care. In many clinical situations it is not readily apparent to the practitioner whether radiographs have a high probability of providing valuable information. In these situations it is up to the practitioner, after weighing patient factors, to decide whether radiographs are indicated. Some of the most common dental diseases will be considered.

Caries. Dental caries affects people of all ages. The caries prevalence rates in developed countries have been decreasing since the 1970s, probably in part because of the widespread use of fluoride.[17] In addition, increasing numbers of older adults are maintaining their teeth throughout their lifetime, leaving these teeth at risk of developing root caries. These factors reinforce the need to individually select the radiographs most appropriate for a patient's age and oral health condition. Occlusal, buccal, and lingual carious lesions are reasonably easy to detect clinically. Interproximal caries and caries associated with existing restorations are much more difficult to detect with only a clinical examination. (See Chapter 15.)

Studies have repeatedly demonstrated that clinicians using radiographs discover caries that is not evident clinically, including both enamel and dentinal caries.[14,25] Although a radiographic examination is very important for diagnosis of dental caries, mitigating factors must be considered in determining the optimal frequency for such an examination: the patient's age, diet, oral hygiene practices, and oral health status and the nature of the carious process.

Carious lesions demonstrate one of three behaviors: progression, arrest, or regression.[20] Only about 50% of lesions progress beyond the initial, just detectable, defect,[8] and in most instances the lesions demonstrate a slow rate of progression through enamel (months to years).[21,22] The rate of caries progression is significantly faster in deciduous than in permanent enamel.[9,19,22] Patients vary widely in their rates of caries formation and progression. Since the presence of caries cannot be determined with confidence by clinical examination alone, it is necessary to expose patients periodically to radiography to monitor for dental caries. The length of exposure intervals will vary considerably because of varying patient circumstances. Most of the parameters mentioned above suggest an infrequent radiographic examination to monitor for dental caries; however, if the patient history and clinical examination suggest a relatively high caries experience, one should shorten the intervals to allow for careful monitoring of disease.

Periodontal diseases. Diseases of the periodontium affect at least half the population by age 50 and almost all by age 65,[2] being responsible for a substantial portion of all teeth lost.[19] There is a consensus among practitioners that radiographic examinations play an important role in the evaluation of patients with periodontal disease. (See Chapter 16.) They serve to demonstrate local factors that complicate the disease (e.g., the presence of gingival irritants like calculus or faulty restorations). Occasionally the length and morphology of roots are a critical factor that will be apparent on periapical films. These observations suggest that when there is clinical evidence of periodontal disease, other than nonspecific gingivitis, it is appropriate to obtain radiographs to aid in establishing the severity of the disease. Use of follow-up radiographs after therapy is completed will help determine whether the destruction of alveolar bone has been halted.

Dental anomalies. Abnormal formation of teeth may present as deviations in number, size, and composition. These abnormalities occur less frequently in the primary than in the permanent dentition. Also the associated problems are less serious in the deciduous dentition than in the permanent dentition.[28] The most frequently encountered anomalies are supernumerary teeth (usually mesiodens) or developmentally absent teeth (usually second premolars). There are some anomalies for which orthodontic treatment or surgical correction or modification must start at an early age.[28]

When the dentist suspects an abnormality that will require treatment, radiographs to confirm and localize it are not required until the time that the surgery is most appropriate. For example, a panoramic examination of a 5-year-old child to determine the presence or absence of permanent teeth may be ill-timed. Even though the examination could provide evidence that one or more second premolars or lateral incisors were developmentally missing, this information usually would not influence the current treatment plan. When examination for dental anomalies is appropriate, both the radiation dose and the anticipated diagnostic benefit should be considered and the projections that will best demonstrate the required diagnostic information should be selected. A panoramic radiograph of the lower face is usually best for disclosing the presence of absence of teeth in all quadrants, although a periapical film would be sufficient for an examination limited to one area.

Occult disease. Occult diseases are those presenting no clinical signs or symptoms. Small carious lesions, cysts, and tumors may go unnoticed until signs and symptoms develop. Although the consequences of some occult diseases may be quite serious, the prevalence of such diseases in the perioral tissues is rare. Usually there is some clinical sign or symptom of intraosseous disease suggesting its presence.[6] For instance, an unusual contour of bone or an absent third molar, not explained by a history of extraction, suggests the possibility of an impaction, with the potential for an associated dentigerous cyst. Because occult disease is so rare (except for caries, as described above), a radiographic examination of the jaws should not be undertaken solely to look for it in dentate individuals when there is no unusual clinical sign or symptom. Caries is an exception, however, because of its much higher prevalence than exists with occult cysts or tumors.

The situation is different for edentulous patients. In these patients the high number of dental problems found usually justifies a radiographic examination to look for occult disease.[16] In addition to having a greater frequency of occult disease, edentulous patients tend to be older and thus have a lower risk of radiation-induced disease.

Radiographic examinations

When it is concluded that a patient requires a radiograph, the dentist should consider which radiographic examination is most appropriate. There are a variety of projections from which to select,

TABLE 4-1. Common dental radiographic examinations and their properties

Type of examination	Coverage	Resolution	Relative patient exposure*	Detectable diseases
Intraoral radiographs				
Individual periapical	Limited	High	1	Caries, periodontal disease, periapical disease, dental anomalies, occult disease
Interproximal bitewings	Limited	High	4	Caries, periodontal bone level
Full-mouth examination	Limited	High	14 to 17	
Occlusal	Moderate	High	1	Dental anomalies, occult disease
Extraoral radiographs				
Panoramic	Broad	Moderate	1-2	Dental anomalies, occult disease, extensive caries, periodontal disease, periapical disease

*Based on the use of E-speed film and rectangular collimation for periapical films, round collimation for bitewings and occlusal views, and rare-earth screens for the panoramic examination. With D-speed film, the intraoral values are doubled; and with round collimation, the periapical values increase by two and a half times.
Information derived from White SC: *Dentomaxillofac Radiol* 21:118-126, 1992.

and the choice involves consideration of the anatomic relationships, size of the field, and radiation dose from each view. Table 4-1 summarizes the more common types of radiographic examinations for general dental patients and factors to consider in choosing the most appropriate one. For example, a panoramic radiograph will provide broad area coverage with moderate resolution (Fig. 4-1). Intraoral films will give more detailed information but a significantly higher radiation dose per unit area exposed. The clinician must use clinical judgment in weighing these factors. Figure 4-1 shows examples of each of the radiographic examinations.

Intraoral radiographs. Intraoral radiographs are examinations made by placing the x-ray film within the patient's mouth during the exposure. They offer the dentist a high-detail view of the teeth and bone in the area exposed and are most appropriate for revealing caries, periodontal disease, or periapical disease in a localized region. A complete-mouth or full-mouth examination (FMX) consists of periapical views of all the tooth-bearing regions as well as interproximal views. (See Chapter 9.)

Periapical radiographs. Periapical views (PAs) show all of a tooth and the surrounding bone. They are very useful for revealing caries, periodontal disease, and periapical lesions.

Interproximal radiographs. Interproximal views (bitewings) show the coronal aspects of both the maxillary and the mandibular dentition as well as the surrounding crestal bone in a region. They are most useful for revealing proximal caries and evaluating the height of the alveolar crest, and they can be made in either the anterior or the posterior region of the mouth.

Occlusal radiographs. Occlusal views are intraoral radiographs in which the film is positioned in the occlusal plane (see Chapter 9). They are often used in children in place of periapical views because of the small size of the patient's mouth. In adults occlusal radiographs may supplement periapical views, providing visualization of a greater area of teeth and bone. They are useful for demonstrating impacted or abnormally placed maxillary anterior teeth or for visualizing the region of a palatal cleft. They may also demonstrate buccal or lingual expansion of bone.

Extraoral radiographs. Extraoral radiographs are examinations made of the orofacial region using films located extraorally. They allow the practitioner to examine areas not completely covered by intraoral films, such as the jaws, skull, or temporomandibular joints (TMJs). Specific guidelines for ordering most extraoral views, as well as the standard technique for making them, will be discussed in Chapter 11. Only the panoramic radiograph will be described here, since it has common use as a radiographic examination for general dental patients.

Panoramic radiographs. Panoramic radiographs provide a broad view of the jaws, teeth, maxillary sinuses, nasal fosse, and TMJs. They show which teeth are present, the relative state of development, the presence or absence of dental

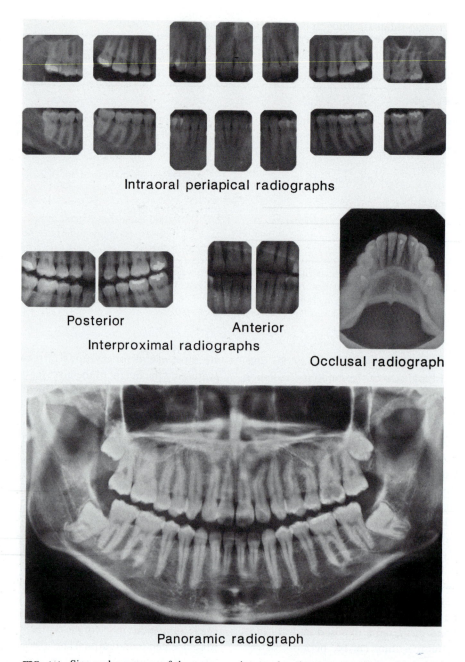

Intraoral periapical radiographs

Posterior   Anterior
Interproximal radiographs

Occlusal radiograph

Panoramic radiograph

FIG. 4-1. Size and coverage of the common intraoral and extraoral radiographs.

abnormalities, and many traumatic and pathologic lesions in bone. They are the initial examination of choice for edentulous patients.

Since panoramic radiography is an extraoral technique and uses intensifying screens, the resolution of images is less than with intraoral non-screen films. (See Chapter 5.) Consequently, it is generally inadequate for the accurate diagnosis of caries, root abnormalities, and periapical changes.[13,24] In the great majority of dental patients, oral disease involving the teeth or jaws lies within the area imaged by periapical radiographs, and thus when a full-mouth set of radiographs is available, a panoramic examination is usually redundant since it does not add additional information that will alter the treatment plan.[30] Panoramic views are most useful when the required field of view is large. Although the selection of a radiographic examination should be based on the extent of information it is likely to provide, the relatively low dose of radiation from a panoramic examination should be one qualifying factor.

Guidelines for ordering radiographs

Ever since radiographs were hailed as a means of detecting disease not evident clinically, the profession has issued guidelines advising dentists as to what radiographs to obtain for patients and how often to repeat them. The profession emphatically recommends that dentists (1) make radiographs only after a clinical examination of the patient and (2) order only those that will directly benefit the patient's diagnosis or treatment plan.

Previous radiographs. Most patients have been seen previously by a dentist and have had radiographs made. The practitioner should attempt to get these radiographs, regardless of when they were exposed. If they are relatively recent, they may be adequate to the diagnostic problem at hand. Even if they were made so long ago that they are not likely to reflect the current status of the patient, they may still prove useful. They may demonstrate whether a condition has worsened, remained unchanged, or shown improvement (e.g., the progression of caries or periodontal disease).

Administrative radiographs. Administrative radiographs are those made for reasons other than diagnosis. Examples include radiographs obtained for an insurance company or for an examining board. We believe that a patient should be exposed only when it benefits his or her health care. Most administrative radiographs do not serve such an objective. Unfortunately, this recommendation is often not adhered to in practice, and dentists are left to sort out the most appropriate set of criteria to use in their practice.[18,26]

Development of guidelines based on patient characteristics. As the number of x-ray examinations available to practitioners has increased (bitewing, occlusal, panoramic, etc.), professional guidelines have concentrated on specifying which examination to order for different types of disease. Recent information regarding changes in the patterns of dental disease and increased fear of the lifelong risk of low levels of x-radiation have led the profession to refine its guidelines further and recommend specific patient factors that could influence the number and type of dental x-rays to order.

In the mid-1980s a branch of the Food and Drug Administration (FDA)[27] convened a panel to develop a set of guidelines (Table 4-2) for making dental radiographs. This committee based its recommendations on the available literature pertaining to the efficacy of dental examinations. The panel addressed the question of what would be the appropriate radiographs for an adequate evaluation of a new or recall asymptomatic patient seeking general dental care. The guidelines described circumstances (patient age, medical and dental history, and physical signs) that would suggest the need for radiographs. These circumstances were called *selection criteria*. The guidelines also suggested the types of radiographic examinations most likely to benefit the patient in terms of yielding diagnostic information. The recommendations were that radiographs not be made unless there was some expectation that they would provide evidence of diseases affecting the treatment plan. The American Dental Association (ADA)[7] recommends use of these guidelines.

Using the FDA guidelines for ordering radiographs

Central to the guidelines recommended by the FDA is the idea that dentists should expose patients to radiation *only* when there is a reasonable expectation that the resulting radiograph will benefit patient care. Accordingly, radiographs should be made only when there is some clinical evidence of an abnormality or when the probability of disease is reasonably high.

The selection criteria for radiographs are any signs or symptoms found in the patient history or clinical examination that suggest a radiographic examination would yield clinically useful information. For example, a clinical examination may disclose a disease that is clinically apparent but whose nature and extent cannot be evaluated clinically. Such situations will frequently require a radiographic examination for adequate assessment. This chapter considers the choice of appropriate radiographic examinations. Other chapters will cover the means for conducting such examinations and interpreting the results.

A key concept in the use of selection criteria is to recognize the need to consider each patient individually. Radiographs should be prescribed on an individual basis according to a demonstrated need. The American Dental Association's recommendations on the use of radiography include two main concepts:

1. That the nature and extent of diagnosis required for patient care constitute the only rational basis for de-

TABLE 4-2. Guidelines for prescribing dental radiographs

The recommendations in this table are subject to clinical judgment and may not apply to every patient. They are to be used by dentists only after reviewing the patient's health history and completing a clinical examination. They do not need to be altered because of pregnancy.

	Child	
	Primary dentition (prior to eruption of first permanent tooth)	**Transitional dentition (following eruption of first permanent tooth)**
New patient		
All new patients to assess dental diseases and growth and development	Posterior bitewing examination if proximal surfaces of primary teeth cannot be visualized or probed	Individualized radiographic examination consisting of periapical and/or occlusal views, posterior bitewing or panoramic examination and posterior bitewings
Recall patient		
Clinical caries or high-risk factors for caries*	Posterior bitewing examination at 6-month intervals or until no carious lesions are evident	
No clinical caries and no high-risk factors for caries	Posterior bitewing examination at 12 to 24-month intervals if proximal surfaces of primary teeth cannot be visualized or probed	Posterior bitewing examination at 12 to 24-month intervals
Periodontal disease or history of periodontal treatment	Individualized radiographic examination consisting of selected periapical and/or bitewing radiographs for areas where periodontal disease (other than nonspecific gingivitis) can be demonstrated clinically	
Growth and development assessment	Usually not indicated	Individualized radiographic examination consisting of a periapical and/or occlusal or panoramic examination

*Clinical situations for which radiographs may be indicated include the following:	Positive clinical signs or symptoms 1. Clinical evidence of periodontal disease 2. Large or deep restorations 3. Deep carious lesions 4. Malposed or clinically impacted teeth 5. Swelling 6. Evidence of facial trauma	7. Mobility of teeth 8. Fistula or sinus tract infection 9. Clinically suspected sinus pathology 10. Growth abnormalities 11. Oral involvement in known or suspected systemic disease 12. Positive neurologic findings in the head and neck 13. Evidence of foreign objects 14. Pain and/or dysfunction of the TMJ
Positive historical findings 1. Previous periodontal or endodontic therapy 2. History of pain or trauma 3. Familial history of dental anomalies 4. Postoperative evaluation of healing 5. Presence of implants		

termining the need, type, and frequency of radiographic examination

2. That, because each patient is different, radiographic examinations be individualized

The ADA[7] specifically cautions against the routine use of radiography as a part of periodic examination of all patients.

There is a description in the guidelines of clinical situations in which radiographs are likely to contribute to the diagnosis, treatment, and prognosis. Two examples highlight the differences between ordering radiographs for dental diseases with clinical signs or symptoms and ordering them for dental diseases with no clinical indicators but a high prevalence.

In the first case would be the patient with a hard swelling in the premolar region of the mandible with expansion of the buccal and lingual cortical plates. The clinical sign of swelling alerts the dentist to the need for a radiograph. The radiograph indicates that the abnormality in the region involves the bone.

A more common example would be the patient who has not seen a dentist for many years who comes seeking general dental care. Even though there may be no clinical evidence of caries involving the posterior teeth, bite-

Adolescent	Adult	
Permanent dentition (prior to eruption of third molars)	**Dentulous**	**Edentulous**
Individualized radiographic examination consisting of posterior bitewings and selected periapicals*; a full-mouth intraoral radiographic examination is appropriate when patient presents with clinical evidence of generalized dental disease or a history of extensive dental treatment		Full-mouth intraoral radiographic examination or panoramic examination
Posterior bitewing examination at 6 to 12-month intervals or until no carious lesions are evident	Posterior bitewing examination at 12 to 18-month intervals	Not applicable
Posterior bitewing examination at 18 to 36-month intervals	Posterior bitewing examination at 24 to 36-month intervals	Not applicable
Individualized radiographic examination consisting of selected periapical and/or bitewing radiographs for areas where periodontal disease (other than nonspecific gingivitis) can be demonstrated clinically		Not applicable
Periapical or panoramic examination to assess developing third molars	Usually not indicated	Usually not indicated

15. Facial asymmetry
16. Abutment for fixed or removable partial prosthesis
17. Unexplained bleeding
18. Unexplained sensitivity of teeth
19. Unusual eruption, spacing or migration of teeth
20. Unusual tooth morphology, calcification or color
21. Missing teeth with unknown reason

†Patients at high risk for caries may demonstrate any of the following:

1. High level of caries experience
2. History of recurrent caries
3. Existing restoration of poor quality
4. Poor oral hygiene
5. Inadequate fluoride exposure
6. Prolonged nursing (bottle or breast)

7. Diet with high sucrose frequency
8. Poor family dental health
9. Developmental enamel defects
10. Developmental disability
11. Xerostomia
12. Genetic abnormality of teeth
13. Many multisurface restorations
14. Chemo/radiation therapy

wings are indicated. Since this patient has not had interproximal radiographs for many years, there is a reasonable possibility that he/she may benefit from them through the detection of interproximal decay. No clinical signs exist suggesting the presence of caries, and yet the dentist's clinical knowledge of the prevalence of caries indicates that this radiograph has a reasonable probability of disclosing disease.

Without some specific indication, it is inappropriate to expose the patient "just to see if there is something there." The major exception to this rule is the use of interproximal films for caries when there may be no clinical signs of early lesions. The probability of finding occult disease in a patient with all permanent teeth erupted and no clinical or historical evidence of abnormality is so low that making a periapical radiographic survey just to look for such disease is not indicated.[6]

Patient examination. Radiographs should be ordered only when there is a reasonable expectation that they will provide information that will be contributory to the diagnostic problem at hand. Accordingly, the first step is a *careful* examination of the patient. The clinical examination will provide indications as to the nature and extent of the radiographic examination that will likely be appropriate. Posterior interproximal radiographs form the foundation of the FDA guidelines. They are useful for the detection of interproximal caries and periodontal disease. Preliminary testing of the use of selection criteria[3,5] has suggested that anterior interproximal radiographs may also prove valuable for detecting interproximal caries in the anterior region. Others[1,15] note, however, that use of selection criteria may not result in 100% coverage of all disease present in a patient's mouth.

A footnote to Table 4-2 outlines some clinical findings that indicate when radiographs will likely contribute to a complete description of the asymptomatic patient. In the guidelines, patients are classified by stage of dental development—whether they are being evaluated for the first time (without previous documentation) or being reevaluated during the clinical examination, and by an estimate of their risk of having dental caries or periodontal disease.

Clinical judgment and an amalgamation of knowledge, experience, and concern should always be used in applying these guidelines to the specific circumstances of each patient. Recognizing situations not described by the guidelines in which patients will need radiographs also requires clinical judgment.

Initial visit. The guidelines recommend that the child with a primary dentition who is cooperative and has closed posterior contacts receive only interproximal radiographs to examine for caries. Additional periapical views are recommended only if there are clinically evident diseases and/or specific historical or clinical indications such as those listed at the bottom of Table 4-2. If the molar contacts are not closed, no radiographs are necessary since the proximal surfaces can be examined directly. The guidelines recommend radiographic coverage of all tooth-bearing areas for the child with a transitional dentition (following eruption of the first permanent tooth, 6 to 8 years of age). This generally consists of bitewings supplemented with either periapical or occlusal views (8 to 12 exposures) or a panoramic view. A panoramic projection is usually the view of choice since it offers the most general information with the lowest dose of ionizing radiation. Some[23] express concern that complete coverage of all tooth-bearing areas is not warranted without a specific indication.

The guidelines group adolescents and dentate adults together to identify the kind and extent of appropriate radiographic examination. It is recommended that these patients receive an individualized examination consisting of interproximal and periapical views selected on the basis of specific historical or clinical indications. The presence of generalized dental disease often indicates the need for a full-mouth examination. Alternatively, the presence of only a few localized abnormalities or diseases suggests that a more limited examination consisting of interproximal and selected periapical views may suffice. When there is no evidence of dental disease, only interproximal views may be necessary for caries examination.

For the edentulous patient it is appropriate to obtain a radiographic examination of all the tooth-bearing areas, by either periapical or panoramic radiographs. If available, the panoramic projection will usually provide the required information at a reduced radiation dose.

Recall visit. It is important always to carefully examine patients who are returning after initial care. As at the initial examination, selected periapical views are obtained if there are any of the historical or clinical signs or symptoms listed in the footnote to Table 4-2.

The guidelines recommend interproximal radiographs for recall patients to detect caries and monitor the status of alveolar bone loss. The optimum frequency for these views will depend on the age of the patient and the probability of finding these two diseases. If the patient has clinically demonstrable caries or is at high risk for caries (poor diet, poor oral hygiene, and the factors listed in the footnote to Table 4-2), then bitewings should be obtained at fairly frequent intervals—such as for children at 6-month intervals until no carious lesions are clinically evident. For the adolescent at high risk of caries, the guidelines recommend bitewings at 6- to 12-month intervals and for the high-risk adult at 12- to 18-month intervals. The recommended intervals are longer for individuals not at high risk for caries: 12 to 24 months for the children, 18 to 36 months for adolescents, and 24 to 36 months for adults. Note that individuals can change their risk category, going from high to low risk or the reverse. Similarly, recall patients with a history or clinical evidence of periodontal disease more serious than nonspecific gingivitis should have a combination of periapical and interproximal radiographs made to allow appropriate monitoring.

Children and adolescents being assessed for growth and development will require an individualized radiographic examination that may include periapicals or a panoramic radiograph to supplement any radiographs ordered for the evaluation of dental disease. In addition, a patient of any age group who is being considered for orthodontic treatment may need other projections (e.g., a lateral or frontal cephalograph or TMJ radiograph, Fig. 4-2). The needs of these patients should always be weighed individually, and the appropriate radiographs selected to allow for a maximum diagnostic yield with minimal radiographic exposure. The clinical findings and study of plaster models and photographs will help in determining the optimum time to initiate treatment.[4,12]

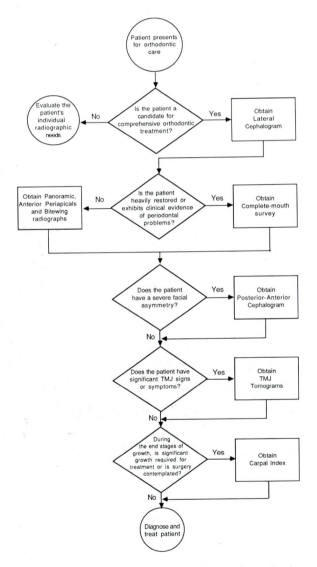

FIG. 4-2. Clinical algorithm for ordering radiographs, in this instance to treat patients seeking orthodontic care. Selected radiographs are ordered following consideration of the patient's history and clinical characteristics.

Special considerations

Pregnancy. Occasionally it is desirable to obtain radiographs on a woman who is pregnant. The x-ray beam is largely confined to the head and neck region in dental x-ray examinations; thus the fetal exposure is only about 1 μGy for a full-mouth examination.[11] This exposure is quite small compared to that received normally from natural background sources. Accordingly, the guidelines can be used with pregnant patients just as with other patients.

Radiotherapy. Patients with a malignancy in the oral cavity or perioral region often undergo radiotherapy for their disease. Some oral tissues will receive 50 Gy or more. Although such patients are often apprehensive about this additional exposure, the dental dose is insignificant compared to what they have already received from radiation therapy. The average skin dose from a dental radiograph is approximately 3 mGy.[10] Furthermore, patients who have received radiotherapy may suffer from radiation-induced xerostomia and thus are at a high risk of developing radiation caries. Accordingly, patients who have had radiotherapy to the oral cavity should be carefully followed because they are at special risk for the development of dental disease.

Examples of how to use the FDA guidelines

Following are some examples of how the FDA guidelines would be applied to different clinical situations:

A 5-year-old boy has his first visit to your office. A careful clinical examination reveals that he is cooperative and his posterior teeth are in contact. Posterior bitewings are recommended to detect caries. If all of such a patient's teeth are present, there is no evidence of decay, a reasonably good diet is being observed, and the parent(s) seem well motivated to promote good oral hygiene, a radiographic examination may not be in order at this time. Radiographs for the detection of developmental abnormalities are also not in order at this age because a complete appraisal cannot be made at 5 years of age and it is too early to initiate treatment if any are found.

A 25-year-old woman is seen for a 6-month checkup following her last treatment for a fractured incisor. No caries is evident on interproximal radiographs made 6 months ago, and currently there are no clinical signs of caries or high-risk factors present. There is also no evidence of periodontal disease or other signs or symptoms associated with the recently fractured tooth. Providing the fractured incisor is vital, no radiographs are recis vital, no radiographs are recommended for this patient. If it is nonvital, then make a periapical view of this tooth.

A 45-year-old man returns to your office after 1 year. At his last visit, you placed two MOD amalgam restorations on premolars and performed root canal therapy on number 30. The patient has a 5 mm pocket in the buccal furcation of number 3 but no other evidence of periodontal disease. The guidelines recommend that this patient receive bitewings (to see if he is still caries active) and periapical views of numbers 3 and 30 (to evaluate the extent of periodontal and periapical disease).

A 65-year-old woman comes to your office for the first time. No previous radiographs are available. There is a history of root canal therapy in two teeth, although the patient is not aware which teeth were treated. Clinical examination reveals multiple carious teeth, multiple missing teeth, and pockets of more than 3 mm involving most of the remaining teeth. The guidelines recommend a full-mouth examination including bitewings for this patient because of the high probability of finding caries, periodontal disease, and periapical disease.

REFERENCES

1. Åkerblom A, Rohlin M, Hasselgren G: Individualised restricted intraoral radiography versus full-mouth radiography in the detection of periradicular lesions, *Swed Dent J* 12:151-159, 1988.
2. American Dental Association Task Force Special Committees: A.D.A. Task Force committee reports, *J Am Dent Assoc* 91:7-9, 1971.
3. Atchison K, White S, Hewlett E, Flack V: Preliminary findings on the impact of using selection criteria to order dental radiographs. Abstract 27, AAPHD 55th annual meeting, 1992.
4. Atchison KA, Luke LS, White SC: An algorithm for ordering pretreatment orthodontic radiographs, *Am J Orthod Dentofacial Orthop* 102(1):29-44, 1992.
5. Brooks SL: A study of selection criteria for intraoral dental radiography, *Oral Surg* 62:234-239, 1986.
6. Brooks S, Joseph L: Basic concepts in the selection of patients for dental x-ray examinations, HHS Publ (FDA) 85-8249, 1985.
7. Council on Dental Materials, Instruments, and Equipment: Recommendations in radiographic practices: an update, 1988, *J Am Dent Assoc* 118:115-117, 1989.
8. Dirks OB: Posteruptive changes in dental enamel, *J Dent Res* 45(suppl):503-511, 1966.
9. Featherstone JDB, Mellberg JR: Relative rates of progress of artificial carious lesions in bovine and human enamel, *Caries Res* 15:109-114, 1981.
10. Frederiksen NL: Health physics. In Goaz PW, White SC: *Oral radiology: principles and interpretation*, ed 2, St Louis, 1987, Mosby.
11. Gonad doses and genetically significant dose from diagnostic radiology: U.S., 1964 and 1970, DHEW Publ (FDA) 76-8034, 1976.
12. Han UK, Vig KWL, Weintraub JA, et al: Consistency of orthodontic treatment decisions relative to diagnostic records, *Am J Orthod Dentofacial Orthop* 100:212-219, 1991.
13. Hansen BF, Johnson JR: Oral radiographic findings in a Norwegian urban population, *Oral Surg* 41:261-266, 1976.
14. Hennon DK, Stooky GK, Muhler JC: A survey of the prevalence and distribution of dental caries in preschool children, *J Am Dent Assoc* 79:1405-1414, 1969.
15. Hollender L: Decision making in radiographic imaging, *J Dent Educ* 56(12):834-843, 1992.
16. Keur JJ: Radiographic screening of edentulous patients: sense or nonsense? A risk-benefit analysis, *Oral Surg* 62:463-467, 1986.
17. Leverett DH: Fluorides and the changing prevalence of dental caries, *Science* 217:26-30, July 1982.
18. National Center for Health Care Technology: Dental radiology: a summary of recommendations from the technology assessment forum, *J Am Dent Assoc* 103:423-425, 1981.
19. Pelton WJ, Pennell EH, Druzina A: Tooth morbidity experience of adults, *J Am Dent Assoc* 17:1-15, 1967.
20. Pitts NB, Kidd EA: Some of the factors to be considered in the prescription and timing of bitewing radiography in the diagnosis and management of dental caries, *J Dent* 20(2):74-84, 1992.
21. Shellis RP: Relationship between structure and the formation of caries-like lesions *in vitro*, *Arch Oral Biol* 29(7):975-981, 1984.
22. Shwartz M, Gröndahl HG, Pliskin JS, Boffa J: A longitudinal analysis from bite-wing radiographs of the rate of progression of approximal carious lesions through human dental enamel, *Arch Oral Biol* 29(7):529-536, 1984.
23. Stephens RG, Kogon SL: New U.S. guidelines for prescribing dental radiographs: a critical review, *J Can Dent Assoc* 56:1019-1024, 1990.
24. Stephens RG, Kogon SL, Reid JA: A comparison of Panorex and intraoral surveys for routine dental radiography, *J Can Dent Assoc* 6:281-286, 1977.
25. Stephens RG, Kogon SL, Wainright RJ, Reid JA: Information yield from routine bitewing radiographs for young adults, *J Can Dent Assoc* 4:247-252, 1981.
26. U.S. Department of Health and Human Services: Administratively required dental radiographs, HHS Publ (FDA) 81-8176, 1981.
27. U.S. Department of Health and Human Services: The selection of patients for x-ray examinations: dental radiographic examinations, HHS Publ (FDA) 88-8273, 1987.
28. Van der Linden PGM, Boersma H: Diagnosis and treatment planning in dentofacial orthopedics, Chicago, 1987, Quintessence Publishing.
29. White SC: 1992 Assessment of radiation risks from dental radiology, *Dentomaxillofac Radiol* 21:118-126, 1992.
30. White SC, Weissman DD: Relative discernment of lesions by intraoral and panoramic radiography, *J Am Dent Assoc* 95:1117-1121, 1977.

5

X-Ray Film, Intensifying Screens, and Grids

A beam of x-ray photons traversing an object is reduced in intensity (attenuated) by absorption and scattering of the photons out of the primary beam. The pattern of the photons that exit the object (those that did not interact with the atoms of the object) carries information pertaining to the structure and composition of the absorber. For this information to be diagnostically useful it must be recorded on an image receptor. The image receptor system most frequently used in dental radiography is x-ray film. This chapter describes x-ray film and its properties, and the use of intensifying screens and grids to modify x-ray images. Digital radiographic systems are described in Chapter 13.

FILM
Composition

X-ray film is a type of photographic film that is composed of two principal components: the emulsion and the base. The emulsion is sensitive to x rays and visible light and records the radiographic image. The base is the supporting material onto which the emulsion is coated (Fig. 5-1).

Emulsion. The two principal components of the emulsion are the silver halide crystals (which are photosensitive) and a gelatin matrix (in which the crystals are suspended). The *silver halide grains* are composed primarily of silver bromide and to a lesser extent silver iodide. The mean diameter of the silver halide crystals in Ektaspeed film (an E-speed film) is about 1 μm). In D-speed film the crystals are somewhat smaller, about 0.7 μm (Fig. 5-2). The presence of silver iodide adds greatly to the sensitivity of the film emulsion, by virtue of iodide's larger diameter than that of bromide, thereby reducing the radiation dose required to produce an adequate diagnostic image. The photosensitivity of the silver halide crystals is dependent

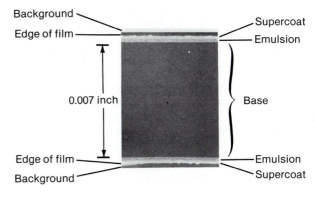

FIG. 5-1. Scanning electron micrograph of Kodak Ultra-Speed dental x-ray film (300×). Note the supercoat, emulsion, and base on this double-emulsion film. (Courtesy Eastman Kodak, Rochester NY.)

upon the incorporation of a sulfur-containing contaminant during manufacture. (See Chapter 7.) The silver halide grains suspended in the *gelatin* matrix are applied to both sides of the supporting base. The gelatin, made from cattle bone, is important for keeping the silver grains evenly dispersed. During film processing the gelatin absorbs the processing solutions, thereby allowing the chemicals to reach and react with the silver halide grains. (See Chapter 7.)

Because an x-ray film receives considerable manipulation during processing, a coating is placed on the surface of the emulsion to serve as a protective barrier. Typically, this protective barrier is an additional layer of gelatin added as a *supercoating* to the film emulsion. This coating helps protect the film from damage by scratching, contamination, and pressure from the rollers when it is being processed in an automatic processor.

The composition of Kodak film emulsion is shown in Table 5-1.

Film emulsions are especially sensitive to either x-ray photons or visible light. Film intended to be exposed by x rays is called *direct exposure* film. All intraoral dental film is direct exposure film. *Screen film* is another type of x-ray film, intended to be used in combination with intensifying screens that emit visible light, which affects most of the exposure for this type of film. Intensifying screens are described later in this chapter.

Base. The function of the film base is to support the emulsion of light-sensitive silver halide grains and gelatin. It is important that the film base have the proper amount of flexibility to allow ease in handling of the film. Excessive rigidity or floppiness would be inconvenient. The film base also should be evenly translucent, casting no pattern on the resultant radiograph. Optimum viewing of diagnostic detail is achieved when the film base has a slight bluish tint. Finally, the film base must be able to withstand exposure to processing solutions without distorting. Dental x-ray film base is composed of polyethylene terephthalate (a polyester) and is about 0.2 mm thick (0.007 inch). To assure good adhesion between the emulsion and the film

base, a thin layer of adhesive material is added to the base before application of the emulsion.

Dental x-ray film

Intraoral dental x-ray film is provided by a number of manufacturers in the United States. In each case the emulsion is double coated; that is, *emulsion is coated on each side of the base*. Double-emulsion film is used because the double layer permits the use of less radiation to make an image. Single-emulsion film provides images with increased sharpness (Fig. 5-3) and is usually used when there is no concern for exposure (e.g., industrial applications or x-ray duplicating film). This film is called *direct exposure* film because it is intended to be exposed by x rays. The only current application of direct film is for intraoral use where only small areas are exposed and high resolution is required. One corner of each dental film has a little raised *dot* that is used for film orientation. The side of the film with the raised dot is always placed toward the x-ray tube, and the side of the film with the depression is oriented toward the patient's tongue. After the film is processed, the dot is used to identify the exposure as being of the patient's left or right side. (See Fig. 7-27.)

The film is packaged as either a single or a double sheet within each packet. When double-film packs are used, the second film serves as a duplicate record. The film is encased in a protective black paper wrapper and then in an outer white paper or plastic wrapping, which should be resistant to moisture (Fig. 5-4). The outer wrapping clearly indicates which side of the film should be directed toward the x-ray tube.

Also included in the film packet, between the wrappers, is a thin lead foil backing. This layer is included in the film packet on the back side of the film away from the tube to shield the film from backscattered (secondary) radiation, which would fog the film. It may also effect some slight reduction in patient exposure. If the film is placed backwards in the patient's mouth so the tube side of the film is not facing the tube, the lead foil will be positioned between the object and the film. This will cause much of the radiation intended for the

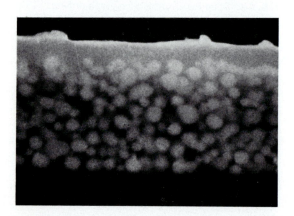

FIG. 5-2. Scanning electron micrograph of an unprocessed emulsion of Kodak Ultra-Speed dental x-ray film (5000×). Note the white-appearing unexposed silver bromide grains. Compare these with the grains in a processed emulsion (Fig. 7-5). (Courtesy Eastman Kodak, Rochester NY.)

TABLE 5-1. Coating weight per film side (mg/cm²)

Film speed	Silver	Bromide	Iodide	Gelatin	Gelatin supercoat
D	1.02	0.74	0.02	0.56	0.16
E	1.14	0.83	0.02	0.66	0.16

film to be absorbed by the lead foil, resulting in a light image. The lead foil has a pattern embossed on it. When the film is reversed and the radiation passes through the foil before striking the film, this pattern is transferred to the film. The combination of a light film with the characteristic pattern indicates that the film was placed backwards in the patient's mouth. This also means that the left side—right side designation (as indicated by the film dot) is reversed.

Intraoral film is generally manufactured in three sizes that facilitate different clinical applications. It should be noted that the films in these size categories do not differ intrinsically but vary only in size and clinical use. The composition of the film is identical.

Periapical film. Periapical film is usually used to record the crowns, roots, and periapical regions of teeth. It comes in three sizes: 0 for small children (about 22 × 35 mm); 1, which is relatively narrow and used for anterior projections (about 24 × 40 mm); and 2, the standard film used for adults (about 32 × 41 mm) (Fig. 5-5).

Bitewing film. Bitewing (interproximal) film is used to record the coronal portions of the maxillary and mandibular teeth in one image. It is useful for the detection of interproximal caries (approximately twofold) compared to clinical examination alone. In addition, the alveolar crests are usually visible, which is valuable in the assessment of periodontal disease. In adults size 2 film is usually used, whereas in children the smaller size 1 is pre-

ferred, and in very small children size 0 film may be used for bitewing projections.

Bitewing films often have a paper tab projecting from the middle of the film, on which the patient bites to support the film (Fig. 5-6). This tab is rarely visualized and does not interfere with the diagnostic quality of the image. Film-holding instruments for bitewing projections are also available.

Occlusal film. Occlusal film is approximately four times larger than size 2 film (about 57 × 76

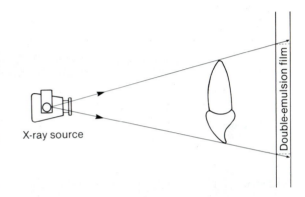

Image shorter on one side of emulsion, longer on other

FIG. 5-3. Parallax "unsharpness" results from the use of double-emulsion film because of the slightly greater magnification on the side of the film away from the x-ray source. In clinical practice, parallax unsharpness is a minor problem.

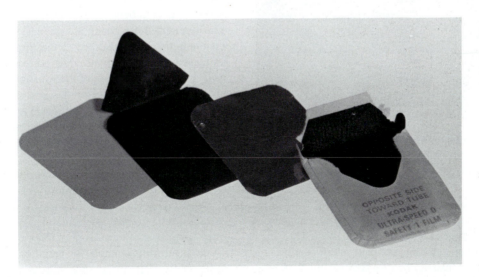

FIG. 5-4. Contents of a film packet revealing *(from left)* the x-ray film, paper film wrapper, sheet of lead foil, and paper package wrapping.

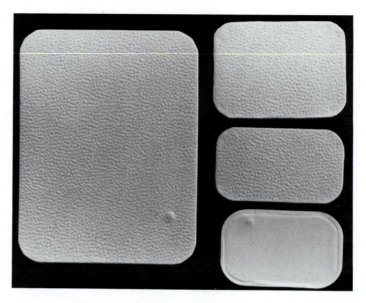

FIG. 5-5. Dental x-ray film is commonly supplied in various sizes. *Left,* Occlusal film; *top right,* adult posterior film; *middle right,* adult anterior film; *bottom right,* child size film (in plastic wrapping).

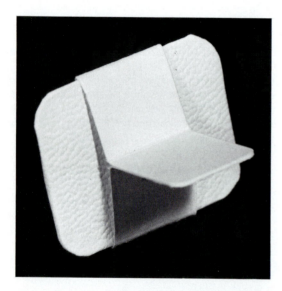

FIG. 5-6. Paper loop placed around a size 2 adult film to support the film when the patient bites on the tab for a bitewing projection. This projection reveals the tooth crowns and alveolar crests.

mm) (Fig. 5-5). It is used to show larger areas of the maxilla or mandible than may be seen on a single periapical film. Its name derives from the fact that it is usually held in position by having the patient bite lightly on the film to support it between the occlusal surfaces of the teeth (See Chapter 9).

Screen film

The extraoral projections used most frequently in dentistry are for panoramic, skull, and cephalometric radiography. For these projections and virtually all other extraoral radiography, *screen film* is used in combination with intensifying screens (described later in this chapter). These films are different from dental film in that they are designed to be particularly sensitive to visible light rather than to x-radiation. This is because they are used by being placed between two intensifying screens. The intensifying screens absorb x rays and emit visible light that exposes the screen film. The emulsion used in screen film has dyes added specifically to increase its absorption of the wavelength of light emitted by the intensifying screens. Because the properties of intensifying screens vary, it is important to use the appropriate screen-film combination recommended by the screen or film manufacturer so the emission characteristics of the screen will be matched to the absorption characteristics (sensitivity) of the film.

Several general types of films are suitable for extraoral radiography, each intended for a specific use. All manufacturers supply high-contrast medium-speed films suitable for panoramic and skull radiography. Often one such film is intended for manual processing and the other for automatic processing. Other films are available that are faster

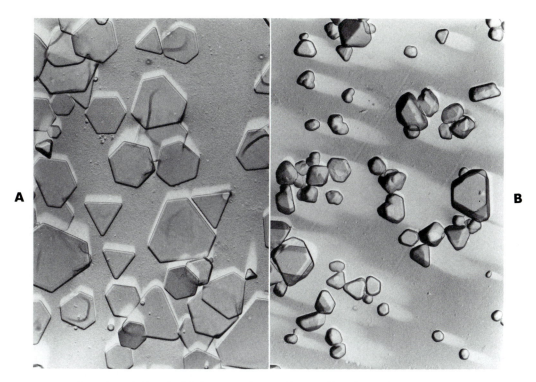

FIG. 5-7. T-grains of silver halide in an emulsion of T-Mat film, **A,** are larger and flatter than the smaller, thicker crystals in an emulsion of conventional film, **B.** Note that the flat surfaces of the T-grains are oriented parallel with the film surface, facing the radiation source. (Courtesy Eastman Kodak, Rochester NY.)

(i.e., that require less radiation exposure) but provide less image detail. Such films should be considered for panoramic radiography, when fine image detail is not available because of movement of the tube head during the exposure. Another type of film provides less contrast and a wider latitude. This type will reveal a wide range of densities and should be considered for cephalometric radiography, in which soft tissue detail is desired.

The design of screen films is constantly changing to optimize their imaging characteristics. Kodak, for instance, has introduced T-Mat films with tabular shaped (flat) grains of silver halide (Fig. 5-7). The tabular (T) grains are oriented with their relatively large flat surfaces facing the radiation source, providing a larger cross section (target) and resulting in increased speed without loss of sharpness. This is achieved because these flat grains collapse on development, forming smaller specks of metallic silver. In addition, green-sensitizing dyes are added to the surface of the tabular grains, which increases their light-gathering capability and reduces the crossover of light from the phosphor layer on one side of the intensifying screen to the

film emulsion on the other. The combined effect of these properties is to increase both the speed of the film and the sharpness of the image. Du Pont also uses tabular grains in its Cronex 10T film. 3M coats both sides of the base of its XD/A and XL/A films with an anticrossover agent.

INTENSIFYING SCREENS
Function

For the information in an x-ray beam to be translated into useful form, the intensities of radiation passing through (out of) the object (remnant radiation) must be recorded as a visual image. Although film is sensitive to radiation, early in the history of radiography it was also discovered that various inorganic salts or phosphors would *fluoresce* (emit visible light) when exposed to an x-ray beam. The intensity of this fluorescence was seen to be proportional to the intensity of the exiting (incident) beam. These phosphors have been incorporated into intensifying screens for use with x-ray film. It is the sum of the effects of the x rays and the visible light emitted by the phosphors that exposes the x-ray film. The combination of film and intensifying screen results in an image receptor system that is 10 to 60 times more sensitive to x rays than the film alone. As a consequence the use of intensifying screens results in substantial dose reduction to the patient.

Intensifying screens are used with films for virtually all *extraoral radiography,* including panoramic, cephalometric, and skull projections. Although there is a range of speeds of intensifying screens, use of a high-speed screen reduces the patient dose required to achieve a standard exposure by a factor of approximately 50. The resolving power of screens is related to their speed: the slower the speed of the screen, the greater its resolving power, and vice versa. Intensifying screens are generally not used intraorally with periapical or occlusal films because of the loss of resolution inherent with their use.

Composition

The components of an intensifying screen are a base of supporting material, a reflecting layer, a phosphor layer, and a protective plastic coat (Fig. 5-8). In practice a pair of screens are used, one on each side of the film.

Base. The base material of most intensifying screens is usually some form of polyester plastic (like that used for the base of the radiographic film) about 0.25 mm thick. The base provides mechanical support for the phosphor layer.

Reflecting layer. The reflecting layer is a white coat of titanium dioxide applied to the base material and lying beneath the phosphor layer. Its purpose is to reflect any light emitted from the phosphor layer back to the x-ray film. This has the effect of increasing the sensitivity of the intensifying screen, but it also results in the production of some image unsharpness because of the divergence of light rays reflected back to the film. Some fine-detail intensifying screens omit this layer.

Phosphor layer. The phosphor layer is composed of light-sensitive phosphorescent crystals suspended in a plastic material. When the crystals are struck by photons, they *phosphoresce* (i.e.,

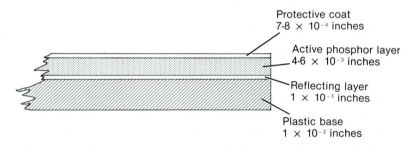

FIG. 5-8. Intensifying screen cross section demonstrating the protective coat (which goes against the film), the active phosphor layer (which fluoresces when exposed to x-ray photons), the reflecting layer (which reflects visible light back to the film), and the supporting plastic base.

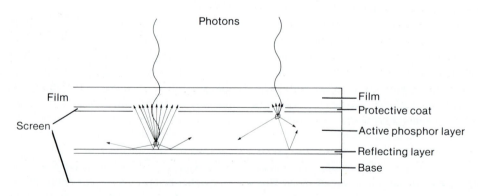

FIG. 5-9. Intensifying screens contain phosphors that emit visible light when struck by x-ray photons. Multiple visible light photons then strike the film, reducing the amount of radiation required to expose the film but resulting in a loss of fine detail in the image because of the dispersion of visible light photons from the phosphor crystals.

emit visible light photons that expose the x-ray film, Fig. 5-9). In recent years the rare earth elements have replaced traditional calcium tungstate as the phosphor. The rare earth elements consist of lanthanum (atomic number 57) through lutetium (atomic number 71). The most commonly used rare earth phosphors are lanthanum and gadolinium. The extent of their phosphorescence or (fluorescence) can be increased (activated) by the addition of small amounts of thulium, niobium, or terbium. Rare earth elements are efficient phosphors. A pair of rare earth intensifying screens absorb about 60% of the photons passing through a patient (remnant radiation). They are about 18% efficient in converting this x-ray energy to visible light, in contrast to calcium tungstate screens (which absorb only 20% to 40% of the beam and are only about 5% efficient in converting x-ray energy into visible light). Once a photon is absorbed, the rare earth screens convert it into about 4000 visible light photons whereas calcium tungstate screens will convert it into only about 1000 visible light photons. These features make the rare elements useful as phosphors.

Different phosphors fluoresce in differing portions of the spectrum. The light emission from 3M Trimax rare earth intensifying screens, for instance, ranges from 375 to 600 nm and peaks sharply at 545 nm. The Du Pont Quanta Detail screen has a major peak at 350 nm and another at 450 nm. This underscores the importance of properly matching the emission characteristics of the screen with the spectral sensitivity of the film. Intensifying screens should be used only with x-ray film designed to be sensitive to the spectral emission of the screen. Figure 5-10 shows the spectral emission of a rare earth screen and the spectral sensitivity of a film designed to be used with that screen. It is important to match blue-emitting screens with blue-sensitive films and green-emitting screens with green-sensitive films. Common phosphor combinations in intensifying screens are shown in Table 5-2.

Each screen-film combination has its own speed. Table 5-3 shows several of the currently used screen and film combinations. Fast screens are very effi-cient in the conversion of x-ray photons to visible light. When combined with fast films (i.e., those very sensitive to light), they have the highest speed ratings. High speed ratings mean lower patient exposure but also reduced detail. As the size of the phosphor crystals increases, the speed of the screen will increase but image sharpness will be reduced. Table 5-3 also shows the approximate speed ratings of some common screen-film combinations. The decision regarding which to use requires consideration of the resolution requirements of the task for which the image will be used. Most dental extraoral diagnostic tasks can be accomplished with screen-film combinations having a speed of 250 or faster. Rare earth screens are advocated for panoramic, cephalometric, TMJ, and all other dental radiography outside the oral cavity.

Coat. A protective coat of plastic (about 8 μm) is placed over the phosphor layer to provide protection for the phosphor and a surface that may be

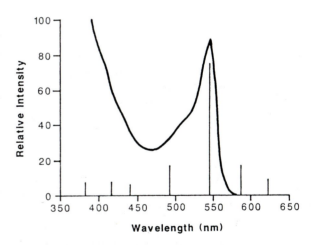

FIG. 5-10. Relative sensitivity of Kodak-T-Mat film *(continuous line)* and emission of a Kodak Lanex Regular screen (gadolinium oxysulfide, terbium activated). Intensifying screens emit light as a series of relatively narrow line emissions. Note how the maximum emission of the screen at the 545 nm corresponds well to a region of high sensitivity of the film. (Data courtesy Eastman Kodak, Rochester NY.)

TABLE 5-2. Rare earth elements used in intensifying screens

Company	Name	Phosphor	Emission
Du Pont	Cronex Quanta Fast Detail	Yttrium tantalate, niobium activated	Blue and UV
Kodak	Lanex Regular	Gadolinium oxysulfide, terbium activated	Green
3M	Trimax 2, 4, 6, 8, 12	Gadolinium oxysulfide, terbium activated	Green

TABLE 5-3. Speed class of various screen-film combinations*

Screens		Films	
Kodak		*TMG, TML*	*TMH*
Lanex	Fine	100	250
	Medium	250	600
	Regular	400	800
	Fast	600	1200
3M		*XD/A, XL/A*	*XM*
Trimax	2	100	
	4	200	
	8	400	800
	12	600	1200
Du Pont		*10T, 10TL*	
Quanta	Detail	100	
	Fast Detail	200	
	Rapid	400	
TMG, XD/A, 10T:		Medium detail, medium speed, high contrast	
TML, XL/A, 10TL:		Medium detail, medium speed, wide latitude	
TMH, XM		Low detail, high speed, high contrast	

*The descriptions of these films should be used only to compare the films with others by the same manufacturer.

cleaned. It is important to keep intensifying screens clean, because any debris, spots (which are opaque to visible light), or scratches will result in light spots (underexposed) on the resultant radiograph.

When intensifying screens are used, they are positioned inside a *cassette* (Fig. 5-11). The purpose of a cassette is to hold the intensifying screen in intimate (firm or tight) contact with the x-ray film to reduce the detrimental effect of divergent light and improve sharpness. Cassettes contain two intensifying screens, one to expose each side of the film. Most cassettes are rigid, but at least one panoramic x-ray machine uses a flexible cassette.*

IMAGE CHARACTERISTICS

Processing of an exposed x-ray film results in its becoming darkened in the exposed area. The degree and pattern of film darkening are dependent on numerous factors—including the quality (energy) and quantity (intensity) of the x-ray beam, the nature of the absorber, and the nature of the film emulsion. The visible response of the film (i.e., the pattern of the image on a film exposed to an x-ray beam) may be evaluated for multiple

*Gendex Panelipse machine.

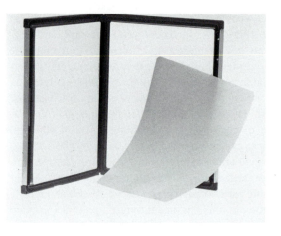

FIG. 5-11. Cassette for holding 8 × 10 inch film. When the cassette is closed, the film is supported between two intensifying screens.

characteristics. In this section are described the major imaging characteristics of x-ray film.

Radiographic density

Description. When a film is exposed to an x-ray beam and is subsequently processed, the silver halide crystals that have been struck by x-ray photons are converted to grains of metallic silver that give the film its black appearance. The net effect of exposure and processing is darkening of an x-ray film. The *overall degree of darkening* of the exposed film is referred to as density. The density of an x-ray film is defined as follows:

$$\text{Density} = \text{Log}\frac{I_0}{I_t}$$

where I_0 is the intensity of incident light (e.g., from a viewbox) and I_t is the intensity of the light transmitted through the film. Thus the measurement of film density is also a measure of *film opacity*. With a density of 0, 100% of the light is transmitted; with a density of 1, 10% of the light is transmitted; with a density of 2, 1% of the light is transmitted; with a density of 3, 0.1% of the light is transmitted, and so on. In routine radiography the useful range of film densities is approximately 0.3 (very light) to 2 (very dark). Beyond these extremes the image is usually too light or too dark to be diagnostically useful.

A plot of the relationship between film density and exposure is called a *characteristic curve* (Fig. 5-12) or an *H and D curve* (after the two early investigators, Hurter and Driffield, who first de-

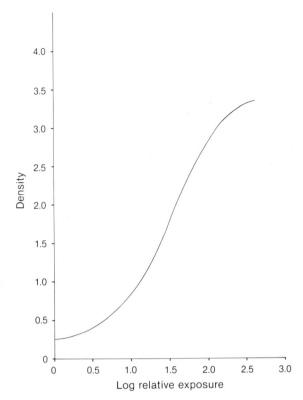

FIG. 5-12. Characteristic curve showing the relationship between exposure of a film and the resultant density. This curve is typical of a screen-film combination.

scribed this relationship in 1890). The characteristic curve is a graphic representation of the film response on exposure to light or x rays. It is usually shown as the relation between the optical density of the film and the logarithm of the corresponding exposure. One can see from this curve that as the exposure is increased the film density increases. A film is of greatest diagnostic value when the structures of interest are imaged on the relatively straight portion of the graph, between 0.3 and 2.0 optical density units. Examination of the characteristic curves of films exposed under standard conditions reveals much information concerning film contrast, speed, and latitude.

Influencing factors

Exposure. The overall film density is dependent on the number of photons absorbed by the film emulsion. The exposure factors that increase the number of photons absorbed by the film also increase the density of the processed film. Increasing the *milliamperage* (mA), *operating voltage* (kVp), or *time* (s) of exposure will each increase the den-

sity of the resultant radiograph. If it is decided to increase the kVp, then the mA or s must be reduced to maintain a film with constant density. Reduction in the amount of added *filtration* in the x-ray beam or in the *distance* between focal spot and film will also increase the film density by increasing the number of x-ray photons striking the film. When exposure factors intended for adults are used on children or edentulous patients, the resultant films are darker because of excessive density resulting from the reduced amount of absorbing tissue in the path of the x-ray beam. The experienced clinician will vary the exposure in accordance with the patient's size to produce radiographs of optimum density. X-ray processing procedures may also have a pronounced influence on film density (as described in Chapter 7).

Subject thickness. As an x-ray beam travels through an object, it is attenuated by absorption and scattering of photons. The thicker the object, the more the beam will be attenuated. When exposing radiographs, one should adjust the exposure time to compensate for varying sizes of patients and the increased or decreased absorption. Figure 5-13 shows that as a step wedge becomes thicker the density of the exposed and processed film is reduced.

Object density. Variations in the density of the structure being radiographed exert a profound influence on the resultant image. The greater the density of an object, or an area within the object, the greater will be the attenuation of the x-ray beam directed through that object or area. In the oral cavity the relative densities of various natural structures, in order of decreasing density, are enamel, dentin and cementum, bone, muscle, fat, and air. Metallic objects (e.g., restorations) are far more dense, and hence better absorbers, than enamel. As an x-ray beam is differentially attenuated by these absorbers, the resultant beam carries information that is recorded on the radiographic film as light and dark areas. Dense objects (which are good absorbers) cause the radiographic image to be light and are said to be *radiopaque;* objects that are not good absorbers cast a dark area on the film that corresponds to the *radiolucent* object.

Radiographic contrast

Description. Radiographic contrast is defined as the difference in densities between various regions on a radiograph. Thus a film that shows very light areas and very dark areas has *high contrast.* This is also referred to as a short gray scale of

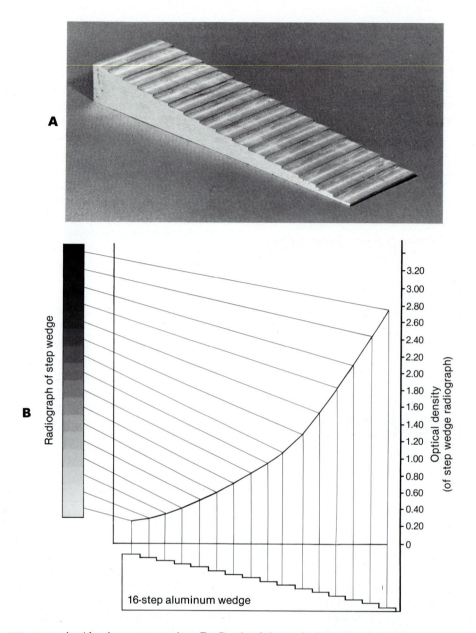

FIG. 5-13. A, Aluminum step wedge. **B,** Graph of the optical density of a radiograph made by exposing the step wedge. Note that as the thickness of the aluminum decreases more photons are available to expose the film and the image becomes progressively darker.

contrast, because there are few shades of gray between the black and white images on the film. Alternatively, a radiographic image that is composed of light gray and dark gray zones is *low contrast,* also referred to as having a long gray scale of contrast (Fig. 5-14).

Influencing factors. The degree of contrast demonstrated on a radiograph is dependent on the following:

- Subject contrast

- Film contrast
- Beam energy and intensity
- Fog and scattered radiation

Subject contrast. Subject contrast is the range of characteristics of the subject being radiographed that influence radiographic contrast. It is influenced by the subject's thickness, density, and atomic number.

The subject contrast of a patient's head and neck exposed in a lateral cephalometric view is very

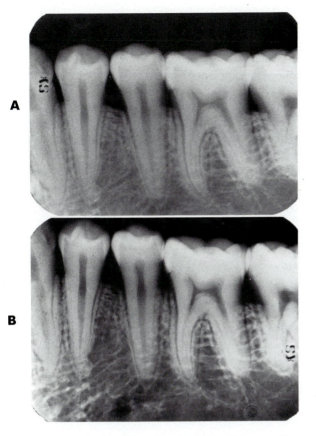

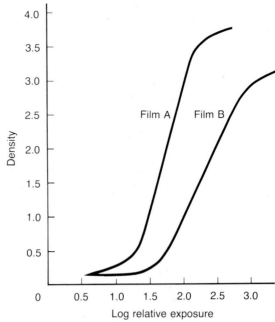

FIG. 5-15. Characteristic curves of two films demonstrating the greater inherent contrast of film *A* than of film *B*, as indicated by the greater slope of the straight-line portion of the curve representing film *A*.

FIG. 5-14. Radiographs of a dried mandible revealing low contrast, **A,** and high contrast, **B.**

high. The dense regions of the bone and teeth will absorb most of the incident radiation while the less dense soft tissue facial profile will transmit most of the radiation.

In general, as the *thickness, density,* and *atomic number* of the part of the subject being irradiated are increased, the absorption of x-ray photons will be increased. Consequently the portion of the x-ray film imaging that part of the subject will appear relatively radiopaque in comparison to other areas, thereby demonstrating an image.

Film contrast. Film contrast describes the capacity of radiographic films to display differences in subject contrast. A high-contrast film will reveal areas of small difference in subject contrast more clearly than will a low-contrast film. Film contrast is usually measured as the slope of the diagnostically useful portion of the characteristic curve. It may be modified by film density, intensifying screens, and film processing.

The slope of the *characteristic curve* of a film in the useful diagnostic range is a measure of its

contrast (Fig. 5-15): the greater the slope of the curve in this region, the greater the film contrast. In this illustration film *A* has a higher contrast than film *B*. When the slope of the curve in the useful range (i.e., the *film gamma*) is greater than 1, the film will exaggerate subject contrast. This desirable feature is found in most diagnostic film and allows visualization of structures of only slightly differing densities. Films used with intensifying screens typically have gammas in the range of 2 to 3. Figure 5-16 shows that film contrast is also dependent on the density range being examined. When dental direct-exposure films are considered, the slope of the curve continually increases with increasing exposure. As a result, properly exposed films have more contrast than under exposed (light) films.

The use of intensifying screens also tends to increase the contrast of the resultant film. Film contrast will be maximum when optimum film processing conditions are used. Incomplete or excessive development of films results in decreased film contrast.

Beam energy and intensity. The effect of *kVp* on subject contrast is illustrated in Figure 5-17. An

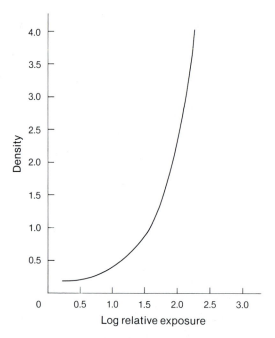

FIG. 5-16. Characteristic curve of direct-exposure film. Note that the contrast (slope of the curve) is greater in the high-density than in the low-density region.

aluminum step wedge has been exposed to x-ray beams of differing energies. Because increasing the kVp will raise the overall density of the image, the time of exposure has been reduced to the point that the density of the middle step in each case is comparable. As the kVp of the x-ray beam is increased and the density of the film is held constant (by reducing exposure time), one can see that the resultant subject contrast will be decreased. Similarly, when relatively low kVp energies are used the resultant subject contrast will be increased. It should also be noted that the energy of an x-ray beam may be modified by changing the added filtration on the x-ray machine (as described in Chapter 2). Most clinicians select a kVp value in the range of 60 to 90. At higher values the exposure time is reduced but the loss of contrast may be objectionable. This reduction in exposure time, however, is often advantageous to reduce possible film blurring caused by inadvertent motion of the patient.

Changing the milliamperage (mAs) of the exposure will also influence the image contrast. If the film is excessively light or dark, the contrast will be reduced. More subtle changes in the mAs may also change the contrast by changing the position on the characteristic curve, as described above.

Fog and scatter. Radiographic contrast will be reduced by the addition of undesirable density from fog and scatter radiation.

Fog on an x-ray film results in increased film density from causes other than exposure to the remnant beam. Common causes of film fog are improper safelighting conditions, storage of film at excessive temperatures, and film development at excessive temperature or for prolonged time. Film fog may be reduced by proper film processing and storage procedures.

Scatter radiation results from Compton interactions. (See Chapter 2.) When scattered radiation strikes a film, it causes an overall darkening and results in loss of image contrast. Scattered radiation may be reduced by (1) use of decreased kVp values, (2) collimation of the beam to the size of the film to prevent scatter from an area outside the region of the image, and (3) use of grids in extraoral radiography (p. 94).

Latitude

Description. Film latitude is a measure of the range of exposures that may be recorded as a series of usefully distinguishable densities on a film. A film with a wide latitude can record an object with a wide range of inherent subject contrast (Fig. 5-18). As a consequence, wide variations in the amount of radiation exiting the object can be usefully recorded, the image representing all the object density variations proportionally and in detail. Accordingly, a film with a characteristic curve that has a long straight-line portion and a shallow slope will have a wide latitude. In practice the variation in radiation reaching the film is a function of the variation in density throughout the object. Therefore, the wider the latitude of a film the greater will be the range of object densities that can be visualized. Typically, films with a wide latitude also tend to show relatively low contrast (long gray scale), because many densities between totally black and totally clear will be recorded. Such films are often useful when both the osseous structures of the skull and the soft tissues of the facial region must be recorded.

Influencing factors. Film latitude may be modified to some extent by the operator. The use of *high kVp* will result in images with a wide latitude and low contrast. Also, if *reduced exposure* is used with dental film, the resultant image will be somewhat lighter and show a slightly wider latitude (but lower contrast). When wide latitude is

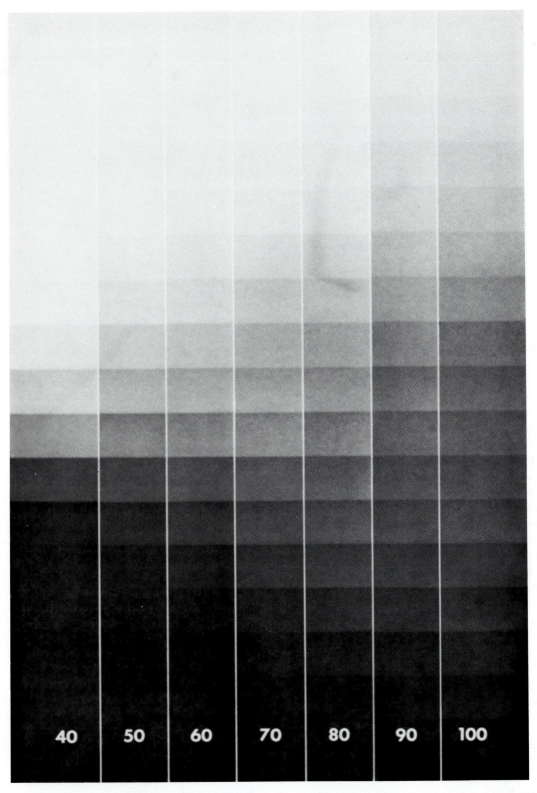

FIG. 5-17. Radiographs of a step wedge made at 40 to 100 kVp. With increasing kVp, the mAs was reduced to maintain the uniform middle-step density. Note the long gray scale (low contrast) with high kVp. (Courtesy Eastman Kodak, Rochester, NY.)

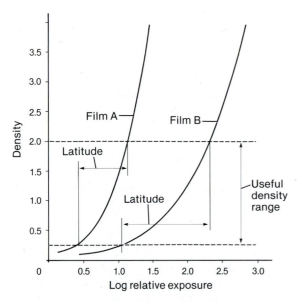

FIG. 5-18. Characteristic curves showing the broader latitude for film *B* than for film *A*.

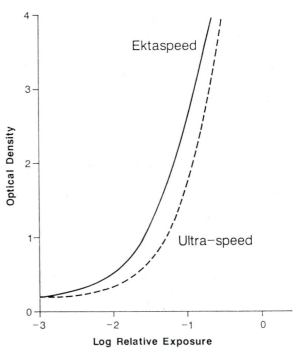

FIG. 5-19. Characteristic curves for Kodak Ultra-Speed and Ektaspeed films. Note that the faster film, Ektaspeed, requires less exposure to achieve the same density as the Ultra-Speed film. (Data courtesy Eastman Kodak, Rochester NY.)

desired for extraoral radiography, it is recommended that a film with this characteristic be selected.

Speed

Description. Speed is the amount of radiation required to produce a radiographic film of standard density (usually 1.0 above base and fog*). It is largely controlled by the size of the silver halide grains. The speed of dental x-ray film is indicated by a letter designating a particular group. The fastest dental film currently available has a speed rating of E. Only films with a D or E speed rating are suitable for intraoral radiography. A small amount of the slower C speed film is being manufactured, but it should not be used because of the greater patient exposure required to obtain radiographs of satisfactory density.

Film speed is frequently expressed as the reciprocal of the exposure (in roentgens) required to cause a standard film density. A fast film requires a relatively low exposure to produce a density of 1.0 above base and fog whereas a slower film will require a longer exposure for the processed film to

have the same density. Currently the most commonly used types of film are Kodak Ultra-Speed film (group D) and Kodak Ektaspeed film (group E). The Ektaspeed film requires about half the exposure of Ultra-Speed film and offers comparable contrast and resolution. The greater speed of Ektaspeed film compared to Ultra-Speed film results from the larger crystal size and the greater amount of AgBr in the emulsion. Figure 5-19 shows that Ektaspeed film (with the characteristic curve on the left) is faster than Ultra-Speed film (on the right) because less exposure is required to produce the same level of density even though the films have similar contrast.

Influencing factors. Because speed is an inherent property of film, little can be done to modify its value. Film can be made slightly faster by processing at higher temperature, but only at the expense of increased film fog and graininess.

Radiographic mottle

Description. Radiographic mottle (or noise) is the appearance of *uneven density* of an exposed radiographic film. It may be seen on a small area

---

*Base and fog is the density encountered when unexposed film is processed. It is due to the inherent density of base composition and the added tint, and to the development of unexposed halogen crystals. It should not exceed a density of 0.05.

of film as small darker spots and some lighter areas.

Influencing factors. On dental film mottle may be seen as *film graininess,* which is due to the visibility of silver grains in the film emulsion, especially when magnification is used to examine an image. Film graininess is most evident when high-temperature processing is used.

Radiographic mottle is also evident when the film is used in combination with intensifying screens. The most important cause of this finding is *quantum mottle,* caused by a fluctuation in the number of photons or quanta (intensity) per unit of the beam cross-sectional area absorbed by the intensifying screen. Thus, with a low-intensity x-ray beam, small variation in beam intensity will be amplified by the intensifying screen and may be visualized as variations in density on the film. Quantum mottle will be most evident when very fast film-screen combinations are used. Under these conditions the nonuniformity of the beam is highest. The longer exposures required by slower film-screen combinations tend to average out the beam pattern and thereby reduce quantum mottle.

Sharpness

Description. Sharpness is the degree to which the image reveals the differential at "density boundaries." The appearance of the radiographic image of a boundary should be proportional to the change in density (or thickness) at the boundary in the object. It is thus the effectiveness of a radiograph to precisely *define an edge,* such as that of an amalgam restoration. Several causes for the loss of sharpness are important in the practice of dentistry.

Influencing factors

Focal spot size. Loss of image sharpness results in part from the fact that photons are not being emitted from a point source (focal spot) on the target in the x-ray tube. The larger the focal spot, the greater the loss of image sharpness will be. Various means of modifying the projection geometry to minimize this problem are discussed in Chapter 6.

Motion. Loss of image sharpness also results from movement of the film, object, or x-ray source during the exposure. Movement, in effect, enlarges the focal spot and decreases image sharpness. This problem may be minimized by stabilizing the patient's head with the headrest of the chair during exposure. The use of higher mA and kVp values and correspondingly shorter exposure times will also help minimize this problem.

Image receptor. Multiple features of an image receptor, the film, and intensifying screens may cause loss of image sharpness. In x-ray film the *size of the silver grains* in the image limits image sharpness. The finer the grain size, the finer the image sharpness will be. In general, slow speed films have fine grains and faster films have larger grains. Grain size is also influenced by processing: at elevated temperatures processing can increase film graininess.

The use of *intensifying screens* will also have an adverse effect on image sharpness. The loss of sharpness results when visible light and ultraviolet radiation emitted from the screen spread out beyond the point of origin and expose a film area that is larger than the cross-sectional area of the beam entering the screen (Fig. 5-9). The spreading light causes a blurring of fine detail on the radiograph. The diffusion of fluorescent light from a screen can be minimized and image sharpness maximized by assuring as close a contact as possible between the intensifying screen and the film.

The selection of an intensifying screen is based on a compromise that relates to the crystal size of the phosphor in the screen. If large crystals are used, fluorescence will be efficient and the screen fast, causing a reduction in patient exposure but a loss of image sharpness. If small crystals are used, the screen will have a low sensitivity because of lessened phosphorescent efficiency but the resulting image will have improved sharpness. The best compromise requires selection of appropriate screens for the specific diagnostic task to be accomplished.

The presence of an image on each side of a double-emulsion film also causes a loss of image sharpness, because of *parallax* (Fig. 5-3). Parallax results from the apparent change in position or size of an object when seen from different perspectives. Because dental film has a double coating of emulsion and the x-ray beam is divergent, the images recorded on each emulsion will vary slightly in size. In general, the effect of parallax on image sharpness is unimportant but is most apparent when wet films are viewed. Under these conditions the emulsion is swollen with water and the loss of image sharpness caused by parallax is more evident. Also parallax is more evident when the bisecting-angle technique is used, because of the shorter target-film distance and the resulting greater divergence of the x rays.

Resolution

Description. Resolution, or resolving power, is the ability of a radiograph to record *separate structures* that are close together. It is usually measured by radiographing an object (referred to as a target but not to be confused with the target in the x-ray tube) made up of a series of thin lead strips (usually four) of prescribed thickness, alternating with radiolucent spaces of the same thickness. The groups of lines and spaces are arranged in the test target in order of increasing numbers of lines and spaces per millimeter (Fig. 5-20). The resolving power is then measured as the highest number of line pairs (a line pair being the image of an absorber and the adjacent lucent space) per millimeter that can be distinguished or resolved on the resultant radiograph when examined with low-power magnification. Typically, panoramic film-screen combinations are capable of resolving about 5 line pairs per millimeter and periapical film, with better resolving power, will clearly delineate at least 10 line pairs per millimeter.

Influencing factors. The same factors that cause loss of image sharpness—focal spot size, motion, and image receptor—cause a loss of image resolution.

Image clarity

Image clarity is the overall appearance of a radiograph and the clinician's subjective judgment of its appearance. The relative importance of density, contrast, latitude, sharpness, and resolution is unknown. There may be other parameters not listed here that also contribute to image clarity. Various mathematical approaches have been used to evaluate these parameters further, but a thorough discussion of them is beyond the scope of this text. The *line spread function* measures the loss of image sharpness by light diffusion from intensifying screens. The *modulation transfer function* (MTF) is a measure of the fraction of information available in the x-ray beam leaving the subject that is recorded (on film) for examination. It is largely an expression of sharpness and resolution. The *Wiener spectrum* is a measure of radiographic mottle (radiographic graininess plus quantum mottle). Even with these sophisticated approaches, however, more information is needed to complete our understanding of all the factors responsible for image clarity.

GRIDS
Function

The quality of a radiographic image is improved by the removal of scattered radiation (which causes fog and reduces film contrast). Under most conditions the intensity of the scattered radiation is 2

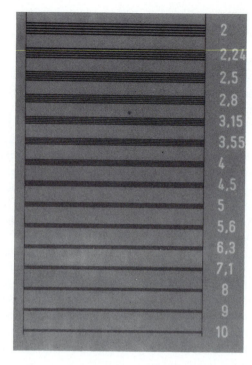

FIG. 5-20. Radiograph of a resolving power target consisting of groups of radiopaque lines and radiolucent spaces. Numbers at each group indicate the line pairs per millimeter represented by the group.

to 4 times that of the remnant beam because of Compton scattering of photons in the object.* Scattered radiation exiting an irradiated object may be largely removed or reduced from the beam reaching the film by placing an x-ray grid between the object and the film. This has the effect of reducing film fog and increasing radiographic (film) contrast.

Composition

A grid is composed of alternate strips of a radiopaque material, usually lead, and strips of radiolucent material, often plastic. Figure 5-21 shows a diagram of a grid and how it interacts with an x-ray beam. When secondary photons generated in the object are scattered toward the film they have a high probability of being absorbed by the radiopaque material in the grid. This is because the direction of the scattered photons deviates from the primary and remnant beam and consequently can-

---

*The amount of scatter radiation increases with increasing object thickness, field size, and kVp (energy of the x-ray beam).

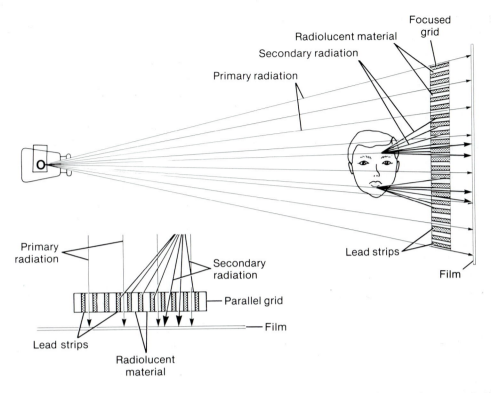

FIG. 5-21. An x-ray grid absorbs scattered x-ray photons from the primary beam and prevents their fogging the film. In a focused grid, the absorber plates are angled toward the anode, whereas in a parallel grid, the absorber plates are parallel.

not pass through the parallel plates of the grid. In practice *focused grids* are used more frequently. In a focused grid the strips of radiopaque material are all directed toward a common point, the focal spot, some distance away. Because a focused grid has the lead strips angulated toward the focal spot, their direction coincides with the direction of the paths of diverging photons in the primary x-ray beam, thereby accommodating their passage through the grid. This arrangement of the elements of the focus grid will eliminate the absorption of more divergent primary photons at the margins of an x-ray beam, where their direction does not coincide with the alignment of the perpendicular lead strips in a linear grid. The focused grid may be used only within a range of distances from the focal spot where the alignment of lead strips closely coincides with the path of the diverging x-ray beam. The range of distances is specified on the grid.

The presence of a grid between an object and the film causes the images of the radiopaque absorbing material to be projected onto the film. The closer together the grid lines are on the film, however, the less objectionable they become. Grids are

manufactured with variable numbers of line pairs of absorbers and radiolucent spaces per inch.

In general, grids with 80 or more line pairs per inch do not show objectionable grid lines. The ratio of grid thickness to the width of the radiolucent spacer is known as the *grid ratio*. The higher the grid ratio, the more effectively will scattered radiation be removed from the x-ray beam. In general, grids with a grid ratio of 8 or 10 are preferred.

The images of the radiolucent grid lines on the film can be deleted by mechanically moving the grid in a direction of 90 degrees to the grid lines (but not moving the object or the film) during exposure. This has the effect of evening (blurring) out the radiolucent lines and resulting in a more uniform exposure. It does not interfere with the absorption of scattered photons. A moving grid is called a *Bucky grid*.

To compensate for the presence of absorbing materials in the grid, the exposure required to produce a radiograph when a grid is used approximately doubles compared to that used in the absence of a grid. Accordingly, one should use grids only when there is sufficient improvement in diagnostic image quality to justify the added exposure. In the case of lateral cephalometric examinations made for assessing growth and development of the facial region (Chapter 11), the use of grids is usually not indicated since the improved contrast does not aid in the identification of anatomic landmarks.

SELECTED REFERENCES
General

Curry TS III, Dowdey JE, Murry RC: Christensen's Physics of diagnostic radiology, ed 4, Philadelphia, 1990, Lea & Febiger.

E-speed film

Domon M, Yoshino N: Factors involved in the high radiographic sensitivity of E-speed films, *Oral Surg* 69:113-119, 1990.

Farman AG, Mendel RW, von Fraunhofer JA: Ultraspeed versus Ektaspeed X-ray film: endodontists' perceptions, *J Endod* 14(12):615-619, 1988.

Frommer HH, Jain RK: A comparative clinical study of group D and E dental film, *Oral Surg* 63:738-742, 1987.

Gratt BM, White SC, Halse A: Clinical recommendations for the use of D-speed film, E-speed film, and xeroradiography, *J Am Dent Assoc* 117(5):609-614, 1988.

Kaffe I, Gratt BM: E-speed dental films processed with rapid chemistry: a comparison with D-speed film, *Oral Surg* 64:367-372, 1987.

Kaffe I, Littner M, Kuspet M: Densitometric evaluation of intraoral x-ray films: Ektaspeed versus Ultraspeed, *Oral Surg* 57:338-342, 1984.

Kleier D, Hicks MJ, Flaitz CM: A comparison of Ultraspeed and Ektaspeed dental x-ray film: in vitro study of the radiographic and histologic appearance of interproximal lesions, *Quintessence Int* 18(9):623-631, 1987.

Kleier DJ, Hicks MJ, Flaitz CM: A comparison of Ultraspeed and Ektaspeed dental x-ray film: in vitro study of the radiographic appearance of interproximal lesions, *Oral Surg* 63:381-385, 1987.

MacDonald JC, Reid JA, Luke M: The spectral sensitivity of dental x-ray film, *Dentomaxillofac Radiol* 16(1):29-32, 1987.

Petersson A, Lindh C, Nilsson M: Is E-speed dental film more sensitive to storage than D-speed dental film? *Swed Dent J* 11(4):159-162, 1987.

Silha RE: Methods for reducing patient exposure combined with Kodak Ektaspeed dental x-ray film, *Dent Radiogr Photogr* 54:80-87, 1981.

Silha RE: The new Kodak Ektaspeed dental x-ray film, *Dent Radiogr Photogr* 54:32-35, 1981.

Thunthy KH, Weinberg R: Sensitometric comparison of dental films of groups D and E, *Oral Surg* 54:250-252, 1982.

Waggoner WF, Ashton JJ: Comparison of Kodak D-speed and E-speed x-ray film in detection of proximal caries, *J Dent Child* 55(6):459-462, 1988.

Intensifying screens

Hurlburt C: Screen-film combinations used for cephalometric radiography, *Oral Surg* 46:721-724, 1978.

Hurlburt C, Coggins L: Rare earth screens for panoramic radiography, *Oral Surg* 57:451-454, 1984.

Kircos LT, Staninec M, Chou L: Comparative evaluation of the sensitometric properties of screen-film systems and conventional dental receptors for intraoral radiography, *Oral Surg* 68:787-792, 1989.

Kircos LT, Vandre RH, Lorton L: Exposure reduction of 96% in intraoral radiography, *J Am Dent Assoc* 113(5):746-750, 1986.

Kogon S, Stephens R, Reid J, Lubus N: A clinical trial of a rare earth screen film system in a periapical cassette, *Oral Surg* 57:455-461, 1984.

Miles DA, Van Dis ML, Peterson MG: Information yield: a comparison of Kodak T-Mat G, Ortho L, and RP X-Omat films, *Dentomaxillofac Radiol* 18(1):15-18, 1989.

Thunthy KH, Manson-Hing L: A study of the resolution of dental films and screens, *Oral Surg* 42:255-266, 1976.

Thunthy KH, Weinberg R: Effect of kilovoltage on the relative speed of rare-earth screens, *Dentomaxillofac Radiol* 15(1):27-30, 1986.

6

Projection Geometry

The image on a radiograph is a two-dimensional representation of a three-dimensional object. To obtain the maximum value from a radiograph, the clinician must mentally reconstruct an accurate three-dimensional image of the anatomic structures of interest from one or more of these two-dimensional images (radiographs). This task is greatly facilitated when the radiographs used are of high quality. The principles of projection geometry describe the effect of focal spot size and its position (relative to the object and the film) on the quality of the resultant image. This chapter describes the manner in which these factors influence image clarity (particularly sharpness and contrast), image magnification, and image distortion. Also described is the application of these imaging principles to periapical radiography and object localization.

IMAGE SHARPNESS AND RESOLUTION

There are several geometric considerations that contribute to image clarity, particularly image sharpness and resolution. *Sharpness* measures how well the minimum details of an object are reproduced on the radiograph. More specifically, it is a measure of how well a boundary between two areas of contrasting radiodensity is delineated. *Image resolution* is a measure of the visualization of relatively small objects that are close together. Although sharpness and resolution are two distinct features, they are to a certain extent interdependent, being influenced by the same geometric variables.

When x rays emanate from the focal spot on the target of an x-ray tube, they originate from all points over the actual target and radiate in all directions. (See Chapter 2.) Some of the rays from each of these point sources will pass tangentially to the edge of the object, forming separate images of the object's edges. Because these rays originate

from different points and travel in straight lines, their projections on the film will not be in exactly the same spot. As a result the image of the edge is not sharp and distinct but broad and fuzzy (blurred). Figure 6-1 depicts these events. For clarification this illustration shows only the course of the photons that originate at the margins of the focal area and image the edges of the object. This broad and fuzzy zone is the penumbra. The blurring causes a loss in image clarity by reducing sharpness

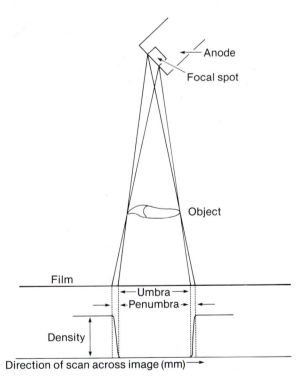

FIG. 6-1. Photons originating at different places on the focal spot result in a penumbra or zone of unsharpness on the radiograph. The density of the image will change from a high background value to a low value in the area of enamel or dentin.

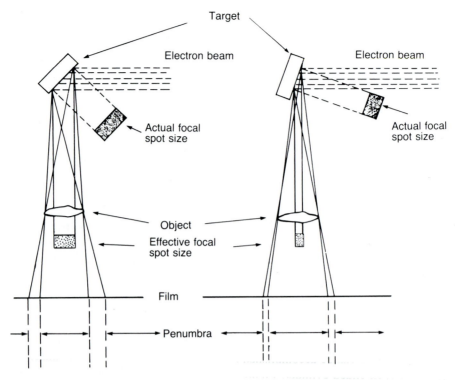

FIG. 6-2. Decreasing the angle of the target perpendicular to the long axis of the electron beam decreases the actual focal spot size and decreases heat dissipation and thereby tube life, but it also decreases effective focal spot size and thus increases sharpness of the image.

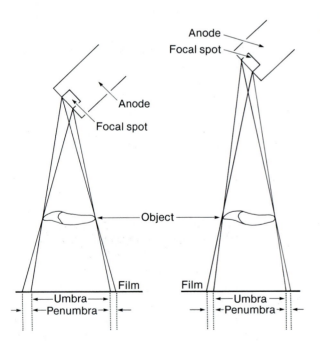

FIG. 6-3. Increasing the distance between the focal spot and the object results in an image with increased sharpness because the size of the penumbra is reduced. Also, there is less magnification of the object.

and resolution. There are three ways to minimize these deleterious effects and improve the quality of the radiographs.

1. *Use as small an effective focal spot as practical.* The size of the effective focal spot is a function of the angle* of the target with respect to the long axis of the electron beam (line focus principle, Chapter 2). The angle selected is a compromise between image quality and tube life (Fig. 6-2). A large angle will distribute the electron beam over a larger surface and decrease the heat generated per unit of target area. This results in a larger effective focal spot and loss of image clarity. A small angle has a greater wearing effect on the target. However, it results in a smaller effective focal spot, decreased penumbra and increased image sharpness and resolution. This angle is ususally between 10 and 20 degrees.

2. *Increase the distance between the focal spot*

―――――――

*The angle is usually measured (and described) perpendicular to the (long axis of the) electron beam.

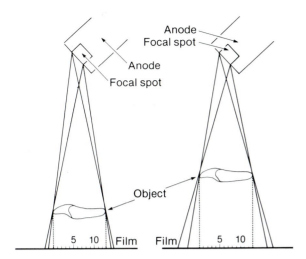

FIG. 6-4. Decreasing the distance between the object and the film increases the sharpness by decreasing the size of the penumbra. Also there is less magnification of the object.

and the object. This can be accomplished by using a long open-ended cylinder. Figure 6-3 shows how increasing the object-to-focal spot distance reduces image blurring (edge gradient or penumbra) and enhances sharpness. It also demonstrates that loss of sharpness is primarily the result of the divergent nature of the x-ray beam. The longer focal spot-to-object distance minimizes this effect by using photons whose paths are almost parallel.

3. *Decrease the distance between the object and the film.* Figure 6-4 shows that as the object-to-film distance is reduced there is an increase in image clarity.

X-ray tube manufacturers use as small a focal spot size (actual and effective) as is consistent with the requirements for heat dissipation. Although focal spot size is not adjustable on dental x-ray machines, the use of high kVp and low mA causes the electron beam to be focused on a small focal spot.*

The requirement for a long focal spot-to-object distance supports the use of long open-ended cylinders as aiming devices on dental x-ray machines. When this technique for intraoral radiographs is

---

*The size of the focal spot increases in direct proportion to the tube current, especially at low kVp. A threefold increase in mA will increase the focal spot size about 15%. In the diagnostic range focal spot size decreases slightly with increased kVp— less than 5%.

used, it results in images whose clarity is increased and whose magnification and distortion are reduced.

To obtain a minimum object-to-film distance, position the film as close to the teeth as consistent with other constraints imposed by the technique being used.

IMAGE SIZE DISTORTION

Image size distortion (magnification) is the increase in size of the image on the film compared to the actual size of the object. The divergent paths of photons in an x-ray beam cause enlargement of the image on a radiograph. Image size distortion results from the relative focal spot-to-film and object-to-film distances (Figs. 6-3 and 6-4). Accordingly, increasing the focal spot-to-film distance and decreasing the object-to-film distance will minimize image magnification.

Note that these two methods for reducing magnification also increase image clarity (sharpness and resolution). Thus the use of a long open-ended cylinder as an aiming device on an x-ray machine reduces the magnification of images on periapical films, because it uses the more parallel rays at the center of the x-ray beam.

IMAGE SHAPE DISTORTION

Image shape distortion is the result of unequal magnification of different parts of the same object. This situation arises when not all the parts of an object are at the same focal spot-to-object distance. The physical shape of the object may often prevent its optimal orientation, resulting in shape distortion. Such a phenomenon will be seen by the differences in appearance of the image on a radiograph compared with the true shape. To minimize shape distortion, it is advisable to make an effort to carefully align tube, object, and film using the following criteria:

1. *Position the film parallel to the object.* Standardize its orientation with the object so it can be duplicated. Figure 6-5 shows that the central ray of the x-ray beam is perpendicular to the film but the object is not parallel to the film. The resultant image is distorted because of the unequal distances of the various parts of the object from the film. This type of shape distortion is *foreshortening* because it causes the radiographic image to be shorter than the object.

2. *Be sure that the central ray is perpendicular*

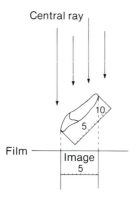

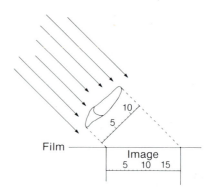

FIG. 6-5. Foreshortening of a radiographic image results when the central ray is perpendicular to the film but the object is not parallel with the film.

FIG. 6-6. Elongation of a radiographic image results when the central ray is perpendicular to the object but not the film.

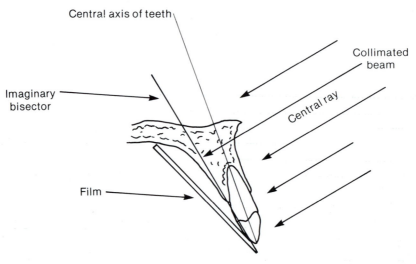

FIG. 6-7. In the bisecting-angle technique the central ray is directed at a right angle to the imaginary plane that bisects the angle formed by the film and the central axis of the object. This method will result in an image that is the same length as the object.

to the object and film. Figure 6-6 shows that when the x-ray beam is oriented at a right angle to the object but not the film there will be shape distortion, resulting in *elongation* of the image.

One can prevent potential distortion problems by aligning the object and film parallel with each other and the central ray perpendicular to both.

BISECTING-THE-ANGLE AND PARALLELING TECHNIQUES

From the earliest days of dental radiography, it has been a clinical objective to produce accurate images of the dental structures that are normally visually obscured. To accomplish this goal, two methods evolved for orientation of the teeth, film, and x-ray beam.

One method that evolved early, and is still in use, was the *bisecting-angle technique,* a term descriptive of the procedure (Fig. 6-7). With it the film was placed as close to the teeth as possible without deforming it. The structure of the teeth and jaws, however, is such that with the film in this position it did not parallel the long axes of the teeth. The arrangement inherently caused distortion. Nevertheless, by directing the central ray perpendicular to an imaginary plane (the bisector) that bisects the angle between the teeth and the film, it was possible to make the length of the tooth's image on the film correspond to the actual length of the tooth. Note

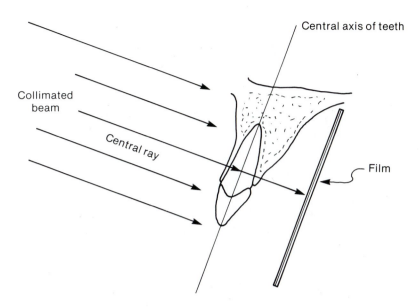

Central axis of teeth

Collimated beam

Central ray

Film

FIG. 6-8. In the paralleling technique the central ray is directed at a right angle to the central axis of the object and film.

that the coronal end of the tooth would then be in contact with the film and the apex a considerable distance from the film, creating the angle "bisected." This angle between a tooth and the film is especially apparent when radiographing teeth in the maxilla or anterior mandible. Even though the projected length of a tooth is correct, the image can still show distortion, because the film and object are not parallel and the x-ray beam is not directed at right angles to them. This distortion tends to increase along the image toward its apical extreme.

When the central ray is not perpendicular to the *bisector,* the length of the image of a projected tooth will change. If the central ray is directed at an angle that is more positive than perpendicular to the bisector, the image of the tooth will be *foreshortened.* Likewise, if it is inclined with more negative angulation to the bisector, the image will be *elongated.* The method for using this bisecting-angle technique is demonstrated in Chapter 9. A short target-to-object distance is generally used although a longer target-to-object distance often gives better results. In recent years the bisecting-angle technique has been used less frequently for general periapical radiography as use of the paralleling technique has increased.

The adoption of the *paralleling technique* (long-cone or right-angle technique) followed the availability of higher-energy x-ray generators and faster films.[3-6] The paralleling technique derives its name from, and produces improved images as the result of, placing the film parallel with the long axis of the tooth (Fig. 6-8).

To achieve this parallel orientation, it is often necessary to position the film toward the middle of the oral cavity, away from the teeth. Although this allows the teeth and film to be parallel, it results in some image magnification (size distortion) and loss of definition (by increasing penumbra). As a consequence, the paralleling technique uses a relatively long open-ended aiming cylinder ("cone") to increase the focal spot to object distance. This has the effect of directing only the most central and parallel rays of the beam to the film and teeth and reduces image magnification while increasing image sharpness and resolution. This technique has benefited from the development of fast-speed film emulsions; an increase exposure time is inherent in the technique because of the increased target-to-object distance.

Although the target-to-film distance used in the paralleling technique is usually about 12 to 16 inches, one normally uses a target-to-tooth distance as great as is practical and possible with the equipment at hand. In many cases absolute parallelism between the film and long axis of the teeth is impossible or at least very difficult to accomplish. In such circumstances, if the film can be placed so it does not diverge more than 20 degrees from the ideal position (parallel to the long axis of the tooth), the image will show little apparent distortion.[1] Be-

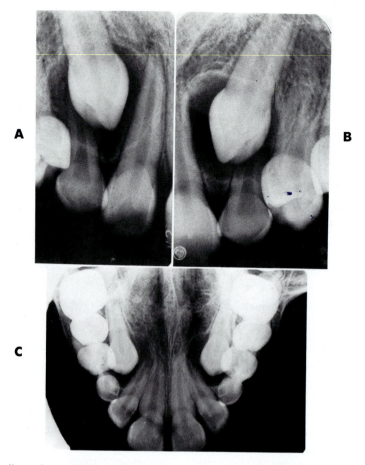

FIG. 6-9. Radiographs exposed at right angles to each other offer valuable information for localization. Periapical radiographs, **A** and **B,** demonstrate impacted the permanent canines in the region of the retained primary canines. An occlusal projection, **C,** is exposed at nearly a right angle to the periapical projections and clearly shows that the impacted canines are palatal to the primary canines.

cause it is desirable to position the film near the middle of the oral cavity with the paralleling technique, film holders should be used to support the film in the patient's mouth. Chapter 9 discusses film-holding instruments and techniques for intraoral radiography using the paralleling technique. The paralleling technique best incorporates the imaging principles described in the first three sections of this chapter and is the preferred method of periapical radiography.

OBJECT LOCALIZATION

In clinical practice it is often necessary to derive three-dimensional information concerning patients from a radiograph. The dentist may wish to use radiographs, for example, to determine the location of a foreign object or an impacted tooth within the jaws. Two methods are frequently used to obtain such three-dimensional information. The first is to employ two films projected at right angles to each other. The second is to employ the so-called tube shift principle.

Figure 6-9 shows the first method, in which *two projections taken at right angles to one another* localize an object in or about the maxilla in three dimensions. In clinical practice an object's position on each radiograph is noted relative to the anatomic landmarks. This allows the observer to determine the position of the object or area of interest. For example, if a radiopacity is found near the apex of the first molar on a periapical radiograph, the dentist may take an occlusal projection to identify its mediolateral position. The occlusal film may reveal a calcification in the soft tissues located laterally or medially to the body of the mandible. This information is important in determining what treat-

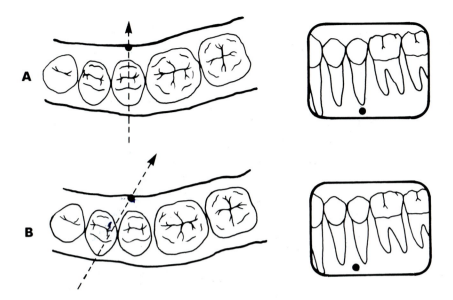

FIG. 6-10. The position of an object may be determined with respect to reference structures by using the tube shift technique. In top pair drawings, **A,** an object on the lingual surface of the mandible may appear apical to the second premolar. When another radiograph is made of this region angulated from the mesial, **B,** the object appears to have moved mesially with respect to the second premolar apex (*same-lingual* in the acronym SLOB).

ment, if any, is required. The right-angle (or cross-section) technique is best for the mandible. On a maxillary occlusal projection the superimposition of features in the anterior part of the skull may frequently obscure the area of interest.

The second technique used to identify the spatial position of an object is the *tube shift technique*.[7] Other names for this procedure are the *buccal object rule*[8] or *Clark's rule* (after C.A. Clark,[2] who described it in 1910). The rationale for this procedure derives from the manner in which the relative positions of radiographic images of two separate objects change when the projection angle at which the images were made is changed. Figure 6-10 shows two radiographs of an object exposed with slightly different angles. Compare the position of the object in question on each radiograph with the reference structures. If the tube is shifted and directed at the reference object (e.g., the apex of a tooth) from a more mesial angulation and the object in question also moves mesially with respect to the reference object, then the object lies lingual to the reference object. Alternatively, if the tube is shifted mesially and the object in question appears to move distally, it lies on the buccal aspect of the reference object (Fig. 6-11). These relations can be easily remembered by the acronym *SLOB:* same-lingual, opposite-buccal. Thus if the object

in question appears to move in the same direction with respect to the reference structures as the x-ray tube, it is on the lingual aspect of the reference object; if it appears to move in the opposite direction as the x-ray tube, it is on the buccal aspect. If it does not move with respect to the reference object, it lies at the same depth (in the same vertical plane) as the reference object.

Examination of a conventional set of full-mouth films with this rule in mind will demonstrate that the incisive foramen is indeed lingual (palatal) to the roots of the central incisors and that the mental foramen is buccal to the roots of the premolars. This procedure will assist in determining the position of impacted teeth, foreign objects, or other abnormal conditions. It works just as well when the x-ray machine is moved in the vertical plane as in the horizontal plane.

As sometimes happens, the dentist may have two radiographs of a region of the dentition that were made at different angles but there is no record of the orientation of the x-ray machine. Comparison of the anatomy displayed on the images will help distinguish changes in horizontal or vertical angulation. A more reliable method, however, is to compare the image fields (i.e., the changed positions of the bony anatomy with respect to the teeth). In the first instance the image of a lateral incisor

FIG. 6-11. The position of an object can be determined with respect to reference structures by using the tube shift technique. In the top pair of drawings, **A,** an object on the buccal surface of the mandible may appear apical to the second premolar. When another radiograph is made of this region angulated from the mesial, **B,** the object appears to have moved distally with respect to the second premolar apex (*opposite-buccal* in the acronym SLOB).

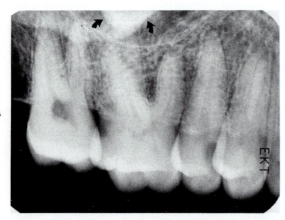

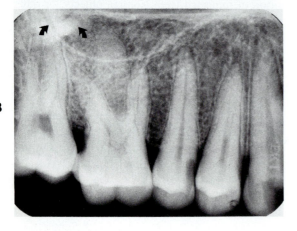

FIG. 6-12. The position of the maxillary zygomatic process in relation to the roots of the molars can help in identifying the orientation of projections. Note that in **A** the inferior border of the process (*arrows*) lies over the palatal root of the first molar whereas in **B** it lies posterior to the palatal root of the first molar. This indicates that when A was made the beam was oriented more from the posterior than when B was made. The same conclusion can be reached independently by examining the roots of the first molar. Notice that in A the palatal root lies behind the distobuccal root but in B it lies between the two buccal roots.

on an incisor view will be projected more from the mesial than it will on a canine view. In the second the relative positions of osseous landmarks—such as the inferior border of the zygomatic process of the maxilla (Fig. 6-12) or the anterior border of the mandibular ramus—with respect to the teeth will help identify changes in horizontal or vertical angulation.[7] These two structures lie buccal to the teeth and will appear to move mesially as the x-ray beam is oriented more from the distal. Similarly, as the angulation of the beam is increased vertically, the zygomatic process will be projected occlusally over the teeth.

SPECIFIC REFERENCES

1. Barr JH, Gron P: Palate contour as a limiting factor in intraoral x-ray technique, *Oral Surg* 12:459-472, 1959.
2. Clark CA: A method of ascertaining the relative position of unerupted teeth by means of film radiographs, *Proc R Soc Med Odontol Sect* 3:87-90, 1910.
3. Fitzgerald GM: Dental roentgenography. II. Vertical angulation, film placement and increased object-film distance, *J Am Dent Assoc* 34:160-170, 1947.
4. Fitzgerald GM: Dental roentgenography. III. The roentgenographic periapical survey of the upper molar region, *J Am Dent Assoc* 38:293-303, 1949.
5. McCormack FW: Dental roentgenology: a technical procedure for furthering the advancement toward anatomical accuracy, *J S Calif Dent Assoc* 13:1-28, 1937.
6. McCormack FW: A plea for a standardized technique for oral radiography, with an illustrated classification of findings and their verified interpretation, *J Dent Res* 2:467-510, 1920.
7. Langlalis RA, Langland OE, Morris CR: Radiographic localization techniques, *Dent Radiogr Photogr* 52:69-77, 1979.
8. Richards AG: The buccal object rule, *Dent Radiogr Photogr* 53:37-56, 1980.

7

Processing X-Ray Film

The recording medium (image receptor) most frequently used in dental radiography is the radiographic film. When a beam of photons exiting an object exposes an x-ray film, it chemically changes the photosensitive silver halide crystals in the film emulsion with which it interacts. These chemically altered crystals constitute the *latent* (invisible) *image* on the film. The idea of the latent image implies that the chemical changes produced by the x rays renders the altered crystals sensitive to the chemical action of the developing process that converts the latent image into the *visible image*.

FORMATION OF THE LATENT IMAGE

Film emulsion consists of photosensitive crystals containing silver bromide and silver iodide suspended in gelatin and layered on a thin sheet of transparent plastic base. These crystals are imperfect in several respects. First, they contain a few *free silver ions* in the spaces between the crystalline lattice positions (Figs. 7-1 and 7-2). These are interstitial silver ions. Second, there are physical *distortions* in the regular array of the silver and bromide ions in the crystals caused by the presence of relatively large iodine atoms occupying some of the bromide sites. Third, the silver halide crystals are *chemically sensitized* by the presence of (added) sulfur compounds bound to their surface. The sulfur compounds are not a detriment to the film but play a critical role in image formation. Along with the physical irregularities in the crystal produced by the iodide ions, they comprise the *latent image sites*. They begin the process of image formation by trapping the electrons generated when the emulsion is irradiated. There are many such latent image sites in each crystal.

When the silver halide crystals are irradiated, x-ray photons interact primarily with the bromide ions by Compton and photoelectric interactions (Fig. 7-2, *B*). These interactions result in the re-

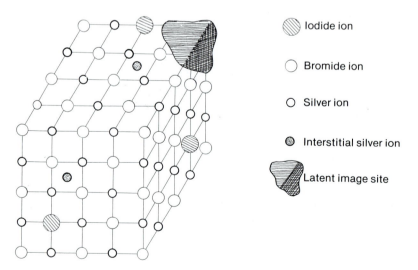

FIG. 7-1. A silver bromide crystal in the emulsion of an x-ray film contains mostly silver and bromide ions with small amounts of iodide ions in a crystal lattice. There are also free interstitial silver ions and areas of trace chemicals that serve as latent image sites.

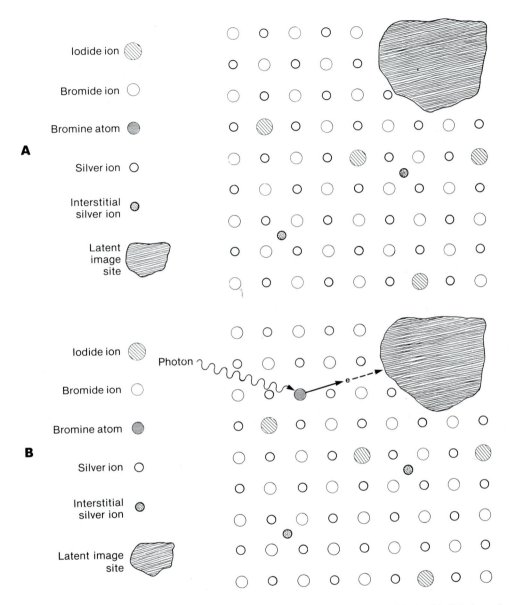

FIG. 7-2. Formation of the latent image: **A,** A crystal contains silver, bromide, and iodide ions; it also has some interstitial silver ions and latent image sites before exposure. **B,** Exposure of the crystal to an x-ray beam results in the release of electrons, usually by interaction with the bromide ions. Bromide ions are thus converted to bromine atoms, and the recoil electrons *(e)* have sufficient kinetic energy to move about in the crystal. When they strike a latent image site, they impart a negative charge to this region.

Continued.

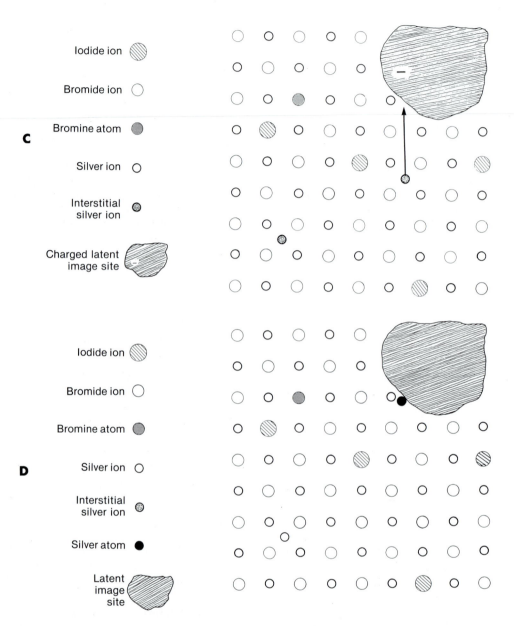

FIG. 7-2, cont'd. C, Free interstitial silver ions (with a positive charge) are attracted to the negatively charged latent image site. **D,** When they reach this site, they acquire an electron and become silver atoms. These silver atoms constitute the latent image. In the presence of developer these silver atoms initiate the conversion of silver ions in the crystal to a grain of metallic silver.

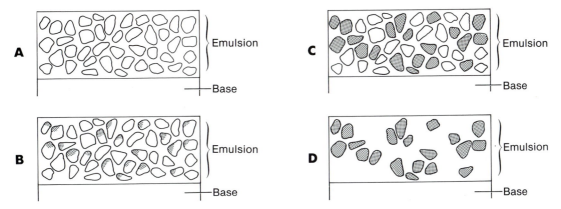

FIG. 7-3. Emulsion changes during film processing. **A,** Before exposure, there are multiple silver bromide crystals in the emulsion. **B,** After exposure, the exposed crystals containing silver particles at latent image sites consitute the latent image (*shaded areas* in the crystals). **C,** After development, the exposed crystals containing silver particles at the latent image sites are converted to metallic silver grains by the developing solution. **D,** After fixing, the unexposed undeveloped silver bromide crystals are dissolved and washed away by the fixing solution and washing procedure. (Courtesy Dr. C.L. Crabtree, Bureau of Radiological Health, Rockville Md.)

moval of an electron from the bromide ions, with the production of high-speed electrons and scattered photons. By the loss of its recoil electrons, a bromide ion is converted to a bromine atom. The recoil electrons move through the crystal, generating additional bromine atoms, secondary recoil electrons, and scattered photons, until they come across a latent image site. Here they become trapped and impart a negative charge to the site. The negatively charged latent image site attracts positively charged free interstitial silver ions (Fig. 7-2, *C*). When a silver ion reaches the charged latent image site, it becomes neutralized and precipitates as an atom of metallic silver at the site (Fig. 7-2, *D*). This process occurs many times at a single site within a crystal whenever photons and recoil electrons strike bromide ions. After exposure of a film to radiation, the aggregate of metallic silver atoms at latent image sites comprises the latent image. It is the metallic silver at each latent image site that renders the crystals sensitive to development and image formation. The larger the aggregate of silver atoms, the more sensitive the crystal is to the effects of the developer. Developer converts crystals with metallic silver deposited at latent image sites into black metallic silver grains that can be visualized. Fixer removes the unexposed, undeveloped silver bromide crystals. This renders the film clear in those areas.

PROCESSING SOLUTIONS

Film processing involves the following procedures:

1. Immersion of exposed films in developer solution
2. Rinsing in running water
3. Immersion in fixing solution
4. Washing
5. Drying and mounting for viewing

This discussion describes the function of each of these solutions. Later the procedures used for performing each of these steps will be described.

Developer solution

The developer reduces all silver ions in the exposed crystals of silver bromide (with a latent image) to metallic silver (Fig. 7-3). To produce a diagnostic image, this reduction process must be restricted to crystals containing a latent image. Thus the reducing agents used as developers are those that are catalyzed by the presence of metallic silver at the latent image sites. The metallic silver appears to act as a bridge by which electrons from the developing solution (reducing agents or chemical electron donors) can reach silver ions in the crystal and convert them to metallic silver. Individual crystals are developed completely or not at all during the recommended developing times. Variations in densities on the processed radiographs are the result of uneven distribution of developed (exposed) and undeveloped (unexposed) crystals in the areas. Areas that have many exposed crystals will be the more dense (blacker) because of their higher concentration of black metallic silver granules after development. If the developer remains in contact with silver bromide crystals that do not contain a latent image, it will slowly reduce them also and thereby overdevelop the image.

When an exposed film is being developed, there is an initial period in which no visible effect of the developer is apparent (Fig. 7-4). After this initial phase the density increases, very rapidly at first and then more slowly. Eventually all the exposed crystals develop (become reduced to black metallic silver) and the unexposed crystals start to be reduced by the developing agent. Development of unexposed crystals results in the production of chemical fog on the film. This interval between maximum density and fogging explains why a properly exposed film does not become overdeveloped even though it may be in contact with the developer longer than the recommended interval. Thus dark films are usually the result of overexposure, not overdevelopment. An overexposed film will develop larger more effective latent image sites, which explains why such a film will develop acceptable density with a shorter developing time than a film that has been properly exposed. Unfortunately this results in unnecessary overexposure of the patient.

The developing solution contains four components: (1) developer, (2) preservative, (3) activator, and (4) restrainer.

Developer. The primary function of the developing agents is to amplify the latent image by *converting the exposed silver halide crystals into metallic silver grains*. This process begins at the latent image sites, where electrons from the developing agents are conducted into the silver halide crystal and reduce the (10^9 to 10^{10}) constituent silver ions to metallic silver. Unexposed crystals without latent images are unaffected during the time required for reduction of the exposed crystals. This emphasizes the importance of carefully controlling the time for development. To control the developing process, two developing agents are usually present in the developing solutions used in dental radiology: Elon (monomethy-para-aminophenol sulfate) and hydroquinone (paradihydroxy benzene). The hydroquinone brings out the contrast of the image. It is quite sensitive to temperature changes, becoming inactive below 60° F and very reactive

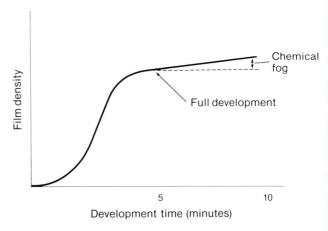

FIG. 7-4. Film density versus development time. The density of a film initially rises quickly and then levels off, increasing more slowly because of chemical fogging.

above 70° F. Thus the temperature of the developing solution is critical. Elon is less temperature sensitive and acts quickly to bring out the gray shades in an image. Photographic developers used with film and photographic paper commonly use this combination of Elon and hydroquinone.

Preservative. The developing solution contains a preservative, usually sodium sulfite (which has a great affinity for oxygen, as do the developing agents). The addition of preservative helps *protect the developers from being oxidized* by atmospheric oxygen. Preservative also combines with the brown oxidized developer to produce a colorless soluble compound. Such oxidation products, if not removed, will interfere with the developing reaction and stain the film. The sulfite preservative helps extend the useful life of the hydroquinone and Elon.

Activator. The developers are active only at high pH values, usually above 11. To maintain this condition, the developing solution contains *alkali,* which serves as an activator (accelerator). The alkalies generally used are sodium carbonate, sodium hydroxide, and sometimes sodium metaborate and tetraborate. The activators also serve to *soften the gelatin* so the developer agents can diffuse more rapidly into the emulsion and reach the silver bromide crystals suspended in the gelatin.

Restrainer. The fourth component added to the developing solution is a restrainer, usually potassium bromide. The manufacturer adds bromide because bromine is a product of the reduction of silver halide crystals and the added bromide serves to depress this by the common ion effect. Although it does depress the reduction of both exposed and unexposed crystals, it is much more effective in depressing the reduction of unexposed crystals. As a consequence it acts as an *antifog agent*.

Developer replenisher

Developer replenisher is a solution made for topping off the developing solution each morning. It is a more concentrated solution of developer constituents designed to replace those depleted from the original solution without unduly increasing its volume. Its high pH compensates for the reduced alkalinity of the used solution and will partially offset the inhibitory effect of the accumulating bromine atoms, a major factor limiting the life of developing solutions.

Rinsing

After development the film emulsion swells and becomes saturated with developer. At this time the films are rinsed in water for 15 to 20 seconds before being placed in the fixer. This dilutes the developer and thereby *slows the development process*. The rinse also *removes the alkali activator,* thus preventing neutralization of the acid fixer.

Fixing solution

The primary function of fixing solution is to *remove (dissolve) the undeveloped silver halide crystals* from the emulsion (Fig. 7-3, *D*). The presence of unexposed crystals causes film to be opaque. If these crystals are not removed, the image on the resultant radiograph is dark and nondiagnostic. A second function of fixing solution is to *harden (fix) the film emulsion.* Figure 7-5 is a photomicrograph of film emulsion showing the silver grains after fixer has removed the unexposed silver halide crystals. Compare it with Fig. 5-2, which shows the unprocessed emulsion.

The fixing solution also contains four components: (1) clearing agent, (2) acidifier, (3) preservative, and (4) hardener.

Clearing agent. After development it is necessary to clear the film emulsion by dissolving and removing the unexposed silver halide. Aqueous solutions of sodium or ammonium thiosulfate (*"hypo"*) dissolve the silver halide. Their action is to *form stable water-soluble complexes with silver ions,* thus effectively removing the ions from solution. As a result the solubility of the unexposed silver halide crystals increases to maintain the solubility product of the silver bromide in solution

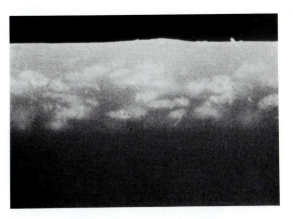

FIG. 7-5. Scanning electron micrograph of a processed emulsion of Kodak Ultra-Speed dental x-ray film (5000×). Note the white-appearing silver grains above the base. (Courtesy Eastman Kodak, Rochester NY.)

and they readily dissolve from the emulsion. The clearing agent has no rapid effect on the metallic silver grains in the film emulsion. Excessive fixation, however, results in a gradual loss of film density because the grains of silver slowly dissolve in the acetic acid of the fixing solution.

Acidifier. The fixing solution, which contains acid (usually acetic), functions to *neutralize any contaminating alkali* from the developing solution and to inhibit any carryover of developing agents. Unneutralized alkali and uninhibited developing agents from the developing solution may cause development of the unexposed crystals to continue in the fixing tank.

Preservative. Sodium sulfite is the preservative in the fixing solution, as it is in the developer, and its action is to *prevent the decomposition of the thiosulfate clearing agent,* which is unstable in the acid environment of the fixing solution. Furthermore, it *complexes with any colored oxidized developer* carried over into the fixing solution, and effectively removes it from solution, because it will stain the film.

Hardener. Hardeners added to the fixer *prevent damage to the gelatin* by subsequent handling. They also shorten the drying time. The most common hardening agents are aluminum potassium sulfate and chromium potassium sulfate. The acidity of the fixing solution enhances their capacity to harden the gelatin.

Washing

After fixing, the processed film is washed in a sufficient flow of water and for an adequate time

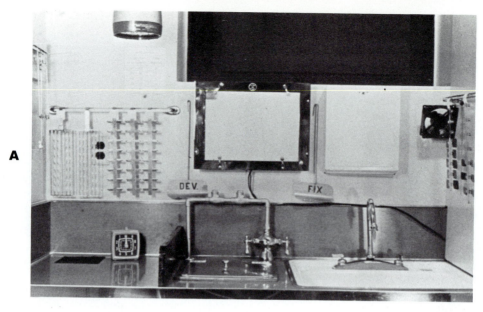

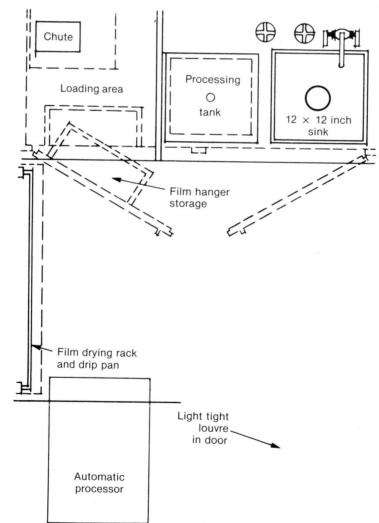

FIG. 7-6. A, Darkroom working area. *Left:* Film-mounting area, timer, film racks, and safelight above; *middle:* developing and fixing tanks below the viewbox and stirring paddles; *right:* sink and drying racks with fan. **B,** Floor plan. (**A** courtesy Dr. C.L. Crabtree, Bureau of Radiological Health, Rockville Md; **B** courtesy Eastman Kodak, Rochester NY.)

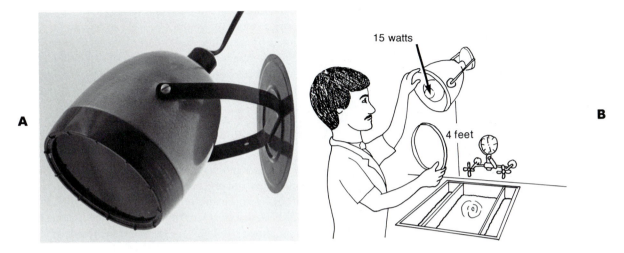

FIG. 7-7. A, A safelight may be mounted on the wall or ceiling in the darkroom and should be at least 4 feet from the working surface. **B,** It uses a GBX-2 filter and 15 W bulb.

assure *removal of all processing chemicals*. Washing efficiency decreases rapidly when the water temperature falls below 60° F. Any remaining silver compounds or thiosulfate resulting from improper washing will discolor and cause stains that are most apparent in the radiopaque (light) areas. This results when the thiosulfate reacts with silver to form brown silver sulfide, which can obscure diagnostic information.

DARKROOM EQUIPMENT

The darkroom should be convenient to the x-ray machines and dental operatories and be at least 4 × 5 feet in area (Fig. 7-6). One of its main requirements is that it be lightproof. To accomplish this, a light-tight door or doorless maze (if space permits) is used. The door should have a lock to prevent accidental opening, which would allow an unexpected flood of light in and ruin opened films. The room must be well ventilated for the comfort of individuals working in the area and to exhaust the heat from the dryer or moisture from the drying films. Also, when the room is at a comfortable temperature, it will be easier to maintain optimum conditions for the developing, fixing, and washing solutions. If supplies (including unexposed x-ray film) are to be stored in the darkroom, ventilation is doubly important, for temperatures of 90° F or higher can cause the film to show a generalized increase in density (film fog).

Safelighting

Equipment. The processing room should have both white illumination and safelighting. Safelighting is low-intensity illumination of relatively long wavelength (red) that does not rapidly affect open film but permits one to see well enough to work in the area. The arrangement of safelight filters (Fig. 7-7) in a manual processing room should provide three zones of illumination: a dimly lit zone for loading and opening the film cassettes, a medium-illumination zone for developing and fixing the films, and a brightly lit zone for washing and drying the films. It is best to place one safelight above the working area on the wall behind the processing tanks and somewhat to the right of the fixing tank. To minimize the fogging effect of prolonged exposure, the safelight should be mounted at least 4 feet above the surface where opened films are handled and use a 15-watt bulb.

X-ray films are very sensitive to the blue-green region of the spectrum and less sensitive to yellow and red wavelengths. Accordingly, the red GBX-2 filter is recommended for the safelight in a darkroom where both intraoral and extraoral films are handled (Fig. 7-8). Film handling under a safelight should be limited to about 5 minutes since film emulsion shows some sensitivity to light from a safelight following prolonged exposure.

Testing for unsafe illumination. Film may become fogged in the darkroom from inappropriate safelight filters, from excessive exposure to safe-lights, or from stray light from other sources. Such films will be dark, show low contrast, and have a muddy gray appearance. Here is a simple test to evaluate for fogging caused by inappropriate safe-lighting conditions: (1) Open a film packet and place the bare test film in the area where the films are usually unwrapped and clipped on the film hanger. (2) Place a penny on the film and leave it in this position for the approximate time required to unwrap and mount a full-mouth set of films, usually

about 5 minutes. (3) Develop the test film as usual. If you see the image of the penny on the resultant film, then the room is not light-safe for the particular film tested (Fig. 7-9). Each type of film used in the office should be tested to measure the dark-room's integrity. Sources of light leaks can be detected by standing in the darkroom for 5 minutes to allow the eyes to accommodate. Then light leaks are marked with chalk or masking tape. Weather stripping is useful for sealing light leaks under doors.

Processing tanks

All dental offices must have the capacity to develop radiographs by tank processing. The tank must have hot and cold running water and a means of maintaining the temperature between 60° and 75° F. A practical size for a dental office is a master tank about 20 × 25 cm (8 × 10 inches) that can serve as a water jacket for two removable inserts that fit inside (Fig. 7-10). The insert tanks usually hold 3.8 L (1 gallon) of developer or fixer and are placed within the outer, larger, master tank. The outer tank holds the running water for maintaining the temperature of the developer and fixer in the insert tanks and for washing films. It is customary to place the developer in the insert tank on the left side of the master tank and the fixer in the insert tank on the right. All three tanks should be made of stainless steel, which will not react with the processing solutions and is easy to clean. The master tank should have a cover to reduce oxidation of the processing solutions, protect the developing film from accidental exposure to light, and minimize evaporation of the processing solutions.

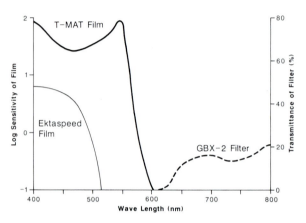

FIG. 7-8. Spectral sensitivities of T-Mat film *(heavy line)* and Ektaspeed film *(thin line)* shown with the transmission characteristics of a GBX-2 filter *(dashed line)*. Note that the films are more sensitive in the blue-green portion of the spectrum (shorter than 600 nm) but the GBX-2 filter transmits primarily red light (longer than 600 nm).

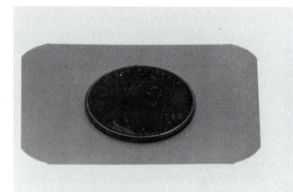 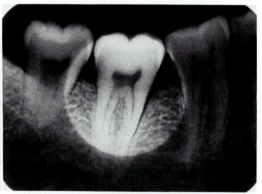

FIG. 7-9. Penny test for unsafe illumination. **A,** Leave a penny on the exposed duplicate film from the double-film pack on the working surface during the time that any film would be opened (usually about 5 minutes). **B,** If the processed radiograph shows an outline of the penny, the film is being fogged by inappropriate safelighting conditions.

Thermometer

It is important to control the temperature of the developing, fixing, and washing solutions closely. A thermometer can be left in the water circulating through the master tank to monitor its temperature. The most desirable thermometers clip onto the side of the tank or float freely in the tank (Fig. 7-11).

Timer

The x-ray film must be exposed to the processing chemicals for specific intervals. To control the time of development and fixation, an interval timer is indispensable in the darkroom (Fig. 7-12).

Drying racks

On a convenient wall two or three drying racks can be mounted for film hangers. Underneath the racks drip trays are placed to catch the water that may run off the wet films. You may also use an electric fan to circulate the air and speed the drying of the films. (Do not aim it directly on the films, however). In addition, cabinet dryers that circulate warm air around the film and accelerate the drying are available. If dryers are in the darkroom, they should be ventilated outside the darkroom to pre-

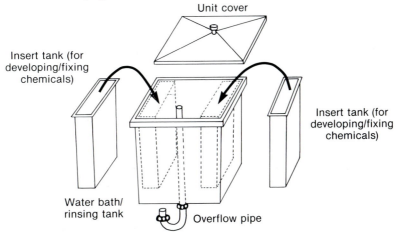

FIG. 7-10. Processing tank. The developing/fixing tanks insert into a bath of running water with an overflow drain.

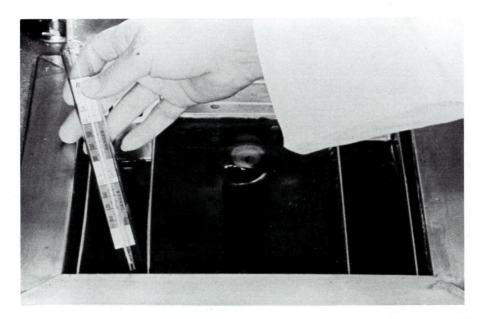

FIG. 7-11. A thermometer may float in the tank or be attached to the tank wall. (Courtesy Dr. C.L. Crabtree, Bureau of Radiological Health, Rockville Md.)

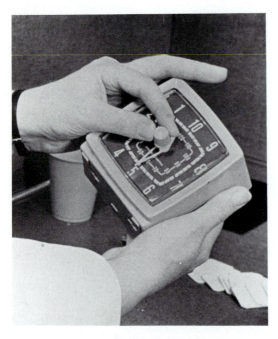

FIG. 7-12. The timer is started when the rack of films is placed in the developer. (Courtesy Dr. C.L. Crabtree, Bureau of Radiological Health, Rockville Md.)

clude high humidity and heat (which would be detrimental to any unexposed film stored in the room).

MANUAL PROCESSING PROCEDURES
Stirring the solutions

The first step in manual tank processing is to stir the developer and fixing solution to mix the chemicals and equalize the temperature throughout the tanks. Because proper developing time varies with the temperature, determine the temperature of the developer after stirring.

Checking the solution levels

Check the levels of the solutions to be certain that the developer and fixer will cover the films on the top clips of the film hangers. Add fresh developer or replenisher to maintain a proper level. Add fresh fixer as necessary.

Mounting films on the hangers

Using only safelight illumination in the darkroom, remove the exposed film from its lightproof packet or cassette. Hold the films only by their edges to avoid damage to the film surface. Take care not to bend the film, scratch the emulsion, or touch it with wet fingers. Clip the bare film onto a film hanger, one film to a clip (Fig. 7-13). To avoid any possible confusion later, label the film racks with the patient's name and exposure date.

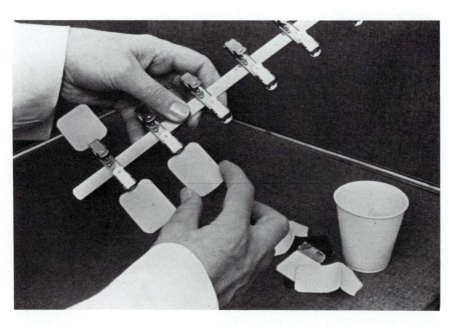

FIG. 7-13. Films are mounted securely on film clips. Always hold a film by its edge to avoid fingerprints on the image. (Courtesy Dr. C.L. Crabtree, Bureau of Radiological Health, Rockville Md.)

Setting the timer

Preset the interval timer to the time indicated for the solution temperature by the manufacturer. For conventional solutions, use the following development times:

Temperature	Development time
65° F	6 minutes
68° F	5 minutes
70° F	4½ minutes
72° F	4 minutes
76° F	3 minutes

Processing films at either higher or lower temperatures and for longer or shorter times than recommended by the manufacturer will reduce the contrast of the processed film. Also, processing too long or at higher than the recommended temperature can lead to increased film fog which will also reduce film contrast.

Developing

Immerse the hanger and films in the developer with mild agitation to sweep air bubbles off the film and bring fresh developer in contact with the entire surface of the emulsion. Start the timer mechanism and leave the films in the developer for the predetermined time.

Rinsing

After development, rinse the hanger and films in the tank running-water bath for about 20 seconds. This will remove excess developer, which would contaminate the fixer. Remember, however, that the film is continuing to develop while it is being washed, albeit at a slower rate.

Fixing

Next, place the hanger and film in the tank of fixer solution and again agitate a few times. This eliminates bubbles and assures complete contact between the solution and the emulsion. A practical rule when fixing is to leave the film in the fixing solution for twice the time it takes to clear the film (to dissolve the unexposed silver bromide). This will ensure that all the silver halide ions have diffused out of the gelatin and that the gelatin has hardened. Excess fixation (several hours) removes some of the metallic silver grains, decreasing the density of the film. The film should generally be in the fixing solution for 10 to 15 minutes—twice the recommended developing time.

Washing and drying

After fixation of the films is complete, place them in running water for at least 20 minutes to

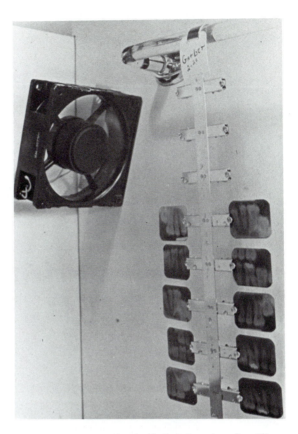

FIG. 7-14. Films dry in circulating air under a fan. (Courtesy Dr. C.L. Crabtree, Bureau of Radiological Health, Rockville, Md.)

remove residual processing solutions. After washing the films, remove the surface moisture by shaking excess water from the films and hanger. Dry the films in circulating moderately warm air (Fig. 7-14). If the films dry rapidly with small drops of water clinging to their surface, the areas under the drops will dry more slowly than the surrounding areas. This uneven drying causes distortion of the gelatin, changing the density of the silver image. The result is spots that are frequently visible and detract from the usefulness of the finished radiograph. After drying, the films are ready to mount.

RAPID PROCESSING CHEMICALS

In recent years a number of manufacturers have made available rapid processing solutions. These solutions typically will develop films in 10 to 30 seconds, sometimes at elevated temperatures, and fix them in 1 to 2 minutes. They have the same general formulation as conventional processing solutions but often are more concentrated. Their use is especially advantageous in endodontics and for

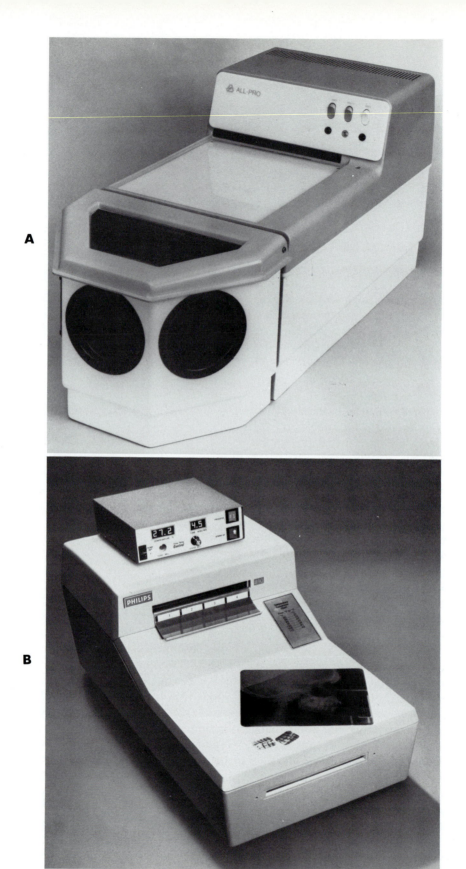

FIG. 7-15. Automatic processors. **A,** All-Pro AR Processor with Intra-Oral Daylight Loader. **B,** Philips 810 Automatic Film Processor. (**A** courtesy Air Techniques, Hicksville, NY; **B** courtesy Philips Dental Systems, Stamford, CT.)

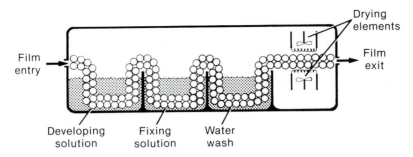

FIG. 7-16. Automatic film processors generally consist of a roller assembly that transports the film between the rollers through developing, fixing, washing, and drying stations.

treating emergency conditions, when the short processing time is quite useful. Although resultant images may be satisfactory, however, they often do not achieve the same degree of contrast as films processed conventionally and they may discolor in the file. After using these rapidly processed films, place them in conventional fixing solution for 10 minutes and wash for 20 minutes. This will improve the contrast and help them remain relatively stable in storage. Regardless, conventional solutions are preferred for most routine use.

CHANGING SOLUTIONS

All processing solutions will deteriorate as the result of continued use and exposure to air. Although the use of replenisher will prolong the useful life of the developer, the eventual buildup of reaction products will cause the developer to cease functioning properly. Exhaustion of the developer results in films that show reduced density and contrast. In addition, solutions should be changed if they become turbid. Under average conditions, solutions may provide about 3 or 4 weeks of service before they must be changed.

A simple procedure will help determine when to change solutions: Expose a double film packet instead of a single film packet on one projection for the first patient radiographed after new solutions are prepared. Place one film in the patient's chart and mount the other on a corner of a viewbox in the darkroom. As successive films are processed, compare them with this reference film (see below). Loss of image contrast and density will become evident as the solutions deteriorate and indicates when it is time to change them. Change the fixer when the developer is changed.

AUTOMATIC FILM PROCESSING

Equipment is available that automates all processing steps (Fig. 7-15). Although there are a number of advantages to automatic processing, the most attractive is the savings in time. Depending on the equipment and the temperature of operation, an automatic processor requires only 4 to 6 minutes to develop, fix, wash, and dry a film. Many of the dental automatic processors have a light-shielded (daylight loading) compartment in which the operator can unwrap films and feed them into the machine without working in a darkroom. This is desirable because the individual doing the developing does not have to work in the dark. When processing extraoral films, remove the light-shielded compartment to provide room for feeding the larger film into the processor. Another attractive feature of the automatic system is that the density and contrast of the resultant radiographs tend to be consistent. Because of the increased temperature and concentration of the developer, however, the quality of films processed automatically is often not as high as for those carefully developed manually. Usually more grain is evident in the final image.

Whether automatic processing equipment is appropriate for a specific practice depends on the dentist and the nature and volume of the practice. The costs of acquisition and maintenance are relatively high. Also a regular and frequent cleaning schedule is mandatory. Furthermore, the automated equipment may break down, thus requiring conventional darkroom equipment as a backup system.

Mechanism

The design of the automatic processor is an in-line arrangement. It typically consists of a transport mechanism that picks up the unwrapped film and passes it through the developer, fixer, and washing and drying sections (Fig. 7-16). The transport system used most is a series of rollers driven by a constant-speed motor operating through gears, belts, or chains. The rollers often consist of independent assemblies, one for each step in the operation. Although these assemblies are designed and positioned so the film crosses over from one to the next, the operator may remove them independently for soaking, cleaning, and repairing. The primary function of the rollers is to move the film through the developing solutions, but they also serve at least two other functions. First, their motion keeps the solutions agitated, which contributes to the uniformity of processing. Second, the top rollers at the crossover point between developer and fixer tank act as wringers to remove developing solution, which minimizes the carryover of developer into the fixer tank. This feature of the system plays a role in maintaining the uniformity of processing chemicals.

Special chemicals that react at higher temperatures than those used for manual processing allow the more rapid rate of development, fixing, washing, and drying characteristic of automatic processing. Hardeners prevent the emulsion from becoming slippery or sticky at these temperatures. Accordingly, the developer contains hardeners and the fixer has an additional hardener. The objective is to reach a compromise in the thickness and stickiness of the emulsion that will facilitate rapid processing while withstanding the physical abuse of the transport system.

Replenishment

It is important to maintain the constituents of the developer and fixer carefully to preserve the optimal physical properties of the film emulsion within the narrow limits imposed by the speed and temperature of automatic processing. As the activities of the developer and fixing solutions lessen, their effect on the film diminishes. To compensate for their loss in activity, some automatic processors include an automatic or manual replenishment system. These systems add replenisher to the developer tank and fixer to the fixer tank. It is often a more concentrated solution of the chemicals than the original developer. Insufficient replenishment and approaching depletion of the developer result in a loss of image contrast. Exhaustion of the fixing solution causes poor clearing of the film, insufficient hardening of the emulsion, and unreliable transport from the fixer assembly on through the drying operation.

USE OF REFERENCE FILMS

A valuable technique that assists in image quality evaluation is the use of *reference films*. A reference film is a "good-quality" radiograph (e.g., bitewing) attached to a viewbox (Fig. 7-17). It provides a standard against which to compare recently processed radiographs for density, contrast, and resolution. It can also serve as a guide to determine whether the anatomic features appropriate for the particular projection are adequately revealed. Additional reference films should be maintained for each type of radiograph used (e.g., panoramic,

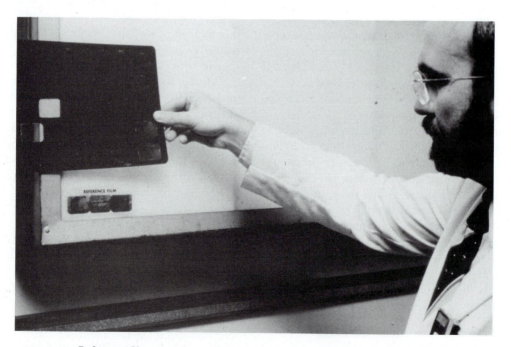

FIG. 7-17. Reference films attached to the viewbox serve as standards for daily film evaluation.

cephalometric). Processing solutions should be changed when current films show a loss of contrast and density caused by chemical exhaustion.

MANAGEMENT OF RADIOGRAPHIC WASTES

To prevent environmental damage, many communities and states have passed laws governing the disposal of wastes. Such laws often derive from the Federal Resource Conservation and Recovery act of 1976. Although waste dental radiographic supplies constitute only a small potential hazard, it is important that they be discarded properly. The primary ingredient of concern in developing solutions is the dissolved silver found in used fixer. Another material of concern is the lead foil found in film packets.

There are several means for properly disposing of the silver and lead. One may recover silver from the fixer by using either metallic replacement or electroplating methods. Metallic replacement utilizes cartridges through which the user pours waste solutions. In this process iron goes into solution and the silver precipitates as a sludge. In the electroplating method the waste solutions are in contact with two electrodes through which there is a current. The cathode captures the silver. In either case, one may then sell the scrap silver to silver refiners and buyers. The lead foil is also a hazardous waste. The lead is separated from the packet and collected until there is enough to sell to a scrap metal dealer. Dental offices should also consider using companies that are licensed to pick up waste materials. The names of such companies are in the telephone directory, or the state hazardous waste management agency can be contacted.

COMMON CAUSES OF FAULTY RADIOGRAPHS

Although film processing can result in radiographs of excellent quality, inattention to detail may lead to many problems and images that are diagnostically suboptimal. Poor radiographs contribute to a loss of diagnostic information and loss of professional and patient time. Following is a list of common causes of faulty radiographs. The steps necessary for correction are self-evident:

1. Light radiographs (Fig. 7-18)
   a. Processing errors
      (1) Underdevelopment
         (a) Temperature too low
         (b) Time too short
         (c) Inaccurate thermometer
      (2) Depleted developer solution
      (3) Diluted or contaminated developer
      (4) Excessive fixation
   b. Underexposure (Fig. 7-19)
      (1) Insufficient mA
      (2) Insufficient kVp
      (3) Insufficient time
      (4) Excessive film-source distance
      (5) Film packet reversed in mouth
2. Dark radiographs (Fig. 7-20)
   a. Processing errors
      (1) Overdevelopment
         (a) Temperature too high
         (b) Time too long
      (2) Developer concentration too high
      (3) Inadequate fixation
      (4) Accidental exposure to light
      (5) Improper safelighting

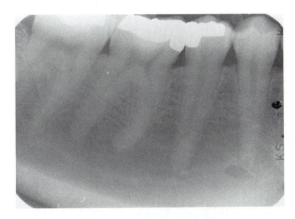

FIG. 7-18. This radiograph is too light because of inadequate processing or insufficient exposure.

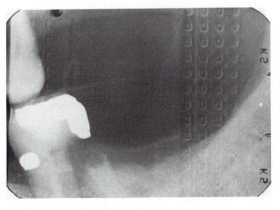

FIG. 7-19. This radiograph is too light because it was placed backward in the mouth. Note the characteristic markings resulting from exposure through the lead foil.

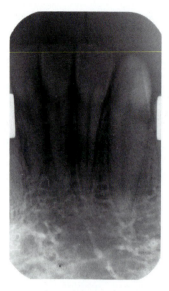

FIG. 7-20. This radiograph is too dark because of overdevelopment or overexposure.

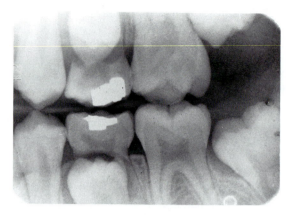

FIG. 7-21. Radiograph with insufficient contrast, showing gray enamel and gray pulp chambers.

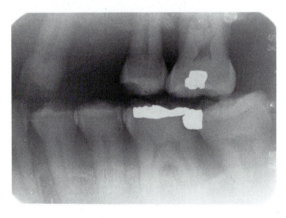

FIG. 7-22. Fogged radiograph showing lack of image detail.

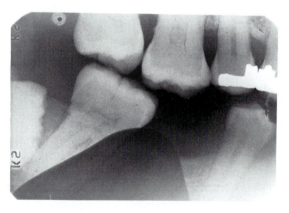

FIG. 7-23. Dark spot on the film resulting from contact with the tank wall during fixation.

  b. Overexposure
    (1) Excessive mA
    (2) Excessive kVp
    (3) Excessive time
    (4) Insufficient film-source distance
3. Insufficient contrast (Fig. 7-21)
  a. Underdevelopment
  b. Underexposure
  c. Excessive kVp
  d. Excessive film fog
4. Film fog (Fig. 7-22)
  a. Improper safelighting conditions
    (1) Improper filter
    (2) Excessive bulb wattage

    (3) Inadequate distance between safelight and working surface
    (4) Prolonged exposure of films to safelight
  b. Light leaks
    (1) Cracked safelight filter
    (2) Lights from doors, vents, etc.
  c. Overdevelopment
  d. Contaminated solutions
  e. Deteriorated film
    (1) Stored at high temperature
    (2) Stored at high humidity
    (3) Exposed to irradiation
    (4) Outdated
5. Dark spots or lines on radiograph (Fig. 7-23)
  a. Fingerprint contamination
  b. Black wrapping paper sticking to film surface

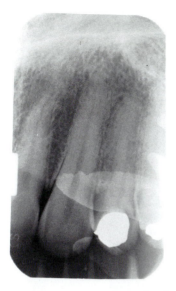

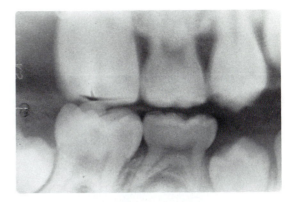

FIG. 7-25. Blurred radiograph caused by movement of the child during exposure.

FIG. 7-24. Light spots on the film resulting from contact with drops of fixer before processing.

c. Film in contact with tank or another film during fixation
d. Film contaminated with developer before processing
e. Excessive bending of films
6. Light spots on radiographs (Fig. 7-24)
a. Film contaminated with fixer before processing
b. Film in contact with tank or another film during development
7. Yellow or brown stains on radiographs
a. Depleted developer
b. Depleted fixer
c. Insufficient washing
d. Contaminated solutions
8. Blurred radiographs (Fig. 7-25)
a. Movement of patient
b. Movement of x-ray tube head
c. Double exposure
9. Radiographs with partial images (Fig. 7-26)
a. Top of film not immersed in developing solutions
b. Misalignment of x-ray tube head ("cone cut")

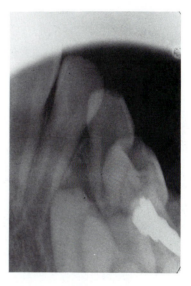

FIG. 7-26. Partial image caused by poor alignment of the tube head with the film.

MOUNTING RADIOGRAPHS

It is important to preserve and maintain radiographs in the most satisfactory and useful condition. Periapical, interproximal and occlusal films are best handled and stored in a film mount (Fig. 7-27). The operator can handle them with greater ease this way and there is less chance of physically

damaging the emulsion. Mounts are made of either plastic or cardboard and may have a clear plastic window that completely covers and protects the film. They may contain scratches or imperfections, however, that interfere with radiographic interpretation. The operator can arrange multiple films from the same individual in a film mount in the proper anatomic relationship. This will facilitate correlation of the clinical and radiographic examinations. Opaque mounts are best because they keep stray light from the viewbox from reaching the viewer's eyes (see Chapter 14).

There are two ways to position periapical and occlusal films in the film mount. The *preferred* method is to arrange them so the images of the

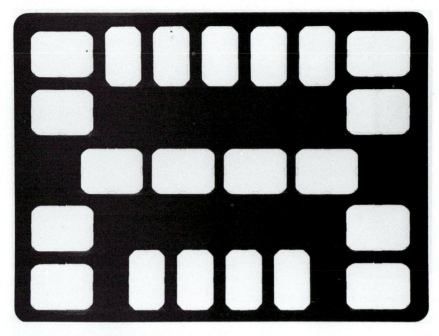

FIG. 7-27. Film mount for holding nine narrow anterior periapical views, eight posterior periapical views, and four bitewing views. (See also Figure 9-1.)

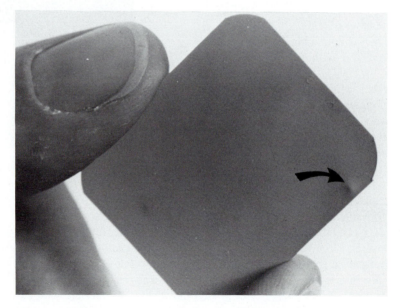

FIG. 7-28. Film dot. This raised dot *(arrow)* indicates the tube side of the film and identifies the patient's right and left sides.

teeth are in the anatomic position and have the same relationship to the viewer as when facing the patient. For this method radiographs of the teeth in the right quadrants should be placed in the left side of the mount, and those of the left quadrants in the right side. This system, advocated by the American Dental Association, permits the examiner to shift gaze from radiograph to tooth without crossing the midline. An *alternative* arrangement is to mount the images of the right quadrants on the right side of the mount and those of the left quadrant on the left. With the films arranged in this manner the teeth on the mounted radiographs will have the same relationship to the viewer as if they were being viewed from the tongue.

IDENTIFICATION DOT

A round impression in a corner of each film, the "dot," allows rapid and proper film orientation (Fig. 7-28). The manufacturer orients the film in the packet so the convex side of the dot is toward the front of the packet and will be facing the source of radiation. Consequently, to mount the films with the images of the teeth in the anatomic position, the operator places the *convex* side of the dot toward the viewer. If the other arrangement is desired, the films are placed in the mount with the *concave* side of the dot toward the viewer. Then, on the basis of the features of the teeth and anatomic landmarks in the adjacent bone, the films can be arranged in their normal sequential relationship in the mount.

DUPLICATING RADIOGRAPHS

On occasion it is necessary to duplicate radiographs. This is best accomplished with duplicating film. The film to be duplicated is placed against the emulsion side of the duplicating film. With the two films held in position by means of a glass-top cassette or photographic printing frame, they are exposed to light, which passes through the clear areas of the original radiograph and exposes the duplicating film. Then the duplicating film is processed in conventional x-ray processing solutions.

Unlike conventional x-ray film, duplicating film gives a positive image. Thus areas exposed to light come out clear as on the original radiograph. Typically duplication results in images with less resolution and more contrast than the original radiographs. To obtain the best images, use a circular ultraviolet light source. In contrast to the usual negative film, too dark or too light images produced on duplicating film are respectively under- or overexposed.

SELECTED REFERENCES
Artifacts

Goodwin PN, Quimby EH, Morgan RH: *Physical foundations of radiology,* ed 4, New York, 1970, Harper & Row, Publishers.

Johns HE, Cunningham JR: *The physics of radiology,* ed 3, Springfield Ill, 1969, Charles C Thomas, Publisher.

Sewerin IP: Mechanically induced images on dental x-ray film, *Oral Surg* 63(2):241–248, 1987.

Successful intraoral radiography. Kodak dental radiography series. Rochester NY, 1990, Eastman Kodak.

Film processing

Fletcher JC: A comparison of Ektaspeed and Ultraspeed films using manual and automatic processing solutions, *Oral Surg* 63(1):94–102, 1987.

Fredholm U, Julin P: Rapid developing of Ektaspeed dental film by increase of temperature, *Swed Dent J* 11(3):121–126, 1987.

Haist G: *Modern photographic processing,* vol 1, New York, 1979, John Wiley & Sons.

Hashimoto K, Thunthy KH, Weinberg R: Automatic processing: effects of temperature and time changes on sensitometric properties of ULTRA-SPEED and EKTASPEED films. *Oral Surg* 71(1):120–124, 1991.

Hedin M: Developing solutions for dental x-ray processors, *Swed Dent J* 13(6):261–265, 1989.

Mees DEK, James TH: *The theory of the photographic process,* New York, 1977, Macmillan.

Sturge JM (ed): *Neblette's Handbook of photography and reprography—materials, processes, and systems,* New York, 1977, Van Nostrand Reinhold.

Thunthy KH, Haskimoto K, Weinberg R: Automatic processing: effects of temperature and time changes on the sensitometric properties of light-sensitive films. *Oral Surg* 72:112–118, 1991.

Waste management

Management of photographic wastes in the dental office. Kodak dental radiography series, Rochester NY, 1990, Eastman Kodak.

Thunthy KH, Fortier AP: Electrolytic recovery of silver from dental radiographic films, *J Ala Dent Assoc* 74(2):13–18, 1990.

Quality control

Thorogood J, Horner K, Smith NJ: Quality control in the processing of dental radiographs: a practical guide to sensitometry, *Br Dent J* 164(9):282–287, 1987.

8

Normal Radiographic Anatomy

The recognition of disease by radiographic techniques requires a sound knowledge of the appearance of normal structures on the radiograph. Intelligent radiologic diagnosis cannot be attempted without an appreciation of the wide range of variation in the appearance of normal anatomic structures. Similarly, it should be recognized that most normal patients demonstrate many of the normal radiographic landmarks, but it is a rare patient who shows them all. Accordingly, the absence of one or even several such landmarks in any individual should not necessarily be considered abnormal.

TEETH

The teeth are composed primarily of dentin, with an enamel cap over the coronal portion and a thin layer of cementum over the root surface (Fig. 8-1). The enamel cap characteristically appears more radiopaque than the other tissues because it is the most dense naturally occurring substance in the body; being 90% mineral, it causes the greatest attenuation of x-ray photons. The dentin is about 75% mineralized, and because of its lower mineral content its radiographic appearance is roughly comparable to that of bone. Dentin is smooth and homogeneous on radiographs because of its uniform morphology. The amelodentinal junction, between enamel and dentin, appears as a distinct interface that separates these two structures. The thin layer of cementum on the root surface has a mineral content (50%) comparable to that of dentin. Cementum is not usually apparent radiographically because the contrast between it and dentin is so low and it is so thin.

Diffuse radiolucent areas with ill-defined borders may be apparent radiographically on the mesial or distal aspects of teeth in the cervical regions between the cervical edge of the enamel cap and the crest of the alveolar ridge (Fig. 8-2). This phenomenon, called *cervical burnout*, is caused by the normal configuration of the affected teeth, which results in decreased x-ray absorption in the areas of question. Furthermore, the perception of these radiolucent areas results from the contrast with the adjacent, relatively opaque enamel and alveolar bone. Such radiolucencies should be anticipated in

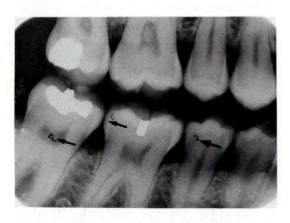

FIG. 8-1. Teeth are composed of enamel (*arrow* on the first molar), dentin (*arrow* on the second premolar), pulp (*arrow* on the second molar), and cementum (usually not visible radiographically).

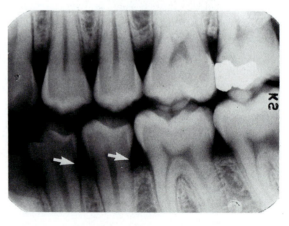

FIG. 8-2. Cervical burnout caused by overexposure of the lateral portions of teeth between the enamel and alveolar crest (*arrows*).

almost any tooth and not be confused with root surface caries, which frequently have a similar appearance.

The pulp of normal teeth is composed of soft tissue and consequently appears radiolucent. The chambers and root canals containing the pulp extend from the interior of the crown to the apices of the roots. Although the shape of most pulp chambers is fairly uniform within morphologic tooth groups, there are great variations among individuals in the size of the pulp chambers and the extent of pulp horns. Such variations in the proportions and distribution of the pulp must be anticipated and verified radiographically when planning restorative procedures.

In normal fully formed teeth the root canal may be apparent extending to the apex of the root and an apical foramen is usually recognizable. In other normal teeth the canal may appear to be constricted in the region of the apex and not discernible in the last millimeter or so of its length (Fig. 8-3). In this case the canal may occasionally exit on the side of the tooth, just short of the radiographic apex. Lateral canals may occur as branches of an otherwise normal root canal. They may extend to the apex and end in a normal discernible foramen or may exit the side of the root. In either case there would be two (or more) terminal foramina that might cause endodontic treatment to fail if not identified (Fig. 8-4).

At the end of a developing tooth root the pulp canal diverges and the walls of the root rapidly taper to a knife edge (Fig. 8-5). In the recess formed by the root walls and extending a short distance beyond is a small rounded radiolucent area in the trabecular bone, surrounded by a thin layer of hyperostotic bone. This is the dental papilla, the formative organ of the dentin and the primordium of the pulp, bounded by its bony crypt. Only as the tooth reaches maturity do the pulpal walls in the apical region begin to constrict and finally come into close apposition, completing the root and establishing a root canal of relatively uniform caliber. Awareness of this sequence and its radiographic pattern is often useful in evaluating the developing tooth's stage of maturation and helps avoid misidentifying the apical radiolucency as a periapical lesion.

In a mature tooth the shape of the pulp chamber and canal may change. With aging there is gradual

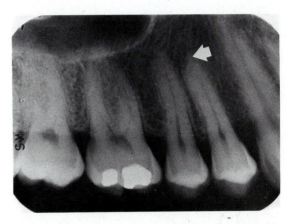

FIG. 8-4. Although the root canal is not radiographically visible in the apical 2 mm of a tooth, anatomically it is present *(arrow)*.

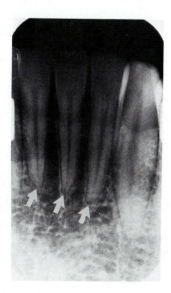

FIG. 8-3. Root canals open at the apices of adult incisors *(arrows)*.

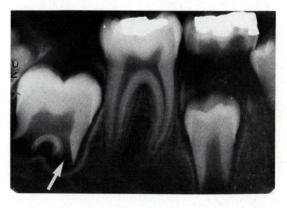

FIG. 8-5. A developing root shown by divergent apex around the dental papilla *(arrow)*, which is enclosed by an opaque bony crypt.

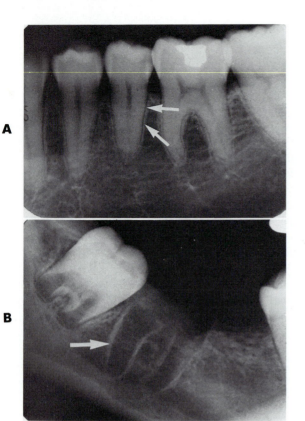

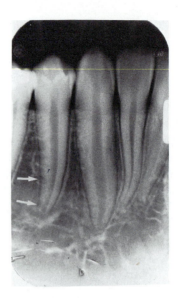

FIG. 8-7. The lamina dura is poorly visualized on the distal surface of this premolar *(arrows)* but is well seen on the mesial surface.

FIG. 8-6. The lamina dura *(arrows)* appears as a thin opaque layer of bone around teeth, **A,** and around a recent extraction socket, **B.**

deposition of secondary dentin and obliteration of the pulp.[14] This process begins apically, proceeds coronally, and may lead to pulp obliteration. Trauma to the tooth (e.g., from caries, a blow, restorations, attrition, or erosion) also may stimulate dentin production, leading to a reduction in size of the pulp chamber and canals. In such cases there will usually be evidence of the source of the pathologic stimulus. In the case of a blow to the teeth, however, only the patient's recollection may suggest the true reason for the reduced pulp chamber size.

SUPPORTING STRUCTURES
Lamina dura

A radiograph of sound teeth in a normal dental arch will show that the tooth sockets are bounded by a thin white or radiopaque shadow, the lamina dura (Fig. 8-6). This image is continuous with the shadow of the cortical bone at the alveolar crest. The radiographic appearance of the lamina dura suggests that it represents a thin layer of dense bone

(the so-called cribriform plate or alveolar bone proper).

On the basis of its appearance, the lamina dura seems to be an extension of the lining of the bony crypt that surrounds each tooth during development. Its name, lamina dura (hard layer), is derived from its radiographic appearance and its various descriptions as a thin layer of compact bone,[5,6,8,11] cortical bone, or bundle bone. It is little thicker and no more highly mineralized than the trabeculae of cancellous bone in the area. Its radiographic appearance is caused by the fact that the x-ray beam passes tangentially through many times the thickness of the thin bony wall, which results in its observed attenuation.[10]

The appearance of the lamina dura on radiographs may be variable. When the x-ray beam is so angled that it projects directly through a relatively long expanse of the structure, the lamina dura will appear radiopaque and well defined. If, however, the beam is directed more obliquely so as not to be so attenuated, the lamina dura will appear more diffuse or may not be discernible at all. In fact, although the supporting bone in a healthy arch is intact, it is frequently difficult to identify a lamina dura completely surrounding every root on each film, even though it is usually evident to some extent about the roots on each film (Fig. 8-7). In addition, small variations and disruptions in the continuity of the lamina dura may represent superimpositions of trabecular pattern and small nu-

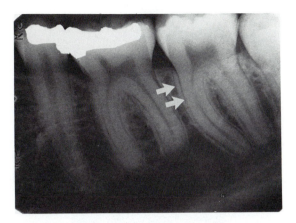

FIG. 8-8. A double periodontal ligament space and lamina dura *(arrows)* may be seen when there is a convexity of the proximal surface of the root.

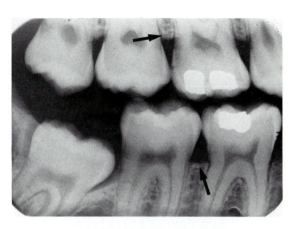

FIG. 8-9. The alveolar crests *(arrows)* are seen as cortical borders of the alveolar bone.

trient canals passing from the mandibular bone to the periodontal ligament.

The thickness and density of the lamina dura on the radiograph vary with the amount of occlusal stress to which the tooth is subjected. The lamina dura is wider and more dense about the roots of teeth in heavy occlusion, and thinner and less dense or even indiscernible about teeth that are not subjected to occlusal function. This phenomenon results from the bones' reaction to stress.

The image of a double lamina dura is not uncommon where the mesial or distal surfaces of roots present two elevations in the path of the x-ray beam. A common example of this is seen on the buccal and lingual eminences on the mesial surface of mandibular first molar roots (Fig. 8-8).

The appearance of the lamina dura is a valuable diagnostic feature. The presence of an intact lamina dura around the apex of a tooth strongly suggests a vital pulp (although acute periapical infections may occasionally occur in which there has not been sufficient time for erosion of the lamina dura to occur). Because of the variable appearance of the lamina dura, however, the absence of its image around an apex on a radiograph may be normal. Rarely, in the absence of disease the lamina dura may be absent from a molar root extending into the maxillary sinus. The clinician is therefore advised to consider other signs and symptoms as well as the integrity of the lamina dura when establishing a diagnosis and treatment.

Alveolar crest

The gingival margin of the alveolar process that extends between the teeth is apparent on properly exposed radiographs as a radiopaque line and is referred to as the alveolar crest (Fig. 8-9). The level of this bony crest is considered normal when it is not more than 1.5 mm from the cementoenamel junction of the adjacent teeth. The alveolar crest may recede apically with age and show marked resorption with periodontal disease. Radiographs can demonstrate only the position of the crest; determining the significance of its level is primarily a clinical problem. (See Chapter 16.)

The length of the normal alveolar crest in a particular region depends on the distance between the teeth in question. In the anterior region the crest is reduced to only a point of bone between close-set incisors. Posteriorly it is flat, aligned parallel with and slightly below a line connecting the cementoenamel junctions of the adjacent teeth. The crest of the bone is continuous with the lamina dura and forms a sharp angle with it. Rounding of these sharp junctions is indicative of periodontal disease.

The image of the crest varies from a dense layer of cortical bone to a smooth surface without cortical bone. In the latter case the trabeculae at the surface are of normal size and density. In the posterior regions this range of radiodensity of the crest is presumed to be normal if the bone is at a proper level in relation to the teeth. The absence of an image of cortex between the incisors, however, is considered by many to be an indication of incipient disease, even though the level of the bone is not abnormal.

Periodontal ligament space

Because the periodontal ligament (PDL) is composed primarily of collagen, it appears as a radio-

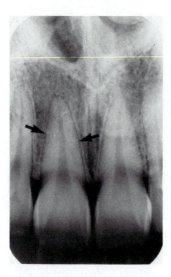

FIG. 8-10. The periodontal ligament space *(arrows)* is seen as a narrow radiolucency between the tooth root and lamina dura.

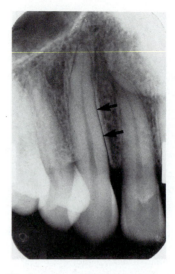

FIG. 8-11. The periodontal ligament space appears wide on the mesial surface of this canine *(arrows)* and thin on the distal surface.

lucent space between the tooth root and the lamina dura. This space begins at the alveolar crest, extends around the portions of the tooth roots that are within the alveolus, and returns to the alveolar crest on the opposite side of the tooth (Fig. 8-10). The PDL varies in width from patient to patient, from tooth to tooth in the same individual, and even from location to location around one tooth (Fig. 8-11). Usually it is thinner in the middle of the root and slightly widened near the alveolar crest and root apex, which arrangement suggests that the fulcrum of physiologic movement is in the region where the PDL is thinnest. The thickness of the ligament relates to the degree of function, because the PDL is thinnest about the roots of embedded teeth and those that have lost their antagonists. The reverse is not necessarily true, however, because an appreciably wider space is not regularly observed in persons with especially heavy occlusion or bruxism.

The appearance of a double PDL space is created by the shape of the tooth. When the x-ray beam is directed so two convexities of a root surface appear on a film, the double PDL space will be seen (Fig. 8-8).

Cancellous bone

The cancellous bone (also called *trabecular bone* or *spongiosa*) lies between the cortical plates in both jaws. It is composed of thin radiopaque plates and rods (trabecula) surrounding many small ra-

diolucent pockets of marrow. The radiographic pattern of the trabeculae shows considerable intra- and interpatient variability, which must be recognized as a normal variation and not a manifestation of disease. To evaluate the trabecular pattern in a specific area, one should examine their distribution, size, and density and compare them throughout both jaws. This will frequently demonstrate that a particularly suspect region is characteristic for the individual.

The trabeculae in the anterior maxilla are typically thin and numerous, forming a fine, granular, dense pattern (Fig. 8-12), and the marrow spaces are consequently small and relatively numerous. In the posterior maxilla the trabecular pattern is usually quite similar to that in the anterior maxilla, although the marrow spaces may be slightly larger.

In the anterior mandible the trabeculae are somewhat thicker than in the maxilla, resulting in a coarser pattern (Fig. 8-13), with trabecular plates that are oriented more horizontally. The trabecular plates are also fewer than in the maxilla, and the marrow spaces correspondingly larger. In the posterior mandible the periradicular trabeculae and marrow spaces may be comparable to those in the anterior mandible but are usually somewhat larger (Fig. 8-14). The trabecular plates are oriented mainly horizontally in this region also. Below the apices of the mandibular molars the number of trabeculae dwindle still more. In some cases the area from just below the molar roots to the inferior

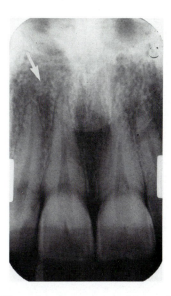

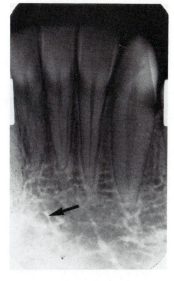

FIG. 8-12. The trabecular pattern in the anterior maxilla is characterized by fine trabecular plates and multiple small trabecular spaces *(arrow)*.

FIG. 8-13. The trabecular pattern in the anterior mandible is characterized by coarser trabecular plates and larger marrow spaces *(arrow)* than in the anterior maxilla.

border of the mandible may appear to be almost devoid of trabeculae.* Occasionally the trabecular spaces in this region will be very irregular with some so large that they mimic pathologic lesions.

Where there is apparent absence of trabeculae that may suggest the presence of disease, it is often revealing to examine previous radiographs of the region in question. This will help determine whether the current appearance represents a change from a prior condition. An abnormality is more likely when the comparison indicates that there has been a change in the trabecular pattern. If prior films are not available, it is frequently useful to repeat the radiographic examination at a reduced exposure, because this will often demonstrate the presence of an expected but sparse trabecular pattern that was overexposed and burned out in the initial projection. Finally, if prior films are not available and reduced exposure does not allay the examiner's apprehension, it may be appropriate to

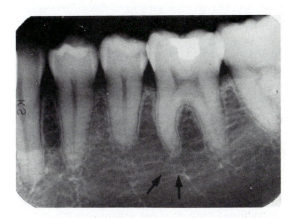

FIG. 8-14. The trabecular pattern in the posterior mandible is quite variable, generally showing large marrow spaces and sparce trabeculation, especially inferiorly *(arrows)*.

expose another radiograph at a later time to monitor for ominous changes. Again, it is emphasized that there may be considerable variation in trabecular pattern between patients so it is important in evaluating a trabecular pattern for any individual that all regions of the jaws be examined. This will enable the dentist to determine what the general nature of the particular pattern is and whether there are any areas that deviate appreciably from that norm.

The buccal and lingual cortical plates of the man-

---

*The distribution and size of the trabeculae throughout both jaws show a relationship to the thickness (and strength) of the adjacent cortical plates. It may be speculated that where the cortical plates are thick (e.g., in the posterior region of the mandibular body) internal bracing by the trabeculae is not required, so they are relatively few except where required to support the alveolae. By contrast, in the maxilla and anterior region of the mandible, where the cortical plates are relatively thin and less rigid, trabeculae are more numerous and lend internal bolstering to the jaw.

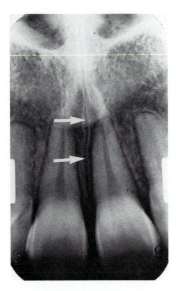

FIG. 8-15. The intermaxillary suture *(arrows)* appears as a curving radiolucency in the midline of the maxilla.

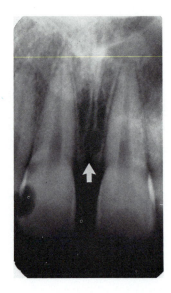

FIG. 8-16. The intermaxillary suture may terminate in a V-shaped widening *(arrow)* at the alveolar crest.

dible and maxilla do not cast a discernible image on periapical radiographs.

MAXILLA
Intermaxillary suture

The intermaxillary suture (also called *median palatal suture*) appears on intraoral periapical radiographs as a thin radiolucent line in the midline between the two portions of the maxilla (Fig. 8-15). It extends from the alveolar crest between the central incisors superiorly through the anterior nasal spine and continues posteriorly between the maxillary palatine processes to the posterior aspect of the hard palate. It is not unusual for this narrow radiolucent suture to terminate at the alveolar crest in a small rounded or V-shaped enlargement (Fig. 8-16). The suture is limited by two parallel radiopaque borders of thin cortical bone in each maxilla. The radiolucent region is usually of uniform width. The adjacent cortical margins may be either smooth or slightly irregular. The appearance of the intermaxillary suture will depend on both anatomic variability and the angulation of the x-ray beam through the suture.

Anterior nasal spine

The anterior nasal spine is most frequently demonstrated on periapical radiographs of the maxillary central incisors (Fig. 8-17). Located in the midline, it lies some 1.5 to 2 cm above the alveolar crest, usually at or just below the junction of the inferior

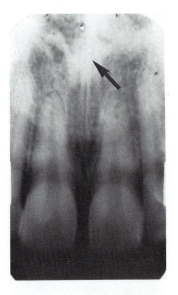

FIG. 8-17. The anterior nasal spine is seen as an opaque V-shaped projection from the floor of the nasal fossa in the midline *(arrow)*.

end of the nasal septum and the inferior outline of the nasal fossa. It is radiopaque because of its bony composition and is usually V shaped.

Nasal fossa

Because the air-filled nasal fossa (cavity) lies just above the oral cavity, its radiolucent image may be apparent on intraoral radiographs of the

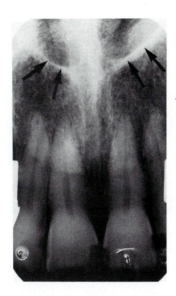

FIG. 8-18. The anterior floor of the nasal fossa *(arrows)* appears as opaque lines extending laterally from the anterior nasal spine.

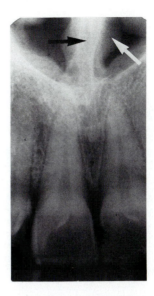

FIG. 8-19. The nasal septum *(black arrow)* arises directly above the anterior nasal spine and is covered on each side by nasal mucosa *(white arrow)*.

maxillary teeth, especially in central incisor projections. On periapical radiographs of the incisors the inferior border of the fossa appears as a radiopaque line extending bilaterally away from the base of the anterior nasal spine (Fig. 8-18). Above this line is the radiolucent space of the inferior portion of the fossa. If the radiograph was made with the x-ray beam directed in the sagittal plane, the relatively radiopaque nasal septum will be seen arising in the midline from the anterior nasal spine (Fig. 8-19). The shadow of the septum may appear wider than anticipated, and not sharply defined, because the image is a superimposition of septal cartilage and vomer bone. Also the septum frequently deviates slightly from the midline, and its plate of bone (the vomer) is somewhat curved.

The nasal cavity contains the hazy shadows of the inferior conchae extending from the right and left lateral walls for varying distances toward the septum. These conchae fill varying amounts of the lateral portions of the fossa (Fig. 8-20). The floor of the nasal fossa and a small segment of the nasal cavity not uncommonly are projected high onto a maxillary canine radiograph (Fig. 8-21). Also, in the posterior maxillary region, the floor of the nasal cavity and a portion of the fossa above it may be

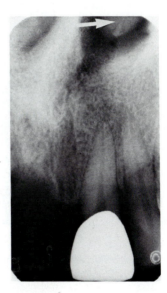

FIG. 8-20. The mucosal covering of the inferior concha *(arrow)* is occasionally visualized in the nasal fossa.

seen in the region of the maxillary sinus.* It may falsely convey the impression of a septum in the sinus or a limiting superior sinus wall (Fig. 8-22).

---

*It is not possible from a single radiograph to determine which of two superimposed structures is in front of or behind the other unless the conclusion is based on an awareness of the anatomic features and relationships.

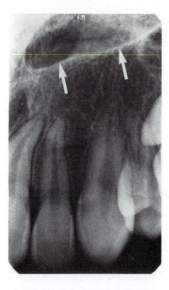

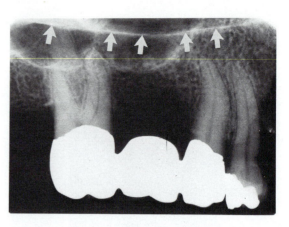

FIG. 8-22. The floor of the nasal fossa *(arrows)* extends posteriorly superimposed with the maxillary sinus.

FIG. 8-21. The floor of the nasal fossa *(arrows)* may often be seen extending above the maxillary lateral incisor and canine.

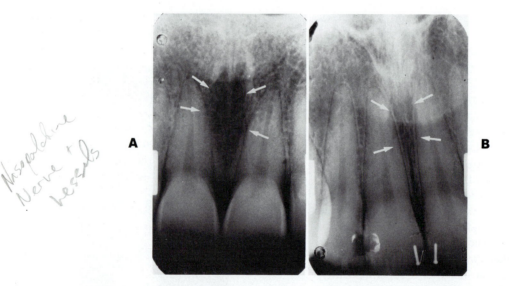

FIG. 8-23. A, The incisive foramen appears as an ovoid radiolucency *(arrows)* between the roots of the central incisors. **B,** Note its borders, which are diffuse but within normal limits.

Incisive foramen

The incisive foramen (also called *nasopalatine* or *anterior palatine foramen*) in the maxilla is the oral terminus of the nasopalatine canal. It transmits the nasopalatine vessels and nerves (which may participate in the innervation of the maxillary central incisors) and lies in the midline of the palate behind the central incisors at approximately the junction of the median palatine and incisive sutures. Its radiographic image is usually projected between the roots, and in the region of the middle and apical thirds, of the central incisors (Fig. 8-23). The foramen varies markedly in its radiographic shape, size, and sharpness. It may appear smoothly symmetric, with numerous forms, or very irregular with a well-demarcated or ill-defined border. The position of the foramen is also variable and may be recognized at the apices of the central incisor roots, near the alveolar crest, anywhere in between, or extending over the entire distance. The

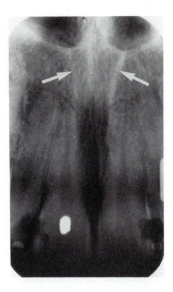

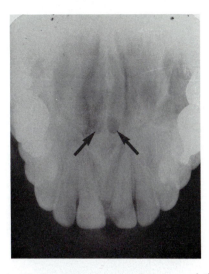

FIG. 8-25. The superior foramina of the nasopalatine canal *(arrows)* appear just lateral to the nasal septum and posterior to the anterior nasal spine.

FIG. 8-24. The lateral walls of the nasopalatine canal *(arrows)* extend from the incisive foramen to the floor of the nasal fossa.

great variability of its radiographic image is primarily the result of (1) the differing angles at which the x-ray beam is directed for the maxillary central incisors and (2) some variability in its anatomic size.

Familiarity with the incisive foramen is important because it is a potential site of cyst formation. An incisive canal cyst is radiographically discernible: it frequently causes an enlargement of the foramen and canal that is readily perceived. The presence of a cyst is presumed where the width of the foramen exceeds 1 cm or when enlargement can be demonstrated on successive radiographs. Also, if the radiolucency of the normal foramen is projected over the apex of one central incisor, it may suggest a pathologic periapical condition. In the absence of pathosis, however, there will be no clinical symptoms and the lamina dura about the central incisor in question will be intact.

The lateral walls of the nasopalatine canal are not usually seen but on occasion can be visualized on a projection of the central incisors as a pair of radiopaque lines running vertically from the superior foramina of the nasopalatine canal to the incisive foramen (Fig. 8-24).

Superior foramina of the nasopalatine canal

The nasopalatine canal originates at two foramina in the floor of the nasal cavity. The openings are on each side of the nasal septum, close to the anteroinferior border of the nasal cavity, and each branch passes downward somewhat anteriorly and medially to unite with the canal from the other side in a common opening, the incisive (nasopalatine) foramen. The superior foramina of the canal occasionally appear in projections of the maxillary incisors, especially when an exaggerated vertical angle is used. When apparent radiographically, they can be recognized as two radiolucent areas above the apices of the central incisors in the floor of the nasal cavity near its anterior border and on both sides of the septum (Fig. 8-25). They are usually round or oval, although they make take a variety of outlines depending on the angle of projection.

Lateral fossa

The lateral fossa (also called *incisive fossa*) is a gentle depression in the maxilla near the apex of the lateral incisor (Fig. 8-26). On periapical projections of this region it may appear diffusely radiolucent. The image will not be misinterpreted as a pathologic condition, however, if the radiograph is examined for an intact lamina dura about the root of the lateral incisor. This finding, coupled with absence of clinical symptoms, suggests normalcy of the bone.

Nose

The soft tissue of the tip of the nose is frequently seen in projections of the maxillary central and

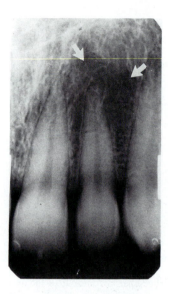

FIG. 8-26. The lateral fossa is a diffuse radiolucency *(arrows)* in the region of the apex of the lateral incisor because of a depression in the maxilla at this location.

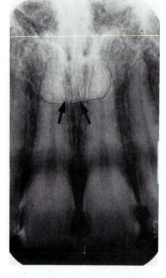

FIG. 8-27. The soft tissue outline of the nose *(arrows)* is superimposed on the anterior maxilla.

lateral incisors, superimposed over the roots of these teeth. The image of the nose has a uniform, slightly opaque appearance with a sharp border (Fig. 8-27). Occasionally the radiolucent nares can be identified, especially when a steep vertical angle is used.

Nasolacrimal canal

The nasolacrimal canal is formed by the nasal and maxillary bones. It runs from the medial aspect of the anteroinferior border of the orbit inferiorly, to drain under the inferior concha into the nasal cavity. Occasionally it can be visualized on periapical radiographs in the region above the apex of the canine, especially when steep vertical angulation is used (Fig. 8-28). The nasolacrimal canals are routinely seen on maxillary occlusal projections (Chapter 11) in the region of the molars (Fig. 8-29).

Maxillary sinus

The maxillary sinus, like the other paranasal sinuses, is an air-containing cavity lined with mucous membrane. It develops by the invagination of mucous membrane from the nasal cavity. Being the largest of the paranasal sinuses, it normally occupies virtually the entire body of the maxilla. Its function is unknown.

The sinus may be considered as a three-sided pyramid, with its base the medial wall adjacent to

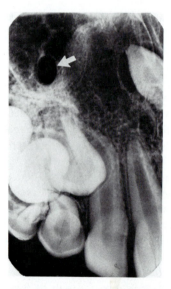

FIG. 8-28. The nasolacrimal canal *(arrow)* is occasionally seen near the apex of the canine when steep vertical angulation is used. Note the mesiodens (supernumerary tooth) superior to the central incisor.

the nasal cavity and its apex extending laterally into the zygomatic process of the maxilla. Its three sides are (1) the superior wall forming the floor of the orbit, (2) the anterior wall extending above the premolars, and (3) the posterior wall bulging above the molar teeth and maxillary tuberosity.[3] The sinus communicates with the nasal cavity via the ostium

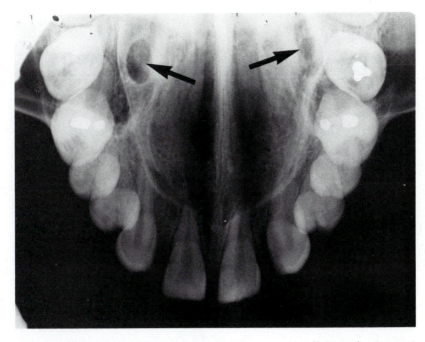

FIG. 8-29. The nasolacrimal canals are commonly seen as ovoid radiolucencies *(arrows)* on maxillary occlusal projections.

some 3 to 6 mm in diameter under the posterior aspect of the middle turbinate.

The borders of the maxillary sinus appear on periapical radiographs as a thin, delicate, tenuous radiopaque line (actually the thin layer of cortical bone) (Fig. 8-30). In the absence of disease it appears continuous, but on close examination it can be seen to have small interruptions in its smoothness or density. These discontinuities are probably illusions caused by superimposition of small marrow spaces. In adults the sinuses are usually seen to extend from the distal aspect of the canine to the posterior wall of the maxilla above the tuberosity.

The maxillary sinuses show considerable variation in size. They enlarge during childhood, achieving mature size by the age of 15 to 18 years.[9] They may change during adult life in response to environmental factors. The right and left sinuses usually appear similar in shape and size, although occasionally there is marked asymmetry. The floors of the maxillary sinus and nasal cavity will be seen on dental radiographs at approximately the same level around the age of puberty. In older individuals the sinus may extend farther into the alveolar process, and in the posterior region of the maxilla its floor may appear considerably below the level of the floor of the nasal cavity. Anteriorly each sinus

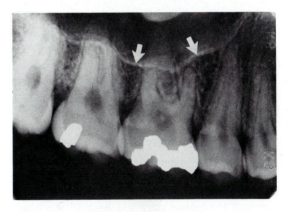

FIG. 8-30. The inferior border of the maxillary sinus *(arrow)* appears as a thin radiopaque line near the apices of the maxillary premolars and molars.

is restricted by the canine fossa and is usually seen to sweep superiorly, crossing the level of the floor of the nasal cavity in the premolar or canine region. Consequently, on periapical radiographs of the canine the floors of the sinus and nasal cavity are often superimposed and may be seen crossing one another, forming an inverted Y in the area (Fig. 8-31). The outline of the nasal fossa is usually heavier and more diffuse than that of the thin, delicate cortical bone denoting the sinus. The degree of

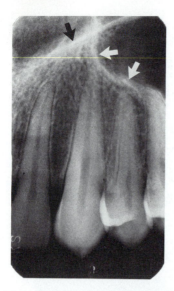

FIG. 8-31. The anterior border of the maxillary sinus *(white arrows)* crosses the floor of the nasal fossa *(black arrow)*.

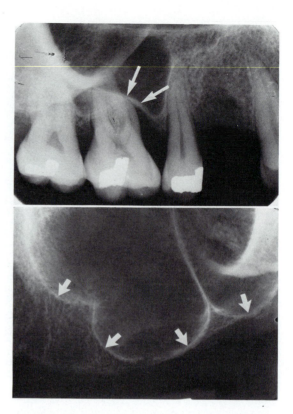

FIG. 8-32. The floor of the maxillary sinus *(arrows)* extends toward the crest of the alveolar ridge in response to missing teeth.

extension of the maxillary sinus into the alveolar process is extremely variable. In some projections the floor of the sinus will be well above the apices of the posterior teeth; in others it may extend well beyond the apices toward the alveolar ridge. In response to a loss of function (associated with the loss of posterior teeth) the sinus may expand farther into the alveolar bone, occasionally extending to the alveolar ridge (Fig. 8-32).

The roots of the molars usually lie in close apposition to the maxillary sinus. Root apices may project anatomically into the floor of the sinus, causing small elevations or prominences. The thin layer of bone covering the root will be seen as a fusion of the lamina dura and floor of the sinus. Rarely there may be defects in the bony covering of the root apices in the sinus floor, and a periapical radiograph will fail to show lamina dura covering the apex. When the rounded sinus floor dips between the buccal and palatal molar roots and is medial to the premolar roots, the projection of the apices will be superior to the floor. This appearance conveys the impression that the roots project into the sinus cavity, which is an illusion. It will be observed that as the positive vertical angle of the projection is increased the roots medial to the sinus appear to project farther into the sinus cavity. In contrast, the roots lateral to the sinus will appear to either move out of the sinus or farther away from it as the angle is increased.

The intimate relationship between sinus and teeth leads to the possibility that clinical symptoms originating in the sinus may be perceived in the teeth, and vice versa. This proximity of sinus and teeth is in part a consequence of the gradual developmental expansion of the maxillary sinus, which thins the sinus walls and opens the canals that traverse the anterolateral and posterolateral walls and carry the superior alveolar nerves. The nerves are then in intimate contact with the membrane lining the sinus. As a result, an acute inflammation of the sinus is frequently accompanied by pain in the maxillary teeth innervated by that portion of the nerve proximal to the insult. Subjective symptoms in the area of the maxillary posterior teeth may require careful analysis to differentiate tooth pain from sinus pain.

Frequently, thin radiolucent lines of uniform width will be found within the image of the maxillary sinus (Fig. 8-33). These are the shadows of nutrient canals or grooves in the lateral sinus walls that accommodate the posterior superior alveolar vessels, their branches, and the accompanying su-

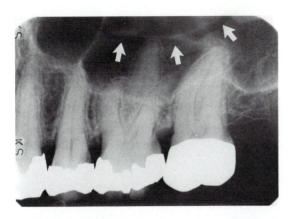

FIG. 8-33. Vascular canals *(arrows)* in the lateral wall of the maxillary sinus.

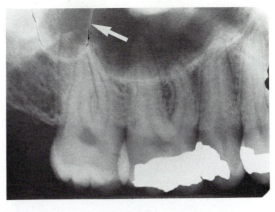

FIG. 8-34. A septum *(arrow)* in the maxillary sinus formed by a low ridge of bone on the sinus wall. (See also Figure 8-32, lower illustration.)

perior alveolar nerves. Although they may be found coursing in any direction (including vertically), they are usually seen running a curved posteroanterior course that is convex toward the alveolar process. On occasion they may be found to branch, and rarely also to extend outside the image of the sinus and continue as an interradicular channel. Because such vascular markings are not seen in the walls of cysts, they may serve to distinguish a normal sinus from a cyst.

Often the image of the maxillary sinus is found to be traversed by an occasional, or several, radiopaque lines (Fig. 8-34). These *septa* represent folds of cortical bone projecting a few millimeters away from the floor and wall of the antrum. They are usually oriented vertically, although horizontal bony ridges also occur, and it is not uncommon for them to vary in number, thickness, and length. Septa are believed by some to have been formed through the uneven resorption of bone as the sinus was pneumatized, but others hold that they are remnants of incompletely fused cavities from which the sinus formed.[4] They appear on many periapical intraoral radiographs, though seldom in extraoral projections, because for this view the x-ray beam is seldom directed tangential to them. Although septa appear to separate the sinuses into distinct compartments, this is seldom the case, because the septa are usually of limited extent. It has been reported however,[13] that in 1% to 10% of examined skulls, complete septa did in fact divide the sinus into individual compartments, each compartment with separate ostia for drainage. Septa deserve attention because they sometimes mimic periapical pathoses, and the chambers they create

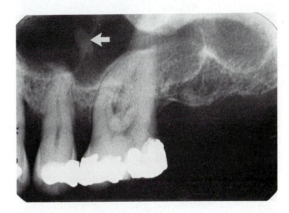

FIG. 8-35. This bony nodule *(arrow)* is a normal variant of the floor of the maxillary sinus.

in the alveolar recess may complicate the search for a root fragment displaced into the sinus.

The floor of the maxillary sinus will occasionally show small radiopaque projections, which are nodules of bone (Fig. 8-35). These must be differentiated from root tips, which they resemble in shape. In contrast to a root fragment, which is quite homogeneous in appearance, the bony nodules often show trabeculation; and although they may be quite well defined, at certain points on their surface they blend with the trabecular pattern of adjacent bone. A root fragment may also be recognized by the presence of a root canal. It is not uncommon to see the floor of the nasal fossa in periapical views of the posterior teeth superimposed on the maxillary sinus (Fig. 8-22). The floor of the nasal fossa is usually oriented more or less horizontally, depending on film placement, and is superimposed

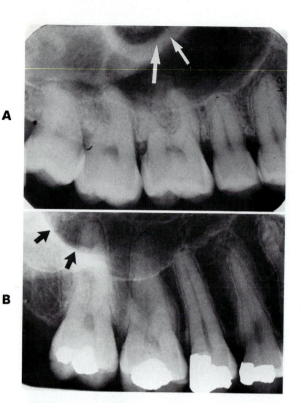

A

B

FIG. 8-36. The zygomatic process of the maxilla *(arrows)* protrudes laterally from the maxillary wall. Its size may be quite variable: small with thick borders, **A**, or large with thin borders, **B**.

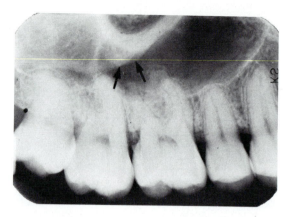

FIG. 8-37. The inferior border of the zygomatic arch *(arrows)* extends posteriorly from the inferior portion of the zygomatic process of the maxilla.

high on maxillary views. The image, a solid opaque line, will frequently appear somewhat thicker than the adjacent sinus walls and septa.

Zygomatic process and zygomatic bone

The zygomatic process of the maxilla is an extension of the lateral maxillary surface that arises in the region of the apices of the first and second molars and serves as the articulation for the zygomatic bone. On periapical radiographs the zygomatic process appears as a U-shaped radiopaque line with its open end directed superiorly. The enclosed rounded end is projected in the apical region of the first and second molars (Fig. 8-36). The size, width, and definition of the zygomatic process are quite variable; and its image may be large, depending on the angle at which the beam was projected. The maxillary antrum may expand laterally into the zygomatic process of the maxilla (and even into the zygomatic bone after the maxillozygomatic suture has fused), thereby resulting in a relatively increased radiolucent region within the U-shaped image of the process. When the sinus

has recessed deep within the process (and perhaps into the zygomatic bone), the image of the air space within the process is dark and typically the walls of the process will be rather thin and well defined (in contrast to the very dark radiolucent air space). When there is relatively little penetration of the maxillary process by the sinus (usually in younger individuals or those who have maintained their posterior teeth and vigorous masticatory function), the image of the walls of the zygomatic process tends to be somewhat thicker, and the appearance of the sinus in this region will be somewhat smaller and more opaque.

The inferior portion of the zygomatic bone may be seen extending posteriorly from the inferior border of the zygomatic process of the maxilla (thereby completing the zygomatic arch between the zygomatic processes of the maxillary and temporal bones). It can be identified as a uniform gray or white radiopacity over the apices of the molars (Fig. 8-37). The prominence of the molar apices superimposed on the shadow of the zygomatic bone, and the amount of detail supplied by the radiograph, will depend in part on the degree of aeration (pneumatization) of the zygomatic bone that has occurred, on the bony structure, and on the orientation of the x-ray beam.

Nasolabial fold

Periapical radiographs of the premolar region are frequently traversed by an oblique line demarcating a region that appears to be covered by a veil of slight radiopacity (Fig. 8-38). The line of contrast is sharp, and the area of increased radiopacity is

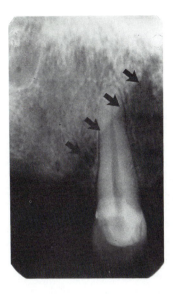

FIG. 8-38. The nasolabial fold *(arrows)* extends across the canine-premolar region.

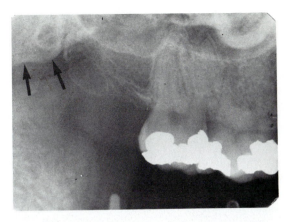

FIG. 8-39. Pterygoid plates *(arrows)* located posterior to the maxillary tuberosity.

posterior to the line. The line is the nasolabial fold, and the opaque veil is the thick cheek tissue superimposed on the teeth and the alveolar process. The image of the fold becomes more evident with age, as the repeated creasing of the skin along the line (where the elevator of the lip, zygomatic head, and orbicularis all insert into the skin) and the degeneration of the elastic fibers finally leads to the formation and deepening of permanent folds. This radiographic feature frequently proves useful in identifying the side of the maxilla represented by a film of the area if it is edentulous and few other anatomic features are demonstrated.

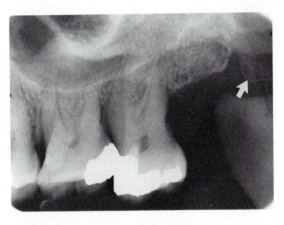

FIG. 8-40. The hamular process *(arrow)* extends downward from the medial pterygoid plate.

Pterygoid plates

The medial and lateral pterygoid plates lie immediately posterior to the tuberosity of the maxilla. The image of these two plates is extremely variable, and on many intraoral radiographs of the third molar area they do not appear at all. When they are apparent, they almost always cast a single radiopaque homogeneous shadow without any evidence of trabeculation (Fig. 8-39). Extending inferiorly from the medial pterygoid plate may be seen the hamular process (Fig. 8-40), which on close inspection can show trabeculae.

MANDIBLE
Symphysis

Radiographs of the region of the mandibular symphysis in infants demonstrate a radiolucent line through the midline of the jaw between the images of the forming deciduous central incisors (Fig. 8-41). This suture usually fuses by the end of the first year of life, after which it is no longer radiographically apparent. It is not frequently encountered on dental radiographs because few young patients have cause to be examined radiographically. If this radiolucency is found in older individuals, it is abnormal and may suggest a fracture or a cleft.

Genial tubercles

The genial tubercles (also called the *mental spine*) are located on the lingual surface of the mandible slightly above the inferior border and in the midline. They are bony protuberances, more or less spine shaped, that often are divided into a right and left prominence and a superior and in-

ferior prominence. They serve to attach the ge-
nioglossus muscles (at the superior tubercles) and
the geniohyoid muscles (at the inferior tubercles)
to the mandible. They usually are well visualized
on standard mandibular occlusal radiographs as one

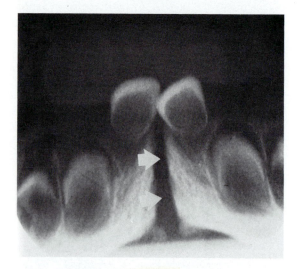

FIG. 8-41. Mandibular symphysis *(arrows)* in a newborn
infant. Note the bilateral supernumerary primary incisors
adjacent to it.

or more small projections (Fig. 8-42). Their appearance on periapical radiographs of the mandibular incisor region may be quite variable: a radiopaque mass (3 to 4 mm in diameter) in the midline
below the incisor roots (Fig. 8-43), of nondescript
shape or suggesting the demonstration of muscle
attachments; or they may not be apparent at all.
When not delineated on periapical films, a small
radiolucent dot (the lingual [spinous] foramen) surrounded by the cortical wall of the termination of
the incisive branch of the mandibular canal, is usually quite apparent (Fig. 8-44).

Mental ridge

On periapical radiographs of the mandibular central incisors the mental ridge may occasionally be
seen as two radiopaque lines sweeping bilaterally
forward and upward toward the midline (Fig. 8-
45). They are of variable width and density and
may be found to extend from low in the premolar
area on each side up to the midline, where they lie
just inferior to or are superimposed on the mandibular incisor tooth roots. The image of the mental
ridge is most prominent when the beam is directed

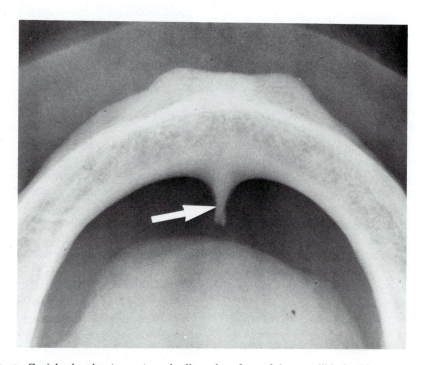

FIG. 8-42. Genial tubercles *(arrow)* on the lingual surface of the mandible in this cross sectional
mandibular occlusal view.

parallel with the surface of the mental tubercle*
(as when using the bisecting technique).

___

*The bony mass on the labial surface of the midline of the
mandible in humans is a mechanical brace that evolved to withstand bending stresses that occur during forceful mastication.
So the jaw can be deformed slightly during mastication, it must
have some flexibility. Consequently, the triangular mental protuberance is not solid cortical bone but a more pliable shell of
dense bone supported by stress-accommodating trabecular bone.

Mental fossa

The mental fossa is a depression on the labial
aspect of the mandible extending laterally from the
midline and above the mental protuberance. Because of the resulting thinness of jawbone in this
area, the image of this depression may be similar
to that caused by the submandibular fossa (see below) and may, likewise, be mistaken for periapical
disease involving the incisors (Fig. 8-46).

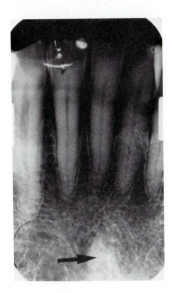

FIG. 8-43. The genial tubercles *(arrow)* appear as a radiopaque mass, in this case without evidence of the lingual foramen.

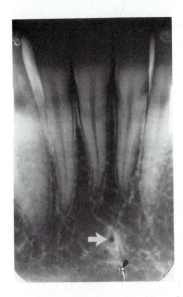

FIG. 8-44. Lingual foramen *(arrow)*, with a sclerotic border, in the symphyseal region of the mandible.

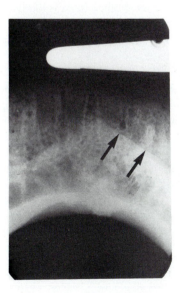

FIG. 8-45. Mental ridge *(arrows)* on the anterior surface
of the mandible seen as a radiopaque ridge.

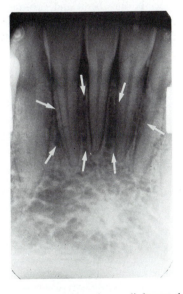

FIG. 8-46. The mental fossa is a radiolucent depression
on the anterior surface of the mandible *(arrows)* between
the alveolar ridge and mental ridge.

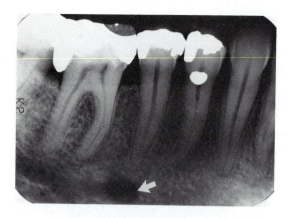

FIG. 8-47. The mental foramen *(arrow)* appears as an oval radiolucency near the apex of the second premolar.

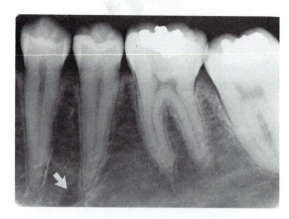

FIG. 8-48. The mental foramen *(arrow)* (over apex of the second premolar) may simulate periapical disease. Continuity of the lamina dura around the apex, however, indicates the absence of periapical abnormality.

Mental foramen

The mental foramen is usually the anterior limit of the inferior dental canal that is apparent on radiographs (Fig. 8-47). Its image is quite variable, and it may be identified only about half the time, because the opening of the mental canal is directed superiorly and posteriorly.* As a result the usual view of the premolars is not projected through the long axis of the canal opening. This circumstance is responsible for the variable appearance of the mental foramen. Although the wall of the foramen is of cortical bone, the density of the foramen's image will vary, as will the shape and definition of its border. It may be round, oblong, slitlike, or very irregular and partially or completely corticated. The foramen is seen about halfway between the lower border of the mandible and the crest of the alveolar process usually in the region of the apex of the second premolar. Also, since it lies on the surface of the mandible, the position of its image in relation to the tooth roots is influenced by projection angulation. It may be projected anywhere from just mesial of the permanent first molar roots to as far anterior as mesial of the first premolar root. The image of two mental foramina, one above the other, has also been observed.

When the mental foramen is projected over one of the premolar apices, it may mimic periapical disease (Fig. 8-48). In such cases evidence of the inferior dental canal extending to the suspect radiolucency or a detectable lamina dura in the area would suggest the true nature of the dark shadow. It is well to point out, however, that the relative thinness of the lamina dura superimposed with the radiolucent foramen may result in considerable "burnout" of the lamina dura image, which will complicate its recognition. Nevertheless, a second radiograph from another angle is likely to show the lamina dura clearly as well as some shift in position of the radiolucent foramen relative to the apex.

Mandibular canal

The radiographic image of the mandibular canal is a dark linear shadow with thin radiopaque superior and inferior borders cast by the lamella of bone that bounds the canal (Fig. 8-49). Sometimes the borders are seen only partially or not at all. The width of the canal shows some interpatient variability but is usually rather constant anterior to

---

*At birth the mental canal exits the mandible at a 90° angle to the surface, or it may even be directed slightly anteriorly. As the mandible grows and shifts anteriorly, however, the canal changes its direction as noted above. This change takes place during infancy and childhood and is caused by forward growth in the body of the mandible. The nerves and accompanying vessels follow at a much slower rate. Also the differential in growth rates of periosteum and bone contributes to this change in direction of the mental canal. The periosteum is firmly attached to the condyles, but relatively loosely attached to the body of the mandible. Consequently the bone slips along beneath the periosteum, changing the direction of the canal.

---

†The mandibular foramen is the proximal opening of the mandibular canal. It is usually located on the lingual surface, near the center, of the mandibular ramus. Its image is customarily described as radiolucent and funnel shaped, although this appearance will be altered if the slightly radiopaque lingula is projected over the shadow of the foramen. The lingula is a bony process that varies in size and partially covers the anteromedial aspects of the foramen, as may be visualized on extraoral radiographs that include the ramus.

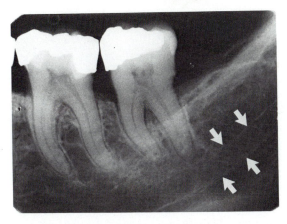

FIG. 8-49. Mandibular canal. *Arrows* denote its radiopaque superior and inferior cortical borders.

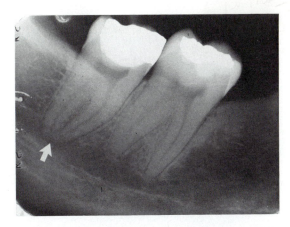

FIG. 8-50. The mandibular canal superimposed over the apex of a molar causes the image of the periodontal ligament space to appear wider *(arrow)*. The presence of an intact lamina dura, however, indicates that there is no periapical disease.

the third molar region. The canal's course may be apparent between the mandibular foramen† and the mental foramen. Only rarely is the image of its anterior continuation toward the midline discernible on the radiograph.

The relationship of the mandibular dental canal to the roots of the lower teeth may vary, from one in which there is close contact with all molars and the second premolar to one in which the canal has no intimate relation to any of the posterior teeth. In the usual picture, however, the canal is in contact with the apex of the third molar and the distance between it and the other roots increases as it progresses anteriorly. When the apices of the molars are projected over the canal, the lamina dura may be overexposed, conveying the impression of a missing lamina or a thickened PDL space that is more radiolucent than apparently normal for the patient (Fig. 8-50). To assure the soundness of such a tooth, other clinical testing procedures must be employed (e.g., vitality testing). Because the canal is usually located just inferior to the apices of the posterior teeth, altering the vertical angle for a second film of the area is not likely to separate the images of the apices and canal.

Nutrient canals

Nutrient canals carry a neurovascular bundle and appear as radiolucent lines of fairly uniform width.[2] They are most often seen on mandibular periapical radiographs running vertically from the inferior dental canal directly to the apex of a tooth (Fig. 8-51) or into the interdental space between the mandibular incisors (Fig. 8-52). They are visible in about 5% of all patients and are more frequent in

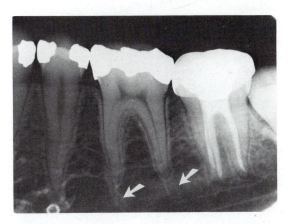

FIG. 8-51. Nutrient canals *(arrows)* demonstrated by radiopaque cortical borders, descend from the mandibular first molar.

blacks, males, older persons, and individuals with high blood pressure or advanced periodontal disease.[7,12] Because they are anatomic spaces with walls of cortical bone, their images occasionally have hyperostotic borders. At times a nutrient canal will appear, perpendicular to the cortex, as a small round radiolucency and be mistaken for a pathologic radiolucency to the inexperienced diagnostician.

Mylohyoid ridge

The mylohyoid ridge (also called the *internal oblique ridge*) is a slightly irregular crest of bone on the lingual surface of the mandibular body. Extending from the area of the third molars to the

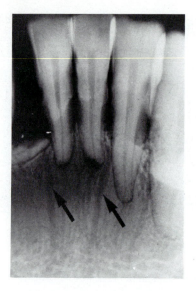

FIG. 8-52. Nutrient canals demonstrated by radiolucencies *(arrows)* in the anterior mandible of a patient with severe periodontal disease.

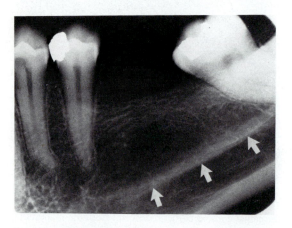

FIG. 8-54. The mylohyoid ridge *(arrows)* may be dense, especially when a radiograph is exposed with excessive negative angulation.

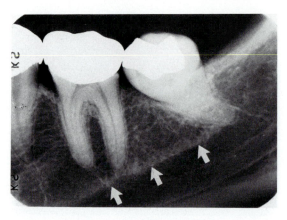

FIG. 8-53. Mylohyoid ridge *(arrows)* running at the level of the molar apices and above the mandibular canal.

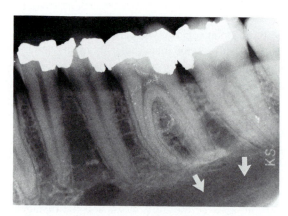

FIG. 8-55. Submandibular gland fossa *(arrows)*, indicated by a poorly defined radiolucency and sparse trabecular bone below the mandibular molars.

lower border of the mandible in the region of the chin, it serves as an attachment for the mylohyoid muscle. Its radiographic image runs diagonally downward and forward from the area of the third molars to the premolar region, at approximately the level of the apices of the posterior teeth (Fig. 8-53). Sometimes this image is superimposed on the images of the molar roots. The margins of the image are not usually well defined but appear quite diffuse and of variable width. The contrary is also observed, however, where the ridge is relatively dense with sharply demarcated borders (Fig. 8-54).

It will be more evident on periapical radiographs when the beam is positioned with excessive negative angulation. In general, as the ridge becomes less well-defined, its anterior and posterior limits blend gradually with the surrounding bone.

Submandibular gland fossa

On the lingual surface of the mandibular body, immediately below the mylohyoid ridge in the molar area, there is frequently a depression in the bone. This concavity accommodates the submandibular gland and often appears as a radiolucent area with the sparse trabecular pattern characteristic of the region (Fig. 8-55). This trabecular pattern is even less defined on radiographs of the area because it is superimposed on the relatively reduced

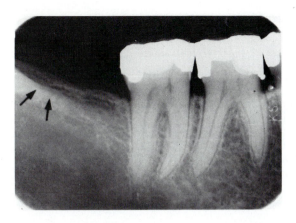

FIG. 8-56. External oblique ridge *(arrows)* seen as a radiopaque line near the alveolar crest in the mandibular third molar region.

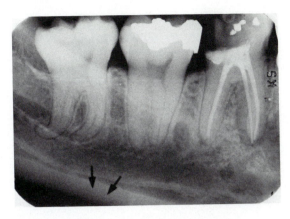

FIG. 8-57. The inferior border of the mandible *(arrows)* is seen as a dense broad radiopaque band.

mass of the concavity. The radiographic image of the fossa is sharply limited superiorly by the mylohyoid ridge, and inferiorly by the lower border of the mandible, but is poorly defined anteriorly (in the premolar region) and posteriorly (at about the ascending ramus). Although the image may appear strikingly radiolucent, accentuated as it is by the dense mylohyoid ridge and inferior border of the mandible, awareness of its possible presence should preclude its being confused with a bony lesion by the inexperienced clinician.

External oblique ridge

The external oblique ridge is a continuation of the anterior border of the mandibular ramus. It follows an anteroinferior course lateral to the alveolar process, being relatively prominent in its upper part and jutting considerably on the outer surface of the mandible in the region of the third molar (Fig. 8-56). This bony elevation gradually flattens, and usually disappears, at about where the alveolar process and mandible join below the first molar. The ridge is a line of attachment of the buccinator muscle. Characteristically, it is projected onto posterior periapical radiographs superior to the mylohyoid ridge, with which it runs an almost parallel course. It appears as a radiopaque line of varying width, density, and length, blending at its anterior end with the shadow of the alveolar bone.

Inferior border of the mandible

Occasionally the inferior mandibular border will be seen on periapical projections (Fig. 8-57) as a characteristically dense, broad, radiopaque band of bone.

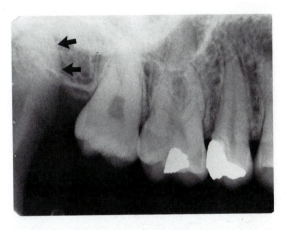

FIG. 8-58. Coronoid process of the mandible *(arrows)* superimposed on the maxillary tuberosity.

Coronoid process

The image of the coronoid process of the mandible is frequently apparent on periapical radiographs of the maxillary molar region as a triangular radiopacity, with its apex directed superiorly and somewhat anteriorly, superimposed on the region of the third molar (Fig. 8-58). In some cases it may appear as far forward as the second molar and be projected above, over, or below these molars depending on the position of the jaw and the projection of the x-ray beam. Usually the shadow of the coronoid process will be homogeneous, although internal trabeculation can be seen in some cases. Its appearance on maxillary molar radiographs results from the downward and forward movement of the mandible when the mouth is open. Consequently, if the opacity reduces the diagnostic

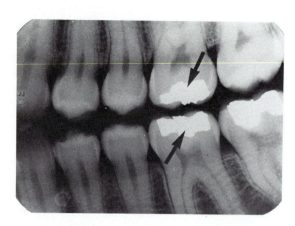

FIG. 8-59. Amalgam restorations appear completely radiopaque *(arrows).*

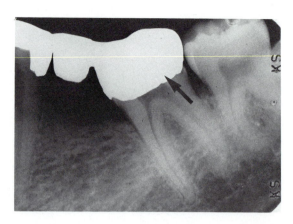

FIG. 8-60. A cast gold crown, appearing completely radiopaque *(arrow)*, serves as the terminal abutment of a bridge.

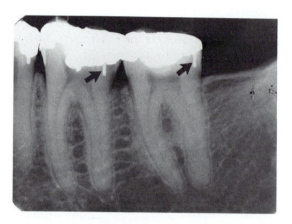

FIG. 8-61. Stainless steel pins *(arrows)* provide retention for amalgam restorations.

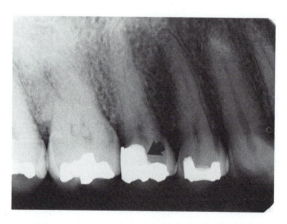

FIG. 8-62. Base material *(arrow)* is usually radiopaque.

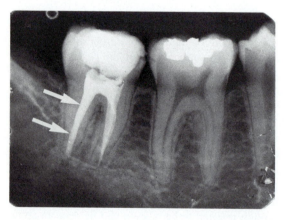

FIG. 8-63. Gutta-percha *(arrows)* is a radiopaque rubberlike material used in endodontic therapy.

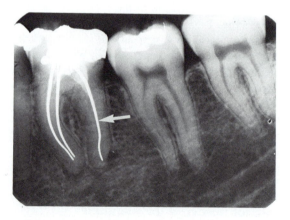

FIG. 8-64. Silver points *(arrow)* were used to fill the root canals in this patient.

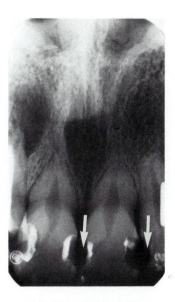

FIG. 8-65. Radiolucent silicate restorations *(arrows)* were placed over a base to protect the pulp in this patient.

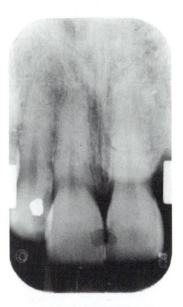

FIG. 8-66. Composite restorations may be radiolucent and may suggest caries but can be recognized by their well-demarcated border with dentin.

value of a film and the film must be remade, the second view should be acquired with the mouth minimally open. (This contingency must be considered whenever this area is radiographically examined.) On occasion, and especially when its shadow is dense and homogeneous, the coronoid process will be mistaken for a root fragment by the neophyte clinician. The true nature of the shadow can be easily demonstrated by obtaining two radiographs with the mouth in different positions and noting the change in position of the suspect shadow.

RESTORATIVE MATERIALS

Restorative materials vary in their radiographic appearance—depending primarily on their thickness, density, and atomic number. Of these, the atomic number is most influential.

A variety of restorative materials may be recognized on intraoral radiographs. The most common, silver amalgam, is completely radiopaque (Fig. 8-59). Gold is equally opaque to x rays, whether cast as a crown or inlay (Fig. 8-60) or condensed as gold foil. Stainless steel pins also appear radiopaque (Fig. 8-61). Often a calcium hydroxide base is placed in a deep cavity to protect the pulp. Although such base material may be radiolucent, most is radiopaque (Fig. 8-62). Another material of comparable radiopacity is gutta-percha, a rubberlike substance used to fill tooth canals dur-

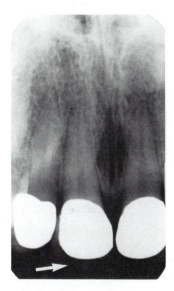

FIG. 8-67. Porcelain appears radiolucent *(arrow)* over a metal coping.

ing endodontic therapy (Fig. 8-63). Silver points were also used during endodontic therapy (Fig. 8-64). Other restorative materials that appear rather radiolucent on intraoral films include silicates, usually in combination with a base but now little used (Fig. 8-65), composite, usually in anterior teeth (Fig. 8-66), and porcelain, now usually fused to a metallic coping (Fig. 8-67). Composite restorative

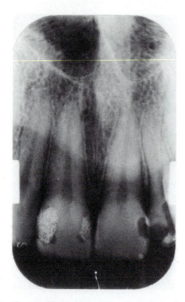

FIG. 8-68. Composite restorations containing particles of barium glass are radiopaque and not likely to be confused with caries.

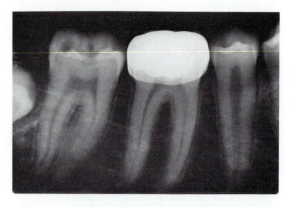

FIG. 8-69. Stainless steel crowns appear mostly radiopaque.

materials may also be opaque (Fig. 8-68). In addition, stainless steel crowns (Fig. 8-69) and orthodontic appliances around teeth (Fig. 8-70) are relatively radiopaque.

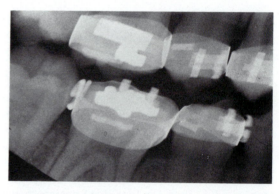

FIG. 8-70. Orthodontic appliances have a characteristic radiopaque appearance.

SPECIFIC REFERENCES

1. Blackman S: *An atlas of dental and oral radiology,* Bristol U.K., 1959, John Wright & Sons.
2. Britt G: A study of human mandibular nutrient canals, *Oral Surg* 44:635-645, 1977.
3. DuBrul EL: *Sicher's Oral anatomy,* ed 7, St Louis, 1980, Mosby.
4. Fairbanks DNE: Embryology and anatomy. In Bluestone CD, Stool SE (eds): *Pediatric otolaryngology,* Philadelphia, 1983, WB Saunders.
5. Elfenbaum A: Alveolar lamina dura, *Dent Radiogr Photogr* 31:21-29, 1958.
6. Goldman HM, Millsap JS, Brenman HS: Origin of registration of the architectual pattern, the lamina dura and the alveolar crest in the dental radiography, *Oral Surg* 10:749-758, 1957.
7. Greer D, Wege W, Wuehrmann A: The significance of nutrient canals appearing on intraoral radiographs, *IADR Abstr,* March 1968.
8. Ingram FL: *Radiology of the teeth and jaws,* London, 1950, Edward Arnold.

9. Killey HC, Kay LW: *The maxillary sinus and its dental implications,* Bristol U.K., 1975, John Wright & Sons.
10. Manson JD: The lamina dura, *Oral Surg* 16:432-438, 1963.
11. Miller SC: *Oral diagnosis and treatment,* New York, 1957, McGraw-Hill.
12. Patel J, Wuehrmann A: A radiographic study of nutrient canals, *Oral Surg* 42:693-701, 1976.
13. Wasson WW, Saunders SH, Cowen DE: *The lung and paranasal sinuses,* Springfield Ill, 1969, Charles C Thomas.
14. Morse DR: Age-related changes of the dental pulp complex and their relationship to systemic aging, *Oral Surg* 72:721-745, 1991.

9

in collaboration with ABDUL H. SHAWKAT

Intraoral Radiographic Examinations

Intraoral examinations are the backbone of dental radiography. There are three categories of intraoral radiographs: periapical, bitewing, and occlusal projections. Periapical radiographs should show all of a tooth, including the surrounding bone. Bitewing radiographs show only the crowns of teeth and the adjacent alveolar crests. Occlusal radiographs reveal an area of teeth and bone larger than periapical films.* A full-mouth set of radiographs consists of periapical and bitewing projections (Fig. 9-1) and, when well exposed and properly processed, can provide considerable diagnostic information to complement the clinical examination. As with any clinical procedure, it is important that the operator have a clear concept of the goal and criteria to evaluate the quality of performance. The operator who demonstrates the skill and pride required to expose a good full-mouth set of radiographs will be amply rewarded when it is time for radiographic interpretation.

Expose radiographs only when there is a clear diagnostic need for the information that the radiograph may provide. Accordingly, the frequency of such examinations will vary with the individual circumstances of each patient. (See Chapter 4.)

CRITERIA OF QUALITY

Every radiographic examination should result in a radiograph of optimum diagnostic quality that incorporates the following features:

1. It records the complete areas of interest on the image. In case of intraoral periapical radiographs, it is essential to obtain the full length of the teeth's roots and at least 2 mm of the periapical bone.[13,17] Should there be evidence of a pathologic condition, the area of the entire lesion plus some surrounding normal bone should show on one radiograph. Sometimes it is impractical to achieve this on a periapical radiograph, and in such an instance an occlusal as well as an extraoral projection may be required. Bitewing examinations should demonstrate each proximal surface at least once.

2. The radiographs should have the least possible amount of distortion. Most distortion results from improper angulation of the x-ray beam rather than from curvature of the structures being examined as well as from inappropriate positioning of the film. Close attention to proper positioning of the film and x-ray tube results in diagnostically useful images.

3. Optimum density and contrast are essential for interpretation. Although tube current (mA), voltage (kVp), and exposure time are the most critical parameters influencing density and contrast, film processing also makes an important contribution to the quality of the radiograph. Faulty processing can adversely affect the quality of a properly exposed radiograph.

PERIAPICAL RADIOGRAPHY

Two intraoral projection techniques may be used for periapical radiography: the paralleling and bisecting-angle techniques. Although each has evolved as the result of efforts to minimize image distortion, most clinicians prefer the paralleling

---

*The term "film" is used in this chapter because the vast majority of intraoral radiographs are made with radiographic film. When intraoral CCD image receptors are used, the radiographic principles are the same as with radiographic film.

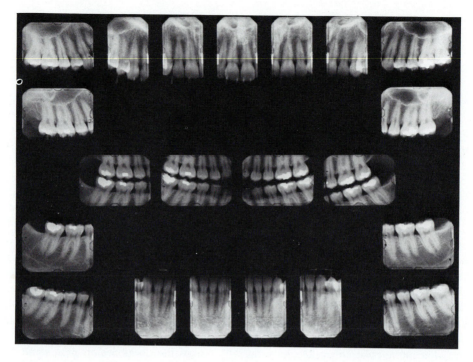

FIG. 9-1. Mounted full-mouth set of radiographs consisting of 17 periapical views and four bitewing views.

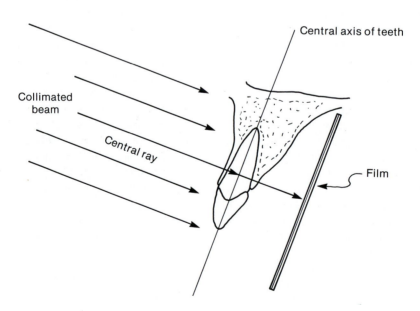

FIG. 9-2. Paralleling technique illustrating parallelism between long axis of tooth and film. Central ray is directed perpendicular to each.

technique because it provides a less distorted view of the dentition.[1] However, morphologic variations from mouth to mouth and even within the same oral cavity pose a variety of geometric problems that repeatedly emphasize that each technique has disadvantages and advantages and must be continually modified to accommodate the immediate circumstances.[1,3] The following discussion describes the principles and uses of the paralleling technique to obtain a full-mouth set of radiographs. When anatomic configuration (e.g., of palate, floor of the mouth) precludes strict adherence to the paralleling concept, one may have to make slight modifications within acceptable (recognized) limits. If the anatomic constraints are extreme, then use some of the principles of the bisecting-angle technique to accomplish the required film placement and to determine vertical angulation of the tube.[9] The bisecting technique is described later in this chapter.

Paralleling technique

The essence of the paralleling technique (also called the right-angle or long-cone technique) is that the x-ray film is supported parallel to the long axis of the teeth and the central ray of the x-ray beam is directed at right angles to the teeth and film (Fig. 9-2). This orientation of the film, teeth, and central ray minimizes geometric distortion.[1,10] To reduce geometric distortions further, it is important that the x-ray source be located relatively distant from the teeth. In addition, the use of a long source-to-object distance reduces the size of the apparent focal spot. These factors result in images with less magnification and increased definition.

Film-holding instruments. Use film-holding instruments to position the film properly in the patient's mouth and to maintain the film in position. To position the film parallel to the teeth and to project the periapical areas onto the film, position the film away from the teeth and toward the center of the mouth to use the maximum height of the palate. The long source-to-object distance used in the paralleling technique minimizes the disadvantages imposed by the increased object-to-film distance. For maxillary projections, the superior border of the film will generally rest at the height of the palatal vault in the midline. Similarly, for mandibular projections use the film to displace the tongue lingually to allow the inferior border of the film to rest on the floor of the mouth away from the mucosa on the lingual surface of the mandible.

A number of available commercial devices will hold the film parallel and at varying distances from the teeth:[2,8,9]

1. The XCP instruments (extension cone paralleling) (Fig. 9-3, *A*)
2. The Precision rectangular collimating instruments, which restrict the beam size at the patient's face to the size of the radiograph (Fig. 9-3, *B*)
3. The Stabe disposable film holder (Fig. 9-3, *C*)
4. The Snap-A-Ray intraoral film holder (Fig. 9-3, *D*)
5. A hemostat inserted through a flattened rubber bite block, which will serve in much the same manner as the Snap-A-Ray film holder (Fig. 9-3, *E*)

The Precision instrument (Isaac Masel, Philadelphia) and the XCP instrument (when used with a rectangular aiming device) (Rinn Corp., Elgin, IL) are recommended because they significantly reduce patient exposure.[4,14,15]

Angulation of tube head. Adjust the position of the x-ray machine tube head in the vertical and horizontal planes. Control the third dimension by bringing the end of the aiming cylinder up to the film-holding instrument or up to within 2 cm of the patient's face. When using the paralleling technique with an instrument that provides an external guide for positioning the aiming cylinder (such as the Precision instrument), it is most important to place the end of the open-ended cylinder flush with the guide.[4] This arrangement helps to eliminate most shield cuts* and assure that the central ray is oriented at right angles to the film.

Positioning the tube head to direct the beam downward from the horizontal, in the vertical plane, is described as positive vertical angulation; directing the beam upward is negative vertical angulation. The vertical angulation is usually described in plus or minus degrees, established by the dial on the side of the tube head. The horizontal direction of the beam primarily influences the degrees of overlapping of the images of the crowns at the interproximal spaces (Fig. 9-4).

---

*A shield cut is an artifact that appears as a clear unexposed area on a film. It is the result of misdirecting the beam so that the radiation does not completely cover the film.

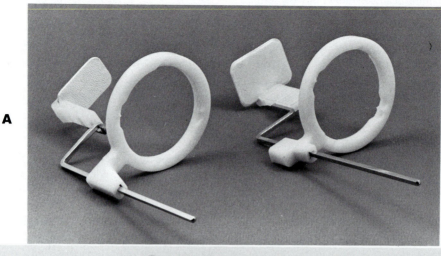

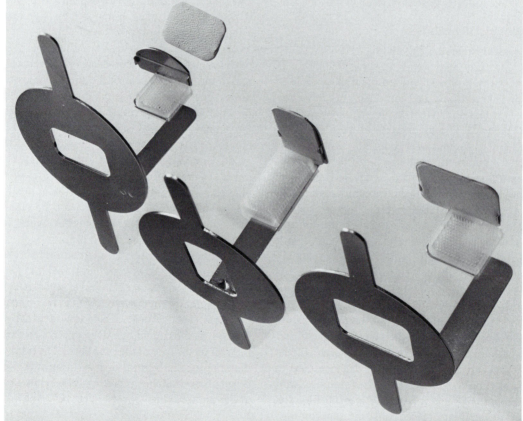

FIG. 9-3. Film-holding instruments. **A,** XCP instruments: instrument for anterior views *(left);* instrument for posterior views *(right)*. Aiming cylinder on x-ray tube head is positioned against localizing ring during use. **B,** Precision x-ray film holders showing instruments for posterior projections *(left* and *right)* and instrument for anterior projections *(middle)*. In use, cylinder on x-ray tube head is positioned against face-shield.

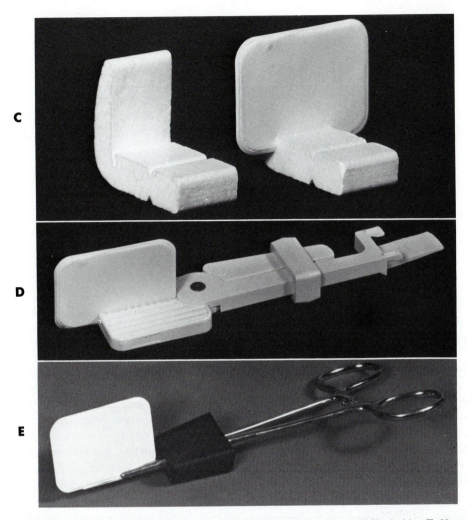

FIG. 9-3, cont'd. C, Stabe disposable film holders. **D,** Snap-A-Ray intraoral film holder. **E,** Hemostat and rubber bite block.

General steps for making an exposure

Greet and seat the patient. Position the patient upright in the chair with his or her back and head well supported and briefly describe the procedures that are about to be performed.* Position the dental chair low for maxillary projections and elevated for mandibular projections. Ask the patient to remove eyeglasses and all removable appliances. Drape the patient with a lead apron whether a single film or a full series is to be made. The supine position is occasionally used in intraoral radiography instead of an upright posture. This may most easily be accomplished by using reclining dental chairs, although an x-ray table may be used.[12] The use of the supine position does not affect the frequency and distribution of technique errors compared to using paralleling instruments in the upright position.[6] In addition, patients' reactions to the supine position are generally favorable, especially apprehensive patients.

Adjust the x-ray unit setting. Set the x-ray machine for the proper kVp, mA, and exposure time

---

*Do not comment on any discomfort the patient may experience during the procedure. The more apologetic the operator is, the more restive most patients will become. If it seems necessary to apologize for any discomfort, do it after the examination. Also, if the patient is experiencing considerable discomfort, probably the film-holding device is not being correctly manipulated.

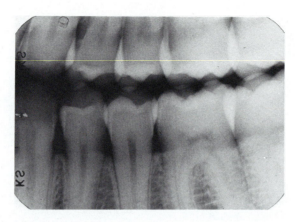

FIG. 9-4. Horizontal overlap of crowns resulting from misdirection of central ray.

according to the recommendations of the film manufacturer or to those experience has demonstrated to produce the highest-quality film with the least radiation.

Position tube head. Bring the tube head to the side to be examined to have it readily available after positioning the film.

Wash hands thoroughly. Wash your hands with soap and water, preferably in front of the patient or at least in an area where the patient can observe or be aware of the washing. Now put on disposable gloves.

Examine the oral cavity. Before placing the film in the mouth, examine the teeth to estimate their axial inclination, which influences the placement of the film. Also note tori or other obstructions that will modify film placement.

Position film. Remove the film from the film dispenser, insert it in the film-holding device, and position the film in the region of the patient's mouth to be examined. Leading with the apical end of the film, rotate the film into the oral cavity. Place the film as far from the teeth as practicable. This contradicts the principle that a short object-to-film distance decreases penumbra and increases sharpness and resolution. However, this compromise provides the maximum space available in the midline of the palate and the greater depth toward the center of the floor of the mouth. This added space permits the film to be oriented parallel with the long axis of the teeth. Make an effort to avoid contact with the very sensitive attached gingiva covering the alveolar processes when placing a film for either a mandibular anterior or posterior projection. Ask the patient to close, gently, holding the instrument and film in place.

When placing films intraorally, first rest the film gently on the palate or floor of the mouth. Next rotate the instrument either up or down until the bite block rests on the teeth to be radiographed. Then ask the patient to close. If the bite block is not on the teeth when the patient closes, the film moves into the palate or floor of the mouth and may cause discomfort. For the mandibular anterior projections, place the film gently on the floor of the mouth in front of the tip of the tongue near the second premolar. Ask the patient to close the mouth slowly. As the patient is closing, tip the instrument upward, and the film will move into the floor of the mouth with ease. Do not permit the film packet to contact the very sensitive attached gingiva on the lingual surface of the mandible.

To position the anterior Precision instrument, center the landmark on the support bar. Do not center on the bite block because it is slightly displaced to one side or the other. When using the XCP anterior instrument, center the landmark on the bite block.

Place a cotton roll between the bite block and the teeth opposite those being radiographed. Hold it in place with an orthodontic elastic. This helps to stabilize the instrument and in many cases contributes to patient comfort.

Position x-ray tube. Adjust the vertical and horizontal angulation of the tube head to correspond to the beam-guiding instrument. The end of the x-ray machine aiming cylinder must be flush or parallel with the face-shield of the Precision instrument or the guide ring of the XCP instrument. The aiming cylinder does not have to be centered on the face-shield. Alignment is satisfactory when the aiming cylinder covers the port and is within the limits of the face-shield. When not using a beam-guiding instrument, aim the central ray at the appropriate entry point on the skin (identified later in this chapter). It is wise to caution the patient not to move.

Make the exposure. After exposure, remove the film from the patient's mouth, dry it with a paper towel, and place it in an appropriate receptacle outside the exposure area.

Projections. A typical full-mouth set of radiographs consists of 21 films (Fig. 9-1):

Anterior periapical (use no. 1 film)
  Maxillary central incisors–1 projection
  Maxillary lateral incisors–2 projections
  Maxillary canines–2 projections
  Mandibular centrolateral incisors–2 projections
  Mandibular canines–2 projections
Posterior periapical (use no. 2 film)
  Maxillary premolars–2 projections
  Maxillary molars–2 projections
  Maxillary distomolar (as needed)–2 projections
  Mandibular premolars–2 projections
  Mandibular molars–2 projections
  Mandibular distomolar (as needed)–2 projections
Bitewing (use no. 2 film)
  Premolars–2 projections
  Molars–2 projections

Establish a regular sequence when making exposures to avoid overlooking individual projections. Make the anterior projections before the posterior projections as they cause less discomfort to the patient. The following description of procedures pertains to the paralleling technique. When using the paralleling technique, use film-holding instruments that also guide the position of the x-ray tube. Position each film-holding instrument to locate the film in the position described. Using a film-holding device with an external guide for film positioning automatically establishes the point of entry. However, if there appears to be a great discrepancy between the point of entry indicated by the device and the point described below, check the placement of the film-holding instrument and the position of the film.

PARALLELING TECHNIQUE

Maxillary central incisor projection

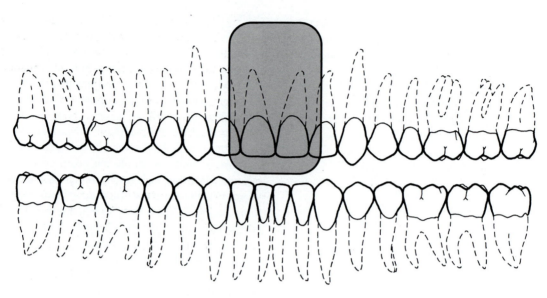

Image field. The field of view on these radiographs *(shaded area)* should include both central incisors and their periapical areas.

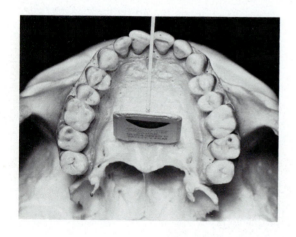

Film placement. Place a no. 1 film at about the level of the second premolars or first molars to take advantage of the maximum palatal height so that the entire length of the teeth can be projected on it. Have the film resting on the palate with its midline centered with the midline of the arch. Position the packet's long axis parallel to the long axis of the maxillary central incisors.

Maxillary central incisor projection

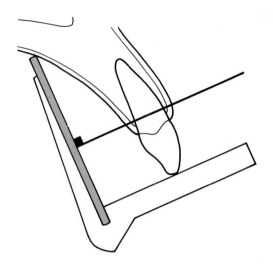

Projection of central ray.* Direct the central ray through the contact point of the central incisors and perpendicular to the plane of the films and roots of the teeth. Because the axial inclination of the maxillary incisors is about 15 to 20 degrees, the vertical angulation of the tube should be at the same positive angle. The tube should have 0 horizontal angulation.

---

*Projection of the central ray and point of entry are described in the discussion of the paralleling technique for instances when using a film-holding device without a tube-alignment ring or face-shield. When using a film-holding device with a tube-aligning ring or face-shield, position the device in the mouth to give the appropriate horizontal and vertical angulation.

Point of entry. Direct the point of entry of the central ray high on the lip, in the midline, just below the septum of the nostril. If there is an unusually low palatal vault or a palatal torus, it may be necessary to tilt the film holder positively and compromise a completely parallel relationship between the film and teeth to ensure including the periapical region on the image.

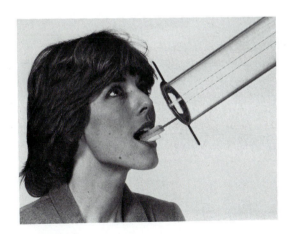

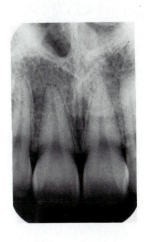

PARALLELING TECHNIQUE

Maxillary lateral projection

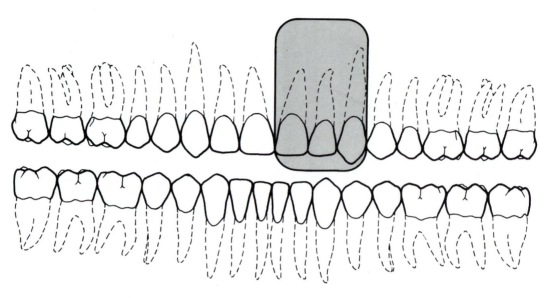

Image field. This projection should show the lateral incisor and its periapical field centered on the radiograph. Include the mesial interproximal area with the distal aspect of the central incisor on the radiograph so that no overlap is evident.

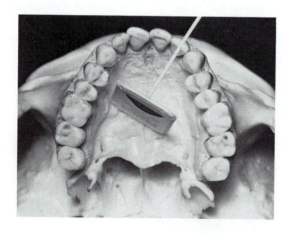

Film placement. Place a no. 1 film deep in the oral cavity parallel with the long axis and the mesiodistal plane of the maxillary lateral incisor.

Maxillary lateral projection

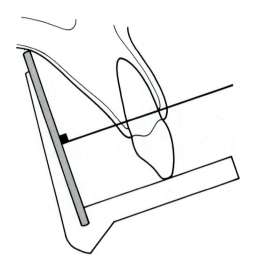

Projection of central ray. Direct the central ray through the middle of the lateral incisor, with no overlapping of the margins of the crowns at the interproximal space on its mesial aspect. Do not attempt to visualize the distal contact with the canine.

Point of entry. Orient the central ray to enter high on the lip about 1 cm from the midline.

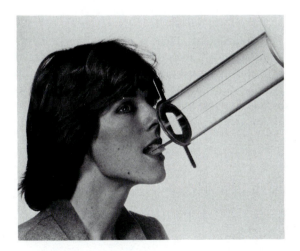

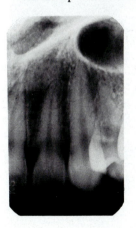

PARALLELING TECHNIQUE

Maxillary canine projection

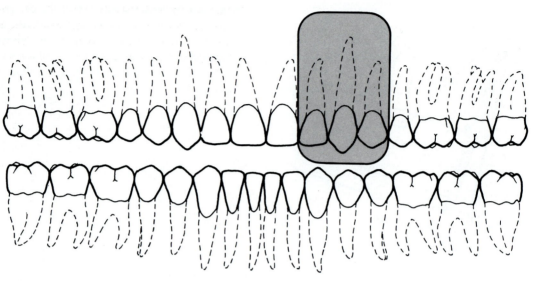

Image field. This projection should demonstrate the entire canine, with its periapical area, in the midline of the radiograph. Open the mesial contact area. Ignore the distal contact because it will be visualized on other projections.

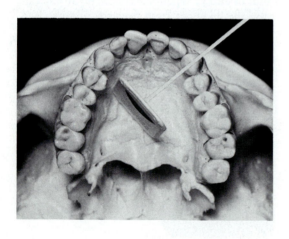

Film placement. Place a no. 1 film against the palate, well away from the palatal surface of the teeth. Orient the film packet with its anterior edge at about the middle of the lateral incisor and its long axis parallel with the long axis of the canine.

Maxillary canine projection

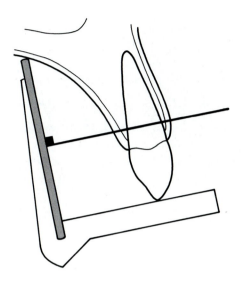

Projection of central ray. Position the holding instrument so it will direct the beam through the mesial contact of the canine. Do not attempt to open the distal contact.

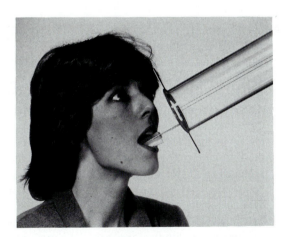

Point of entry. Direct the central ray through the canine eminence. The point of entry will be at about the intersection of the distal and inferior borders of the ala of the nose.

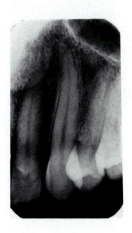

Maxillary premolar projection

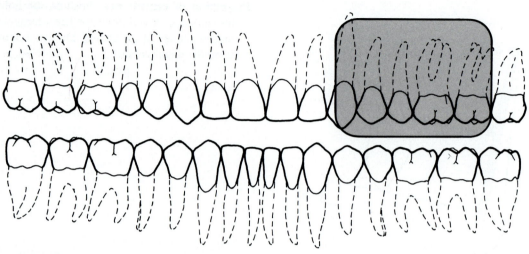

Image field. The radiograph for this region should include the images of the distal half of the canine and the premolars, and there will be room for at least the first molar.

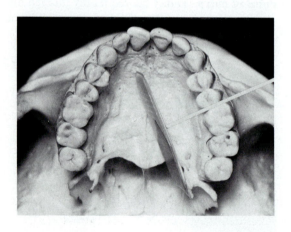

Film placement. Place a no. 2 film in the mouth with the long dimension parallel with the occlusal plane and in the midline. The packet should cover the distal half of the canine, the premolars, and the first molar; it will probably reach to the mesial portion of the second molar. Orient the Precision posterior instrument so that the tip of the canine is in the anterior groove of the bite block. This will ensure that the image includes the distal half of the canine. The exact position of the canine tip in this groove will depend on the size of the individual's mouth. The plane of the film should be nearly vertical to correspond with the long axis of the premolar teeth. Position the film-holding device so the long axis of the film is parallel with the mean buccal plane of the premolars. This will establish the proper horizontal angulation.

Maxillary premolar projection

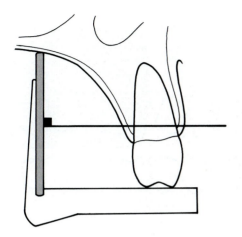

Projection of central ray. Direct the central ray perpendicular to the film. The horizontal angulation of the holding instrument should be adjusted to permit the beam to pass through the interproximal area between the first and second premolars.

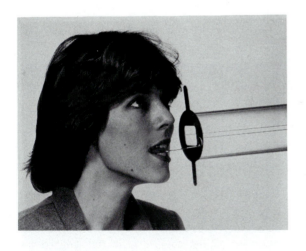

Point of entry. Place the holding instrument so the central ray will pass through the center of the second premolar root. This point is usually below the pupil of the eye.

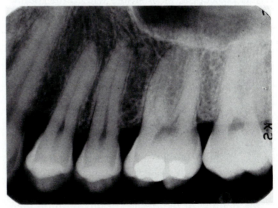

PARALLELING TECHNIQUE

Maxillary molar projection

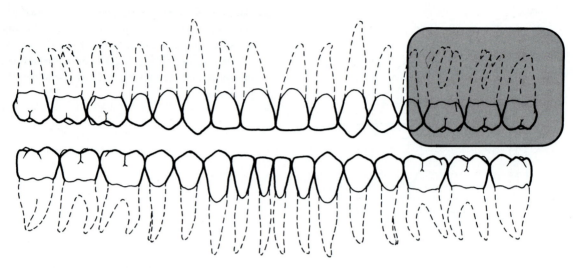

Image field. The radiograph of this region should show the images of the distal half of the second premolar, the three maxillary permanent molars, and some of the tuberosity. Include the same area on the film even if some or all molars are missing. If the third molar is impacted in an area other than the region of the tuberosity, a distal oblique or extraoral projection, such as panoramic or oblique lateral jaw, may be required.

Film placement. When placing the no. 2 film for this projection, position the wide dimension of the film nearly horizontal to minimize brushing the palate and dorsum of the tongue. When the film is in the region to be examined, rotate it into position with a firm and definite motion. This maneuver is important in avoiding the gag reflex, and resolute action by the operator enhances the patient's confidence. Place the film far enough posterior to cover the first, second, and third molar areas and some of the tuberosity. The anterior border should just cover the distal aspect of the second premolar. To cover the molars from crown to apices, place the film at the midline of the palate. In this position there should be room to orient the film parallel with the molar teeth. The mesial or distal rotation of the film-holding device should assure that the long axis of the film is parallel with the mean buccal plane of the molars (to establish the proper horizontal angulation). A shallow palate may require slightly tipping the holding instrument to avoid bending the film.

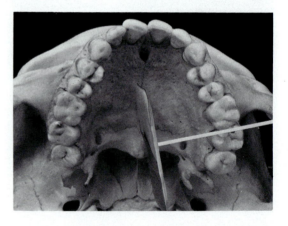

NOTE: In some cases the size of the mouth (length of the arch) will not permit positioning the film (holding device) as far posterior as recommended for the molar projection. However, by placing the film-holding device so that half of the tube-alignment ring or face-shield is behind the outer canthus of the eye, the molars and part of the tuberosity will usually be included in the image of the molar projection.

Maxillary molar projection

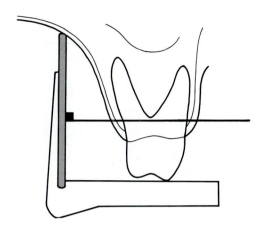

Projection of central ray. Direct the central ray perpendicular to the film. Adjust the horizontal angulation of the film-holding instrument to direct the beam at right angles to the buccal surfaces of the molar teeth. Orient the horizontal angulation of the Precision instrument so the lateral groove on the bite block is parallel with the mean buccal plane of the molars.

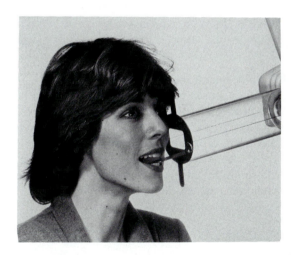

Point of entry. The point of entry of the central ray should be on the cheek below the outer canthus of the eye and the zygoma at the position of the maxillary second molar.

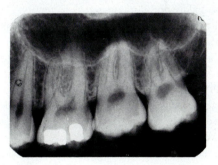

Maxillary distal oblique molar projection

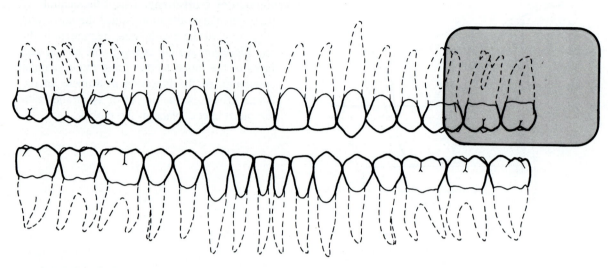

Image field. This projection provides a view of the maxillary tuberosity region more posterior than is usually seen in the molar projection. It allows detection or evaluation of impacted teeth or pathologic conditions in the bone of this area.

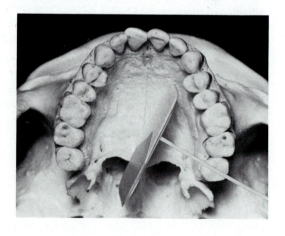

Film placement. Position the holding device with a no. 2 film in the molar region of the maxilla and rotate distally, angling the film across the midline so that the posterior border is away from the teeth of interest and the anterior border is near the molars on the side being radiographed. Position this film with a definite movement to minimize patient discomfort.

Maxillary distal oblique molar projection

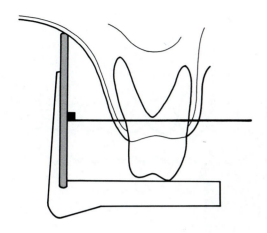

Projection of central ray. Direct the central ray from the posterior aspect through the third molar region and perpendicular to the angled film, projecting the more posterior objects anteriorly onto the film.

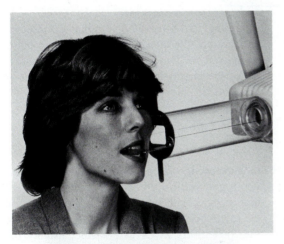

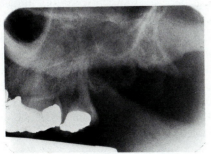

Point of entry. The central ray enters the maxillary third molar region just below the middle of the zygomatic arch, distal to the lateral canthus of the eye.

NOTE: Occasionally a hypersensitive patient gags when a film is placed for the usual maxillary molar projection. However, if a modified distal oblique projection is used, moving the posterior border of the film more medially is frequently less irritating to the patient, and the film is obtained with comfort. The patient's reaction of relief will indicate when a sufficient rotation has been achieved. Although this maneuver may result in some overlapping of the molar contact areas, these surfaces will be apparent on the bitewing projection. Slight overlapping of contact areas is preferable to no radiograph of the region.

PARALLELING TECHNIQUE

Mandibular centrolateral projection

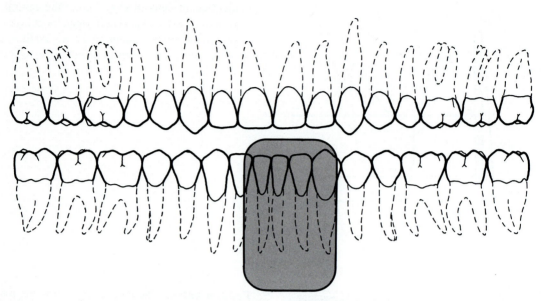

Image field. Center the image of the mandibular central and lateral incisors and their periapical areas on the film. Because the space in this area is frequently restricted, use two of the narrower anterior periapical films for the incisors to provide good coverage with minimal discomfort. In addition, the incisor contact areas are better visualized on two narrower anterior films because the angulation of the central ray can be adjusted for the contact area on each side.

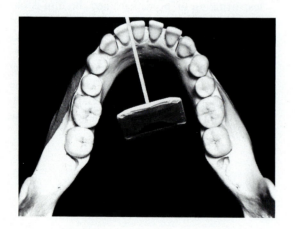

Film placement. Place the long dimension of the no. 1 film vertically behind the central and lateral incisors with the contact area centered and the lower border below the tongue. Position the film posteriorly as far as possible, usually between the premolars. With the film resting gently on the floor of the mouth as the fulcrum, tip the instrument downward until the film-holder bite block is resting on the incisors. Instruct the patient to close the mouth slowly. As the patient is closing slowly and the floor of the mouth is relaxing, rotate the instrument with the teeth as the fulcrum to align the film to be more parallel with the teeth.

Mandibular centrolateral projection

Projection of central ray. Orient the central ray through the interproximal space between the central and lateral incisor.

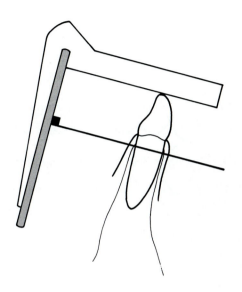

Point of entry. The central ray enters below the lower lip and about 1 cm lateral to the midline.

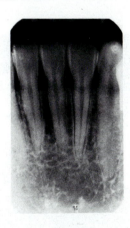

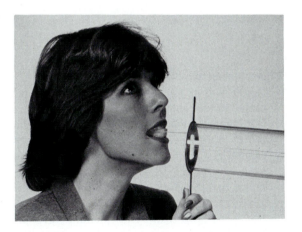

Mandibular canine projection

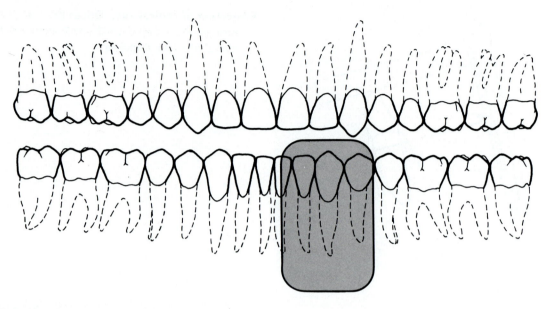

Image field. This image should show the entire mandibular canine and its periapical area. Open its mesial contact area. The distal contact will be included on other projections.

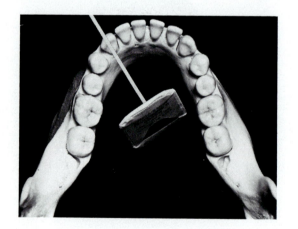

Film placement. Place a no. 1 film packet in the mouth with its long dimension vertical and the canine in the midline of the film. Position it as far lingual as the tongue and contralateral alveolar process will permit, with its long axis parallel and in line with the canine. The instrument must be tipped with the bite block on the canine before the patient is asked to close.

Mandibular canine projection

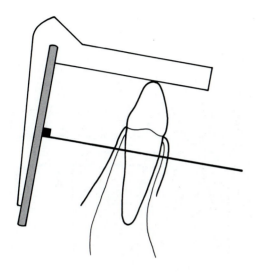

Projection of central ray. Direct the central ray through the mesial contact of the canine without regard to the distal contact.

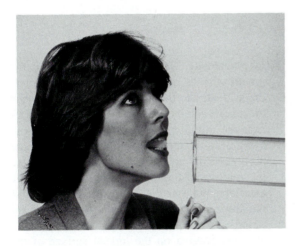

Point of entry. The point of entry will be nearly perpendicular from the ala of the nose, over the position of the canine, and about 3 cm above the inferior border of the mandible.

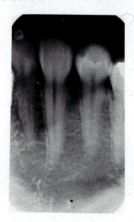

Mandibular premolar projection

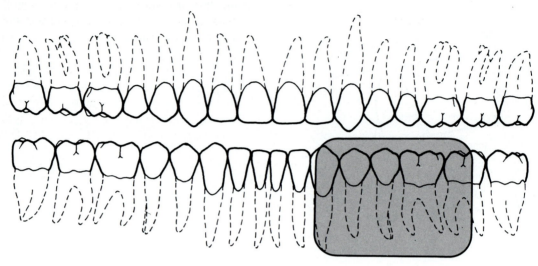

Image field. The radiograph of this area should show the distal half of the canine, the two premolars, and the first molar.

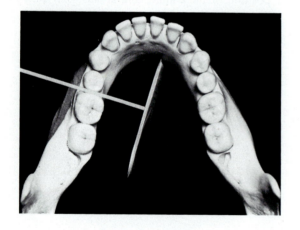

Film placement. Bring the no. 2 film into the mouth with its plane nearly horizontal. Rotate the lead edge to the floor of the mouth between the tongue and the teeth with the anterior border near the midline of the canine. Place the film away from the teeth to position it in the deeper portion of the mouth. Placing the film toward the midline also provides more room for the anterior border of the film in the curvature of the jaw as it sweeps anteriorly. Prevent the anterior border from contacting the very sensitive attached gingiva on the lingual surface of the mandible.

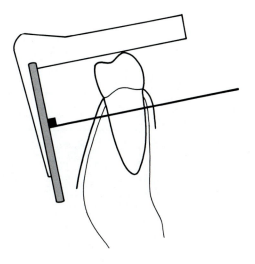

Mandibular premolar projection

Projection of central ray. Position the film-holding instrument to project the central ray through the second premolar-molar area. The vertical angulation should be small, nearly parallel to the occlusal plane, to keep the film as nearly parallel with the long axis of the teeth as possible. Adjust the horizontal angulation and the placement of the film-holding device to direct the beam through the premolar contact points.

Point of entry. The point of entry of the central ray is below the pupil of the eye and about 3 cm above the inferior border of the mandible.

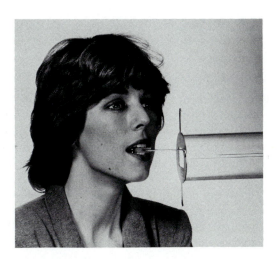

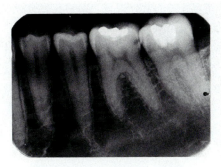

Mandibular molar projection

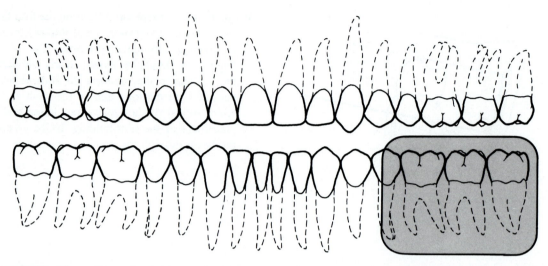

Image field. The radiograph of this region should include the distal half of the second premolar and the three mandibular permanent molars. In the case of an impacted third molar or a pathologic condition distal to the third molar, a distal oblique molar projection or even additional extraoral projections (panoramic or lateral ramus) may be required to demonstrate the area adequately. If the molar area is edentulous, place the film far enough posterior to include the retromolar area in the examination.

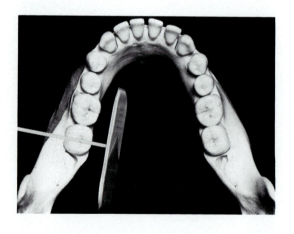

Film placement. Place the no. 2 film into the mouth with its plane nearly horizontal. Rotate the inferior edge downward beneath the lateral border of the tongue, displacing it medially. The anterior edge of the film should be at about the middle of the second premolar. Orient the lateral groove of the bite block used with the Precision instrument parallel with the mean plane of the molars' buccal surfaces. In most cases the tongue will force the film near the alveolar process and molars, aligning it parallel with the long axis of the teeth and the line of occlusion.

Mandibular molar projection

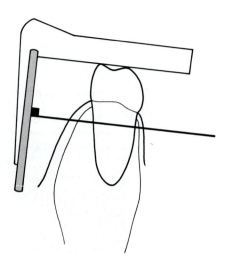

Projection of central ray. The proper placement of the holding instrument will direct the central ray through the second molar. Adjust the horizontal angulation to project the beam through the contact areas. Because of the slight lingual inclination of the molars, the central ray may have some slight positive angulation (approximately 8 degrees).

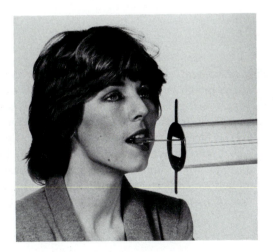

Point of entry. Direct the point of entry of the central ray below the outer canthus of the eye about 3 cm above the inferior border of the mandible.

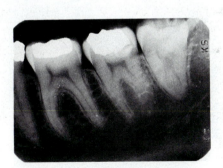

PARALLELING TECHNIQUE

Mandibular distal oblique molar projection

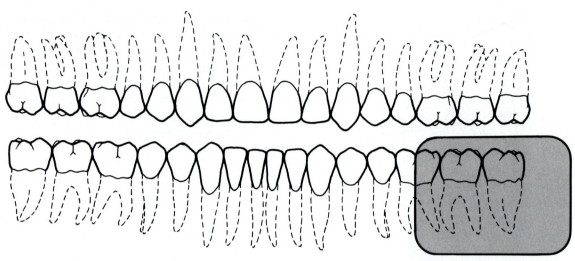

Image field. The distal oblique projection provides a view of the third molar and the retromolar area of the mandible that is usually not included in the molar radiograph. It is primarily intended for the detection or examination of impacted teeth and pathologic conditions in the bone in this area rather than the teeth themselves; the images of the teeth are distorted and overlapped as a result of the oblique path of the x-rays. This projection may eliminate the requirement for an extraoral radiograph of the area.

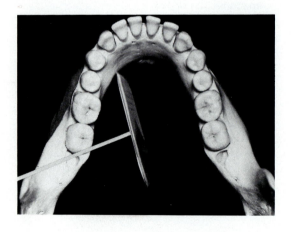

Film placement. Place the film holder in the floor of the mouth between the tongue and alveolar process and parallel to the long axis of the molars. Position the instrument as far posteriorly as possible, and then rotate the film-holding device distally, moving the posterior margin of the film toward the midline. This causes the beam to be directed posteroanteriorly and the projection of more distal objects anteriorly onto the film.

Mandibular distal oblique molar projection

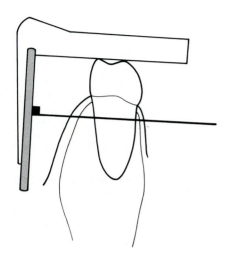

Projection of central ray. The position of the holding instrument will project the central ray from a more posterior aspect through the third molar area to the film.

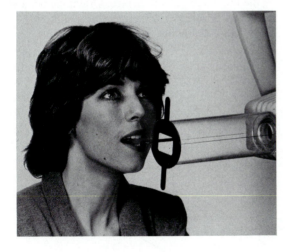

Point of entry. Orient the point of entry about 3 cm above the antegonial notch on the inferior border of the mandible, in line with the anterior border of the ramus.

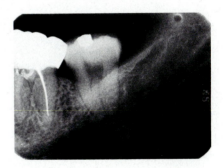

Bisecting-angle technique

The bisecting-angle technique is based on a simple geometric theorem, Cieszynski's rule of isometry, which states that two triangles are equal when they share one complete side and have two equal angles. (In addition, their corresponding sides are equal.) Dental radiography applies the theorem as follows: Position the film as close as possible to the lingual surface of the teeth, resting in the palate or in the floor of the mouth (Fig. 9-5). The plane of the film and the long axis of the teeth form an angle with its apex at the point where the film is in contact with the teeth. When an imaginary plane bisects this angle, it forms two congruent angles, with a common side (the imaginary bisector). A line, representing the central ray (of the x-ray beam), completes the third sides of two triangles when it is directed (through the apices of the teeth) perpendicular to the bisecting plane. The two triangles will be right-angle triangles and congruent, with the corresponding sides equal. Two of the corresponding sides, the hypotenuse of each imaginary congruent triangle, are represented by the long axis of the tooth and the long axis of the film. Consequently, the images cast on the film when these conditions are satisfied is theoretically the same length as the projected object. (To reproduce accurately the length of each root of a multirooted tooth, a different angulation of the central beam would have to be considered for each root.)

Film-holding instruments. There are several methods for supporting films intraorally. The preferred method is to use a film-holding instrument such as the Rinn Snap-A-Ray or bisecting-angle instruments.[9] Both instruments provide an external device for localizing the x-ray beam. The bisecting-angle instrument uses a fixed average bisecting angle. The most common method is to use the patient's forefinger to support the film from the lingual surface. This method has several drawbacks. Often patients use excessive force, thus bending the film and causing distortion of the resultant image. Second, the film might slip without the operator's knowledge, resulting in an improper image field. Finally, without an external guide to the position of the film, there is the possibility that the x-ray beam will miss part of the film, resulting in a partial image (cone cut).

Positioning the patient. To radiograph the maxillary arch, position the patient's head upright with the sagittal plane vertical and the occlusal plane horizontal. When the mandibular teeth are being radiographed, tilt the head back slightly to compensate for the changed occlusal plane when the mouth is opened.

Film placement. Use the same projections described for the paralleling technique. Often the anterior region is covered by using a no. 2 film behind the central incisors in the midline and one lingual to each canine. Position the film behind the area of interest, with the apical end against the mucosa on the lingual or palatal surface. Orient the occlusal or incisal edge against the teeth and with an edge of the film extending just beyond the teeth. It is sometimes necessary for the comfort of the patient to soften the anterior corner of the film by bending

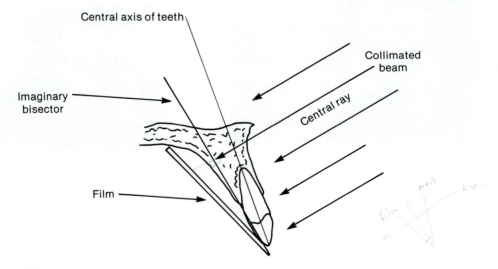

FIG. 9-5. Bisecting-angle technique showing central ray directed at right angle to plane bisecting angle between long axis of tooth and film.

it before placing it against the mucosa. Care must be taken not to bend the film excessively, which may cause considerable image distortion and pressure defects in the emulsion that will be apparent on the processed film.

Angulation of tube head

Horizontal angulation. When using a film-holding device with a beam-localizing ring, position the instrument horizontally so that when the tube is aligned with the ring the central ray is directed through the contacts in the region being examined. When the film-holding device is without a beam-localizing feature, point the tube to direct the central ray through the contacts. In this situation also center the radiation beam on the film. This angulation will usually be at right angles (in the horizontal projection) to the buccal or facial surfaces of the teeth in each region.

Vertical angulation. In practice, the goal of the clinician is to aim the central ray of the x-ray beam at right angles to a plane bisecting the angle between the film and the long axis of the tooth. This principle works well with flat two-dimensional structures, but teeth that have depth or are multi-rooted will show evidence of distortion. Excessive vertical angulation will result in foreshortening of the image, whereas insufficient vertical angulation will result in image elongation. The angle that directs the central ray perpendicular to the bisecting plane will vary with the individual's anatomy. When the occlusal plane is parallel with the floor, use the following table as a general guide.

Projection	Maxilla	Mandible
Incisors	+40 degrees	−15 degrees
Canine	+45 degrees	−20 degrees
Premolar	+30 degrees	−10 degrees
Molar	+20 degrees	−5 degrees

BISECTING-ANGLE TECHNIQUE

Maxillary central incisor projection

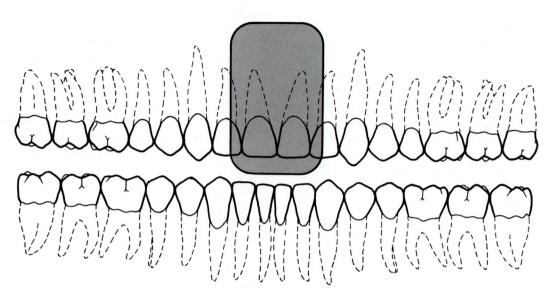

Image field. The field of view on this radiograph should include both central incisors and their periapical areas.

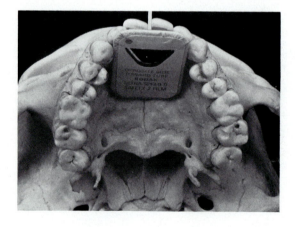

Film placement. Place a no. 1 film directly behind the maxillary central incisors in line with the midline of the arch. Position the superior border of the film on the palate and the inferior border extending just beyond the incisal edges of the teeth.

Maxillary central incisor projection

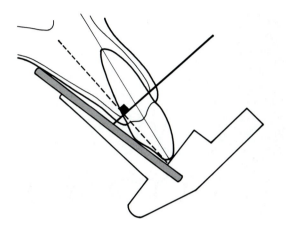

Projection of central ray. Direct the central ray through the contact point of the central incisors and perpendicular to the plane bisecting the angle between the long axis of the film and roots of the teeth. Because the axial inclination of the maxillary incisors is about 15 to 20 degrees, the vertical angulation of the tube should be about +40 degrees. The tube will have a 0 horizontal angulation at the tip of the nose.

Point of entry. The point of entry will be in the midline about through the tip of the nose.

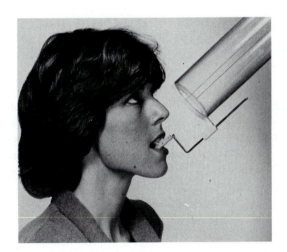

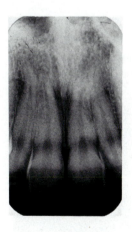

BISECTING-ANGLE TECHNIQUE

Maxillary lateral projection

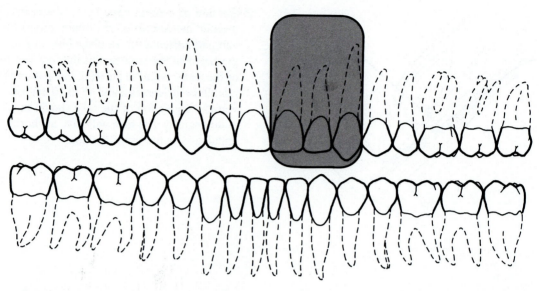

Image field. This projection should show the lateral incisor and its periapical structures centered on the radiograph. The mesial contact area between the lateral incisor and the distal aspect of the central incisor should not be overlapped.

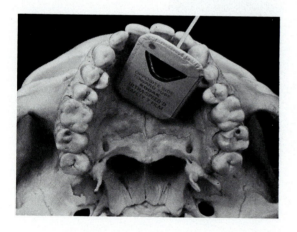

Film placement. Place a no. 1 film directly behind the maxillary lateral incisor with the superior border on the palate and the inferior border extending just beyond the incisal edges of the teeth.

Maxillary lateral projection

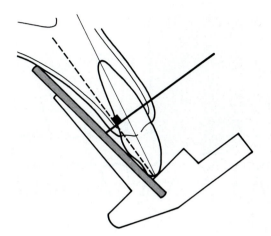

Projection of central ray. Direct the central ray to pass through the middle of the lateral incisor and open the mesial contact area. The vertical angulation should direct the central ray perpendicular to the plane bisecting the angle between the long axes of the film and tooth and will be about +40 degrees.

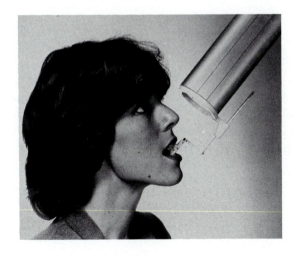

Point of entry. Orient the central ray to enter through the ala of the nose about 1 cm from the midline.

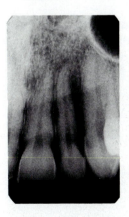

BISECTING-ANGLE TECHNIQUE

Maxillary canine projection

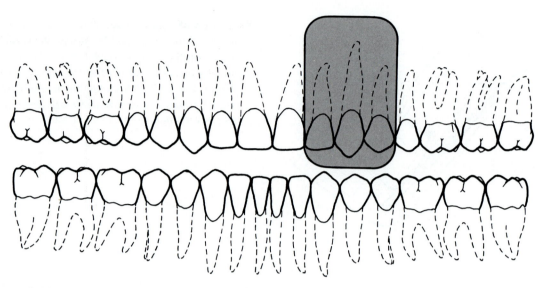

Image field. This projection should demonstrate all the canine and its periapical area centered on the film. The mesial contact area with the distal aspect of the lateral incisor should be "opened" without any overlapping of the two teeth.

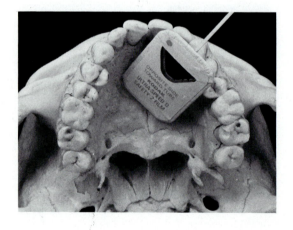

Film placement. Place a no. 1 film with its superior border against the palate and the inferior border extending just below the cusp of the canine, with the long axis of the tooth superimposed on the central long axis of the film.

Maxillary canine projection

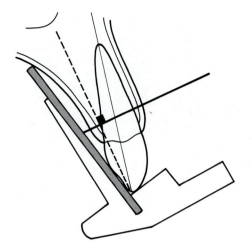

Projection of central ray. Direct the central ray to the center of the film packet perpendicular to the imaginary bisector and with a vertical angulation of about +45 degrees. The horizontal angulation of the tube should cause the beam to pass through the mesial contact of the canine. Do not attempt to open the distal contact.

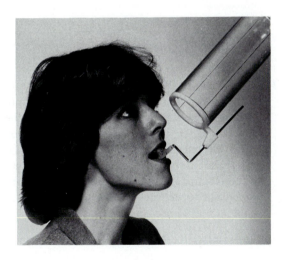

Point of entry. Orient the central ray through the canine eminence. The point of entry is through the ala of the nose.

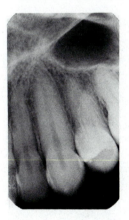

BISECTING-ANGLE TECHNIQUE

Maxillary premolar projection

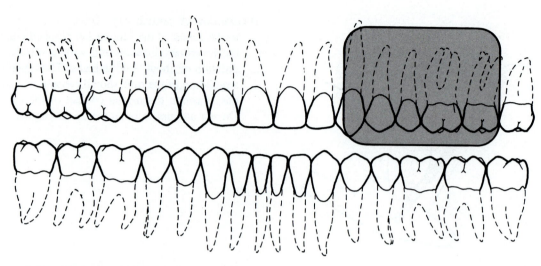

Image field. The radiograph for this region should include the images of the distal half of the canine, the premolars, and the first molar.

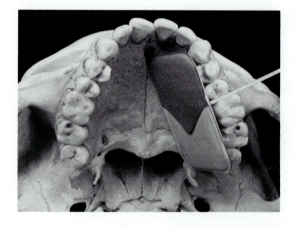

Film placement. Place a no. 2 film in the mouth with the long dimension parallel with the occlusal plane, with the superior border on the palate, and the inferior border extending just below the buccal cusps of the premolars. The packet should cover the distal half of the canine, the premolars, and the first molar and will probably reach to the mesial aspect of the second molar.

BISECTING-ANGLE TECHNIQUE
Maxillary premolar projection

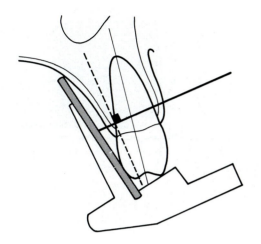

Projection of central ray. Direct the central ray perpendicular to the bisector, which will require a vertical angulation of about $+30$ degrees. Aim the beam through the interproximal area between the first and second premolars.

Point of entry. Orient the point of entry below the pupil of the eye, close to the level of the ala-tragus line.

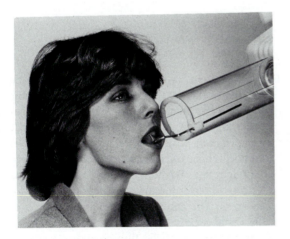

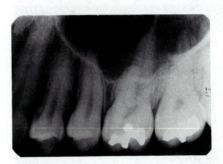

Maxillary molar projection

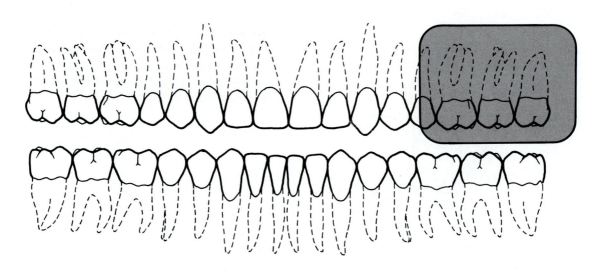

Image field. The radiograph of this region should show the images of the distal half of the second premolar and the three maxillary permanent molars. If the third molar is missing, the outline of the tuberosity should be on the radiograph.

If the third molar is impacted in an area other than the tuberosity, additional extraoral films, such as a panoramic or an oblique lateral jaw projection, may be required.

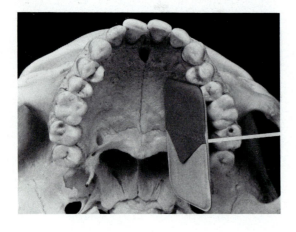

Film placement. When placing this film in the mouth, hold the film horizontal to minimize brushing the palate and dorsum of the tongue. When the film is in the region to be examined, rotate it into position with a firm and definite motion. This maneuver is important in avoiding the gag reflex. Position the film far enough posteriorly to cover the first, second, and third molar areas. The anterior border should just cover the distal aspect of the second premolar. The superior border of the film should rest against the palate, and the inferior border should extend below the buccal cusps of the maxillary molars.

Maxillary molar projection

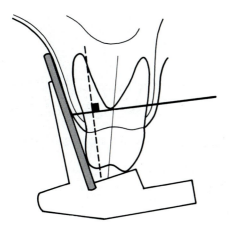

Projection of central ray. Direct the central ray at a vertical angulation of about +20 degrees through the center of the film. Orient the horizontal angulation of the beam to the interproximal spaces between the molar teeth.

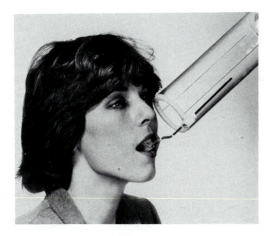

Point of entry. Position the point of entry of the central ray on the cheek in line with the outer cantus of the eye, below the zygoma, and on an anteroposterior level with the second molar.

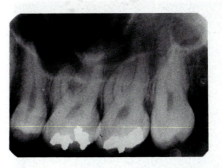

Mandibular centrolateral incisor projection

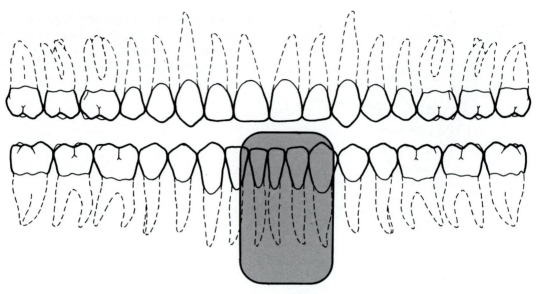

Image field. This projection should show crowns, roots, and periapical areas of the mandibular central and lateral incisors centered on the radiograph. The contact between these two teeth should be open.

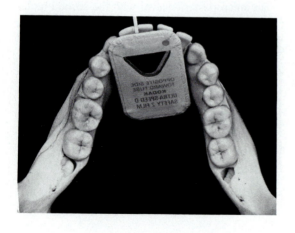

Film placement. Place a no. 1 film directly behind the mandibular central and lateral incisors with the superior border on the incisal edge of these teeth and the inferior border displaced distally, on the lingual mucosa.

Mandibular centrolateral incisor projection

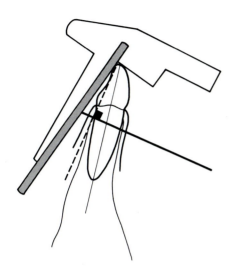

Projection of central ray. Angle the central ray perpendicular to the bisector through the contact area of the central and lateral incisors. The vertical angulation should be about − 15 degrees.

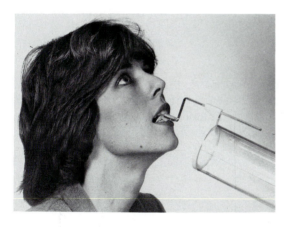

Point of entry. The central ray should enter just below the vermilion border of the lip approximately 1 cm from the midline.

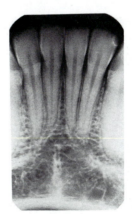

BISECTING-ANGLE TECHNIQUE

Mandibular canine projection

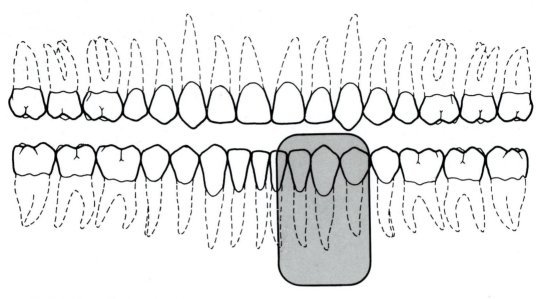

Image field. This projection should center on the canine and its periapical area. The mesial contact area should be open.

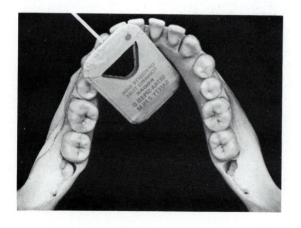

Film placement. Place a no. 1 film with the superior border just above the cusp of the canine and the inferior border resting on the lingual mucosa of the mandible.

Mandibular canine projection

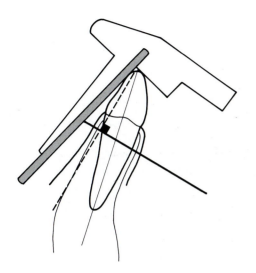

Projection of central ray. Direct the central ray to the center of the film packet through the middle of the canine with a vertical angulation of about -20 degrees. The horizontal angulation of the tube should cause the beam to pass through the mesial contact of the canine.

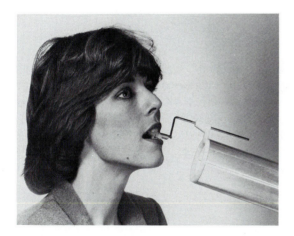

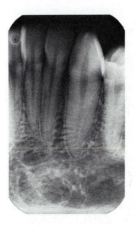

Point of entry. Direct the central ray through the canine approximately 3 cm from the midline.

Mandibular premolar projection

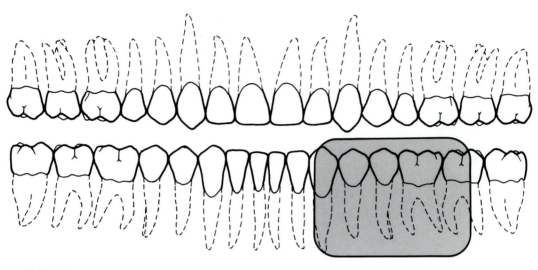

Image field. The radiographic image of this region should cover the distal half of the canine, the premolars, and the first molar.

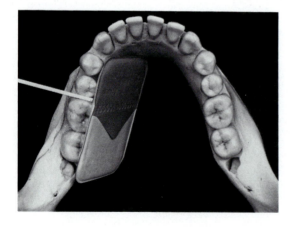

Film placement. Place a no. 2 film in the mouth with the inferior border positioned beneath the lateral border of the tongue. The superior border of the film should extend just above the cusps of the premolars. Extend the anterior border of the film forward to cover the distal half of the canine.

Mandibular premolar projection

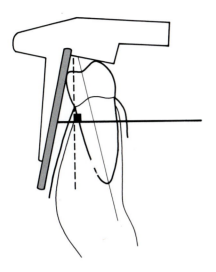

Projection of central ray. Direct the central ray toward the middle of the film with a vertical angulation of about − 10 degrees. Position the horizontal angulation of the central ray to pass between the interproximal areas between the first and second molars.

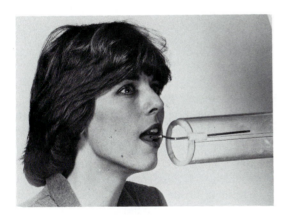

Point of entry. Direct the point of entry so that the central ray passes through the interproximal space between the first and second premolar teeth. This point is usually below the pupil of the eye and approximately 3 cm above the inferior border of the mandible.

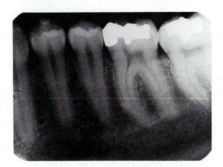

Mandibular molar projection

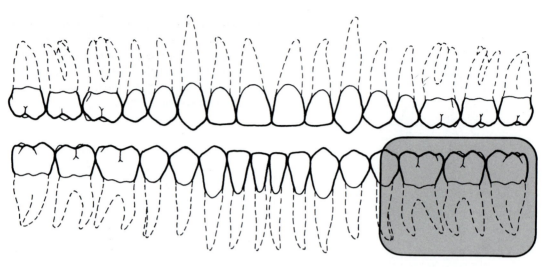

Image field. The radiograph of this region should show the images of the distal half of the second premolar and the three mandibular permanent molars. If the third molar is impacted, additional films such as the mandibular distal oblique projection or extraoral projections may be required to demonstrate the area about the third molar to formulate proper treatment.

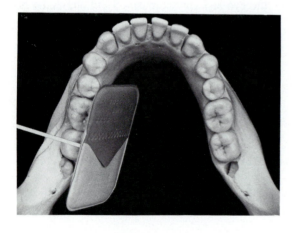

Film placement. Position the inferior border of the no. 2 film beneath the lateral border of the tongue and against the lingual surface of the mandible. The superior border of the film should extend just above the cusps of the mandibular molar teeth, secured in place with a film-holding instrument or the patient's finger. The anterior border of the film should extend to the middle of the second premolar.

Mandibular molar projection

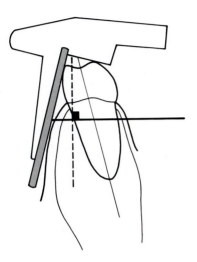

Projection of central ray. Direct the central ray at a vertical angulation of about + 5 degrees and to the center of the film. Orient the horizontal angulation to direct the beam through the interproximal spaces between the molar teeth.

Point of entry. Position the point of entry of the central ray on the cheek below the lateral canthus of the eye, approximately 3 cm above the inferior border of the mandible.

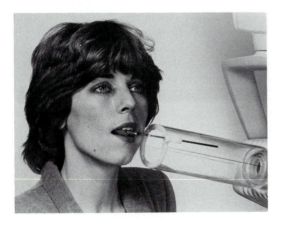

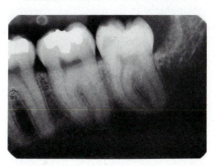

BITEWING EXAMINATIONS

Bitewing (also called *interproximal*) radiographs include the crowns of the maxillary and mandibular teeth and the alveolar crest on the same film. Bitewing films are of particular value in detecting interproximal caries in the early stages of development before they are clinically apparent. Because of the horizontal angle of projection, they may also reveal secondary caries below restorations that may escape recognition in the periapical views. Bitewing projections are also useful for evaluating the periodontal condition. They provide a good perspective of the alveolar bone crest, and change in bone height can be accurately assessed by comparison with the adjacent teeth. In addition, because of the angle of projection directly through the interproximal spaces, the bitewing film is especially effective and useful for detecting calculus deposits in interproximal areas. (As a result of its relatively low radiodensity, calculus will also be better visualized on radiographs made with reduced exposure.)

To obtain these desirable characteristics of the bitewing examination, carefully align the beam between the teeth and parallel with the occlusal plane. As the film or film-holding instrument is placed in the mouth, the portion of the mandibular quadrant that is being radiographed will be in view. Evaluate the position of the teeth in this segment of the mandibular quadrant and direct the beam through the contacts. There may be some difference in the curvature of the mandibular and maxillary arch. However, when the x-ray beam is accurately directed through the mandibular premolar contacts, overlapping is minimal or absent in the maxillary premolar segment. There are a few degrees of tolerance in the horizontal angulation before overlapping becomes critical.[11] The contact between the maxillary first and second molars is often angled a few degrees more anteriorly than between the mandibular first and second molars. Position the aiming cylinder about +10 degrees to project the beam parallel with the occlusal plane (occlusal DEJ). This will minimize overlapping the opposing cusps onto the occlusal surface and thus improve the probability of detecting early occlusal lesions at the DEJ.

The XCP bitewing instrument has an external guide ring for positioning the tube head. This reduces the possibility of cone-cutting the film (Fig. 9-6). To properly position the XCP instrument, place the guide bar parallel with the direction of the beam that will open the contacts of the dentition being examined.

A film fitted with a bitewing tab or loop may be used instead of a holding device (Fig. 9-7). Place the film in a comfortable position lingual to the teeth to be examined. Orient the aiming cylinder in the predetermined direction that will pass the x-ray beam through the interproximal spaces. To help prevent cone cutting, direct the central ray to the center of the bitewing tab that is protruding to the buccal. Orient the beam with a +7 to 10 degrees vertical angulation to preclude overlap of the cusps onto the occlusal surface.

Two posterior bitewing views are recommended for each quadrant, a premolar and a molar. However, for the individual 12 years old or younger, one bitewing film (no. 2) usually suffices. The premolar projection should include the distal half of the canines and the crowns of the premolars. Because the mandibular canines are usually more mesial than the maxillary canines, use the mandibular canine as the guide for the placement of the premolar bitewing film. Place the molar bitewing film a millimeter or two beyond the most distally erupted molar (maxillary or mandibular).

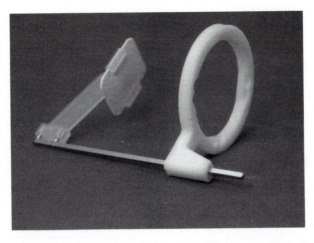

FIG. 9-6. Film-holding device for bitewing radiographs. Note external localizing ring used for positioning aiming tube of x-ray machine to ensure that entire film is in the x-ray beam.

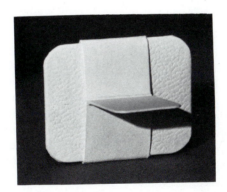

FIG. 9-7. Bitewing loop around film with tab for patient to bite on to support film during exposure.

Premolar bitewing

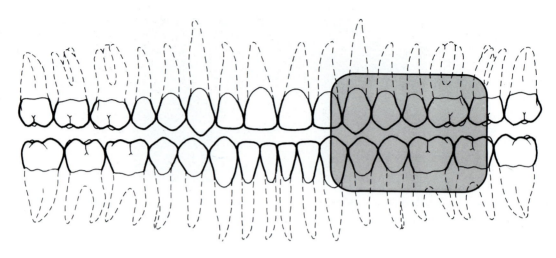

Image field. This projection should cover the distal of the mandibular canine anteriorly and show equally the crowns of the maxillary and mandibular premolar teeth.

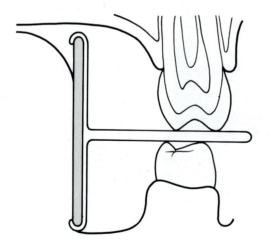

Film placement. Place the film for the bitewing examination of the premolar area between the tongue and the teeth, far enough from the lingual surface of the teeth to prevent interference by the palate on closing and parallel to their long axis. The anterior border of the film should extend anteriorly beyond the contact area between the mandibular canine and the first premolar. Hold the film in place until the patient's mouth is completely closed. Holding the film while closing prevents it from being displaced distally.

Premolar bitewing

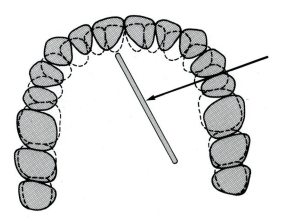

Projection of central ray. Adjust the horizontal angulation of the cone to project the central ray to the center of the film through the premolar contact areas. To compensate for the slight inclination of the film against the palatal mucosa, the vertical angulation should be about +5 degrees. (In the drawing at right the mandibular teeth are in dashed lines.)

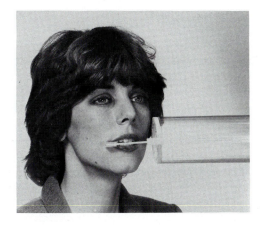

Point of entry. Identify the point of entry by retracting the cheek and determining that the central ray will enter the line of occlusion at the point of contact between the second premolar and first molar.

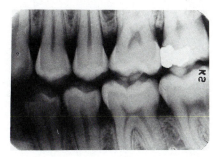

Molar bitewing

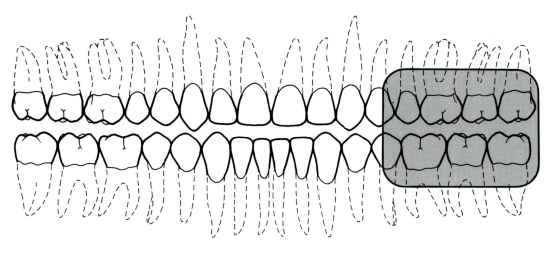

Image field. This projection should show the distal surface of the most posterior erupted molar and equally the crowns of the maxillary and mandibular molars. Because the maxillary and mandibular molar contact areas may not be open from the same horizontal angulation, they may not be visible on one film. In this case it may be desirable to open the maxillary molar contacts because the mandibular molar contacts are usually open on the periapical films.

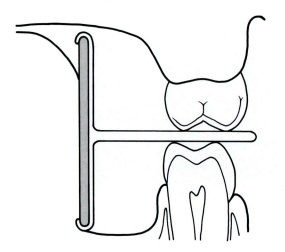

Film placement. Place the film between the tongue and the teeth, as far lingual as practical to avoid contacting the sensitive attached gingiva. The distal margin of the film should extend 1 to 2 mm distal of the most posterior erupted molar. When using the XCP, adjust the horizontal angulation by placing the guide bar parallel with the direction of the central ray that will open the contact area between the first and second molars.

Molar bitewing

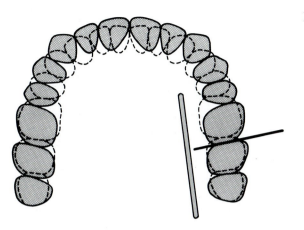

Projection of central ray. Project the central ray to the center of the film and through the contact of the first and second maxillary molars. Angle the central ray slightly from the anterior because the molar contacts usually are not oriented at right angles to the buccal surfaces of these teeth. A vertical angulation of +10 degrees is recommended. (In the drawing at right, the mandibular teeth are in dashed lines.)

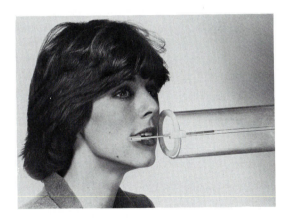

Point of entry. The central ray should enter the cheek below the lateral canthus of the eye at the level of the occlusal plane.

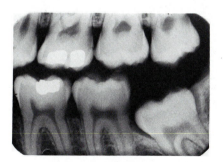

OCCLUSAL RADIOGRAPHY

An occlusal radiograph displays a relatively large segment of a dental arch. It may include the palate or floor of the mouth and a reasonable extent of the contiguous lateral structures. In addition, occlusal radiographs are frequently useful when patients are unable to open wide enough for periapical radiographs or who for other reasons cannot accept periapical radiography. Because occlusal radiographs are exposed at a steep angulation, they may be used with conventional periapical radiographs to determine the location of objects in all three dimensions. Typically, the occlusal radiograph is especially useful in the following cases:

1. To precisely locate roots and supernumerary, unerupted, and impacted teeth. This technique is especially useful in the case of impacted canines and third molars.
2. To localize foreign bodies in the jaws and stones in the ducts of sublingual and submandibular glands.
3. To demonstrate and evaluate the integrity of the anterior, medial, and lateral outlines of the maxillary sinus.
4. To aid in examining patients with trismus who can open their mouths only a few millimeters, thereby precluding the use of intraoral radiography, which may be impossible or at least extremely painful for the patient.
5. In providing information relative to the location, nature, extent, and displacement of fractures of the mandible and maxilla.
6. To determine the medial and lateral extent of disease (e.g., cysts, osteomyelitis, malignancies) and to detect their presence in the palate or floor of the mouth.

To make an occlusal radiograph, insert the relatively large, 7.7×5.8 cm ($3 \times 2\frac{1}{4}$ inch) film between the occlusal surfaces of the teeth. The film lies in the plane of occlusion, thus its name. Position the "tube" side of this film toward the jaw to be examined and direct the x-ray beam through the jaw to the film. The size of the film accommodates examination of relatively large portions of the jaw. Standardized projections are used, stipulating a desired relation between the central ray, film, and region being examined. The clinician should feel free, however, to modify these relations as indicated by a specific clinical requirement.

Anterior maxillary occlusal projection

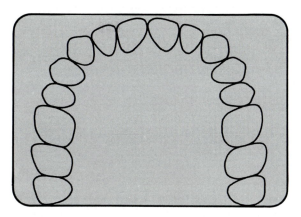

Image field. The primary field of this projection includes the anterior maxilla and its dentition. It will also include the anterior floor of the nasal fossa and teeth from canine to canine.

Film placement. Adjust the head so that the sagittal plane is perpendicular and the occlusal plane is horizontal to the floor. Place the film in the mouth with the exposure side toward the maxilla, with the posterior border touching the rami and the long dimension of the film perpendicular to the sagittal plane. The patient stabilizes the film by gently closing the mouth or using gentle bilateral thumb pressure.

Projection of central ray. Orient the central ray through the tip of the nose toward the middle of the film with a vertical angle of approximately +45 degrees and 0 degrees horizontal angulation.

Point of entry. The central ray enters the patient's face approximately through the tip of the nose.

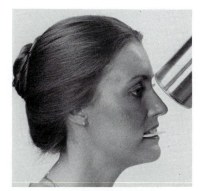

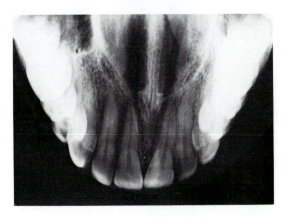

Cross-sectional maxillary occlusal projection

Image field. This projection shows the palate, the zygomatic processes of the maxilla, anteroinferior aspects of each antrum, nasolacrimal canals, teeth from second molar to second molar, and nasal septum.

Film placement. Seat the patient upright with the sagittal plane perpendicular to the floor and the occlusal plane horizontal. Place the film with its long dimension perpendicular to the sagittal plane, crosswise into the mouth. Gently push the film in backward until it contacts the anterior border of the mandibular rami. The patient stabilizes the film by gently closing the mouth.

Projection of central ray. Direct the central ray at a vertical angulation of +65 degrees and a horizontal angulation of 0 degrees, to the bridge of the nose just below nasion, toward the middle of the film.

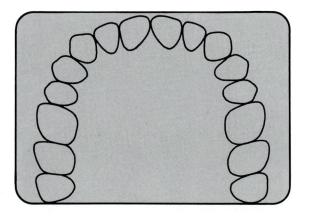

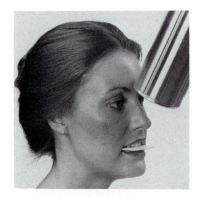

Point of entry. In general, the central ray will enter the patient's face through the bridge of the nose.

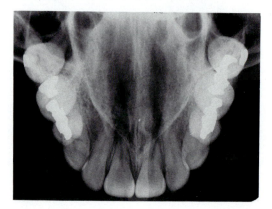

Lateral maxillary occlusal projection

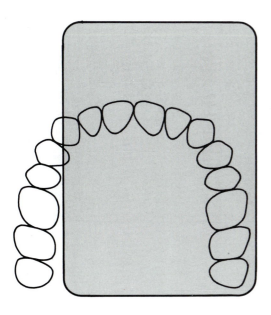

Image field. This projection shows a quadrant of the alveolar ridge of the maxilla, inferolateral aspect of the antrum, the tuberosity, and the teeth from lateral incisor to the contralateral third molar. In addition, the zygomatic process of the maxilla superimposes over the roots of the molar teeth.

Film placement. Place the film with its long axis parallel with the sagittal plane and on the side of interest, with the tube side toward the side of the maxilla in question. Push the film posteriorly until it touches the ramus. Position the lateral border parallel to the buccal surfaces of the posterior teeth and extending laterally approximately 1 cm past the buccal cusps. Ask patient to close gently to maintain the film in position.

Projection of central ray. Orient the central ray with a vertical angulation of +60 degrees, to a point 2 cm below the lateral canthus of the eye, directed toward the center of the film.

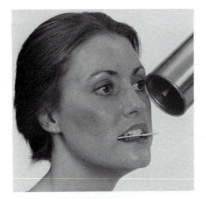

Point of entry. The central ray enters at a point approximately 2 cm below the lateral canthus of the eye.

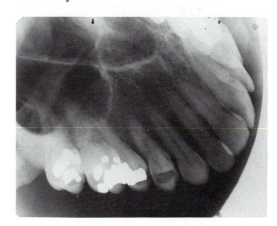

Anterior mandibular occlusal projection

Image field. This projection includes the anterior portion of the mandible, the dentition from canine to canine, and inferior cortical border of the mandible.

Film placement. Seat the patient tilted backward so that the occlusal plane is 45 degrees above horizontal. Place the film in the mouth with the long axis perpendicular to the sagittal plane and posteriorly until it touches the rami. Center the film with the pebbled side (tube side) down, and ask the patient to bite lightly to maintain the film position.

Projection of central ray. Orient the central ray with a − 10 degree angulation through the point of the chin toward the middle of the film, and it will have − 55-degree angulation to the plane of the film.

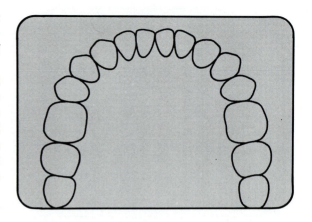

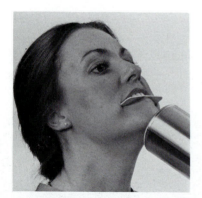

Point of entry. The point of entry of the central ray is in the midline and through the tip of the chin.

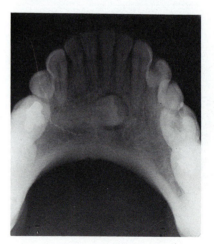

Cross-sectional mandibular occlusal projection

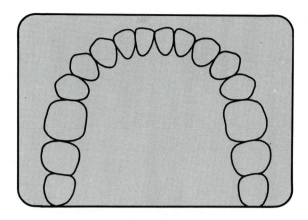

Image field. This projection includes the soft tissue of the floor of the mouth and reveals the lingual and buccal plates of the mandible from second molar to second molar.

Film placement. Seat the patient in a semireclining position with the head tilted backward so that the ala-tragus line is almost perpendicular to the floor. Place the film in the mouth with its long axis perpendicular to the sagittal plane and with the tube side toward the mandible. The anterior border of the film should be approximately 1 cm anterior to the mandibular central incisors. Ask the patient to bite gently on the film to maintain its position.

Projection of the central ray. Direct the central ray at the midline through the floor of the mouth approximately 3 cm below the chin, at right angles to the center of the film.

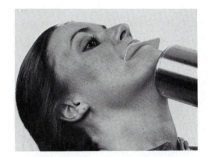

Point of entry. The point of entry of the central ray is in the midline through the floor of the mouth approximately 3 cm below the chin.

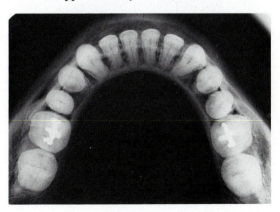

Lateral cross-sectional mandibular occlusal projection

Image field. This projection covers the soft tissue of half the floor of the mouth, the buccal and lingual cortical plates of half of the mandible, and the teeth from the lateral incisor to the contralateral third molar.

Film placement. Seat the patient in a semi-reclining position with the head tilted back so that the ala-tragus line is almost perpendicular to the floor. Place the film in the mouth with its long axis initially parallel with the sagittal plane and the pebbled side down toward the mandible. Place the film as far posterior as possible. Then shift the long axis buccally (right or left) so that the lateral border of the film is parallel to the buccal surfaces of the posterior teeth and extending laterally approximately 1 cm.

Projection of central ray. Direct the central ray perpendicular to the center of the film through a point beneath the chin, approximately 3 cm posterior to the point of the chin and 3 cm lateral to the midline.

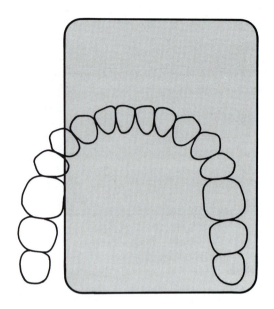

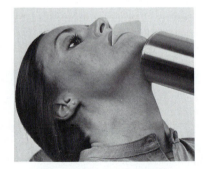

Point of entry. The point of entry of the central ray is beneath the chin approximately 3 cm posterior to the chin and approximately 3 cm lateral to the midline.

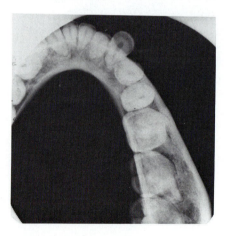

RADIOGRAPHIC EXAMINATION OF CHILDREN

Concerns for radiation protection are most acute in children because of their greater sensitivity to irradiation. The most important means of reducing unnecessary exposure is for the dentist to make the minimum number of films necessary as determined individually for each patient. Make these judgments based on careful clinical examination and consideration of the patient's age, history, presence of caries, growth consideration, general oral health, and time since previous examinations.[16] There are no simple formulas describing frequency and extent of optimal radiographic examinations. Prudence suggests making bitewing examinations for caries assessment at periodic intervals after the patient's contacts have closed. The frequency should be determined in part by the patient's caries rate. A periapical survey is often recommended for children early in the mixed dentition stage. Pay special care to those procedures that reduce exposure. (See Chapter 3.) In particular, use fast film, proper processing, beam-limiting devices, and leaded aprons and thyroid shields.

Radiography in the child may be an interesting and challenging experience. Although the principles of periapical radiography for children are the same as for adults, in practice the child presents special considerations because of small anatomic structures and potential behavioral problems. The smaller size of the arches and dentition obligates the use of smaller periapical film. The relatively shallow palate and floor of the mouth may further require some modification of film placement.[8] Special radiographic examinations using the occlusal film for extraoral projections have been suggested.[7]

Patient management

Children are often apprehensive about the radiographic examination, much as they are of many other types of dental procedures. The radiographic examination is usually the first manipulative procedure performed on the young patient. When the examination is nonthreatening and comfortable, the following dental experiences are usually accepted with little or no apprehension. The best way of allaying this apprehension is to make children familiar with the procedure by explaining it in a manner that they can comprehend. It is often wise to describe the x-ray machine as a camera to take pictures of teeth. Allow the child to be more comfortable with the film and x-ray machine by touching them before the examination. The operator should carry on conversation with children to distract them and gain their confidence. It may be advantageous for the child to watch an older sibling being radiographed or to have the parent or dental assistant serve as a model. For children who experience a gagging sensation, have them breathe through their nose, curl their toes, make a fist, or follow other such devices to distract their attention from the radiographic procedure. If the procedure is postponed until the following appointment, however, the gag reflex may not be encountered or many times is much easier for the patient to control. It is especially important to explain to the patient that it will be much easier the next time—plant the positive thought. In any case, if the dentist is adamant about completing the examination, the problem is likely to become chronic and even progressive.

Examination coverage

When a complete radiographic survey is necessary it should show the periapical region of all teeth, the proximal surfaces of all posterior teeth, and the crypts of the developing permanent teeth. The number of projections required depends upon the child's size. Also use an exposure appropriate to the child's size. For example, a reduction in the mAs of 50% of that used for the usual young adult gives the proper density for patients under 10 years. Decrease the exposure about 25% for those between 10 and 15 years.

Primary dentition (3 to 6 years). A combination of projections can be used to provide an adequate coverage for the pedodontic patient. This examination may consist of two anterior occlusal films, two posterior bitewing films, and up to four posterior periapical films as indicated (Fig. 9-8). For the maxillary and interproximal projections, seat the child upright with the sagittal plane perpendicular and the occlusal plane parallel with the floor (horizontal plane). For mandibular projections, except the occlusal, seat the child upright with the sagittal plane perpendicular. Orient the tragus corner of the mouth line parallel with the floor. Others find that a panoramic film in place of the four periapical films is more informative and results in less exposure to the child. (See Chapter 3.)

Maxillary anterior occlusal projection. Place a no. 2 size film in the mouth with its long axis perpendicular to the sagittal plane with the pebbled surface toward the maxillary teeth. Center the film on the midline with the anterior border extending

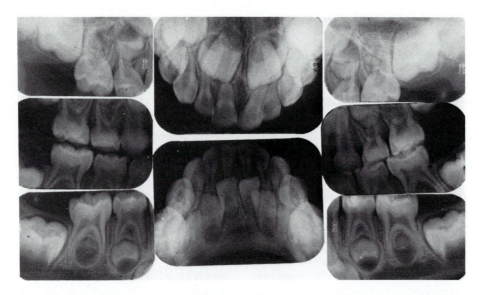

FIG. 9-8. Radiographic examination of primary dentition consisting of two anterior occlusal views, four posterior periapical views, and two bitewing views.

just beyond the incisal edges of the anterior teeth. Direct the central ray at a vertical angulation of +60 degrees through the tip of the nose toward the center of the film.

Mandibular anterior occlusal projection. Seat the child with the head tipped backward so the occlusal plane is about 25 degrees above the plane of floor.* Place a no. 2 film with the long axis perpendicular to the sagittal plane and the pebbled surface toward the mandibular teeth. Orient the central ray at −30 degrees vertical angulation and through the tip of the chin toward the film.

Bitewing. Use a no. 0 size film with a paper loop film holder. Place the film in the child's mouth as in the adult premolar bitewing projection. The image field should include the distal half of the canine and the deciduous molars. Use a positive vertical angulation of +5 to +10 degrees. Orient the horizontal angle to direct the beam through the interproximal spaces.

Deciduous maxillary molar periapical. For this projection use a no. 0 size film in a modified Rinn XCP or BAI bite block, either with or without the aiming ring and indicator bar. Position the film

in the midline of the palate with the anterior border extending up to the maxillary primary canine. The image field of this projection should include the distal half of the primary canine and both primary molars.

Deciduous mandibular molar. Position a no. 0 size film in modified Rinn XCP or BAI bite block, with or without the aiming ring and indicator bar, between the posterior teeth and the tongue. The exposed radiograph should show the distal half of the mandibular primary canine and the primary molar teeth.

Mixed dentition (7 to 12 years). A complete examination of the mixed dentition, if indicated, consists of two incisor periapical films, four canine periapical films, four posterior periapical films, and two or four posterior bitewing films (Fig. 9-9). For the maxillary and interproximal projections, seat the child upright with the sagittal plane perpendicular and the occlusal plane parallel with the floor. For the mandibular projections, seat the child upright with the sagittal plane perpendicular and the ala-tragus line parallel with the floor. Use the Precision Pedodontic or Rinn XCP instruments for these larger children. For smaller individuals, the Rinn BAI bite blocks may be more comfortable.

Maxillary anterior periapical. Center a no. 1 film on the embrasure between the central incisors in the mouth behind the maxillary central and lateral incisors. Center the film on the midline.

Mandibular anterior periapical. Position a no. 1 film behind the mandibular central and lateral incisors.

*Another technique that can be used to project the beam at −55 degrees with the film: visually align the aiming cylinder with the film (occlusal plane) and note the positive angle indicated on the protractor on the side of the head of the unit. Subtract 55 degrees from this reading, and the result is the proper negative angle on the protractor to which the aiming cylinder is tipped (upward) to give a −55 degree angle of projection to the film.

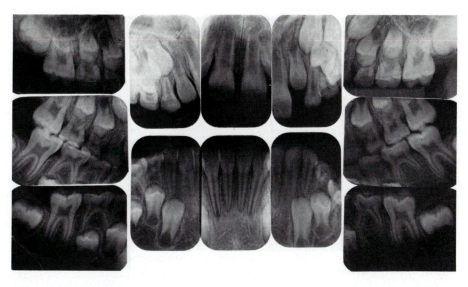

FIG. 9-9. Radiographic examination of mixed dentition consisting of two incisor views, four canine views, four posterior periapical views, and two bitewing views.

Canine periapical. Position a no. 1 film behind each of the canines.

Deciduous and permanent molar periapical. Position a no. 1 or no. 2 film (if child is large enough) with the anterior edge behind the canine.

Posterior bitewing. Expose bitewing projections in the premolar region with no. 1 or no. 2 film as previously described, using either bitewing tabs or the Rinn bitewing instrument. Expose four bitewing projections when the second permanent molars are erupted.

SPECIAL CONSIDERATIONS

The radiographic procedures described are for the "well" patient. Modification of these procedures may be necessary for patients who manifest certain unusual difficulties. The specific modifications depend on the physical and emotional characteristics of the patient. As in the case of any dental procedure, however, the dental assistant initiates the examination with appreciation of the patient's condition and with sympathy for any problems that might occur for either of them. If the assistant is kind but firm, the confidence of the patient increases, which will help the patient relax and cooperate. The following are a few conditions and circumstances that may be encountered, with some recommendations and suggestions that may facilitate an adequate radiographic examination.

Infection

Infection in the orofacial structures may result in edema and lead to trismus of some of the muscles of mastication. As a result of such conditions, intraoral radiography may be painful to the patient and difficult for both the patient and radiologist. Under such circumstances, extraoral or occlusal techniques may offer the only possibility for an examination. The choice of a specific extraoral projection is dependent on the condition and areas to be examined. Although the resulting radiograph may not be ideal in many respects, it usually provides more useful information than the diagnostician would have without it. In the case of edema in an area to be examined, increased exposure is required to compensate for the tissue swelling. Such increase in exposure may be accomplished by increasing the kVp, mA, or duration of exposure. In the case of dental x-ray machines, exposure time is usually the easiest and most convenient variable that will provide the most consistent results (except in those cases where the patient has difficulty remaining motionless for a few seconds).

Patients with communicable diseases such as AIDS, tuberculosis, herpes, hepatitis, or syphilis may require a dental radiographic examination. Strict observance of infection control procedures will prevent the operation from acquiring the disease or passing the infection to subsequent patients. Chapter 10 discusses these infection control procedures in detail.

Trauma

The patient who has suffered trauma and has a suspected fracture of the facial skeleton may be bedridden because of involvement of several other areas of the skeleton. Consequently, an extraoral radiographic examination with the patient in the supine condition is necessary. However, the circumstances will not compromise the techniques, and satisfactory radiographs can be produced if the proper relative positions of the tube, patient, and film are observed.

Frequently, intraoral periapical radiographs are not large enough to delineate the size and extent of oral neoplasms. In these cases it is often necessary to use occlusal and extraoral projections, as these examinations have a greater chance of revealing all of these lesions. When examining such conditions, it is always desirable to have all the borders of the lesion recorded on a single film.

Mentally handicapped patients

Mentally handicapped patients with various nervous disorders may cause some difficulty for the radiologist who is attempting an examination. The difficulty is usually the result of the patient's lack of coordination or inability to comprehend what is expected. However, by performing the radiographic examination speedily, one may avoid unpredictable moves by the patient. Use of increased kVp, mA or fast film and intensifying screens will reduce the exposure time and the possibility that involuntary movement by the patient will make the film unsuitable. If coordination is a major difficulty, sedation may be required. If heavy sedation is used, perform the radiographic examination with the patient in the supine position. When performing intraoral radiographic examination with the patient supine, use film-holding and beam-aiming devices to obtain proper film placement and tube angulation.

Physically handicapped patients

Physically handicapped patients (e.g., those with loss of vision, loss of hearing, loss of the use of any or all extremities, congenital defects such as cleft palate) may require special handling during a radiographic examination. Usually these patients are cooperative and eager to assist. They may well have or have had so much discomfort and inconvenience that their tolerance level is high, and they are not challenged by the relatively slight irritation represented by the x-ray procedures. It is generally the case that intraoral and extraoral radiographic examination may be performed for these patients when a good rapport between the patient and the radiology technician is established and maintained. Members of the handicapped patient's family are frequently very helpful in assisting the patient into and out of the examination chair and in film positioning and holding, inasmuch as they are usually familiar with the patient's condition and accustomed to coping with it.

Occasionally patients requiring a radiographic examination manifest a gag reflex on the slightest provocation. These patients are usually very apprehensive and frightened by the unknown procedures; others simply seem to have very sensitive tissue that precipitates a gag reflex when stimulated. This sensitivity is manifested when the film is placed in the oral cavity. To overcome this disability, the radiologist should make an effort to relax and reassure the patient. One way of doing this is to describe and explain the procedures that are about to be performed. There is little doubt that gagging may frequently be controlled by the operator bolstering the patient's confidence through demonstration of technical competence and through authoritarianism tempered with compassion. It frequently appears that the gag reflex is worse when the patient is tired, so it is advisable to perform the examination in the morning when the individual is well rested, rather than in the afternoon or evening, especially in the case of children. Stimulating the posterior dorsum of the tongue or the soft palate usually initiates the gag reflex. Consequently, during the placement of the film, the tongue should be very relaxed and positioned well to the floor of the mouth. This can be accomplished by asking the patient to swallow deeply just before opening the mouth to place the film. (Never mention the tongue. Do not ask the patients to relax the tongue; this usually makes them more conscious of it and precipitates involuntary movements.) Carry the film into the mouth parallel with the occlusal plane: when it is at the desired area, rotate it with a decisive motion, bringing it into contact with the palate or in the floor of the mouth. Sliding it along the palate or tongue is likely to stimulate the gag reflex. Also, keep in mind that the longer the film stays in the mouth, the greater the possibility that the patient will start to gag. Advise the patient to breathe rapidly through the nose because mouth breathing usually aggravates this condition.

Any little exercise that can be devised that will not interfere with the x-ray examination but will cause the patient to shift attention from the film and the mouth is likely to relieve the gag reaction. Such a distraction can frequently be created by asking the patient to hold his or her breath or to keep a foot or arm suspended during film placement and exposure. In extreme cases, administer topical anesthetic agents in mouth washes or spray to produce temporary numbness of the tongue and palate to reduce gagging. However, in our experience this procedure gives limited results. The most effective approach is to reduce apprehension, minimize tissue irritation, and encourage rapid breathing through the nose. If all measures fail, an extraoral examination may be the only means, short of administering general anesthesia, to examine the patient radiographically.

Radiographic techniques for endodontics

Radiographs are essential to the practice of endodontics. Not only are they indispensable for determining the diagnosis and prognosis of pulp treatment but also they are the most reliable method of managing endodontic treatment. The presence of a rubber dam, rubber dam clamp, and root canal instruments may complicate an intraoral periapical examination by impairing proper film positioning and aiming cylinder angulation. In spite of these obstacles, there are certain requirements to observe:

- Center the tooth being treated in the image.
- Position the film as far from the tooth and apex as the region permits to assure that the apex of the tooth and some periapical bone are apparent on the radiograph.

Projection technique. For maxillary projections, seat the patient so that the sagittal plane is perpendicular and the occlusal plane is parallel to the floor. For mandibular projection, the patient is seated upright with the sagittal plane perpendicular and the tragus corner of the mouth line parallel with the floor. Use a hemostat as a film holder as it occupies minimal space and is easy to manage by the operator and patient (Fig. 9-10).

Use a no. 2 periapical film for all projections. For anterior projections, grasp the film along the edge of the short dimension of the film. For posterior projections, engage the long side of the film. Insert the film in the hemostat into the mouth with the film parallel to the occlusal plane. Place the film into proper position by rotating the hemostat and film into a position as near parallel as possible to the long axis of the tooth to be radiographed.

Align the aiming cylinder to direct the central ray perpendicular to the center of the film. The plane of the end of the aiming cylinder should be parallel with the hemostat handle. After positioning the film, guide the patient's hand with instructions

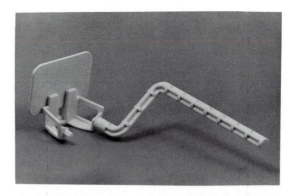

FIG. 9-10. Endo-Ray film holder used for endodontic radiographs. (Courtesy Demac, Ltd., St. Charles, IL.)

to hold and stabilize the hemostat against the teeth in the same arch during exposure. Alternatively, insert the hemostat through a bite block onto which the patient can bite and provide stabilization of the instrument and film.

Frequently a single radiograph of a multirooted tooth made at the normal vertical and horizontal projection will not display all the roots. In these cases where it is prudent to separate the roots on multirooted teeth, a second projection may be made. Alter the horizontal angulation 20 degrees mesially to the hemostat handle for the maxillary premolars, 20 degrees mesially or distally for the maxillary molars, or 20 degrees distally for an oblique projection of the mandibular molar roots.

If a sinus tract is encountered, trace its course by threading a no. 40 gutta-percha cone through the tract before the radiograph is made. It is also possible to localize and determine the depth of periodontal defects with this gutta-percha tracking technique.

Make a final radiograph of the treated tooth to demonstrate the quality of the root canal filling and the condition of the periapical tissues after the removal of the clamp and rubber dam. Use an oblique projection if there is a possibility of superimposing any of the canals.

Pregnancy

The unborn child is very sensitive to ionizing radiation. (See Chapter 3.) Limit radiographic exmination during pregnancy to cases with a specific diagnostic indication. Postpone elective procedures until the termination of the pregnancy. However, with the protection afforded by the lead apron, an intraoral or extraoral examination can be performed whenever there is a reasonable diagnostic requirement. (See Chapter 4.) Although there has been no reported incidence of damage to an unborn child from dental radiography, prudence suggests such radiographic examinations be kept to a minimum consistent with the mother's dental needs.

Edentulous patients

The radiographic examination of edentulous patients, whether the area is one tooth in extent or an entire arch, is important. These areas may contain roots, residual infection, impacted teeth, cysts, or other pathologic entities that may adversely affect the usefulness of prosthetic appliances or the health of the patient. Once it has been determined that these entities are not present, repeated examinations to detect their presence are not warranted. Edentulous patients typically represent an older age group, and their potential for development of malignant tumors is higher. However, the low probability of developing a malignancy does not constitute a continuing indication for periodic radiographic examination in the absence of other clinical signs or symptoms. Once it has been determined that the jaws are free of disease, periodic radiographs are not warranted in the absence of symptoms.

Radiographic techniques for edentulous patients. If available, a panoramic examination of the edentulous jaws is most convenient. If abnormalities of the alveolar ridges are identified, use the increased resolution of periapical film to make intraoral projections to supplement the panoramic examination.

For intraoral radiography of the alveolar ridges in an edentulous or partially edentulous patient, use a film-holding device. Placement of the film-holding instrument may be complicated by its tipping into the voids normally occupied by the crowns of the missing teeth. To manage this difficulty, place cotton rolls between the ridge and the film holder, thereby supporting the holder in a horizontal position. An orthodontic elastic to hold cotton rolls to the bite block on the film holder is frequently useful when several such projections must be exposed. With elastics, it is simple to maneuver the cotton rolls into the areas that require support. The patient may steady the film-holding instrument with a hand or an opposing denture.

When panoramic equipment is not available, an examination consisting of 14 intraoral films will provide an excellent survey.[5] The exposure required for an edentulous ridge is approximately 25% less than that for dentulous ridge. This examination consists of seven projections (adult no. 2 size) in each jaw as follows:

Central incisors (midline)	1 projection
Lateral-canine	2 projections
Premolar	2 projections
Molar	2 projections

REFERENCES

1. Bean LR: Comparison of bisecting angle and paralleling methods of intraoral radiology, *J Dent Educ* 33:441-445, 1969.
2. Jones PE, Warner B: A teaching method for the paralleling technique, *Oral Surg* 42:126-134, 1976.
3. Manson-Hing LR: On the evaluation of radiographic techniques, *Oral Surg* 27:631-634, 1969.
4. Medwedeff FM, Elcan PD: A precision technique to minimize radiation, *Dent Surv* 43:45-53, 1967.
5. Scandrett FR, Tebo HG, Miller JT, et al: Radiographic examination of the edentulous patient: 1, review of the literature and preliminary report comparing three methods, *Oral Surg* 35:266-274, 1973.
6. Shawkat AH, Nolting FW, Phllips JD, et al: Evaluation of the utilization of the supine position in intraoral radiology, *Oral Surg* 43:963-970, 1977.
7. Silha RE: Special radiographic surveys, *Dent Radiogr Photogr* 45:23-33, 1972.
8. Silha RE: Paralleling technique with a disposable film holder, *Dent Radiogr Photogr* 48:27-35, 1975.
9. Updegrave WJ: Right-angle dental radiography, *Dent Clin North Am* 12:571-579, 1968.
10. Updegrave WJ: Simplified and standardized intraoral radiography with reduced tissue irradiation, *J Am Dent Assoc* 85:861-869, 1972.
11. van der Stelt PF, Ruttiman VE, Webber RL, et al: In vitro study into the influence of x-ray beam angulation on the detection of artificial defects on bitewing radiographs. *Caries Res* 23:334-341, 1989.
12. Venokur PC, Einbender S, Myers BS: Modified x-ray technique for dentistry with patients in the supine position, *Oral Surg* 32:148-150, 1974.
13. Walton RE: Endodontic radiographic techniques, *Dent Radiogr Photogr* 46:51-59, 1973.
14. Weissman DD, Longhurst GE: Clinical evaluation of a rectangular field collimating device for periapical radiography, *J Am Dent Assoc* 82:580-582, 1971.
15. Weissman DD, Sobkowski FJ: Comparative thermoluminescent dosimetry of intraoral periapical radiography, *Oral Surg* 29:376-386, 1970.
16. White SC: Radiation exposure in pediatric dentistry: current standards in pedodontic radiology with suggestions for alternatives, *Pediatr Dent* 3:441-447, 1982.
17. Wuehrmann AH, Manson-Hing LR: *Dental radiology,* ed 4, St Louis, 1977, Mosby.

10

Radiographic Infection Control

It has been common knowledge for years that dental personnel and patients alike have been at increased risk of acquiring tuberculosis, syphilis, herpes viruses, and upper respiratory infections, as well as the hepatitis A through E viruses.[7] However, only after the recognition of AIDS in 1981 as a new and distinct clinical entry[6] did rigorous hygienic procedures in the dental office become a reality. The evolution of infection control procedures to prevent cross-contamination in the dental setting was spurred by several factors, including the concern for patients and self because of the 100% case fatality of AIDS, the epidemic proportion of AIDS, the litigious bent of society, and the threat of penalties by the Occupational Safety and Health Administration (OSHA). Because of these concerns, there has been a decided increase in the use of infection control techniques in all areas of the dental office.

This chapter focuses on the preparation of the radiographic areas and equipment. Although radiographic procedures are not invasive, saliva is a potentially infectious medium due to its frequent contamination with blood.[4] Further, the oral radiographic procedures used in the dental office are likely performed in the same dental units that are used for all the different types of procedures, including invasive procedures. Because a medical history and clinical examination do not guarantee identification of patients with HIV infection or other serious infectious diseases such as hepatitis, treat all patients as potentially infected. Radiographic infection control procedures are now an important and integral part of a dental practice.

OVERVIEW

The primary goal of infection control procedures is to prevent cross-contamination between patients as well as between patients and health care providers. In radiographic practice this goal is addressed by using surface disinfectants on all relevant surfaces and by using barriers. Although descriptions of infection control procedures for the dental office repeatedly refer to the use of surface disinfectants and covers or barriers on *only* those working areas that were either contaminated during the treatment of a previous patient or presumed to be used during the anticipated procedure, such advice is contrary to the concept of infection control.[9] An infection control procedure is no more effective than the least effective feature or step. Trying to anticipate what surfaces will be contacted during a procedure is adding an unacceptable degree of probability that in reality invalidates the intent of the total effort. Consequently, it is important to disinfect all accessible surfaces in the unit.[1] This effort is facilitated if the surfaces are clear. Most items that accumulate on working surfaces in the operatory should be in a central preparation (cleaning/sterilizing) room and brought as necessary to the treatment area on trays. This eliminates the probability of touching items and surfaces that have not been properly prepared and defeating all the precautions that have been observed.

Although barriers greatly aid infection control,[2,3] they do not replace the need for effective surface cleaning and disinfection. Experience has demonstrated that, during the daily activity of treatment, failure of mechanical barriers is not uncommon. It is advantageous and reassuring to the operator to know that whenever this happens the surfaces that may become accidently exposed are clean and disinfected.

INFECTION CONTROL PROCEDURES

The following techniques will facilitate infection control during radiography. They are presented in the order in which they should be applied. The sequence of the steps in the following guidelines is important as adherence to this order should contribute significantly to their effectiveness in preventing disease transmission. Perform the preparation and cleanup work described here while wearing disinfected, thick, general purpose, utility gloves. After use, wash the gloves with soap and water; then rinse and dry them and apply a disinfectant. Discard the utility gloves weekly. All individuals who participate in the disinfection routines should have their own gloves.

The infection control sequence for radiography is as follows:
1. Prepackage x-ray film and sterilize film-holding instruments.
2. Disinfect environmental working surfaces.
3. Disinfect the apron.
4. Disinfect and cover PID, x-ray head, and support.
5. Cover disinfected environmental working surfaces.
6. Process contaminated x-ray films.
7. Remove all barriers and respray or wipe all working surfaces and apron.
8. Disinfect panoramic machine and cephalostat.

Sterilization and disinfection

1. Prepackage x-ray film and sterilize film-holding instruments. To prevent contamination of bulk supplies of film, dispense them in procedure quantities. Prepackage the required number of films for a full-mouth or interproximal series in coin envelopes or paper cups in the central preparation room. Dispense these envelopes of films with the film-holding instruments. If Kodak ClinAsept Dental Barrier protective plastic envelopes* are used, the films may be inserted into these envelopes at the time they are packaged in the coin envelopes (Fig. 10-1). For those unanticipated occasions when an unusual number of films may be required, a small container of films can be on hand in the central preparation/sterilizing room. No one wearing contaminated gloves should retrieve a film from this supply. They should be dispensed by someone with clean hands or wearing clean gloves.

The film-holding instruments described in Chapter 9, the Precision and the XCP, can both be steam autoclaved. The Precision instrument may also be dry-heat sterilized, but not the plastic XCP instruments. Both should be mechanically cleaned and well rinsed in running tap water to remove saliva before sterilizing. The bite blocks used with the Precision instruments are disposable and should be discarded. After sterilizing, place the instruments in 16 × 10⅜ inch plastic bags† (with new dis-

*Eastman Kodak Company, Rochester, NY 14650-9547.
†North America Film Corporation, Spartanburg, SC.

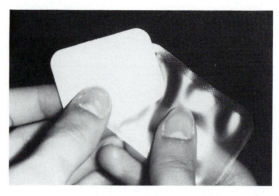

FIG. 10-1. Place films in plastic barrier envelopes in stockroom prior to radiographic examination.

posable bite blocks in the case of the Precision instrument) for storage and subsequent transport to the radiography area. Place the instruments in the bags with clean, ungloved hands, working on a clean, disinfected surface.

When the instruments are taken to the radiographic area, it is good technique to use them out of the bag. After using an instrument, replace it in the plastic bag to reinforce cleanliness in the area. Use the same plastic bag to transport the contaminated instruments back to the cleaning/sterilizing room.

2. Disinfect environmental working surfaces. First, liberally spray all exposed environmental working surfaces (counter tops) with a disinfecting solution. Even though it is not anticipated that all the surfaces will be used for the procedures at hand, it is not always apparent which areas have been contaminated during the last treatment or which surface may suddenly become convenient to use during the current procedure.

Good surface disinfectants include the iodophors, chlorines, or synthetic phenolics.[5] The American Dental Association's guide to chemical agents for disinfection and sterilization lists the iodophores Biocide, Surf-A-Cide, and Pro-Medyne-D. In addition, Wescodyne has been used as a surface disinfectant and sterilizing agent in the laboratory and dental clinic and office for 40 years, and it has been completely satisfactory when applied in the manner described here. Hypersensitivity to iodine or contamination to areas in which critical iodine tests are being conducted (hospital laboratories) are the only contraindications to the use of iodophores for disinfection. The iodophores are generally less expensive than the phenolic com-

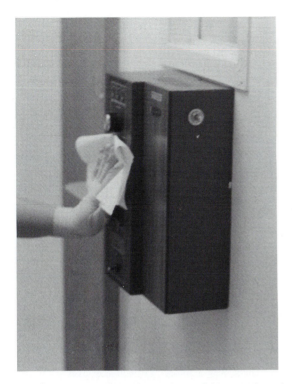

FIG. 10-2. Vigorously wipe the front of the console and the exposure switch with a folded, double paper towel moistened with disinfectant. Note utility gloves to protect hands.

pounds because they can be diluted with more water. They are also less corrosive then hypochlorite, the least expensive of all, but perhaps the least pleasant to use.

Spray the top of the x-ray control console and sides with the disinfectant, but not the front, as it may damage the switches, dials, and meters.[10] Wipe the front of the console and the exposure switch vigorously with a folded, double paper towel that has been well moistened with disinfectant (Fig. 10-2).

Spray or wipe the headrest, headrest adjustment, the arms, backrest, and seat of the chair with disinfectant. If the positioning of the chair is electrically controlled, wipe the switches with a double-folded towel liberally moistened with the disinfectant. Foot controls for the positioning of the chair, which are available for many models, should be considered as infection-control equipment. Radiographic procedures are not likely to contaminate the chair, but a unit that was used previously for an operative procedure is apt to have been contaminated by splatters, drips, or aerosols. Even if the chair was not contaminated during the previous

procedure, it is a thoughtful gesture to wipe the chair between patients and maintain the posture of cleanliness—the equipment is at hand and the procedure requires only seconds.

To ensure that the disinfecting action of the solution will continue for as long as possible on these surfaces, leave them "wet" with the solution while performing the next infection control steps in the area. Although it is usually recommended that the liquid disinfectants be in contact with the surface to be disinfected for at least 10 minutes, the procedure and rationalization described here will permit some moderation of this schedule. Considering that the environmental surfaces are repeatedly sprayed throughout a working day and that those surfaces most at risk to contamination are covered when they are most likely to be contaminated, it is reasonable that these procedures are effective even though the pace of treatment does not always permit a full 10 minutes of contact[2] between the disinfectant and the surface before the gross excess is removed by wiping. Those surfaces that are not wiped remain in contact with the disinfectant until it dries, after which some disinfecting action continues.

Although exposing dental intraoral radiographs does not usually require use of a dental overhead treatment light, it is well to include it in the prophylactic routine. Because spraying the light may represent an electrical hazard, wipe its handles with a double-folded paper towel amply moistened with disinfecting solution. Then cover the handles. A very handy and inexpensive cover for the handles is the common sandwich bag (5.5 × 6.75 inches).* Also a cover-all, universal film with an adhesive on one side is produced in a roll that is perforated to provide 1200 4 × 6 inch sheets.† The adhesive is unique in that it adheres only to itself with any tenacity and leaves no residue.

3. Disinfect the apron. Also clean, disinfect, and cover the leaded apron between patients. Not only is it frequently contaminated with saliva as the result of handling (readjusting its position) during a radiographic procedure but also it is occasionally showered with vomit. Suspend the apron on a heavy coat hanger to permit turning front to back. Spray it with the detergent containing disinfectant, then wipe, and cover with the same type of plastic garment bag used for the x-ray head and chair back (Fig. 10-3).

*Presto Products, Inc., P.O. Box 2399, Appleton, WI 54913.
†COVER-ALL, Pinnacle Products, Inc., 624 South Smith Avenue, St. Paul, MN 55107.

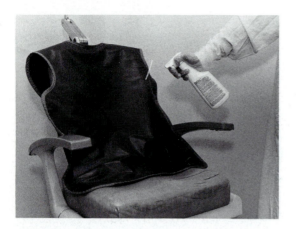

FIG. 10-3. Spray hanging apron with disinfectant; then dry and cover with a garment bag.

4. Disinfect and cover PID, x-ray head, and support. The last areas to be treated with a disinfecting solution are the surfaces of the x-ray machine. Depending upon the floor covering, spray or wipe disinfectant on the x-ray PID, tube head, yoke, and the swivel just proximal to the yoke. Spraying can be used without concern if the floor in the area is covered with a vinyl or a hard vinyl-like covering. In this case, apply the disinfectant to the point just short of dripping. If dripping is encountered, the excess can be blotted with a paper towel wipe that can be used later on other surfaces. If the design of the area is such that an area is not subject to traffic, move the x-ray head to that area and the drips will not be a cause for concern. One does not have to be apprehensive about the disinfectant seeping into the head and corroding the electrical system because the head is sealed against the leakage of the cooling-insulating oil. Cover the PID and head while they are still "wet" with disinfectant with a barrier to stop any dripping. A plastic garment bag serves as an effective, relatively inexpensive, easily applied microbial barrier for this application (Fig. 10-4). A commercially available, disposable plastic sleeve made to cover the x-ray head and cone is also available.* Slide either barrier over the PID and the head and as far proximally onto the support arm as the bag permits. Secure it with a heavy, no. A6A 564 rubber band stretched over the head and placed just proximal

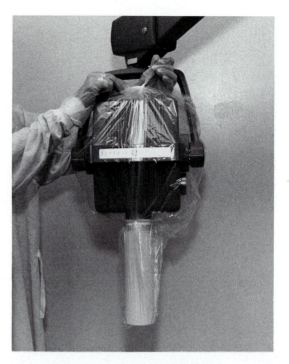

FIG. 10-4. Slip a plastic garment bag over x-ray tube head. Place a large rubber band just proximal to the swivel or tie ends as shown here. Pull the plastic tight over the PID and secure with a lighter rubber band slipped over the PID and placed next to the head.

to the swivel. Pull the plastic over the PID tight and secure it with a lighter No. A6A 532 rubber band slipped over the PID and placed next to the head.†

If the floor is carpeted, fold a doubled paper towel and use it as a backup to intercept the spray that bypasses the equipment and to blot immediately any spray that may run and drip. Another alternative is to fold and liberally spray doubled paper towels and wipe all the areas of the x-ray machine up to the distal end of the support arm. After wiping, apply the plastic barrier as described previously.

5. Cover environmental working surfaces. Wipe the surfaces that were previously sprayed and apply barriers. Wipe the areas in sequence from those that are the least heavily infected to the most heavily infected; the x-ray console, the counter tops, then the chair. Barriers protect the underlying surface from becoming contaminated. An effective barrier for the counter tops and x-ray control console is plastic wrap that can be obtained in 1200-foot rolls that are 18 inches wide.‡ It is convenient to store this plastic in a butcher's paper dispenser mounted on a wall out of heavy traffic

*X-RAY SLEEVE, Pinnacle Products, Inc., 624 South Smith Avenue, St. Paul, MN 55107.
†Associated Rubber Bands via Boise Cascade Corp., P.O. Box 50, Boise, Idaho 83728.
‡Reynolds Food Service Packaging, Richmond, VA 23261.

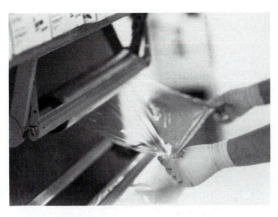

FIG. 10-5. Obtain plastic wrap from dispenser to cover counter tops and x-ray machine console.

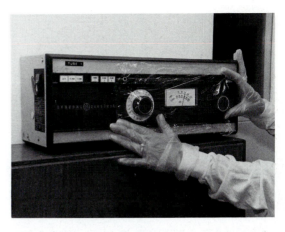

FIG. 10-6. Cover console with plastic wrap on parts that will be touched during the radiographic examination.

patterns to preclude it being repeatedly brushed by passing patients and staff (Fig. 10-5). Use these sheets to cover the counters and x-ray console. They may be secured to the counter tops quite effectively (by electrostatic attraction) if they are pulled tight, lapped over the edges, and rubbed down. When covering the x-ray control console, be sure to include the exposure switch and the exposure time control if they are an integral part of the unit (Fig. 10-6). There has been at least one report that the application of plastic wrap over the kVp meter may cause electrostatic deflection of the meter needle and result in an erroneous voltage reading.[8] Experiment with your equipment to determine if the application of plastic wrap influences the meter reading. Cover an x-ray exposure switch that is independent of the console with a sandwich bag or food storage bag, or wrap it with plastic wrap.

Wipe the headrest and chair back adjustments, the chair back, and the seat of the chair with a paper towel. Check the seat of the chair to be sure that some disinfectant was not inadvertently overlooked that may subsequently cause some damage to a patient or a patient's clothes. Cover the headrest, headrest adjustments, and chair back adjustments with the same type of plastic garment bag* used to cover the x-ray head (Fig. 10-7); an alternative is a product called Chair Sleeve.†

The operatory is now prepared for radiography. After seating the patient, wash your hands and put

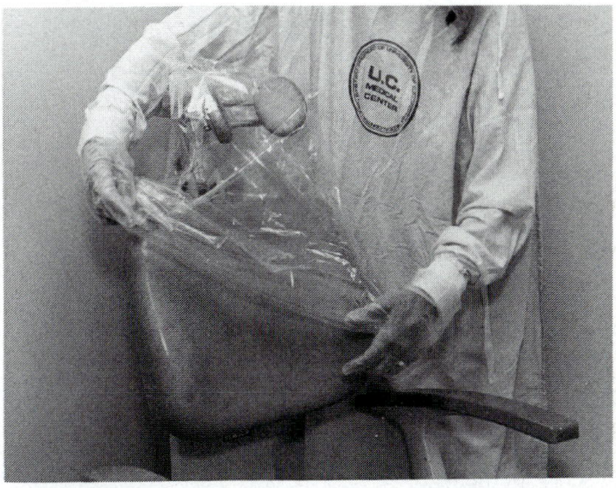

FIG. 10-7. Place garment bag over chair and headrest between patients.

on disposable gloves in sight of the patient if the operatory arrangement permits. All the objects that will be touched from this point on have been disinfected or sterilized.

6. Process contaminated x-ray films. Film packets are exposed to saliva and possibly blood during exposure in the patient's mouth. To prevent saliva from seeping into the film packet, place a paper towel beside the container for exposed films. Use this towel to wipe each film as you remove it from the patient's mouth and before placing it with the other exposed films. After making all exposures, take the contaminated films to the darkroom. Lay out two towels on the darkroom working surface. Place the container of contaminated films on one of these towels. Film is removed from its

---

*W.P. Ballard, Inc., 8929 Diplomacy, Dallas, TX 75247.
†CHAIR SLEEVE, Pinnacle Products, Inc., 624 South Smith Avenue, St. Paul, MN 55107.

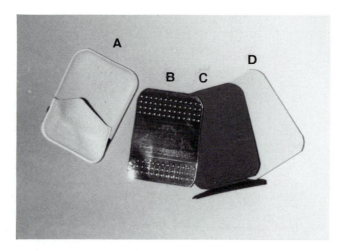

FIG. 10-8. A moisture- and light-proof film packet **(A)** contains an opening tab on the side opposite the tube. Inside is a sheet of lead foil **(B)** and a black light-proof interleaf paper wrapper folded **(C)** around the film **(D).**

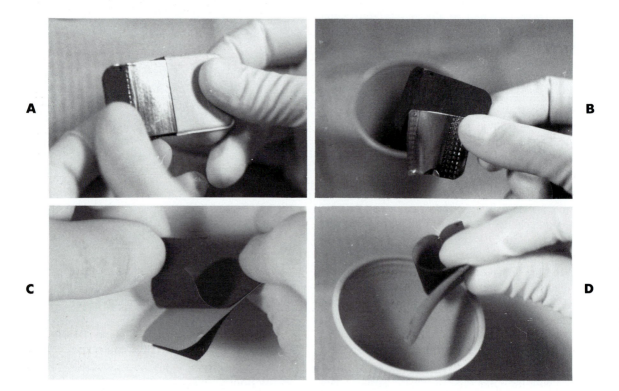

FIG. 10-9. Method for removing films from packet without touching them with contaminated gloves. **A,** Open packet tab and slide lead foil and black interleaf paper from wrapping. Picture illustrating the steps used to open a no. 2 film packet without contaminating film. **B,** Rotate foil away from black paper and discard. **C,** Open paper wrapping. **D,** Allow film to fall into a clean cup.

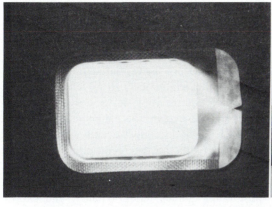 **A**

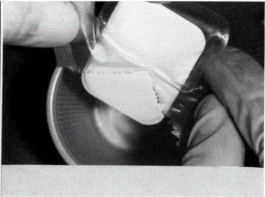 **B**

FIG. 10-10. Dental film with a ClinAsept Barrier to protect film from contact with saliva. **A,** Note notch on side of plastic envelope for opening. **B,** During opening, the plastic is removed and the clean film allowed to drop into a container.

packet and placed on the other towel. The film packaging will be discarded on the first towel with the container.

Removing film from a packet without touching (contaminating) is a relatively easy procedure if specific steps are observed, steps based on knowing how the film is wrapped within the packet (Fig. 10-8). Figure 10-9 illustrates the method for opening a contaminated film packet, while wearing contaminated gloves, without touching the film. Hold the film packet by the color-coded end and grasp the tab. Pull the tab upward and away from the packet to reveal the black paper tab wrapped over the end of the film. Now, holding the film over the second towel, carefully grasp this black paper tab that wraps the film and pull the film from the packet. When the film is pulled from the packet, it will fall from the paper wrapping onto the clean towel. The paper wrapper may need to be shaken lightly to cause the film to fall free. Place the packaging materials on the first paper towel. After opening all films, gather the contaminated packaging and container and discard them along with the contaminated gloves. Process the clean films in the usual manner. After processing the films, while wearing disinfected utility gloves, clean and disinfect all contaminated work surfaces.

A recent commercial development has simplified the handling of contaminated, exposed films. Eastman Kodak has introduced intraoral D- and E-speed films sealed in a plastic envelope (Kodak dental film with ClinAsept barrier) (Fig. 10-10). This plastic barrier protects the film from contact with saliva and blood during exposure.[2] These pro-

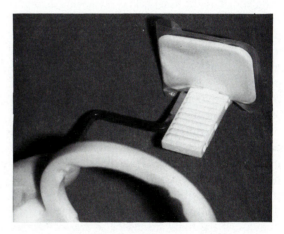

FIG. 10-11. Film-holding instrument with barrier envelope protecting film from saliva.

tected films are relatively expensive, but the empty polyester envelopes (ClinAsept barriers) may be purchased separately and used to seal and protect the conventional film.[2] Although the barrier envelopes are large enough to accommodate no. 2 film, a no. 1 can be placed in the envelope and the excess plastic folded over the film. Both sizes of barrier-protected film fit in the Precision and XCP film-holding instruments (Fig. 10-11). An attractive feature of the protective envelopes is the ease with which they may be opened and the film extracted. Wipe the barrier-protected film as an added precaution against contamination during opening. The envelope has a small V cut in the margin of one side that facilitates opening the envelope, and the film drops out with little chance of contacting the contaminated surfaces of the envelope. The barrier envelopes can be conveniently opened in a lighted area, the film dropped onto a clean work area or into a clean paper or plastic cup, and the film transferred to the daylight loader or darkroom for processing. Use of these envelopes provides the only uncomplicated method of using a daylight loader and maintaining the integrity of an infection-control procedure.

An ideal procedure, when exposing six or more films in plastic packaging, is to place the exposed film, still in the protective plastic envelope, in an approved disinfecting solution when it is removed from the mouth and after wiping with a paper towel. It should remain in the disinfectant following the exposure of the last film for the recommended time, usually about 10 minutes. To increase the time available for the action of the disinfectant on the film packets, clean and disinfect the radiography area before proceeding with film processing. The envelope containing the film can then be dried with a clean paper towel, opened in the light or in the dark, and the film removed and processed without gloves and without transferring infectious material to the daylight loader or darkroom equipment.

A busy practitioner may object to the 10-minute delay between the completion of exposure and the initiation of processing. However, during the exposure of a full-mouth series, only the last few films exposed will not have been in contact with the disinfecting solution for the recommended 10 minutes. If the films are placed in two containers with disinfectant, the first half of the films exposed may be placed in one of the containers with the disinfectant, and the remaining films in the second. Take the containers to the daylight loader or darkroom and dry and process the films that were exposed first. The film packets in the second container have at this point had sufficient contact with the disinfectant and can be dried and processed, either with the daylight loader or in the darkroom.

7. Remove all barriers and respray or wipe all working surfaces and apron. After completing the patient exposures, remove the barriers and spray or wipe all working surfaces and the apron with disinfectant as described previously.

8. Disinfect panoramic machine and cephalostat. The panoramic machine should receive the same concern for contamination and disinfection as other equipment. However, in the use of the panoramic machine, fewer areas are contacted and contaminated by the patient, saliva, or operator. Clean the bite blocks, chin rest, and patient handgrips with the detergent-iodine disinfectant. Cover the chin rest and bite blocks with a 5 1/8 × 7 1/16 inch plastic bag.* Carefully wipe the head-positioning guides, control panel, and exposure switch with a paper towel that is well moistened with disinfectant. The radiographer should wear disposable gloves while positioning and exposing the patient. Remove the gloves before removing the cassette from the machine for processing because the cassette and film remain extraoral and should not be handled while wearing contaminated, disposable gloves.

Clean and disinfect cephalostat ear posts, ear post brackets, and forehead support or nasion pointer by vigorous wiping with a paper towel generously moistened with the iodine-detergent disinfectant.

REFERENCES

1. American Academy of Oral and Maxillofacial Radiology infection control guidelines for dental radiographic procedures, *Oral Surg Oral Med Oral Pathol* 73:248-249, 1992.
2. American Dental Association, Council on Dental Materials, Instruments and Equipment, Council on Dental Practice, and Council on Dental Therapeutics: Infection control recommendations for the dental office and dental laboratory. *Am Dent Assoc* 116:241-248, 1988.
3. Centers for Disease Control: Recommended infection-control practices for dentistry, *MMWR* 35:237-242, 1986.
4. Centers for Disease Control: Guidelines for prevention of transmission of human immunodeficiency virus and hepatitis B virus to health-care and public-safety workers, *MMWR* 38:S-6, 1989.
5. Cattone JA, Milinari JA: State-of-the-art infection control in dentistry *J Am Dent Assoc* 123:33-41, 1991.
6. DeVita VT, Hellman S, Rosenberg SA, editors: AIDS, Philadelphia, 1985, Lippincott.
7. Hovius M: Disinfection and sterilization: duties and responsibilities of dentists and dental hygienists, *Int Dent J* 42:241-244, 1992.
8. Jefferies D, Morris J, White V: KVp meter errors induced by plastic wrap, *J Dent Hygiene* 65:91-93, 1991.
9. Katz JO, Cattone JA, Hardman PK, et al. Infection control protocol for dental radiology, *General Dentistry* 38:261-264, 1990.
10. Miller CH: Sterilization and disinfection: what every dentist needs to know. *J. Am Dent Assoc* 123:46-54, 1992.

---

*Johnson Bag, 200 Scott Street, Elk Grove Village, IL. 60001; 17 × 18 garbage bag, Albertson's Inc., Boise, ID 83726; 11.5 × 12.5 food storage bag, Topco Assoc., Skokie, IL 60076.

11

In collaboration with Abdul H. Shawkat

Extraoral Radiographic Examinations

Extraoral radiographic examinations include all views made of the orofacial region with films positioned extraorally. The dentist often uses these views to examine areas not fully covered by intraoral films or to visualize the skull and facial structures. When there are appropriate clinical signs or symptoms, it may be valuable to examine the mandible, maxilla, and other facial bones for evidence of disease or injury. Orthodontists often use extraoral projections to evaluate skeletal growth. This chapter describes the standard views used for these purposes. Panoramic radiography is considered in Chapter 12, and specific radiographic techniques for examining the temporomandibular joint are described in Chapter 25.

Film and intensifying screens

To achieve the best images with the lowest exposures, it is important to make all extraoral radiographic projections using appropriate combinations of film and intensifying screens (Table 5-8). Medium- or high-speed rare-earth screen-film combinations provide the optimum balance between loss of image detail and reduction of patient exposure. For lateral oblique views of the mandible it is sufficient to use a 13 × 18 cm (5 × 7 inch) film and cassette. Skull film will require at least a 20 × 25 cm (8 × 10 inch) film and cassette. Extraoral films can usually be processed in either conventional wet tanks or an automatic processor. It is wise to place an "R" or "L" on the appropriate corner of the cassette to indicate the patient's right and left side on the resultant radiograph. The use of grids will reduce fog from scattered radiation, which in turn increases contrast. Because the use of grids approximately doubles patient exposure, however, they should be used only when the highest contrast is necessary. The most common extraoral

projection (the lateral cephalometric) can be made quite satisfactorily without a grid.

X-ray machines

It is possible to make extraoral skull projections using conventional dental x-ray machines, advanced types of panoramic x-ray machines, or larger x-ray units designed specifically for extraoral radiography. When using a conventional dental x-ray machine for skull radiography (e.g., in an orthodontic practice), it is important to provide some means for fixing the tube head in a standardized position. Often wall-mounted brackets are used for this purpose. Similarly, it is important that a device for positioning the head (a *cephalostat*) be available for reproducible positioning of the patient. By these means one can achieve consistent and accurate positioning of the patient in relation to the tube head and film cassette. The more specialized types of equipment available for extraoral radiography provide the means for consistent positioning of the patient.

SKULL PROJECTIONS

Radiographic examination of the skull requires patience, attention to detail, and practice to produce satisfactory results. Proper patient positioning requires the use of skeletal landmarks. The *Frankfort plane* (connecting the superior border of the external auditory meatus with the infraorbital rim) is the classic reference line. The *canthomeatal line* (joining the central point of the external auditory meatus to the outer canthus of the eye) forms an angle of about 10 degrees with the Frankfort plane. Radiologists prefer using the canthomeatal line for patient positioning because it is more easily visualized. Obtaining consistent results requires use of a cephalostat.

227

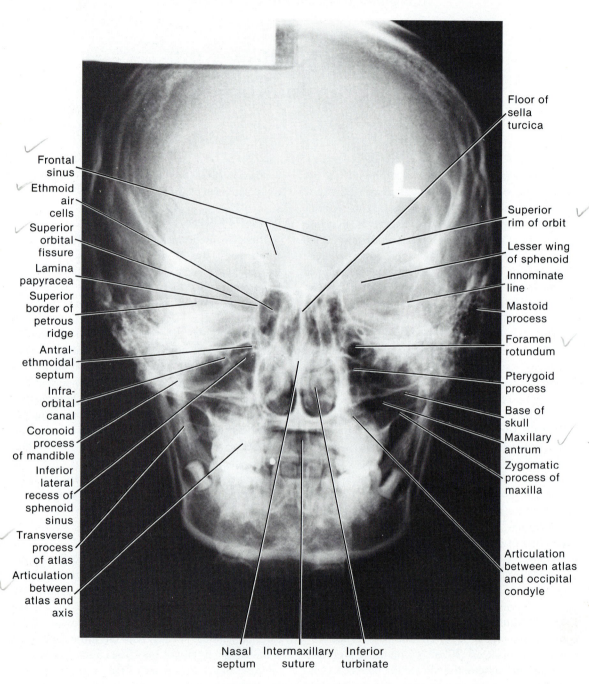

Floor of
sella
turcica

Frontal
sinus

Ethmoid
air
cells

Superior
orbital
fissure

Lamina
papyracea

Superior
border of
petrous
ridge

Antral-
ethmoidal
septum

Infra-
orbital
canal

Coronoid
process
of mandible

Inferior
lateral
recess of
sphenoid
sinus

Transverse
process
of atlas

Articulation
between
atlas and
axis

Superior
rim of orbit

Lesser wing
of sphenoid

Innominate
line

Mastoid
process

Foramen
rotundum

Pterygoid
process

Base of
skull

Maxillary
antrum

Zygomatic
process of
maxilla

Articulation
between atlas
and occipital
condyle

Nasal   Intermaxillary   Inferior
septum   suture   turbinate

FIG. 11-1. Posteroanterior cephalometric projection of the skull.

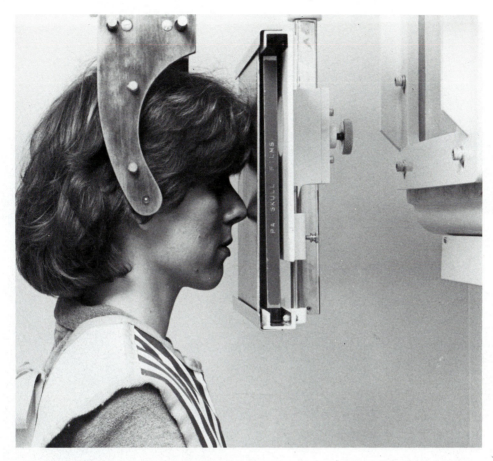

FIG. 11-2. Patient positioning for a posteroanterior cephalometric projection of the skull.

Posteroanterior projection

The straight posteroanterior (PA) projection is so named because the x-ray beam passes in a posterior-to-anterior direction through the skull (Fig. 11-1). It is used to examine the skull for disease, trauma, or developmental abnormalities and provides a good record to detect progressive changes in the mediolateral dimensions of the skull, including asymmetric growth. It also offers good visualization of facial structures—including the frontal and ethmoid sinuses, nasal fossae, and orbits. Cephalometric examinations use a slight variation of this technique.

Film placement. The cassette is positioned vertically in a holding device.

Head position. For the straight PA projection the head is centered in front of the cassette with the canthomeatal line parallel to the floor. For cephalometric applications the nose should be a little higher so the anterior projection of the canthomeatal line is 10 degrees above the horizontal and the Frankfort plane is perpendicular to the film (Fig. 11-2). On the resultant radiograph the superior border of the petrous ridge should lie in the lower third of the orbit. This orientation places the occlusal plane horizontal.

Projection of the central ray. The central ray is directed perpendicular to the plane of the film in the horizontal and vertical dimensions from a source at a distance of 91 to 102 cm (36 to 40 inches). It should be coincident with the midsagittal plane of the head at the level of the bridge of the nose. For cephalometric applications there should be a distance of 152.4 cm (60 inches) between the x-ray source and midcoronal plane of the patient.

Exposure parameters. The exposure parameters will vary considerably—depending on the type of x-ray machine, the distance from the source to the patient, and the screen-film combination. When a film and screen combination having a speed class of 250 is used, and with a kVp of 70, the mAs should be about 30 to 50.

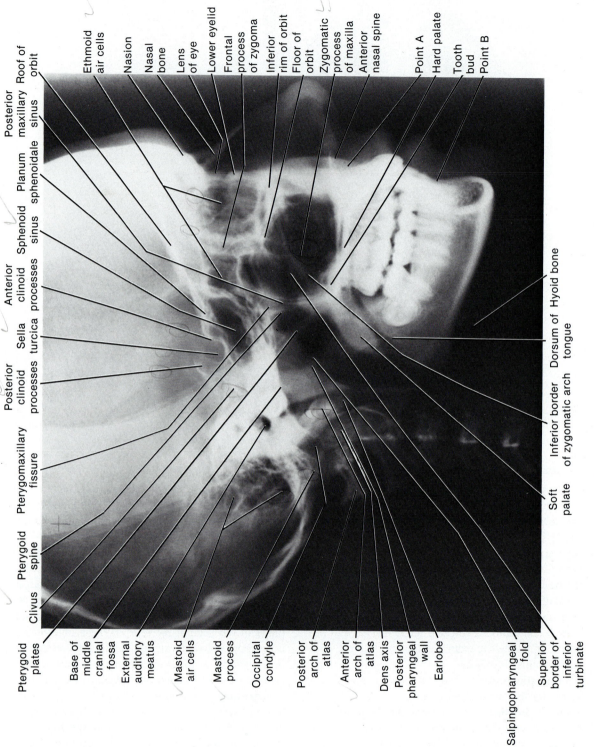

FIG. 11-3. Lateral cephalometric projection of the facial bones.

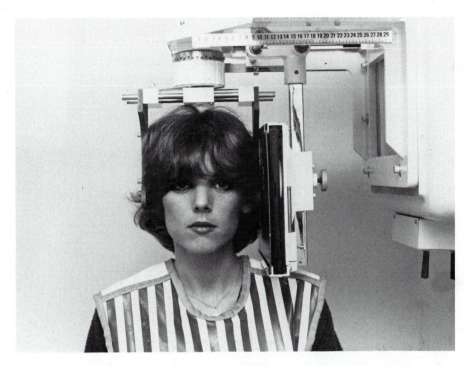

FIG. 11-4. Patient positioning for a lateral cephalometric projection of the facial bones.

Lateral skull projection (lateral cephalometric)

The lateral skull projection is used to survey the skull and facial bones for evidence of trauma, disease, or developmental abnormality. This view reveals the nasopharyngeal soft tissues, paranasal sinuses, and hard palate. Orthodontists use it to assess facial growth (Fig. 11-3), and in oral surgery and prosthetics it establishes pretreatment and posttreatment records. The lateral cephalometric projection reveals the facial soft tissue profile but otherwise is identical to the lateral skull view.

Film placement. The film is positioned vertically in a cassette-holding device.

Head position. The head should be positioned with the left side of the face near the cassette and the midsagittal plane parallel to the plane of the film (Fig. 11-4). A wedge filter is placed over the anterior side of the beam at the tube head. This will cause it to absorb some of the radiation striking the nose, lips, and chin. The filter thus reduces the intensity of radiation in the anterior region and helps reveal the soft tissue outline of the patient's face on the resultant radiograph.

Projection of the central ray. For cephalometric applications the distance between the x-ray source and the midsagittal plane is 152.4 cm (60 inches). The central ray is directed toward the external auditory meatus and perpendicular to the plane of the film and the midsagittal plane.

Exposure parameters. The exposure parameters will vary considerably depending on the type of x-ray machine, the distance from the source to the patient, and the screen-film combination used. When a film and screen combination having a speed class of 250 is used and with a kVp of 70, the mAs should be about 15 to 25.

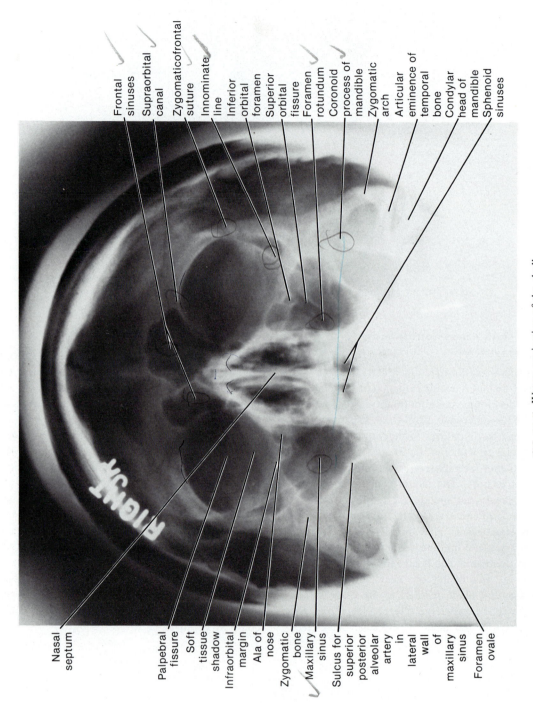

Frontal sinuses
Supraorbital canal
Zygomaticofrontal suture
Innominate line
Inferior orbital foramen
Superior orbital fissure
Foramen rotundum
Coronoid process of mandible
Zygomatic arch
Articular eminence of temporal bone
Condylar head of mandible
Sphenoid sinuses

Nasal septum
Palpebral fissure
Soft tissue shadow
Infraorbital margin
Ala of nose
Zygomatic bone
Maxillary sinus
Sulcus for superior posterior alveolar artery in lateral wall of maxillary sinus
Foramen ovale

FIG. 11-5. Waters projection of the skull.

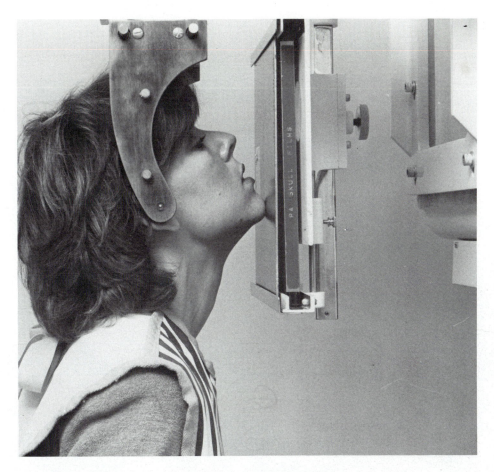

FIG. 11-6. Patient positioning for a Waters projection of the skull.

Waters projection

The Waters projection (also called *occipitomental projection*) is a variation of the PA view. It is particularly useful for evaluation of the maxillary sinuses. In addition, it demonstrates the frontal and ethmoid sinuses, the orbit, the zygomaticofrontal suture, and the nasal cavity (Fig. 11-5). It also demonstrates the position of the coronoid process of the mandible between the maxilla and the zygomatic arch.

Film placement. The cassette is positioned vertically.

Head position. The head should be oriented with the sagittal plane perpendicular to the plane of the film. The chin is raised high to elevate the canthomeatal line 37 degrees above horizontal (Fig. 11-6). If the petrous portion of the temporal bone lies over the apex of the maxillary sinus, then the patient's chin needs to be further elevated. If the patient's mouth is open, the image of the sphenoid sinus will project onto the palate.

Projection of the central ray. The central ray should be perpendicular to the film, through the midsagittal plane, and at the level of the maxillary sinus.

Exposure parameters. The exposure parameters will vary considerably depending on the type of x-ray machine used, the distance from the source to the patient, and the screen-film combination and grid chosen. When a film and screen combination having a speed class of 250 is used, and with a kVp of 70, the mAs should be about 100.

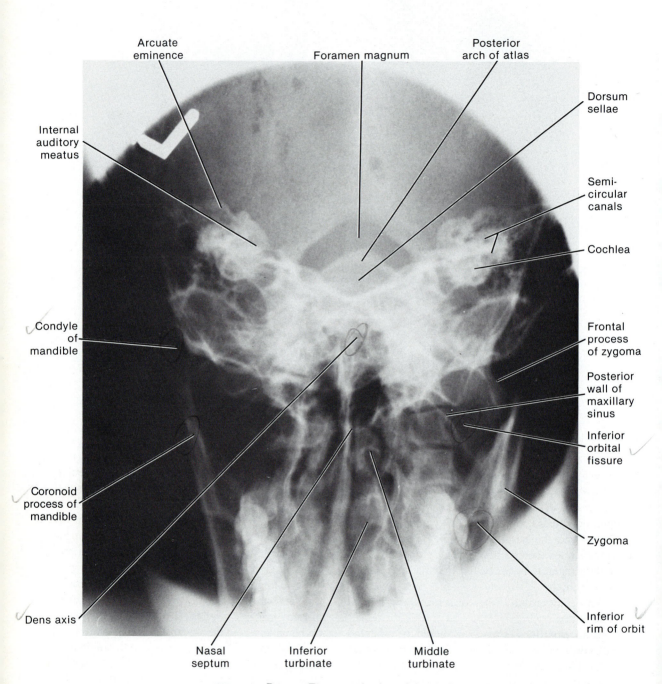

FIG. 11-7. Reverse-Towne projection of the skull.

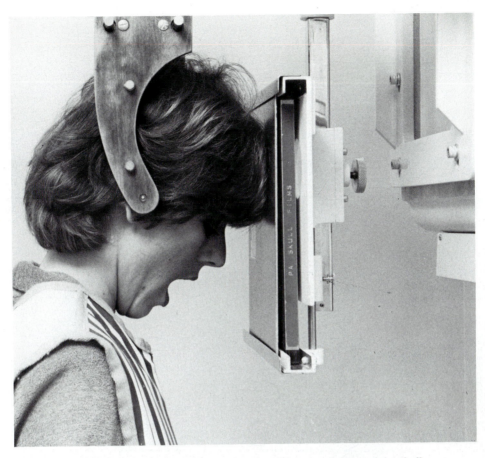

FIG. 11-8. Patient positioning for a reverse-Towne projection of the skull.

Reverse-Towne projection

The reverse-Towne projection is used to examine a patient with a suspected fracture of the condylar neck (Fig. 11-7). It is particularly suitable for revealing a medially displaced condyle. This projection also reveals the posterolateral wall of the maxillary antrum.

Film placement. The cassette is positioned in a holding device.

Head position. The head should be centered in front of the cassette with the canthomeatal line oriented downward 25 to 30 degrees (Fig. 11-8). To help visualize the condyles, it is advisable to have the patient open his or her mouth as wide as possible.

Projection of the central ray. The central ray is directed to the film in the sagittal plane through the occipital bone, with the beam collimated to the areas of interest to reduce patient exposure and film fog.

Exposure parameters. The exposure parameters will vary considerably depending on the type of x-ray machine used, the distance from the source to the patient, and the screen-film combination and grid chosen. When a film and screen combination is used having a speed class of 250 and with a kVp of 70, the mAs should be about 100.

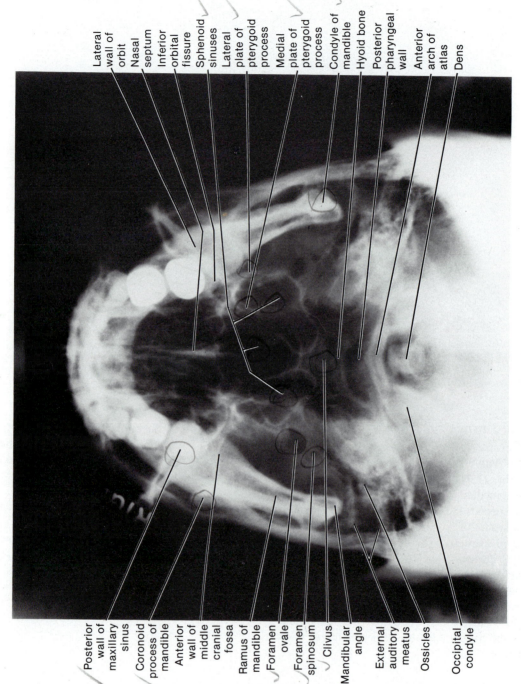

Lateral wall of orbit
Nasal septum
Inferior orbital fissure
Sphenoid sinuses
Lateral plate of pterygoid process
Medial plate of pterygoid process
Condyle of mandible
Hyoid bone
Posterior pharyngeal wall
Anterior arch of atlas
Dens

Posterior wall of maxillary sinus
Coronoid process of mandible
Anterior wall of middle cranial fossa
Ramus of mandible
Foramen ovale
Foramen spinosum
Clivus
Mandibular angle
External auditory meatus
Ossicles
Occipital condyle

FIG. 11-9. Submentovertex projection of the skull.

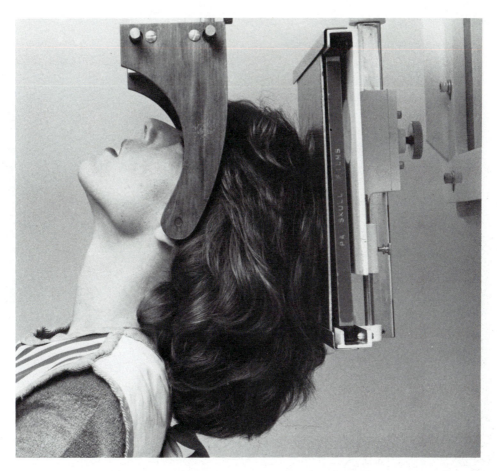

FIG. 11-10. Patient positioning for a submentovertex projection of the skull.

Submentovertex projection

The submentovertex projection (also called *base* or *full axial projection*) is used to demonstrate the base of the skull, the position and orientation of the condyles, the sphenoid sinus, the curvature of the mandible, the lateral wall of the maxillary sinuses, or any displacement of a fractured zygomatic arch (Fig. 11-9). This view will often also display the medial and lateral pterygoid plates and foramina in the base of the skull.

Film placement. The film cassette is placed vertically in a holding device.

Head position. The patient's head and neck should be extended backward as far as possible, with the vertex of the skull on the center of the cassette. It is usually helpful to lean the patient's chair back as far as it will go to help the patient orient his head. The midsagittal plane of the head, however, must remain perpendicular to the floor.

The canthomeatal line should extend 10 degrees past vertical so the Frankfort line is vertical and parallel with the film (Fig. 11-10).

Projection of the central ray. The central ray is directed from below the mandible upward, toward the vertex of the skull, and is positioned far enough anterior to pass about 2 cm in front of a line connecting the right and left condylar processes.

Exposure parameters. The exposure parameters will vary considerably depending on the type of x-ray machine used, the distance from the source to the patient, and the screen-film combination and grid chosen. When a film and screen combination having a speed class of 250 is used, and with a kVp of 70, the mAs should be about 100. To view the zygomatic arches specifically, reduce the exposure time to one third that used to visualize the skull (Fig. 11-11).

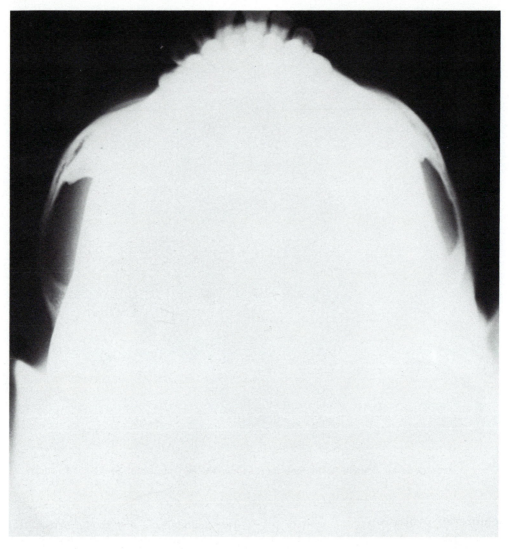

FIG. 11-11. Submentovertex projection of the zygomatic arches.

MANDIBULAR LATERAL OBLIQUE PROJECTIONS

There are two lateral oblique projections commonly used to examine the mandible: one for the body and one for the ramus. A dental x-ray machine with an open-ended aiming cylinder is best for these projections. The film is usually a 13 × 18 cm (5 × 7 inch) screen film or larger. (Use either fast or moderate-speed film and screens.) The cassette should be hand held by the patient. Although these views have been largely replaced by panoramic radiographs, dentists still use them when an image with greater resolution is needed than can be provided by a panoramic view or when a panoramic machine is not available.

Mandibular body projection

The mandibular body projection demonstrates the premolar-molar region and the inferior border of the mandible (Fig. 11-12). It provides much broader coverage than is possible with periapical projections.

Head position. The head is tilted toward the side being examined and the mandible is protruded.

Film placement. The cassette is placed against the patient's cheek and centered over the first molar, its lower border parallel with the inferior border of the mandible and extending at least 2 cm below it. The patient can hold the cassette in place (Fig. 11-13).

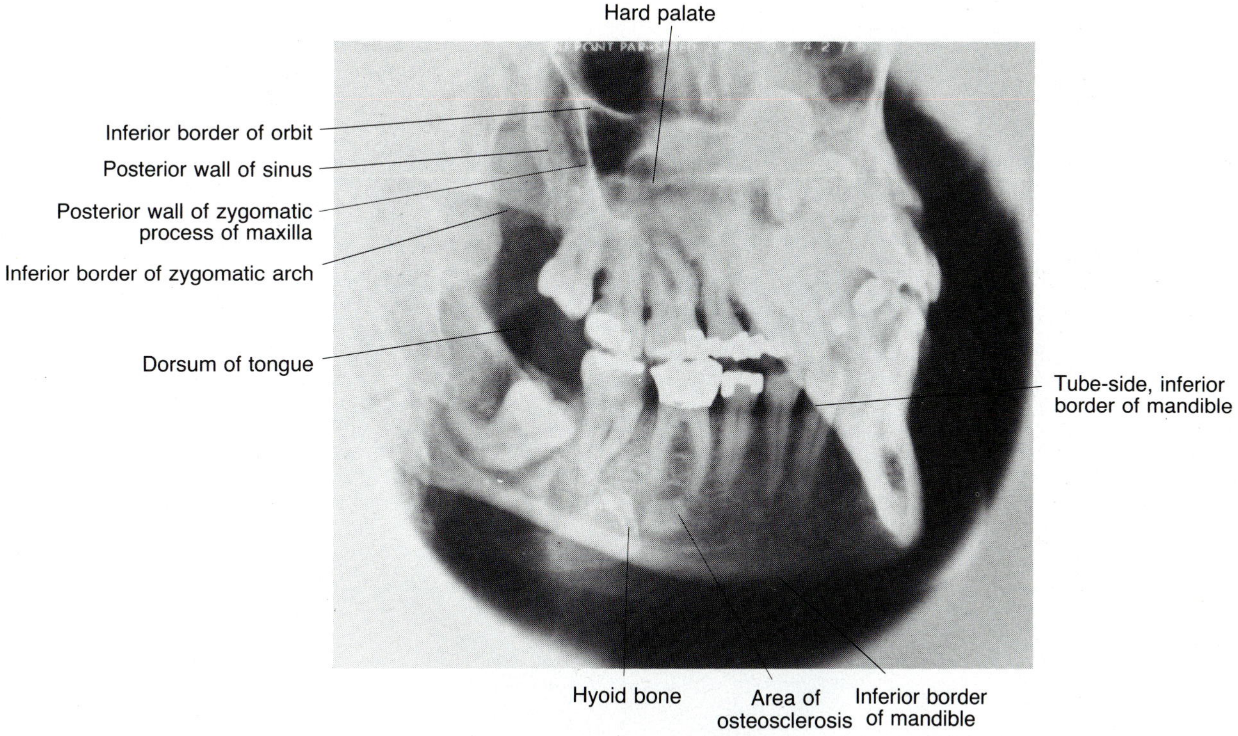

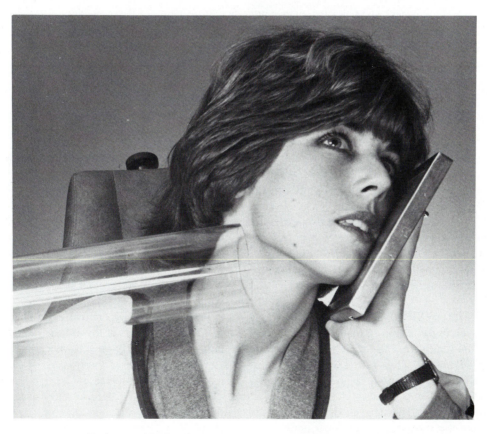

Hard palate

Inferior border of orbit

Posterior wall of sinus

Posterior wall of zygomatic
process of maxilla

Inferior border of zygomatic arch

Dorsum of tongue

Tube-side, inferior
border of mandible

Hyoid bone   Area of   Inferior border
osteosclerosis of mandible

FIG. 11-12. Lateral oblique projection of the body of the mandible.

FIG. 11-13. Patient positioning for a lateral oblique projection of the mandibular body.

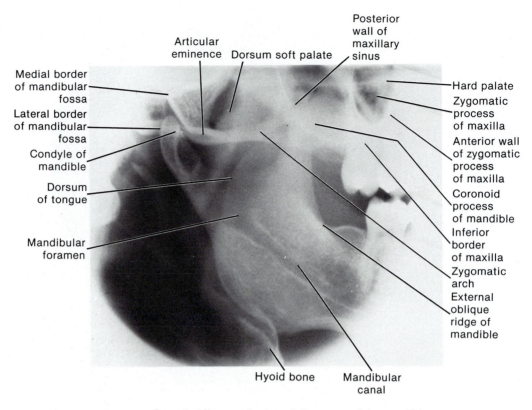

Articular eminence

Dorsum soft palate

Posterior wall of maxillary sinus

Medial border of mandibular fossa

Lateral border of mandibular fossa

Condyle of mandible

Dorsum of tongue

Mandibular foramen

Hard palate

Zygomatic process of maxilla

Anterior wall of zygomatic process of maxilla

Coronoid process of mandible

Inferior border of maxilla

Zygomatic arch

External oblique ridge of mandible

Hyoid bone

Mandibular canal

FIG. 11-14. Lateral oblique projection of the ramus of the mandible.

Projection of the central ray. The central ray is directed toward the first molar region of the mandible from a point 2 cm below the angle on the tube side. The central ray should be as close to perpendicular to the plane of the film as possible.

Exposure parameters. Although exposure parameters will vary, it is customary to use 65 kVp, 10 mA, and about ¼ second for medium-speed screens and film.

Mandibular ramus projection

The mandibular ramus projection will give a view of the ramus from the angle of the mandible to the condyle (Fig. 11-14). It is often very useful for examining the third molar regions of the maxilla and mandible.

Head position. The head is tilted toward the side of the mandible being examined until a line between the mandibular angle next to the tube and

the condyle away from the tube is parallel with the floor. To prevent the cervical spine from being superimposed on the ramus, the patient should protrude his/her mandible.

Film placement. The cassette is placed over the ramus and far enough posteriorly to include the condyle. The lower border of the cassette should be approximately parallel with the inferior border of the mandible and extend at least 2 cm below the border (Fig. 11-15).

Projection of the central ray. The central ray is directed posteriorly toward the center of the ramus on the side of interest from a point 2 cm below the inferior border of the first molar region of the mandible on the tube side.

Exposure parameters. The usual exposure factors for this projection are 65 kVp, 10 mA, and about ¼ second for medium-speed screens and film.

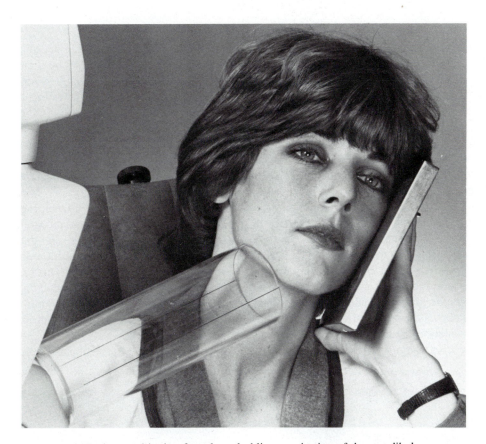

FIG. 11-15. Patient positioning for a lateral oblique projection of the mandibular ramus.

12

BARTON M. GRATT

Panoramic Radiography

Panoramic radiography (also called *pantomography* or *rotational radiography*) is a radiographic technique for producing a single image of the facial structures that includes both maxillary and mandibular arches and their supporting structures (Fig. 12-1). Its principal *advantages* are (1) broad anatomic coverage, (2) low patient radiation dose, (3) convenience of the examination, and (4) the fact that it can be used in patients unable to open their mouth.

The time required to complete a panoramic radiographic examination is quite short, usually in the range of 3 to 4 minutes. This includes the time necessary for positioning the patient and the actual exposure cycle. In addition to providing broad coverage of the oral region for radiographic interpretation, panoramic films are readily accepted by patients. This allows them to be used as a visual aid in case presentations and for patient education.

The main *disadvantage* of panoramic radiography is that the resultant image does not resolve the fine anatomic detail that may be seen on intraoral periapical radiographs. Thus, it is not as useful as periapical radiography for detecting small carious lesions or periapical disease.[17,18] The availability of a panoramic radiograph for an adult patient does not reduce the need for intraoral films in developing a final treatment plan.[9] Other problems associated with panoramic radiography are magnification, geometric distortion, and overlapped images of teeth, especially in the premolar region. Furthermore, objects whose recognition may be important for interpretation of the radiograph may be situated outside the section or plane of focus (called the focal trough). This results in their images being distorted or obscured on the resultant radiograph. The cost of a panoramic dental x-ray machine is 2 to 4 times that of an intraoral x-ray machine.

Experience indicates that panoramic radiographs

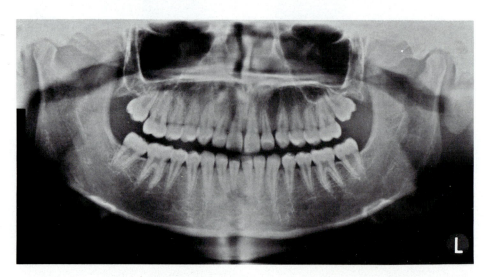

FIG. 12-1. Maxilla, mandible, and dentition in a 12-year-old child (panoramic view).

can be very useful in assisting the dentist with a number of specific diagnostic tasks, particularly when broad coverage of the jaws is desirable. These *indications* include the evaluation of trauma, third molars, extensive disease, tooth development (especially in the mixed dentition), retained teeth or root tips (in edentulous patients), and developmental anomalies. Panoramic radiographs are also useful for patients who do not tolerate intraoral procedures well or those with a large known (or suspected) lesion.

These are evaluations of general structural relationships of teeth and bone, and they do not require high resolution and sharp details seen on intraoral radiographs. The panoramic radiograph is often used as initial survey film that may provide the required insight or assist in determining the need for other projections. Panoramic films are not suitable for diagnostic examinations requiring high image resolution (e.g., the detection of early alveolar bone loss or incipient dental caries or the analysis of trabecular bone changes associated with early periapical lesions).[1,2,7] For such evaluations intraoral periapical and bitewing radiographs, made with direct-exposure film and providing much greater resolution, are required. Various studies[3,11,20] have shown that when a full-mouth series of radiographs is available for a patient receiving a general screening examination little or no additional useful information will be gained from a panoramic examination.

PRINCIPLES OF PANORAMIC RADIOGRAPHY

To interpret panoramic radiographs competently requires a thorough understanding of the following:
- Principles of panoramic image formation
- Techniques for patient positioning with head alignment and their rationale
- Radiographic appearance of normal anatomic structures

All three factors are closely related and must be comprehended before effective interpretation of panoramic radiographs can be achieved.

Principles of panoramic image formation

The principle of panoramic radiography was first described by Numata,[13] and independently by Paatero.[14,15] Their work led to the development of a number of panoramic x-ray machines employing similar radiographic principles. The operation of a panoramic machine can be understood by considering the following illustrations. Two adjacent

disks are rotating at the same speed in opposite directions as an x-ray beam passes through their centers of rotation (Fig. 12-2). Lead collimators in the shape of a slit located at the x-ray source and at the film limit the central ray to a narrow vertical beam. Radiopaque objects *A, B, C,* and *D* on disk *1* rotate past the slit, and their images are recorded on the film, which also moves past the slit at the same time. The objects are displayed sharply on the film because they are moving past the slit at the same rate as the film, which in effect causes their moving images to appear stationary in relation to the moving film.

Figure 12-3 shows that the same relationship of moving film to image is achieved if the x-ray source is rotated so the central ray constantly passes through the center of rotation of disk *1* and, simultaneously, both disk *2* and the film collimator *(Pb)* rotate about the center of disk *1*. Note that, while disk *2* moves, the film on this disk rotates past the slit. To obtain optimum image definition,

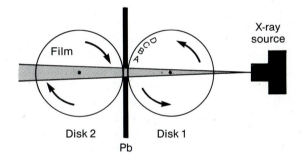

FIG. 12-2. Movement of the film and objects (*A, B, C,* and *D*) about two fixed centers of rotation.

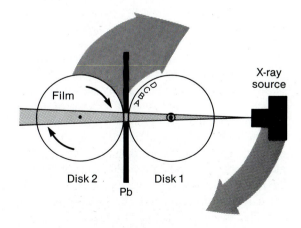

FIG. 12-3. Movement of the film and x-ray source about one fixed center of rotation.

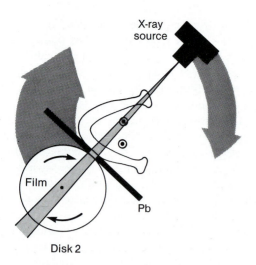

FIG. 12-4. Movement of the film and x-ray source about a shifting center of rotation. *Pb,* Lead collumator.

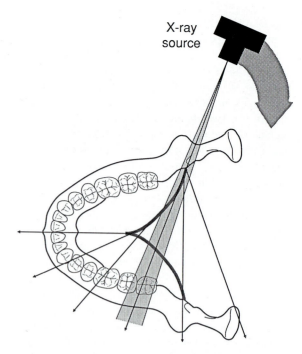

FIG. 12-5. Movement of the x-ray source and beam. The *dark line* shows a continuously moving center of rotation. As the source moves behind the patient's neck and the anterior teeth are imaged, the center of rotation moves forward along the arc *(dark line)* toward the sagittal plane. The x-ray source continues to move around the patient to image the opposite side.

it is critical that the speed of the film passing the collimator slit *(Pb)* be maintained equal to the speed at which the x-ray beam sweeps through the objects of interest.

Figure 12-4 shows that disk *1* may be replaced by a patient. In practice, its center of rotation will be located off to one side. During the exposure cycle the machine will automatically shift to other rotation centers. The movement of the film behind the slit is regulated to be the same as that of the central ray sweeping through the dental structures on the side of the patient near the film. Structures on the opposite side of the patient (near the x-ray tube) are distorted and out of focus because the x-ray beam sweeps through them in the direction opposite that in which the film cassette is moving. In addition, structures near the x-ray source are so magnified (and their borders so blurred) that they are not seen as discrete images on the resultant radiograph. Because of both these circumstances, only structures near the film will be usefully imaged on the resultant radiograph. Many panoramic machines now use a continuously moving center of rotation rather than fixed locations.

Figure 12-5 shows a continually moving center of rotation. This center of rotation is near the lingual surface of the right body of the mandible when the left TMJ is imaged. It moves forward along an arc that ends just lingual to the symphysis of the mandible when the midline is imaged. The arc is reversed as the opposite side of the face is imaged.

Focal trough. The focal trough is a three-dimensional curved zone or image layer in which structures are reasonably well defined on panoramic radiographs. The image seen on a panoramic radiograph consists largely of the anatomic structures located within the focal trough. Objects in front of or behind the focal trough are blurred, magnified, or reduced in size and are sometimes distorted to the extent of not being recognizable. The focal trough is the region in which structures will be revealed most sharply. The shape of the focal trough varies with the brand of equipment used. Figure 12-6 shows the general shape of the focal trough used in panoramic machines. The factors that affect its size are variables that influence image definition: arc path, velocity of the film and x-ray tube head, alignment of the x-ray beam, and collimator width. In practice the location of the focal trough can change with use of the machine,[16] so recalibration may be indicated if consistently suboptimal images are produced.

As the position of an object is moved within the focal trough, the size and shape of the resultant

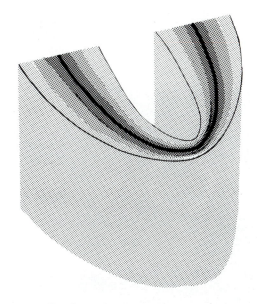

FIG. 12-6. Focal trough. The closer to the center of the trough *(dark zone)* an anatomic structure is positioned, the more clearly it will be imaged on the resulting radiograph.

image will change. Figure 12-7, *A* to *F,* illustrates a comparison of the variable image *magnification* of objects that are within the focal trough. Figure 12-7, *A* and *B,* shows a mandible supporting a brass ring properly aligned in the middle of the focal trough. Note the even magnification of the ring and the images of the anterior teeth in proper proportion. Figure 12-7, *C* and *D,* shows the same mandible positioned 5 mm anterior to the middle of the focal trough. This position will cause distortion of the ring in the horizontal dimension with decreased width of the images of the teeth. Figure 12-7, *E* and *F,* shows the same mandible positioned 5 mm posterior to the middle of the focal trough. Note the horizontal magnification of the ring and the increased width of the projected teeth. On these radiographs the vertical dimension, in contrast to the horizontal dimension, is not as significantly altered. These distortions result from the horizontal movement of the film and x-ray source. When the object is displaced posteriorly from its optimum position in the focal trough toward the x-ray source, the beam passes more slowly through the anterior mandible than it normally would. Consequently the image of the structures in this region is elongated horizontally on the film, which is moving at the normal rate. Alternatively, when the mandible is displaced anteriorly toward the film the beam

passes at a rate faster than normal through the anterior structures. Because the film is moving at the proper rate, the image of the anterior teeth is compressed horizontally on the film. Special attention must be paid to these considerations in following the progress of a bony lesion, especially in the anterior region. As a result of improper patient positioning the lesion may appear greater (enlarging) (Fig. 12-7, *F*) or reduced (healing) (Fig. 12-7, *D*) on successive radiographs. Thus it is apparent how important careful alignment and positioning of the patient's dental arches within the area of the focal trough can be. Malalignment will result in suboptimal images that either are unacceptable to the experienced clinician or cause misinterpretation by the less experienced.

Panoramic machines. The imaging principles described above are employed in many panoramic machines. The Orthopantomograph 10E (Siemens) (Fig. 12-8) uses principles similar to those demonstrated in Figure 12-5 to produce its image. The Panelipse II (Gendex) (Fig. 12-9) uses an elliptic path simulating the shape of the dental arches. The resultant radiograph is a continuous image of the jaws with relatively constant horizontal and vertical magnification because of its capability to adjust the size of the ellipse to correspond to the size of a patient's arch (Fig. 12-10). The Panorex 2 (Keystone X-ray) (Fig. 12-11) uses two fixed centers of rotation to image the posterior regions of the jaws and a moving center of rotation to image the anterior region (Fig. 12-12).

Several panoramic machines have the capability of providing improved images of the temporomandibular joints. This is usually accomplished by having special tube head and film movements programmed into the machine. These views provide orientation of the x-ray beam through the long axis of the condyle rather than obliquely through it as with conventional panoramic machines. In addition to conventional panoramic radiography, the Orthophos (Siemens), Planmeca (Planmeca) (Fig. 12-13), and Ortholix SD (Gendex) perform specialized examinations of the TMJs and maxillary sinuses.

Recently a new line of computer-controlled multimodality machines has become available. In these machines the direction and speed of movement of the tube head and film are highly variable, in some cases including multidirection tomography. This allows the machines to be programmed to make tomographic views through many areas of the head. For instance, they can be programmed to image frontal or lateral views of the TMJs, coronal or

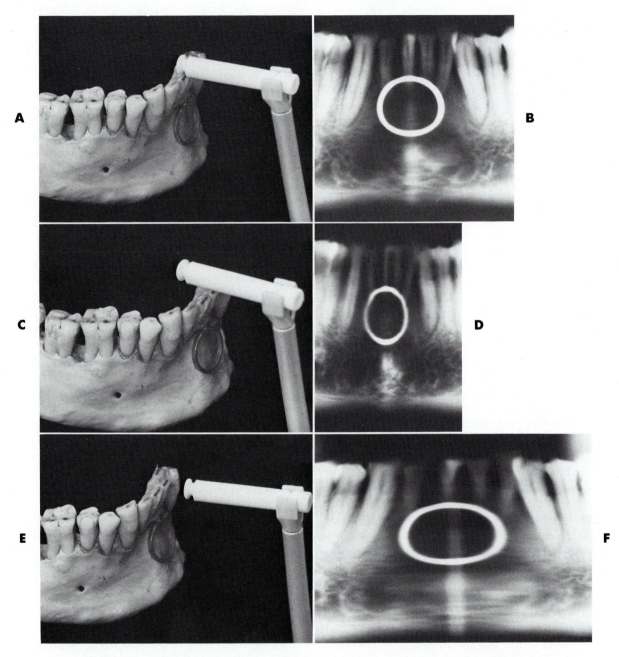

FIG. 12-7. A, Mandible supporting a metal ring positioned at the center of the focal trough. The incisal edges of the mandibular teeth are indexed by a bite rod positioning device. The mandible is positioned at the center of the trough. **B,** Resultant panoramic radiograph. **C,** Mandible and ring positioned 5 mm anterior to the focal trough. The incisal edges of the teeth are anterior to the trough. **D,** Resultant panoramic radiograph demonstrating the horizontal minification of both ring and mandibular teeth. **E,** Mandible and ring positioned 5 mm posterior to the focal trough. The incisal edges of the teeth are also posterior to the trough. **F,** Resultant panoramic radiograph demonstrating the horizontal magnification of both ring and mandibular teeth.

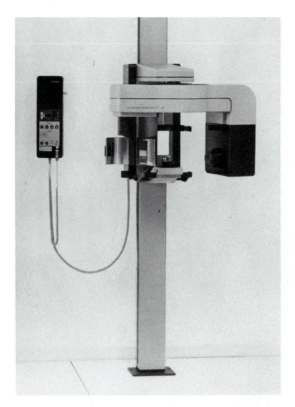

FIG. 12-8. Orthopantomograph 10 panoramic machine. (Courtesy Siemens Corp., Iselin NJ.)

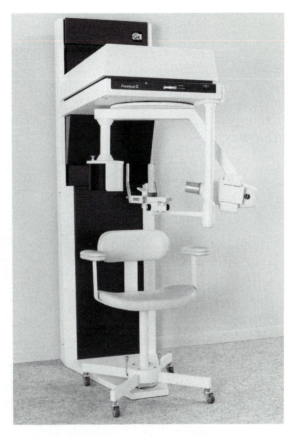

FIG. 12-9. Panelipse II panoramic machine. (Courtesy Gendex Corp., Milwaukee.)

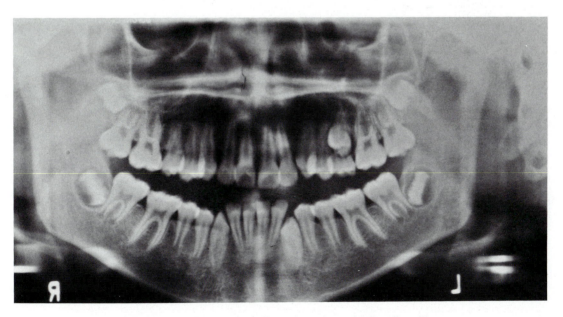

FIG. 12-10. Panoramic radiograph made on the Panelipse II.

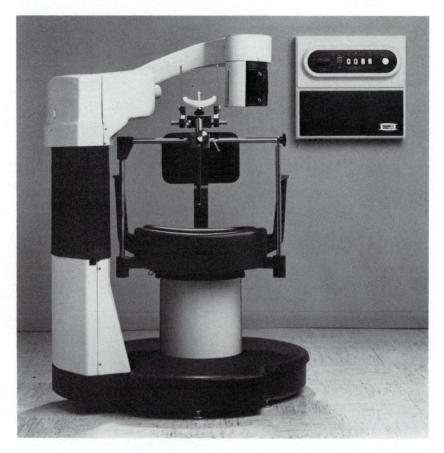

FIG. 12-11. Panorex 2 panoramic machine. (Courtesy Keystone X-Ray Inc., Neptune NJ.)

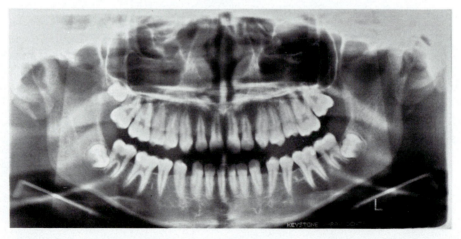

FIG. 12-12. Panoramic radiograph made by the Panorex 2. (Courtesy Keystone X-Ray Inc., Neptune NJ.)

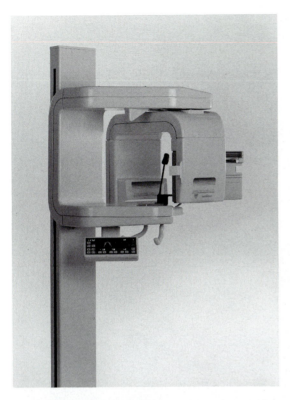

FIG. 12-13. Planmeca 2002 cc Panoramic machine. (Courtesy Planmeca Inc., Wood Dale, IL.)

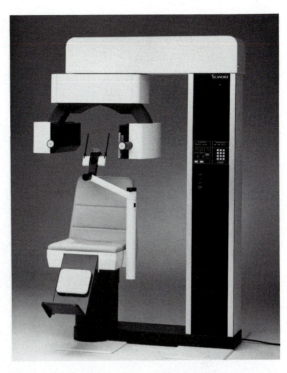

FIG. 12-14. Scanora multimodality machine. (Courtesy Soredex Medical Systems Inc., Conroe Tx.)

sagittal sections through the maxillary sinuses, and cross-sectional cuts through a predetermined portion of the maxilla or mandible. These machines have much greater versatility than the conventional panoramic machines, and they are much more expensive.

The Scanora (Soredex) (Fig. 12-14) has the capability of making conventional panoramic images as well as many special-purpose examinations of the facial skeleton. Most of the special examinations made on this machine use circular tomography. (See Chapter 13.)

Patient positioning and head alignment

To attain adequate panoramic radiographs, one must properly prepare and position the patient with the head carefully aligned in the focal trough. *Preparation* of adult patients and children includes the removal of dental appliances, earrings, necklaces, hairpins, or any other metallic objects in the head and neck region. It is also wise to demonstrate the machine by cycling it while explaining the need to

remain still during the procedure. This is particularly true for children, who may be anxious. Children should be instructed to look forward and not follow the tube head with their eyes. All patients should be draped with a leaded apron.

Proper *patient positioning* requires placing the patient so the dental arches are located in the middle of the focal trough. The details of this procedure vary with different machines. There are, however, some general principles that apply to most machines. The anteroposterior position of the patient is achieved by having the patient place the incisal edges of his maxillary and mandibular incisors into a notched positioning device (the bite block). As discussed above, if the dental arches are placed out of the focal trough, their image will be distorted.

When the patient's head is aligned, the midsagittal plane must be positioned within the exact center of the focal trough of the particular x-ray unit. Failure to position the midsagittal plane in the midline will result in a radiograph whose right and left sides are unequally magnified in their horizontal

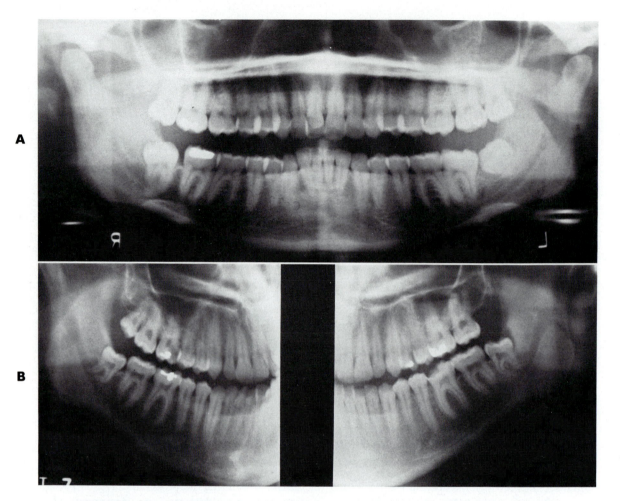

FIG. 12-15. Panoramic radiographs demonstrating poor patient head alignment. **A,** The chin and occlusal plane are rotated upward, resulting in overlapping images of the teeth and an opaque shadow (the hard palate) obscuring the roots of the maxillary teeth. **B,** The chin and occlusal plane are rotated downward, cutting off both condyles and the symphyseal region on the radiograph.

dimension. Poor midline positioning is a common error, causing horizontal distortion in the posterior regions and, on occasion, clinically unacceptable radiographs. A simple method for evaluating the degree of horizontal distortion of the image is to compare the apparent width of the mandibular first molars bilaterally. If one tooth is more than 20% wider than the other, the radiograph may have to be remade. The smaller side is the side closer to the film.

The patient's chin and occlusal plane must be properly positioned to avoid distortion. The occlusal plane is aligned so it is lower anteriorly, angled 20 to 30 degrees below the horizontal. If it is tipped too high, the occlusal plane on the radiograph will appear flat or inverted and the image of the mandible will be distorted (Fig. 12-15, *A*). In addition,

a radiopaque shadow of the hard palate will be superimposed on the roots of the maxillary teeth. If the chin is tipped too low, the teeth will become severely overlapped, the symphyseal region of the mandible may be cut off the film, and both mandibular condyles may be projected off the superior edge of the film (Fig. 12-15, *B*). A general guide for chin positioning is to place the patient so the Frankfort plane is parallel with the floor.

Proper patient positioning also requires that the patient's back and spine be erect, with the neck extended. Slumping causes a large opaque artifact in the midline created by the superimposition of an increased mass of cervical spine. This shadow will obscure the entire symphyseal region of the mandible and may require that the radiograph be retaken (Fig. 12-16). Proper positioning in seated units

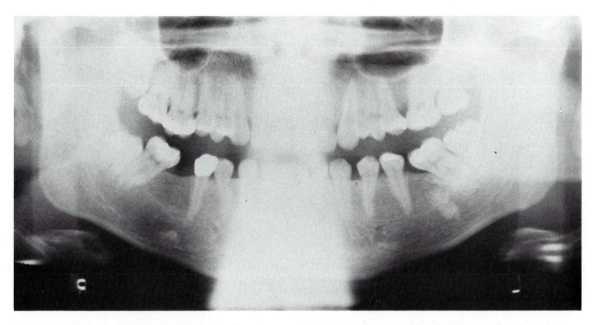

FIG. 12-16. Panoramic radiograph of an improperly positioned patient. Note the large radiopaque region in the middle. This artifact ("spine-shadow ghost") could have been eliminated by having the patient sit straight and align or stretch the neck.

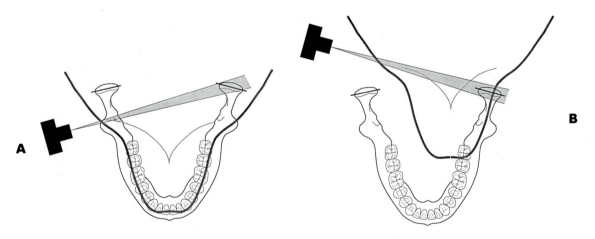

FIG. 12-17. TMJ panoramic imaging. **A,** A conventional panoramic machine orients the x-ray beam obliquely through the condyle (shown with a *line* through its long axis). **B,** In advanced panoramic machines, when the patient's head is displaced forward and to the side or the alignment of the x-ray source is altered, the beam may be oriented along the long axis of the condyle. This provides an improved image of the mandibular condyle. (Courtesy Dr. I. Chilvarquer, Sao Paulo, Brazil.)

may be facilitated by having the patient place his or her feet on a foot support[8] and by using a cushion back support. These devices help straighten the spine, reducing the artifact produced by a shadow of the spine.

A special technique has been described[5,6] specifically for imaging the temporomandibular joints with a panoramic machine. To obtain the best im-

ages of the TMJs it is recommended that the patient be displaced forward and laterally away from the side under examination (Fig. 12-17). This technique has the advantage of orienting the central ray along the long axis of the condyle instead of obliquely through the condyle as in the conventional panoramic technique.

Intensifying screens. Intensifying screens

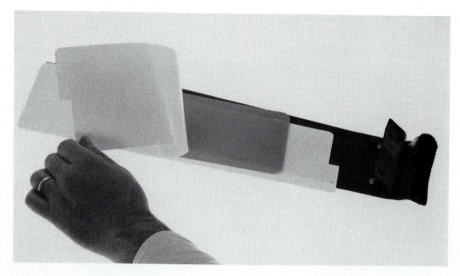

FIG. 12-18. White flexible intensifying screen surrounding a sheet of film *(gray)*, all lying on a *black* flexible cassette used with the Gendex Panelipse II machine.

(Chapter 5) are routinely used in panoramic radiography because they significantly reduce the amount of radiation required for properly exposing a radiograph. In most cases panoramic machines are provided with intensifying screens by the manufacturer (Fig. 12-18). The type of screen (manufacturer and model) is printed in black letters on each screen and clearly projected onto the radiograph. The selection of a film-screen combination depends on the diagnostic application for the panoramic radiograph in question. Fast films combined with high-speed (rare-earth) screens are indicated for most examinations. It is generally wise to use rare-earth intensifying screens with appropriate films (Chapter 5) to reduce patient radiation exposure. Figure 12-19 shows the result of an attempt to expose a panoramic radiograph without the use of intensifying screens. When a detailed view of a region is required, nontomographic (plane) films, such as those used for periapical, occlusal, or extraoral projections, will provide superior definition. A new experimental panoramic system replaces the film-screen combination with a charged-coupled device (CCD) sensor. This system produces an immediate digital image.[12]

Identification markings. All panoramic radiographs should have notations made for "left" and "right" sides using lead markers projected onto the image. Also the patient's name and age and the date the film was exposed should be indicated by markers, photographic imprinting, or glued labels. The dentist's name must show on the film.

No significant anatomic structures should be obscured by any of these labels or markings.

Panoramic film darkroom techniques. Special darkroom procedures are needed when panoramic film is being processed. These films are far more light sensitive than intraoral films, especially after they have been exposed. A reduction in darkroom lighting from that used for conventional intraoral film is necessary. A Kodak GBX-2 filter can be installed with a 15 W bulb at least 4 feet from the working surface. Although an ML-2 filter may be used when processing periapical films, the wavelengths of light it transmits will fog panoramic film. Develop panoramic film either manually or in automatic film processors using the manufacturer's recommendations. To obtain optimum results, the same care must be taken to develop, rinse, fix, and wash panoramic films as is taken with intraoral films.

Dose reduction. Panoramic radiographs subject the patient to a dose approximately equivalent to that received from four bitewing films.[19] This low exposure results largely from the use of intensifying screens with panoramic radiography. To assure that the dose is as low as possible, only rare-earth intensifying screens and corresponding film should be used. Some older panoramic machines do not allow the mA setting to be reduced sufficiently to allow use of rare-earth screens. It is not desirable to reduce the kVp below 65, for then the mean beam energy is below the optimum sensitivity of the screens. To reduce the output, it is best

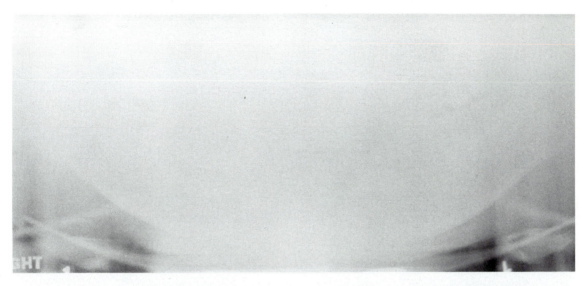

FIG. 12-19. Panoramic radiograph taken with the film in the cassette without use of an intensifying screen. Note that it lacks density and is not clinically acceptable.

to filter the beam. One inexpensive filter that has been found to be effective is a piece of Lanex screen.[10] A single or double thickness of Lanex screens (Kodak dental x-ray beam filter kit) added to the front of a panoramic x-ray tube will reduce the beam output enough to allow use of the faster films and screens. For facilities using panoramic machines already equipped with rare-earth screens, the addition of the Lanex screens (with an increase in the kVp of about 6) will further reduce patient exposure.

Radiographic appearance of normal anatomy

The recognition of normal anatomic structures on panoramic radiographs is frequently challenging because of the complex anatomy of the region, the multiple superimposition of various anatomic structures, and the changing projection orientation. A systematic approach is useful in interpreting panoramic radiographs so as not to overlook structures. We suggest the following method for examining panoramic radiographs:

1. Place the radiograph on a viewbox as if you were looking at the patient, with the structures on the patient's right side positioned on your left side (Fig. 12-20, *A*). Mask out any extraneous light from around the film and dim the room lights. When possible, work seated in a quiet room.
2. Begin viewing the radiograph at the superior aspect at the head of the right mandibular condyle (Fig. 12-20, *B*). Follow the posterior border of the condylar head down past the condylar neck along the posterior border of the mandible and down toward the mandibular angle. Note that the condyle may be positioned downward and forward in the mandibular fossa because the patient is biting on the bite block. Is the cortical border intact? Is the image of the cortical bone of normal width? Scalloped? Expanded? Can you account for the radiolucent and radiopaque shadows superimposed over the border? Carefully assess the outline of the border. Usually only fairly gross structural changes of the condyles can be seen. A corrected frontal and lateral tomographic examination is recommended for detailed examination of the osseous structures of the TMJ.
3. From the angle of the mandible, continue viewing anteriorly toward the symphyseal region (Fig. 12-20, *C*). Is there a history of trauma, and are there discontinuities in the border? Is the width of the cortical bone at the inferior border of the mandible thicker than that seen on the posterior borders of the rami? The bone may be thinned locally by an expansile lesion such as a cyst or thinned generally by systemic disease such as hyperparathyroidism or osteoporosis.
4. Continue viewing toward the opposite site of

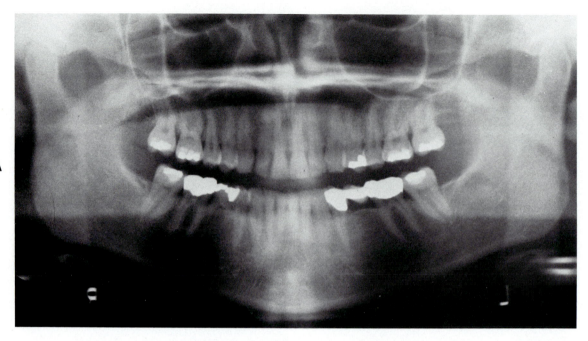

FIG. 12-20. A, Normal panoramic radiograph viewed as if looking at the patient.   *Continued.*

the mandible, noting the symphyseal region anteriorly and the symmetry of the outlined mandible, the left mandibular angle, the posterior border of the ramus, and the condyle. Compare the outlines of both sides for symmetry, noting any changes (Fig. 12-20, *C*). Remember that asymmetry of size may result from improper patient positioning. Conditions such as hemifacial hypertrophy or atrophy can affect facial symmetry.

5. Assess the entire medullary bone of the mandible. Examine for expected structures such as the mandibular canals, mental foramina, and various superimpositions frequently encountered. Examine the entire bone for radiolucencies or opacities in the peripheral, central, or periapical areas (Fig. 12-20, *D*). The midline is more opaque because of the mental protuberance and superimposition of the cervical spine. The regions of the submandibular gland fossae will be more radiolucent. Trabeculation is most evident within the alevolar process, less so inferiorly.

6. Examine the cortical outline of the maxilla. Note the right side first and then compare it with the left side (Fig. 12-21). Trace the border of the maxilla, beginning from the superior portion of the pterygomaxillary fissure down to the tuberosity region and around to the other side. The posterior border of the pterygomax-

illary fissure is the pterygoid spine of the sphenoid bone. Occasionally, the lateral sphenoid air cells extend into this structure.[4] Examine the trabecular bone for evidence of abnormalities.

7. Examine both maxillary sinuses, first by identifying each of the borders and then by noting whether they are entirely outlined with cortical bone, roughly symmetrical, and comparable in radiographic density (Fig. 12-21). It is often useful to compare both right and left maxillary sinuses when looking for abnormalities. The sinuses are more opaque in the region of the zygoma. Is there evidence of a mucous retention cyst or mucoperiosteal thickening, or are there radiopacities within either sinus? Are all the borders intact? Examine next the nasal fossa, noting the midline septum.

8. Assess the zygomatic process of the maxilla arising over the maxillary first or second molar (Fig. 12-22). Note the inferior border of the zygomatic arch, extending posteriorly from the inferior portion of the zygomatic process of the maxilla to the articular eminence and glenoid fossa. Note also its superior border. The zygomaticotemporal suture often lies in the middle third of the zygomatic arch. Do not confuse it with a fracture line in patients with a recent history of trauma.

9. The margins of a number of soft tissue struc-

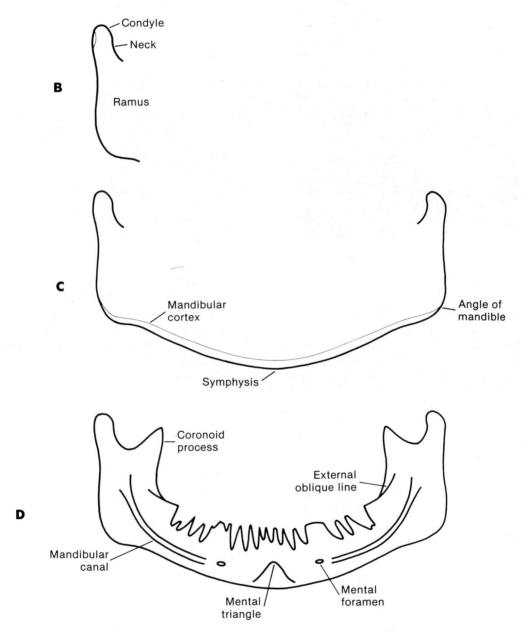

FIG. 12-20, cont'd. B to **D,** Outlines of the structures shown. In **B,** note the right condylar head and neck and the posterior border of the mandible. Follow the outline of the mandibular ramus on the radiograph. Continue following the outline, **C,** from the right condyle to the left, noting its thickness and the density of the mandibular cortex. In **D,** note the symmetry of the mandible and its structures—including the mandibular canals, mental foramina, and coronoid processes.

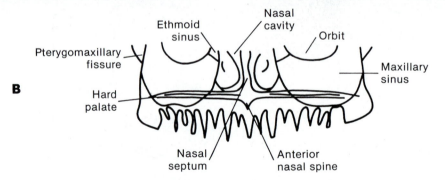

FIG. 12-21. A, Normal panoramic radiograph for interpreting the maxilla. **B,** Outline of the maxillary sinus, the nasal fossa, and the maxilla.

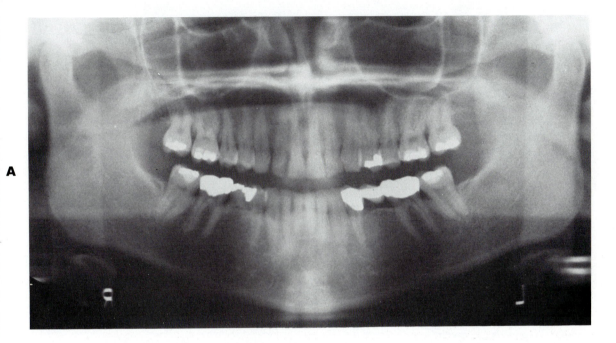

A

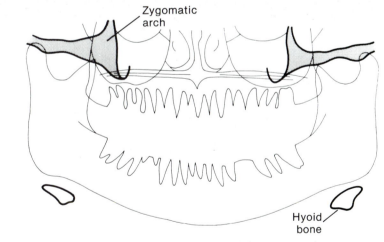

Zygomatic
arch

B

Hyoid
bone

FIG. 12-22. A, Normal panoramic radiograph for interpreting the zygomatic arches. **B,** Outline of the right and left arches. Note the relationship between them and the posterior border of the maxilla.

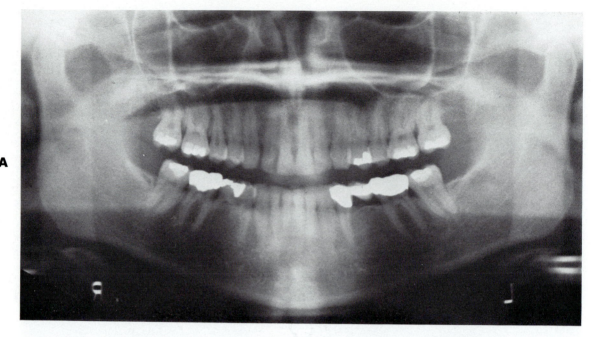

A

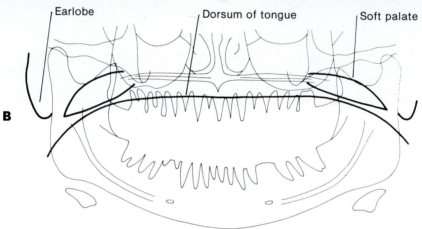

Earlobe   Dorsum of tongue   Soft palate

B

FIG. 12-23. A, Normal panoramic radiograph for interpreting soft tissue structures of the oral region. **B,** Outline of the structures shown—tongue, soft palate, and earlobe—all routinely observed on panoramic radiographs.

tures may be identified on panoramic radiographs (Fig. 12-23). These tissues appear radiopaque and include the tongue (arching across the film under the hard palate, roughly from the region of the right angle of the mandible to the left angle), lip markings (in the middle of the film), the soft palate over each ramus, the posterior wall of the oral and nasal pharynx, the nasal septum, and the earlobes. Figure 12-24 demonstrates soft tissue outlines of the nose, lips, nasolabial folds, and earlobes; note the soft tissue mucous retention

cyst in the right maxillary sinus. Radiolucent airway shadows also become superimposed on normal anatomic structures and may be demonstrated by the borders of adjacent soft tissues. They include the nasal fossa, nasal pharynx, oral cavity, and oral pharynx. Occasionally the air space between the dorsum of the tongue and the soft palate will simulate a fracture through the angle of the mandible.

10. Many radiopaque shadows superimposed on normal anatomic structures are called "ghosts" and are artifactual. They result when the x-ray

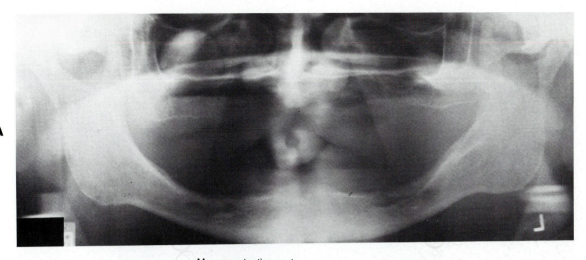

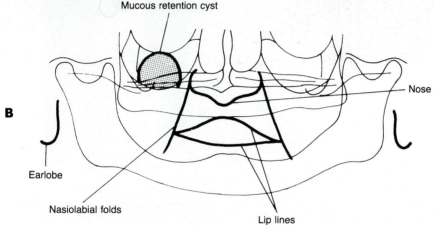

Mucous retention cyst

Nose

Earlobe

Nasiolabial folds

Lip lines

B

A

FIG. 12-24. A, Panoramic radiograph demonstrating normal soft tissue detail. **B,** Outline of the structures shown—earlobes, lip lines, nasolabial folds, and nose. In addition, note the soft tissue changes in the right maxillary sinus on the radiograph, which contains a mucous retention cyst.

beam projects through a dense object (e.g., an earring, the spinal column, the mandibular ramus, or the hard palate) and the opaque shadow of the object (the ghost) projects onto the opposite side of the radiograph. These ghostlike opaque artifacts can be a problem in radiographic interpretation. Figure 12-25, *A,* demonstrates a sectioned dry skull positioned and aligned on a panoramic unit. The resultant radiograph shows half the normal bony structures, as expected, on the right side and, in addition, the resultant ghosted artifacts on the left (Fig. 12-25, *B*). Figure 12-26 demonstrates a sectioned cadaver head positioned and aligned on a panoramic unit. The radiograph images half of the normal body and soft tissue structures, as expected, on the right side and,

in addition, artifactual radiolucent and radiopaque ghosts on the left. Along with bony structures that may create ghostlike artifacts, metal objects allowed to remain on the patient can result in opaque shadows (Fig. 12-27) caused by earrings left in place. The midline opacity in this figure is a leaded marker.

11. Finally, evaluate the *teeth*. The maxillary and mandibular cusp tips should be separate, and there should be a gentle curve (or "smile") to the occlusal plane (Fig. 12-28). Assess, first, the anterior teeth. Are they wider or narrower than normal (magnified or minimized in the horizontal dimension)? Are both the incisal edges and the root ends clearly visualized, or are they blurred from being positioned (or inclined) out of the focal trough? Use only peri-

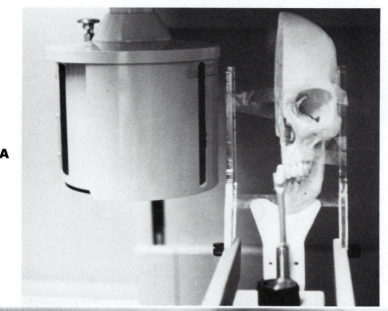

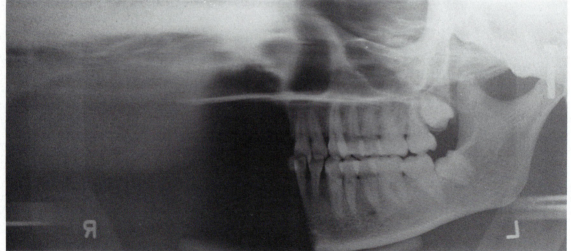

FIG. 12-25. A, Hemisectioned skull positioned on a panoramic x-ray machine. **B,** The resultant radiograph demonstrates opaque shadowlike "ghosts" on the right side.

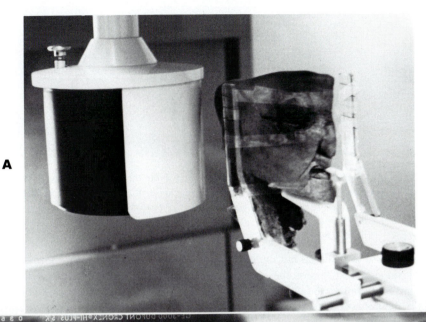

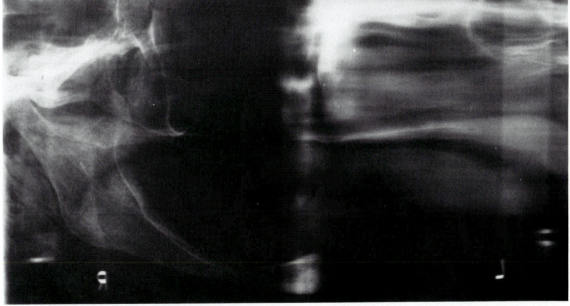

FIG. 12-26. A, Hemisectioned cadaver head positioned on a panoramic machine. **B,** The resultant radiograph demonstrates both radiopaque and radiolucent shadows on the left side of the film that are totally artifactual (or "ghostlike"). (The light-colored bands across the head are tape supporting the cadaver head.)

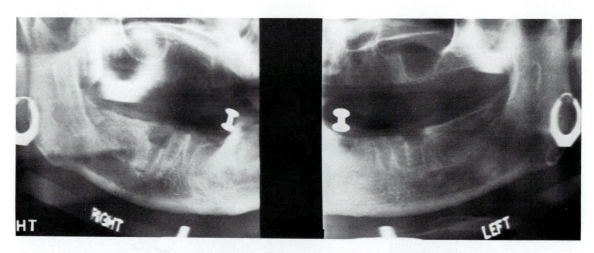

FIG. 12-27. Radiograph taken with large earrings in place. Note the opaque shadows present in the maxillary right and left tuberosity regions. These obscuring artifacts could have been eliminated by having the patient remove her earrings before the x-ray procedure.

apical radiographs to evaluate all but the most gross tooth changes. Next, assess the premolars, which are commonly overlapped on panoramic radiographs because of the geometric orientation of the x-ray beam. Are the premolars on both sides of equal dimension? Are any missing? Fractured? Grossly decayed? Do the premolars have single or multiple roots? Evaluation of these teeth for subtle features such as incipient caries, root morphology, and pulpal changes requires intraoral radiographs. Finally, assess the molars. Are the contralateral maxillary and mandibular molars of equal dimension? Are any unerupted, impacted, or missing? Are any supererupted? Does there appear to be adequate intraocclusal space for the construction of prosthetic appliances? In children, are all permanent molars present and developing normally? Gross tooth changes, gross caries, large fractured or missing restorations, and large areas of disease can be visualized. Other radiographs—including periapical, bitewing, and occlusal projections—must be obtained to complete a radiographic interpretation of the teeth.

The above assessment system is only one of many for panoramic radiographic interpretation. Other methods could be equally useful, provided a thorough and systematic approach is followed. The clinician must constantly strive to avoid missing an important radiographic feature that may be critical to diagnosis and treatment in the dental patient.

Figures 12-29 and 12-30 identify the commonly recognized panoramic radiographic landmarks.

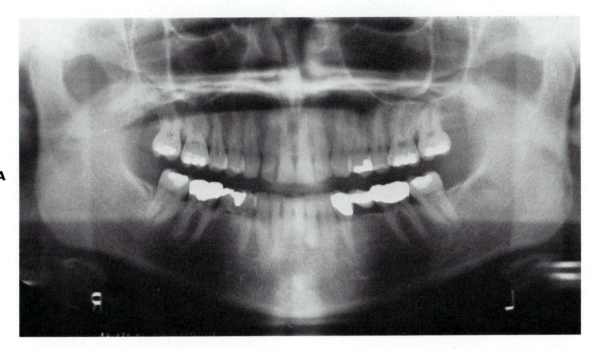

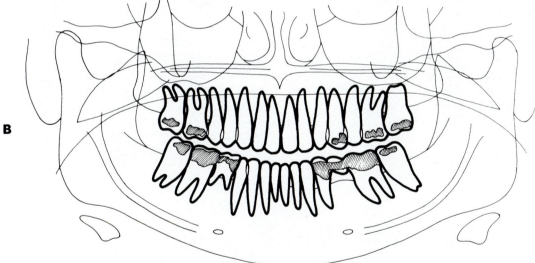

FIG. 12-28. A, Panoramic radiograph of the maxillary and mandibular teeth. **B,** Outline of the structures shown—demonstrating the gentle curve of the occlusal plane, the missing third molars, and the presence of metallic restorations. Note also the overlapping of the premolars.

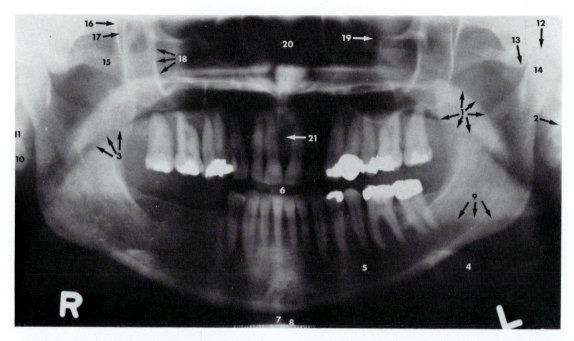

FIG. 12-29. Commonly recognized panoramic landmarks: *1*, soft palate; *2*, stylohyoid ligament (calcified); *3*, dorsum of the tongue; *4*, hyoid bone; *5*, submandibular gland fossa; *6*, bite block; *7*, superimposition of the cervical spine; *8*, chin rest; *9*, superimposition of the contralateral angle; *10*, earlobe; *11*, styloid process; *12*, mandibular fossa; *13*, articular eminence; *14*, mandibular condyle; *15*, zygomatic arch; *16*, pterygoid process; *17*, pterygomaxillary fissure; *18*, zygomatic process of the maxilla; *19*, infraorbital canal; *20*, nasal septum; *21*, incisive foramen.

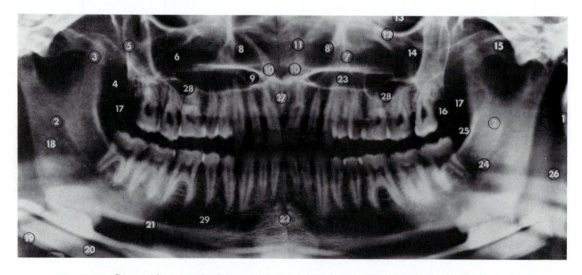

FIG. 12-30. Commonly recognized panoramic landmarks: *1*, earlobe; *2*, lingula (mandibular foramen); *3*, coronoid process; *4*, lateral pterygoid plate (region); *5*, posterior wall of the antrum; *6*, maxillary sinus; *7*, medial wall of the sinus; *8*, inferior turbinate; *9*, floor of the nasal fossa; *10*, anterior nasal spine; *11*, nasal septum; *12*, infraorbital ridge; *13*, orbital cavity; *14*, zygomatic process of the maxilla; *15*, zygomatic arch; *16*, maxillary tuberosity; *17*, hamulus (region); *18*, ramus of the mandible; *19*, superimposition of the chin rest; *20*, chin rest; *21*, inferior border of the mandible; *22*, mental protuberance; *23*, hard palate; *24*, mandibular canal; *25*, external oblique line; *26*, superimposition of the right mandible; *27*, incisive foramen; *28*, floor of the sinus; *29*, mental foramen (region).

SPECIFIC REFERENCES

1. Ahlqwist M, Halling A, Hollender L: Rotational panoramic radiography in epidemiological studies of dental health. Comparison between panoramic radiographs and intraoral full mouth surveys, *Swed Dent J* 10(1-2):73-84, 1986.

2. Åkesson L, Rohlin M, Håkansson J: Marginal bone in periodontal disease: an evaluation of image quality in panoramic and intra-oral radiography, *Dentomaxillofac Radiol* 18:105-112, 1989.

3. Barrett AP, Waters BE, Griffiths CJ: Critical evaluation of panoramic radiography as a screening procedure in dental practice, *Oral Surg* 47:673-677, 1984.

4. Bishop MG, Smith NJ: Pneumatisation of the pterygoid plates of the sphenoid bone as a normal finding on dental panoramic tomographs, *Br Dent J* 162(9):341-342, 1987.

5. Chilvarquer I, McDavid WD, Langlais RP, et al: A new technique for imaging the temporomandibular joint with a panoramic x-ray machine. I. Description of the technique, *Oral Surg* 65:626-631, 1988.

6. Chilvarquer I, Prihoda T, McDavid WD, et al: A new technique for imaging the temporomandibular joint with a panoramic x-ray machine. II. Positioning with the use of patient data, *Oral Surg* 65:632-636, 1988.

7. Douglass CW, Valachovic RW, Wijesinha A, et al: Clinical efficacy of dental radiography in the detection of dental caries and periodontal diseases, *Oral Surg* 62(3):330-339, 1986.

8. Gratt BM, Parks CR, Hall GL, Sickles EA: Use of an inclined footrest for panoramic dental radiography, *Oral Surg* 47:569-571, 1979.

9. Kantor ML, Slome BA: Efficacy of panoramic radiography in dental diagnosis and treatment planning, *J Dent Res* 68:810-812, 1989.

10. Kapa SF, Tyndall DA: Patient exposure reduction in panoramic radiography, *Gen Dent* 39:169-171, 1991.

11. Kogon SL, Stephens RG: Selective radiography instead of screening pantomography: a risk/benefit evaluation, *Can Dent Assoc* 48:271-275, 1982.

12. McDavid WD, Dove SB, Welander U, Tronje G: Electronic system for digital acquisition of rotational panoramic radiographs [published erratum appears in *Oral Surgery,* vol 71, p 762], *Oral Surg* 71:499-502, 1991.

13. Numata H: Consideration of the parabolic radiography of the dental arch, *J Shimazu Stud* 10:13-21, 1933.

14. Paatero YV: The use of a mobile source of light in radiography, *Acta Radiol* 29:221-227, 1948.

15. Paatero YV: A new tomographic method for radiographing curved outer surfaces, *Acta Radiol* 32:177-184, 1949.

16. Razmus TF, Glass BJ, McDavid WD: Comparison of image layer location among panoramic machines of the same manufacturer, *Oral Surg* 67:102-108, 1989.

17. Rohlin M, Kullendorff B, Ahlqwist M, et al: Comparison between panoramic and periapical radiography in the diagnosis of periapical bone lesions, *Dentomaxillofac Radiol* 18:151-155, 1989.

18. Valachovic RW, Douglass CW, Reiskin AB, et al: The use of panoramic radiography in the evaluation of asymptomatic adult dental patients, *Oral Surg* 61:289-296, 1986.

19. White SC: 1992 assessment of radiation risk from dental radiography, *Dentomaxillofac Radiol* 21:118-126, 1992.

20. White SC, Forsythe AB, Joseph LP: Patient selection criteria for panoramic radiography, *Oral Surg* 57:681-690, 1984.

SELECTED REFERENCES

Chomenko AG: *Atlas for maxillofacial pantomographic interpretation,* Chicago, 1985, Quintessence Publishing.

Langland OE, Langlais RP, McDavid WD, DelBalso AM: *Panoramic radiology,* ed 2, Philadelphia, 1989, Lea & Febiger.

13

NEIL L. FREDERIKSEN

Specialized Radiographic Techniques

The techniques described in this chapter are used to address specific diagnostic tasks. Some have been available to the clinician for years; others are more recent innovations made possible by advances in computer technology. Whereas the majority are not routinely used by general dental practitioners, it is the responsibility of all involved in providing oral health care to have a basic knowledge of their operating principles and clinical applications.

FILM RADIOGRAPHY

Tomography. Conventional film-based tomography is a special radiographic technique designed to image more clearly objects lying in a plane of interest. This is accomplished by blurring the image of structures lying superficial and deep to the plane of interest.[12,16] With the introduction of computed tomography and magnetic resonance imaging (p. 275 and 280), both of which have superior low contrast resolution, film-based tomography has been used less frequently. Conventional tomography is now applied primarily to high-contrast anatomy, such as encountered in dental implant diagnostics.

Essential equipment for tomography includes an x-ray tube and radiographic film rigidly connected and capable of rotating about a fixed fulcrum (Fig. 13-1). The examination starts with the x-ray tube and film positioned on opposite sides of the fulcrum, which is located within the plane of interest (focal plane). As the exposure begins, the tube and film move in opposite directions simultaneously through a mechanical linkage. With this coordinated movement of tube and film, the image of an object lying at the fulcrum and within the focal plane will remain in a fixed position on the radiograph throughout the length of tube and film travel and will be clearly imaged. On the other hand, images of objects located superficial or deep to the

focal plane will have constantly changing positions on the radiograph that will cause the images of these objects to be blurred beyond recognition because of motion unsharpness.

The objective of tomography, then, is to blur the images of structures not located in the focal plane both as much as possible and as uniformly as possible. The blurring is greater the farther the structure lies from the focal plane, either superficial or deep; in addition, it is greater with greater distance of the structure from the film, greater amplitudes of tube travel, and the more closely the long axis of the structure to be blurred is oriented perpendicular to the direction of tube travel. Of these factors, the last (orientation of the object to be blurred to the travel of the tube) is the easiest to control.

There are at least five types of tomographic movements: linear, circular, elliptical, hypocycloidal, and spiral (Fig. 13-2). With linear motion, tomographs often appear streaked (Fig. 13-3). These streaks or parasite lines appear when the long axis of a structure lying outside the focal plane is oriented parallel with the movement of the tube. As a result, linear motion fails to satisfy the requirement for optimum blurring. In addition, because the distance from the tube to the patient and the angulation of the x-ray beam through the focal plane change during exposure with linear motion, a nonuniform density may be seen across the tomographic image. Although for some applications this may be acceptable, if sharper tomographs of uniform density are required a multidirectional motion is necessary (Fig. 13-4).

The thickness of tissue in the focal plane is called the tomographic layer. The location of the tomographic layer within the object is determined by the position of the fulcrum and its width (described

266

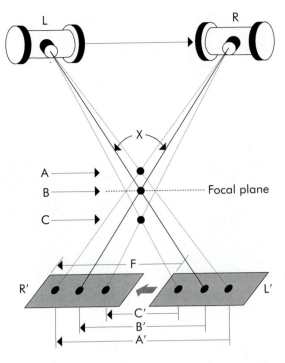

FIG. 13-1. Tomographic techniques. As the x-ray tube moves from *left* to *right,* the film moves in the opposite direction. In the figure points *A* and *C* lie outside the focal plane (the plane that lies parallel with the film and contains the center of rotation) whereas object B lies at the center of rotation. Only objects that lie in the focal plane (e.g., B) remain in sharp focus, because the image of B moves exactly the same distance (B′) as the film travels (F) and thus its image remains stationary on the film. The image of point A moves more than the film (distance A′) and the image of C less than the film (distance C′) so the images of both are blurred. *X* is the tomographic angle. The greater the tomographic angle, the thinner will be the plane of focus.

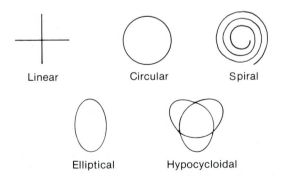

FIG. 13-2. The more complex the motion, the smaller is the likelihood that the x-ray beam will strike an object of importance at the same tangent through the entire exposure. (Therefore, blurring will be less dependent on orientation, of the object under study.)

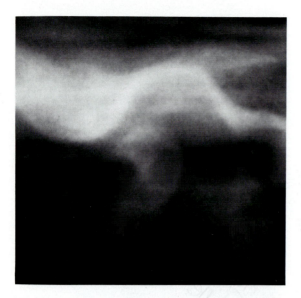

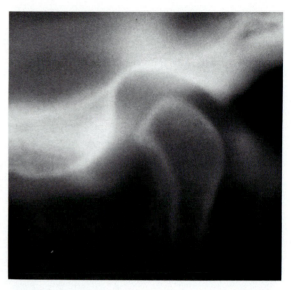

FIG. 13-3. Linear tomogram of the temporomandibular joint. Note the horizontal radiopaque streaks in this image. These streaks, called parasite lines, represent the blurred image of objects lying outside the focal plane. They are evident in the image when the long axes of objects superficial or deep to the focal plane lie parallel with the path of the x-ray tube and film movement. Compare with Figure 13-4.

FIG. 13-4. Spiral tomogram of the temporomandibular joint. Complex tomographic movements result in maximum blurring of the images of objects lying superficial and deep to the plane of focus and the absence of streaking parasite lines. Compare with Figure 13-3.

numerically as the thickness of cut) and by the tomographic angle or arc (Fig. 13-1). The greater the tomographic angle, the thinner the thickness of cut will be. Selection of the tomographic angle, and hence the thickness of cut, depends on the objective of the diagnostic task and the type of tissue being examined.

Wide-angle tomography allows for the visualization of fine structures that would normally be obscured by superimposition in conventional radiography. By this technique, layers as thin as 1 mm can be imaged. A disadvantage of the technique, however, is that it produces images of decreased contrast. Subject contrast results partly from the different thickness of adjacent structures. Because wide-angle tomography reduces these differences by the thinness of its cut, subject contrast is decreased. Wide-angle tomography is most useful when tissues of greatly differing physical densities (another contributor to subject contrast) such as bone are studied. This makes it an excellent technique for evaluating the maxilla and mandible prior to the placement of dental implants (Fig. 13-5).

Narrow-angle tomography is a technique that employs an angle of less than 10 degrees. Called

zonography because a relatively thick zone of tissue is sharply imaged (up to 25 mm), it is particularly useful when subject contrast is low because of little differences in physical density between adjacent structures (Fig. 13-6). Since subject contrast is low in soft tissue, zonography is the preferred tomographic technique.

Stereoscopy. Stereoscopy is not a new technique. It was introduced in 1898 by J. MacKenzie Davidson, only 3 years after Roentgen's discovery of x rays. Over the next 30 to 40 years it grew in popularity among radiologists because of its educational value; understanding normal anatomy is simplified with stereoscopic images. Stereoscopy was also widely used to determine the location of small intracranial calcifications and multiple foreign bodies in dense or thick body sections, where the interpretation of images produced at right angles might be difficult, and to evaluate the relationships of margins of bony fractures. In spite of these advantages, stereoscopy fell from favor for several reasons—incuding the introduction of more sophisticated and less time-consuming imaging techniques and an increased awareness, by the 1930s, of the possible adverse biologic effects of x rays (stereoscopy requires two exposures and thus delivers twice the amount of radiation to the patient). Today stereoscopy has enjoyed renewed interest for cerebral angiography,[18] digital subtrac-

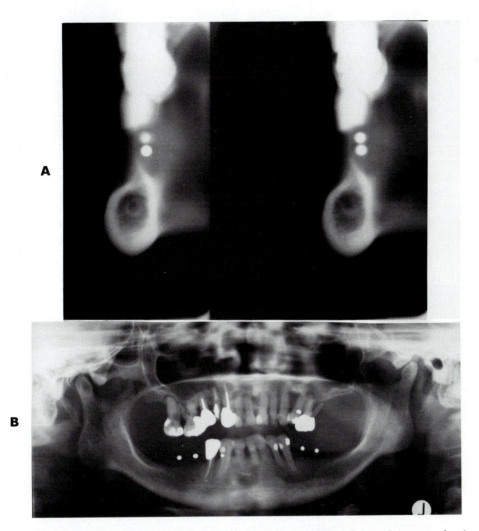

FIG. 13-5. Wide-angle tomograms made to evaluate the mandible prior to placement of a dental implant. They demonstrate the mandibular right premolar–molar area in cross section at the radiopaque markers on both the panoramic radiograph and the tomograms. Note the clarity with which the inferior alveolar canal is imaged in the tomograms. In **A** each slice is 4 mm thick. In **B** the metallic markers are for orientation of the cross-sectional images.

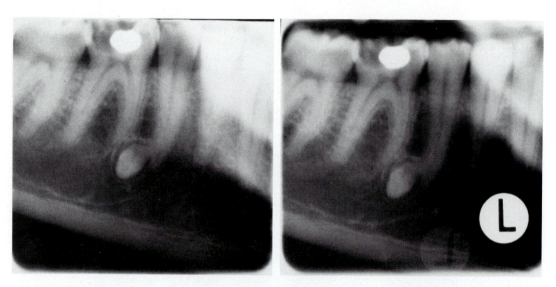

FIG. 13-6. Narrow-angle tomograms (zonograms). This pair, whose plane of focus is tangent to the mandible, was made with narrow-angle tomographic techniques. The thick plane of focus (25 mm) allowed the supernumerary tooth and adjacent permanent teeth to be imaged clearly in one depth of the field. The diagnostic value of these images is increased by their having been made stereoscopically, allowing for localization of the supernumerary tooth relative to clinically erupted teeth. (See also Figure 13-7.)

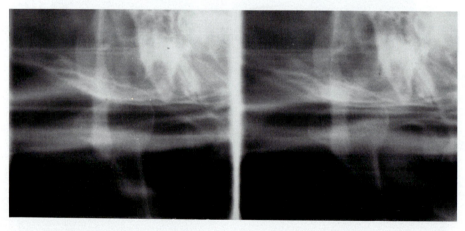

FIG. 13-7. Posteroanterior (PA) rotational stereoscopic scanogram of the right temporomandibular joint. As compared with a standard PA view of the condyle, this view demonstrates higher contrast and greater detail. The diagnostic value of such images is increased by their having been made stereoscopically, which allows for the perception of depth. (See also Figure 13-6.)

tion angiography,[107] and magnification angiography.[84] Additionally, there has been renewed interest in it as a technique for the evaluation of bony pockets in patients with periodontal disease, the determination of root configuration of teeth requiring endodontic therapy, and the assessment of bone shape when considering the placement of dental implants.[19]

Stereoscopic imaging requires two films to be exposed: one for each eye. Between exposures the patient is maintained in position, the film is changed, and the tube is shifted from the right eye to the left eye position. Although the magnitude of the tube shift is empiric, it must be sufficient to form slightly different or discrepant images. A tube shift equal to 10% of the focal-film distance has

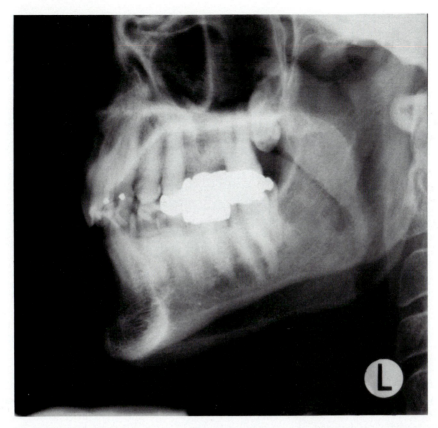

FIG. 13-8. Lateral linear scanogram of the maxillofacial area. Maximum image contrast is obtained by using linear scanning techniques as compared to standard radiography.

been reported[16] to produce satisfactory results. After processing, the films are commonly viewed with a stereoscope that uses either mirrors or prisms to coordinate the accommodation and convergence of the viewer's eyes so the brain can fuse the two images (Figs. 13-6 and 13-7).

Scanography. Scanography is a technique that utilizes a narrowly collimated fan-shaped beam of radiation to scan an area of interest and sequentially project image data relative to this area onto a moving film, much the same as panoramic radiography. Compared to images produced by standard radiography using round or rectangular collimation, scanograms demonstrate higher contrast with the perception of greater detail.[6] Increased image contrast in scanography results from a reduction in the amount of radiation scattered to the film during exposure because of collimation of the x-ray beam. Thus the major advantage of scanography over standard radiography is found in image quality.

The Soredex Scanora (Orion/Soredex, Helsinki Finland) (Fig. 12-13) is a commercially available x-ray unit capable of performing both rotational and linear scanography. In rotational scanography the beam of radiation rotates about a fixed axis that is predetermined based on the area to be imaged. The imaging sequence used by this unit results in the production of two or four scanograms, each made with the x-ray tube in a different position. Thus multiple images are made, any two of which can be viewed as stereoscopic pairs (Fig. 13-7). In linear scanography the x-ray beam and film move in a linear fashion scanning the area of interest. Linear scanography can be thought of as panoramic radiography that has been "straightened out." The Scanora system is capable of both posteroanterior and lateral linear scanning of the maxillofacial complex. Although these views are not produced stereoscopically, they have the advantage of optimum image contrast (Fig. 13-8).

Recently the development of a prototype x-ray imaging system using linear scanning and direct digital image acquisition with a solid-state detector has been reported.[60] It is anticipated that this system will ultimately demonstrate the advantages of both scanography and digital radiography (see p. 272).

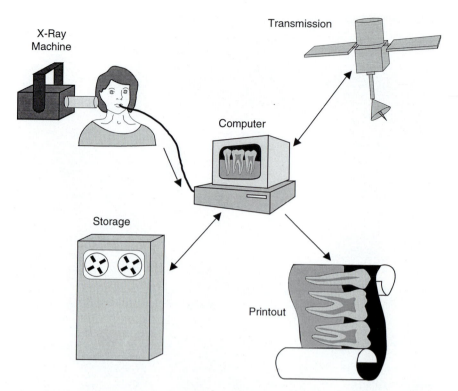

FIG. 13-9. Digital image acquisition and display. In this instance the image is captured directly on a charged-coupled device (CCD) in the patient's mouth. The signal from the CCD is sent to the computer where it is digitized into 256 gray levels. The image may then be displayed on a monitor where it may be enhanced by varying the density and contrast. The image may also be stored for future use, printed when a hard copy is required, or transmitted electronically to a remote site.

DIGITAL IMAGING

The application of computer technology to radiography has allowed for image acquisition, manipulation, storage, retrieval, and transmission (teleradiography) to remote sites in a digital format. Digital imaging requires a number of components including some form of electronic sensor or detector, an analog to digital converter, a computer, and either a monitor or a printer (or both) for image display[16] (Fig. 13-9). The recording of data in digitized form pertaining to an image is utilized in several techniques including computed tomography and magnetic resonance imaging. The techniques described below, however, relate to those that are available today (or will be in the near future) to the general practitioner. It should be kept in mind that the methods by which digital images are produced, manipulated, stored, retrieved, and transmitted are similar for all techniques—from computed tomography to intraoral radiography—differing only in the means by which they are acquired.

The computer is in charge of all components of the digital imaging system. It instructs the x-ray generator when to start and stop the exposure, controls the digitizer (analog to digital converter), constructs the image by mathematical algorithm, determines the method of image display, and provides for storage and transmission of the acquired data.

Images may be acquired by radiographic film or by detectors, which are solid-state electronic devices. The most common detector is the charged-coupled device (CCD). A CCD consists of a chip of pure silicon with an active area that has been divided into a two-dimensional array of elements called *pixels*. When electromagnetic energy in the range of either visible light or x rays interacts with pixels of a CCD, an electric charge is created that the pixels are able to store in much the same fashion as a capacitor does. The total charge developed and stored by a pixel is proportional to the energy incident on the pixel. Following exposure of the CCD to radiation, charges stored by the individual pixels are sequentially removed electronically, creating an analog output signal whose voltage is proportional to the charge on each of the pixels in succession.

Analog information, such as the output signal from the CCD, is any data represented in a continuous fashion. For this information to be useful, it must be converted into discrete units, since computers function only with digital information represented by either a 0 or a 1. Computer "language" is based on the binary number system, in which two digits (0 and 1) are used to represent information. These two characters are called bits, for *BI*nary digi*T*. In a typical computer language the characters form words eight or more bits in length called *bytes*. With every bit of an 8-bit word being either 0 or 1, the number of possible words or bytes in this language is 2^8 (256).

The analog to digital converter (A/D converter or digitizer) is used to change the analog output signal from the CCD detector to a numeric representation, based on the binary number system, that is recognizable by the computer. This task is accomplished by measuring the voltage of the output signal at discrete intervals and then by assigning a number (0 to 255) to the intensity of the voltage. Thus 256 voltage levels may be discriminated that ultimately will be displayed in image form following computer manipulation as 256 shades of gray. The sensitivity of this system can be appreciated when it is considered that the human eye is able to distinguish only 32 shades of gray!

In the context of this section, digital radiography may be considered as either direct or indirect. In direct digital radiography the image is acquired by a CCD detector that is sensitive to electromagnetic energy in the range of visible light or x rays. Indirect digital radiography uses radiographic film as the image receptor, the image digitized from the output signal of a video camera or scanner that views the processed radiograph.

Direct digital radiography. Digital intraoral radiography became a reality when Trophy Radiologie (Vincennes, France) introduced Radio-VisioGraphy (RVG).[64] As suggested by its name, RVG consists of three components. The *Radio* component is a conventional x-ray generator with a timer capable of very short exposure times. The detector or image receptor consists of a rare-earth intensifying screen that is optically coupled with a CCD 26 × 17 mm in size. The *Visio* portion converts the output signal from the CCD to a digital format and displays the image on a monitor. The *Graphy* component consists of a data storage unit connected to a video printer.

Advantages of this digital technique include immediate image display with no waiting for darkroom processing, the ability to manipulate the image by contrast enhancement or gray scale reversal, and patient dose reductions of 60% as compared to E-speed film and 77% compared to D-speed film.[96] This significant reduction in patient dose, however, must be balanced by the fact that the magnitude of exposure reduction refers to an individual film–digital image comparison. Because each digital image may include only one molar or two anterior or premolar teeth, more images may in fact be required for a full mouth examination with this technique than with radiographic film, diminishing the effect of exposure reduction. Major disadvantages of the system can be found in its decreased image resolution and contrast as compared with radiographic film.[26] Currently a third generation of RVG equipment is available; and although resolution has been improved to a reported 11 line pairs per millimeter,[7] this is still considerably lower than the 20 line pairs per millimeter capability of radiographic film (Fig. 13-10).

Recently Regam Medical Systems AB (Sundsvall, Sweden) has introduced a digital system called the Sens-A-Ray,[65,100] and Gendex Dental Systems (Monza, Italy) has introduced the Visualix[63] system. Both of these appear to differ from the RVG system only in detector construction. Each utilizes a CCD that is sensitive to the direct action of x rays whereas in the RVG system the CCD responds to light generated by the intensifying screen. In spite of this, there is apparently no gain in image resolution since each is capable of resolving 8 to 10 line pairs per millimeter.

Current evidence[24,102] suggests that digital systems perform comparably with film radiography for the detection of periodontal bone lesions and occlusal caries in noncavitated teeth. Additionally, rapid image acquisition and reduced radiation exposure per image may prove to be advantageous for imaging during the course of endodontic therapy.

Several panoramic radiographic imaging systems that produce digital images have been described. One uses a linear CCD array,[61] another an imaging plate that consists of a flexible polyester base coated with a crystalline halide composed of europium-activated barium fluorohalide.[44,45] Following exposure, a special laser image reader converts the latent image in the crystalline halide to a luminescent and then to an electric signal that is digitized.

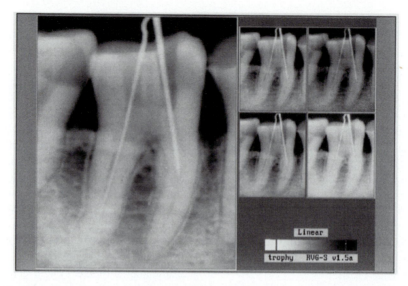

FIG. 13-10. Direct digital intraoral radiographs made on RVG unit. Advantages of digital radiography include rapid image acquisition, the ability to manipulate image contrast and density, and a significant dose reduction as compared with direct exposure film. (Courtesy Trophy Radiology, Marietta Ga.)

Indirect digital radiography. Digital processing of images recorded by radiographic film may serve several useful puposes. First, because of its ability to manipulate digital images, digitization allows for the optimization of image quality in terms of contrast and density, which embodies the potential for enhanced perception of detail and improved diagnosis. Second, as does direct digital radiography, digitization of radiographic images provides for the storage of information. Third, this information can be transmitted to remote sites for consultation. Unfortunately, digital image processing of direct exposure nonscreen films may result in loss of information because the digitized image represents a second generation.[23]

Indirect digital radiography, or the digitization of images recorded by radiographic film, may be accomplished in one of several ways that differ from each other only in the method by which data are acquired and/or displayed. One system (Fuji Photo, Tokyo, Japan) uses a photomultiplier tube (see "Nuclear Medicine," p. 284) with a small aperture (100 × 100 μm) to scan an illuminated radiograph. The analog output signal from the photomultiplier is digitized by an analog to digital converter and the digital data are processed by computer and fed into a digital to analog converter whose output is used to modulate the light intensity of a glow tube. The light output from the glow tube is directed to a sheet of radiographic film and

an image is recovered following standard processing procedures.[22,23] Other systems available employ a television camera as a sensor and a television monitor and/or video printer as the display.[41,46] Regardless of the method of acquisition or display, the result is the same: digital information pertaining to the image is obtained that can be manipulated and stored.

The ability to digitize information contained in the remnant x-ray beam relative to the subject has made possible digital subtraction radiography and the possibility of digitized image interpretation.

Digital subtraction radiography. Subtraction radiography requires two identical images. The subtracted image is a composite of these two, representing their differing densities[31] (Fig. 13-11). Although visual examination of standard radiographs is unable to detect an 0.85 mm change in cortical bone thickness, this technique is so sensitive it can detect a 0.12 mm change.[75] The ability of digital subtraction to record minute differences is dependent on the degree of matching of the two images. Techniques have been developed, however, to correct for differences in image contrast,[66,76] projection geometry,[91] and hardening of the x-ray beam caused by tissues through which the x rays travel.[98,99]

Digital subtraction radiography has been reported[32,67,70,101] to be useful in the diagnosis of periodontal and carious lesions, both of which may be

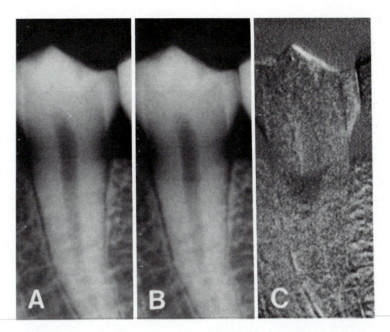

FIG. 13-11. Digital subtraction radiographs. Subtraction radiography requires two images, **A** and **B,** that are exposed with the same geometry. In this instance there is loss of alveolar bone on image **B** that is too subtle to be seen. The subtracted image, **C,** however, displays the differences between **A** and **B,** and now the bone loss is seen as a dark structure superimposed over the pulp. (Courtesy Dr. H.G. Gröndahl, Göteborg, Sweden.)

characterized by their sometimes insidious and relatively slow rate of progression. Contrast enhancement of the subtracted image with color has been suggested[71] to aid in the observation of small periodontal defects. Subtraction radiography has also been reported[20,54,82,87] to have potential for the evaluation of small changes in mandibular condyle position and the integrity of the articular surface and for the assessment of osseous remodeling around granular hydroxyapatite implants. In clinical practice digital subtraction radiography is very demanding because of the requirement for identical alignment of the x-ray machine, teeth, and film on each occasion.

Digitized image interpretation. With the advent of digital imaging has come the possibility for computer interpretation of the image. Systems and programs have been developed for the recognition of anatomy as imaged radiographically, the detection of carious and periodontal lesions, and the assessment of periapical regions of teeth and bone quality. Computer interpretation may prove to play a significant role in diagnoses of the future.[90]

COMPUTED TOMOGRAPHY

In 1972 Godfrey Hounsfield[42] announced the invention of a revolutionary imaging technique (which he referred to as computerized axial transverse scanning). With this technique he was able to produce an axial cross-sectional image of the head by narrowly collimating a moving beam of x rays. The remnant radiation of this beam was detected by a scintillation crystal; the resulting signal was fed into a computer and analyzed by a mathematical algorithm, and the data were reconstructed as an axial tomographic image. The image produced by this technique was like no other x-ray image. Claimed to be 100 times more sensitive than conventional x-ray systems, it demonstrated differences between various soft tissues never before seen with x-ray imaging techniques. Since 1972, computed tomography has had many names, each of which referred to at least one aspect of the technique: computerized axial tomography, computerized reconstruction tomography, computed tomographic scanning, axial tomography, and computerized transaxial tomography. Currently the preferred name is computed tomography, abbreviated CT.

In its simplest form a CT scanner consists of a radiographic tube emitting a finely collimated fan-shaped x-ray beam directed to a series of scintillation detectors or ionization chambers.[16] Depending on the geometry of the scanner, both the radiographic tube and the detectors may rotate synchronously about the patient or the detectors may form a continuous ring about the patient and the x-ray tube may move in a circle within the detector ring (Fig. 13-12). Regardless of the mechanical geometry, the transmission signal recorded by the detectors represents a composite of the absorption characteristics of all elements of the patient in the path of the x-ray beam.

The CT image is reconstructed by computer, which mathematically manipulates the transmission data obtained from multiple projections (Fig. 13-13). For example, if one projection is made every third of a degree, then 1080 projections will result during the course of a single 360-degree rotation of the scanner about the patient. Data derived from these 1080 projections (1080 projections = one scan) contain all the information necessary to construct one image. The CT image is recorded and displayed as a matrix of individual blocks called *voxels* (volume element). Each square of the image matrix is termed a pixel (picture element). Whereas the size of the pixel (about 0.1 mm) is determined in part by the computer program used to construct the image, the length of the voxel (about 1 to 20 mm) is determined by the width of the x-ray beam, which in turn is controlled by the pre- and postpatient collimators. Voxel length is analogous to the tomographic layer in film tomography. For image display, each pixel is assigned a CT number representing density. This number is proportional to the degree to which the material within the voxel has attenuated the x-ray beam. It represents the absorption characteristics, or linear attenuation coefficient, of that particular volume of tissue within the patient. CT numbers, also known as Hounsfield units (named in honor of the inventor Godfrey Hounsfield), range from -1000 to $+1000$, each constituting a different level of optical density. This scale of relative densities is based on air (-1000), water (0), and dense bone ($+1000$).

There are several advantages to CT over conventional film radiography and film tomography. First, CT completely eliminates the superimposition of images of structures superficial or deep to the area of interest within the patient. Second, because of the inherent high contrast resolution of CT, differences may be distinguished between tissues that differ in physical density by less than 1%[72]; a 10% difference in physical density is required to distinguish between tissues by conventional radiography. Third, data from a single CT imaging procedure consisting of multiple contig-

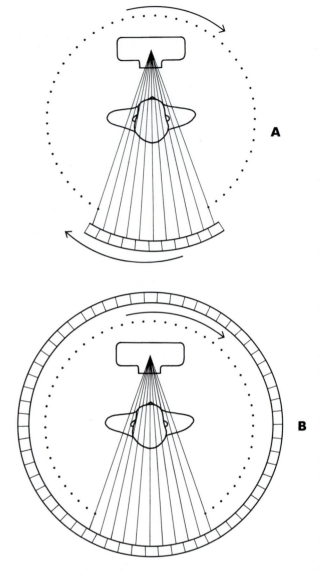

FIG. 13-12. Mechanical geometry of CT scanners. In **A** both the x-ray tube and the detector array revolve around the patient. In **B** only the x-ray tube rotates, radiation detection being accomplished by the use of a fixed circular array of as many as 1000 detectors.

uous scans of a patient may be viewed as images in the axial, coronal, or sagittal planes depending on the diagnostic task, referred to as multiplanar imaging.

Primarily because of its high contrast resolution and ability to demonstrate small differences in soft tissue density, CT has become useful for the diagnosis of disease in the maxillofacial com-

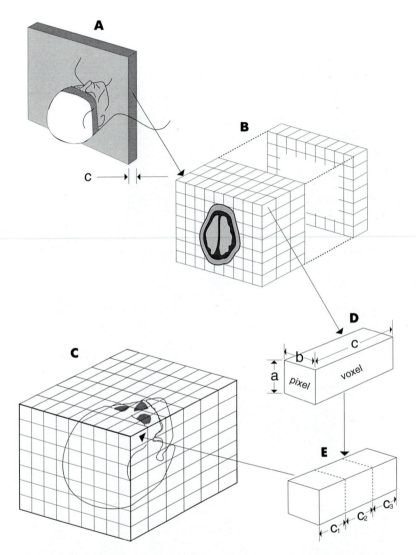

FIG. 13-13. CT image formation. **A,** Data for a single plane image are acquired from multiple projections made during the course of a 360-degree rotation about the patient. Dimension *C* is controlled by pre- and postpatient collimators. **B,** A single-plane image is constructed from absorption characteristics of the subject and displayed as differences in optical density ranging from -1000 to $+1000$ Hounsfield units. Several planes may be imaged from multiple contiguous scans. **C,** The image consists of a matrix of individual pixels representing the face of a volume termed a "voxel." Although dimensions *a* and *b* are determined in part by the computer program used to construct the image, dimension *c* is controlled by the collimators as in **A. D,** Cuboid voxels can be created from the original rectangular voxel by computer interpolation. This allows for the formation of multiplanar and three-dimensional images (**E**).

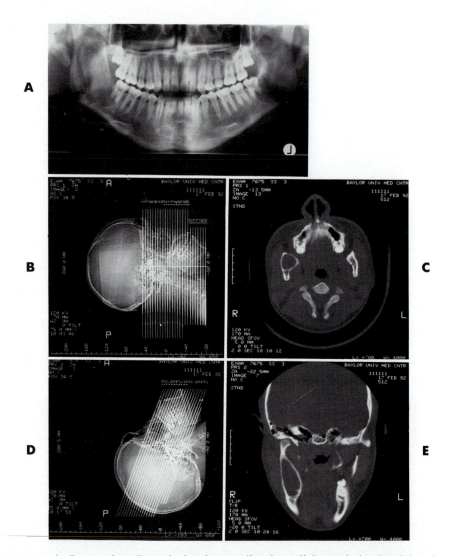

FIG. 13-14. A, Panoramic radiograph showing a unilocular radiolucent lesion involving the right mandibular ramus. **B,** Lateral scout radiograph for planning the location of contiguous CT scans. **C,** Reconstructed axial image at the level of scan *13* in **B.** Note the faciolingual extent of the radiolucent lesion on the right side. **D,** Patient repositioned for oblique scans through the area of the lesion. **E,** Reconstructed oblique image at the level of scan *7* in **B.** Note the superior extent of the lesion. (**B** to **E** courtesy Radiology Department, Baylor University Medical Center, Dallas Tex.)

plex[17,47,80] (Fig. 13-14), including the salivary glands[55,89] (see Chapter 30) and the temporomandibular joint[1,15,35] (see Chapter 25). With the advent of MR imaging, which has proved to be superior to CT for depicting soft tissue, the use of CT scanning in assessment of internal derangements of the TMJ has decreased significantly.[48] Additionally, CT has been shown to be useful for evaluation of patients prior to the placement of endosseous oral implants.* Despite the fact that similar information regarding maxillary and mandibular anatomy may be obtained with film tomography, CT allows for the reconstruction of cross-sectional images of the entire maxilla and/or mandible from a single imaging procedure.

Multiplanar CT imaging has made a significant contribution to diagnosis. These images, however, remain two-dimensional and require a certain degree of mental integration by the viewer for interpretation, which limitation has led to the development of computer programs to reformat data acquired from axial CT scans into three-dimensional images (3D CT).[3,21,40]

Three-dimensional computed tomography requires that each voxel, shaped as a rectangular parallelepiped or rectangular solid, be dimensionally altered into multiple cuboidal voxels.[73] This process, called *interpolation,* creates sets of evenly spaced cuboidal voxels (cuberilles) that occupy the same volume as the original voxel[39] (Fig. 13-13). The CT numbers of the cuberilles represent the average of the original voxel CT numbers surrounding each of the new voxels. Creation of these new cuboidal voxels allows for reconstruction of the image in any plane without loss of resolution by locating their position in space relative to one another. In construction of the 3D CT image, only cuberilles representing the surface of the object scanned are projected onto the viewing monitor. The surface formed by these visible pixels (or cuberilles) then appears as if illuminated by a light source located behind the viewer. In this manner the visible surface of each pixel is assigned a gray level value depending on its distance from, and orientation to, the light source. Thus pixels appear brighter if they face the light source and/or are closer to it than those whose surface is turned from the source and/or is further away. The effects of this shading and the resulting image perceived by the viewer have been described as similar to an artist's three-dimensional rendering of an object

---

*References 50, 74, 77-79, 81.

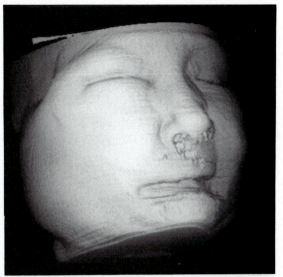

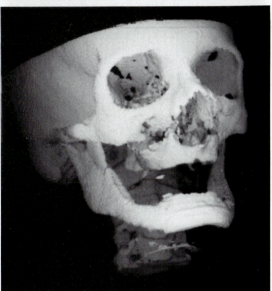

FIG. 13-15. Three-dimensional image reconstruction of a patient following facial trauma. By computer manipulation of the data acquired from a CT scanner, both soft tissue and hard tissue three-dimensional images can be constructed. Note the facial swelling in **A** and the Le Forte I fracture in **B** (with the maxillary alveolar ridge separated from the midface). (Courtesy Columbia Scientific, Columbia Md.)

within a two-dimensional medium. Once constructed, 3D CT images may be further manipulated by rotation about any axis to display the structure imaged from multiple angles (Fig. 13-15). Additionally, external portions of the image may be removed to reveal concealed deeper anatomy.

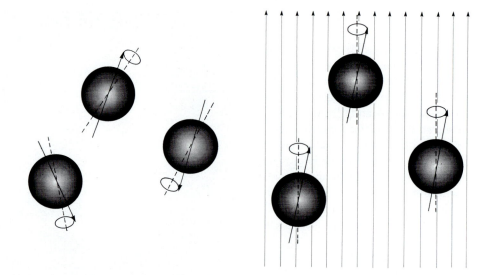

FIG. 13-16. Magnetic resonance imaging. **A,** The axes of spinning hydrogen nuclei (protons) are normally randomly oriented. **B,** When a patient is placed in an MR imager and subjected to a strong external magnetic field, the axes of many protons attempt to align themselves with the direction of the field. The axes oscillate at a specific frequency (Larmor frequency), with a slight tilt (precession) from absolute parallel with the flux of the imaging magnet. The addition of their magnetic moments forms a net magnetization. *Continued.*

One of the first applications of 3D CT was in 1980 for the study of patients with suspected intervertebral disk herniation and spinal stenosis.[38] Since that time 3D CT has been applied to craniofacial reconstructive surgery, for the treatment of congenital and acquired deformities, and the evaluation of intracranial tumors, benign and malignant lesions of the maxillofacial complex, cervical spine injuries, pelvic fractures, and deformities of the hands and feet.* Availability of data in a three-dimensional format has also made possible the construction of life-sized models that can be used to perform trial surgeries, construct surgical stents, and fabricate accurate prostheses for implantation.[9,52]

CT technology is being continuously advanced. Recently, Imatron (San Francisco) has introduced a CT scanner capable of acquiring data up to 10 times faster than conventional CT. Its Ultrafast CT, with scan times on the order of 50 msec, is able to freeze cardiac and pulmonary motion, enhancing the quality without motion artifacts. Several other manufacturers have developed spiral CT scanners. With these, while the gantry containing the x-ray tube and detectors revolves around the patient, the table on which the patient is lying continuously

advances through the gantry. This results in the acquisition of a continuous spiral of data as the x-ray beam moves down the patient. As compared to conventional CT scanners, it is reported[62] that spiral scanners provide for improved multiplaner image reconstructions, reduced examination time (12 seconds vs 5 minutes), and reduced radiation dose (up to 75%).

MAGNETIC RESONANCE[11,16]

In contrast to the techniques described above, which utilize x rays for the acquisition of information pertaining to an object studied, magnetic resonance imaging (MRI) uses nonionizing radiation. To produce an MR image, the patient is placed inside a large magnet, which induces a relatively strong static magnetic field. This causes the nuclei of many atoms in the body, including hydrogen, to align themselves with the magnetic field.

Physical basis for magnetic resonance Fig. 13-16). The nuclei of at least one third of the elements have an odd number of nucleons (protons and neutrons) and, as a result, a mechanical moment known as spin. Although any nucleus with an unpaired nucleon could be used for MRI, hydrogen is used because of its abundance in body tissues. The spin of hydrogen nuclei, plus the fact that they have a charge (hydrogen nuclei consist

*References 2, 34, 37, 56-58, 86, 92-94.

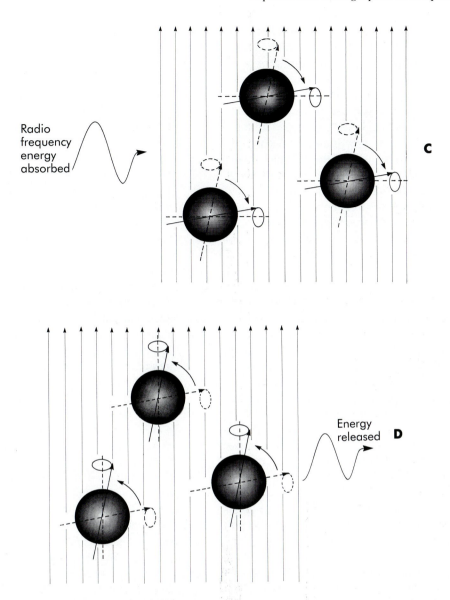

FIG. 13-16, cont'd. C, When electromagnetic energy in the form of radio waves oscillating at the Larmor frequency is directed to protons aligned in the magnetic field, the protons absorb energy and rotate away from the flux of the imaging magnet. **D,** As soon as the radio waves are turned off, some energy that the protons have absorbed is released and the protons attempt to realign within the magnetic field. The energy released is in the form of a radio wave of the same frequency as the incident radio wave. This emitted radio wave or signal is received, stored, and processed to produce the MR image.

of only one proton), causes them to behave like little magnets; they have a north and a south pole as well as magnetic moment. The poles of these nuclear magnets (protons) are normally randomly oriented; but when a patient is placed in an MR imager and subjected to the external magnetic field, they align themselves with the direction of the field. Since each proton has a microscopic magnetic mo-

ment, the alignment of all protons results in the addition of their microscopic moments to form a macroscopic moment of magnetization, referred to as the *net magnetization;* and when aligned parallel with the external magnetic field, the net magnetization is said to be *longitudinally oriented.*

Because of the spin of the nucleus, the alignment of protons in the magnetic field is not perfect. The axes of spinning protons actually oscillate or wobble with a slight tilt from absolute parallel with the flux of the imaging magnet. This tilting or wobbling is called *precession* and is similar to that of a spinning toy top, which does not spin in a perfectly upright position because of the effect of the earth's gravitational field. The axis of the spinning top wobbles about the direction of the local gravitational field, and the axis of the spinning proton wobbles (or precesses) about the applied magnetic field. The rate of frequency of precession is called the *resonant* or *Larmor frequency;* it is dependent on the species of nucleus and proportional to the strength of the external magnetic field. The Larmor frequency of hydrogen is 42.58 MHz in a magnetic field of 1 tesla (T). One tesla is 10,000 times the earth's magnetic field. The magnetic field strengths used for MR imaging range from 0.15 to 1.5 T.

Excitation. When energy in the form of an electromagnetic wave in the radio frequency (RF) range, from an RF antenna coil, is directed to tissue whose protons are aligned by an external static magnetic field (by the imaging magnet), the protons in the tissue whose resonant frequency matches that of the electromagnetic wave will absorb energy and shift or rotate away from the direction induced by the imaging magnet. The longer the RF is applied, the greater the angle of rotation. If the pulse is of sufficient intensity (duration), it will rotate the net tissue magnetization into the transverse plane, which is perpendicular to longitudinal alignment, and cause all the protons to precess in phase. This is referred to as a 90 degree RF pulse. The net magnetization of the tissue in the transverse plane and the amount of transverse magnetization that exists at the termination of the RF pulse is equal to the amount of longitudinal magnetization that existed just before the pulse. Both are directly proportional to the strength of the static magnetic field and the number of hydrogen nuclei present in the tissue.

Free induction decay (FID). When a 90-degree RF pulse is terminated, the macroscopic magnetic moment of excited hydrogen nuclei (net transverse magnetization) is oriented at 90 degrees to the external magnetic field and all nuclei are precessing in phase. At this moment a radio signal is induced in the receiver coil. The initial amplitude of the signal is proportional to the magnitude of the transverse magnetization, which is itself proportional to the number of excited nuclei in the tissue. As soon as the radio waves (90-degree RF

pulse) are turned off, two events begin simultaneously:

First, the nuclei in transverse alignment start to realign themselves with the main magnetic field (i.e., to relax) and net magnetization regrows to the original longitudinal orientation. This relaxation is accomplished by a transfer of energy from individual hydrogen nuclei (spin) to the surrounding molecules (lattice). The time constant that describes the rate at which net magnetization returns to equilibrium by this transfer of energy is termed the "T1 relaxation time" or spin-lattice relaxation time. T1 varies with different tissues and the ability of nuclei to transfer their excess energy to their environment.

Second, the magnetic moments of adjacent hydrogen nuclei begin to interfere with one another; this causes the nuclei to dephase, with a resultant loss of transverse magnetization. The time constant that describes the rate of loss of transverse magnetization is termed the "T2 relaxation time" or transverse (spin-spin) relaxation time. The transverse magnetization rapidly decays (exponentially) to zero, and so do the amplitude and duration of the detected radio signal. The decaying radio signal, which is the fundamental MR signal, has the form of a damped cosine and is referred to as *free induction decay* (FID).

The FID relates signal intensity to time. A mathematical technique called the Fourier transform converts the relationship of signal intensity versus time to signal intensity versus (resonant) frequency, transforming the oscillating FID signal to a pulse of energy (current), the MR signal. When radio signals (FIDs) are received from a mixture of tissues, as would be the case when a section of the body is examined, each volume of tissue generates a different radio signal at different frequencies. The individual signals are not separated by the antenna but are summed to form a complex FID signal. The Fourier transformation will also separate the complex FID signal from the different tissues into its various frequency components. This procedure is coupled with reconstruction techniques utilized in computed tomography to produce diagnostic images.

Spatial localization. Localization of the MR image to a specific part of the body (selecting a slice) and the ability to create a three-dimensional image are dependent on the fact that the resonant or Larmor frequency of a specific nucleus is governed in part by the strength of the external magnetic field. When this strength is changed in a gradient across a body of tissue (selectively exciting the image slice), the Larmor frequency of individual nuclei or groups of nuclei (voxels) in the gradient also changes.

This magnetic gradient is produced by three electromagnetic coils within the bore of the imaging magnet. The coils surround the patient and produce magnetic fields that oppose and redirect the magnetic flux in three orthogonal or right-angle directions to delineate individual volumes of tissue (voxels), which are subjected to magnetic fields of unique strength. Partitioning the local magnetic fields tunes all the hydrogen protons in a particular voxel to the same resonant frequency. This is termed "selective excitation." When an RF pulse with a range of frequencies is applied, a voxel of tissue tuned to one of the frequencies is excited; and when the RF radiation is terminated, the excited voxel reradiates that distinctive frequency, identifying and localizing it. The bandwidth or spectrum of frequencies of the RF pulse and the magnitude of the slice-selecting gradient determine the slice thickness. Slice thickness can be reduced by increasing gradient strength or decreasing the RF bandwidth (frequency range).

MRI parameters. The interpretation of an MR image is dependent on understanding how three parameters influence the strength of the MR signal and thus the appearance of the image. The strength of the MR signal is proportional to proton or spin density and nuclear motion and to T1 (spin-lattice) and T2 (spin-spin) relaxation times.

Proton density and nuclear motion. The MR signal is dependent not only on the presence or absence of hydrogen but also on the degree to which hydrogen is bound within a molecule. Tightly bound hydrogen atoms, such as those present in bone, will not align themselves with the external magnetic field and will not produce a usable signal. Lossely bound or mobile hydrogen atoms, such as those present in liquids, will tilt and align and produce a detectable signal. The measure of the concentration of loosely bound hydrogen nuclei available to create the MR signal is referred to as the *spin density* of the tissue in question. The higher the concentration of these nuclei, the stronger will be the net magnetization at equilibrium and at all degrees of excitement and the more intense the MR signal and brighter the MR image.

T1 relaxation. T1, also called the *spin-lattice* or *longitudinal relaxation time,* is the measure of time required for protons to realign themselves with the field of the imaging magnet following an RF pulse. After the pulse is terminated, the nuclei and their net magnetization return to maximum longitudinal orientation (the vector of longitudinal magnetization changing from zero at transverse alignment to maximum at longitudinal alignment). Longitudinal magnetization returns to equilibrium by transferring the energy the protons (spin) absorbed to the adjacent molecular structure (lattice). This longitudinal relaxation proceeds at an exponential rate. The time constant that describes the rate at which net magnetization returns to equilibrium by this transfer of energy is termed the "T1 relaxation time" or spin-lattice relaxation time. A T1-weighted image is produced by a short repetition time between RF pulses and a short signal recovery time. Since T1 is an exponential growth time constant, a short T1 will produce an intense MR signal, displayed as white in a T1-weighted image. A tissue with a long T1 will produce a low-intensity signal and appear dark in the MR image.

T2 relaxation. T2, also called *spin-spin* or *transverse relaxation time,* is the time required for the tissue protons to dephase following an RF pulse caused by magnetic interactions when they are oriented perpendicular to the external magnetic field. As a result of a pulse of RF energy to tissue magnetized longitudinally, the net longitudinal magnetization is converted to transverse magnetization. When the RF signal is terminated, the net transverse magnetization decays or relaxes exponentially with a time constant T2. A T2-weighted image is acquired using a long repetition time between RF pulses and a long signal recovery time. A tissue with a long T2 will produce a high-intensity signal and be bright in the image. One with a short T2 will produce a low-intensity signal and be dark in the image.

Image contrast between the various tissues in the body is manipulated in MRI by varying the rate at which the RF pulses are transmitted. A short repetition time (TR = 500 msec) between pulses and a short echo or signal recovery time (TE = 20 msec) will produce what is referred to as a T1-weighted image whereas a long TR (2000 msec) and long TE (80 msec) will produce a T2-weighted image. For every diagnostic task the operator must decide which imaging sequence will bring out optimum image contrast. T1-weighted images are

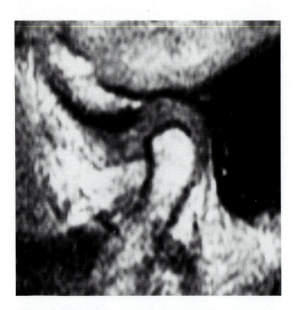

FIG. 13-17. Magnetic resonance image of the temporomandibular joint. The MR signal is dependent not only on the presence or absence of hydrogen (protons) but also on the degree to which hydrogen is bound within a molecule. Tightly bound hydrogen atoms, such as those in bone, will not align themselves with the external magnetic field and will not produce a usable signal (the cortical outlines of the condyles appear black). Loosely bound or mobile hydrogen atoms, such as those in soft tissues and liquids, will tilt and align and produce a detectable signal (varying shades of gray). (Courtesy Radiology Department, Baylor University Medical Center, Dallas Tex.)

called "fat images" because fat has the shortest T1 relaxation time and the highest signal relative to other tissues, and thus appears bright in the image. High anatomic detail is possible in this type of image because of good image contrast. T1-weighted images are thus useful for depicting small anatomic regions (e.g., the TMJ) where high spatial resolution is required[43] (Fig. 13-17). T2-weighted images are called "water images" because water has the longest T2 relaxation time and thus appears bright in the image. In general, T1 and T2 relaxation times of tumors, abscesses, and edema are prolonged. In practice, images often must be acquired using both T1 and T2 weighting to separate the several tissues by contrast resolution.

Magnetic resonance imaging (MRI) has several advantages over other diagnostic imaging procedures. First, it offers the best resolution of tissues of low inherent contrast. Although the x-ray attenuation coefficient may vary by no more than 1% between soft tissues, the MR parameters spin density and T1 and T2 relaxation times may vary by

up to 40%. Second, no ionizing radiation is involved with MRI. Third, because the region of the body imaged in MRI is controlled electronically, direct multiplanar imaging is possible without reorienting the patient. Disadvantages of MRI include relatively long imaging times and the potential hazard imposed by the presence of ferromagnetic metals in the vicinity of the imaging magnet. This latter disadvantage serves to exclude from MR imaging any patient with a medical device (e.g., cardiac pacemaker, cerebral aneurysm clips) or metallic foreign object implanted in his body.

Because of its excellent soft tissue contrast resolution, MRI has proved to be useful in a variety of circumstances: for diagnosing suspected internal derangements of the TMJ[43,53] and postsurgically evaluating treatment of those derangements,[33,103] for identifying and localizing orofacial soft tissue lesions,[36,51] and for imaging salivary gland parenchyma.[89]

NUCLEAR MEDICINE

Film radiography, computed tomography, magnetic resonance imaging, and ultrasound are considered to be morphologic imaging techniques; that is to say, each requires some specific structural difference or anatomic change for information to be recorded by an image receptor. In film radiography, for example, the perception of an image is dependent on contrast, which in turn is partially dependent on the differential absorption of x rays. The dependence of x-ray imaging on differential absorption essentially limits this technique to a single variable (tissue electron density), which in turn is presented as structural or anatomic differences. Human disease, however, may present with no specific anatomic changes. Those seen may simply be later effects of some earlier biochemical process that has remained undetected until physical symptoms developed. Radionuclide imaging, or functional imaging, techniques are the only means by which physiologic change that is a direct result of biochemical alteration may be assessed.

Radionuclide imaging is based on the radiotracer method, which assumes that radioactive atoms or molecules in an organism behave in the same identical manner as their stable counterparts because they are chemically indistinguishable. Radionuclide-labeled tracers are used in quantities well below amounts that are lethal to cells. They allow measurement of tissue function in vivo and provide an early marker of disease by measuring biochemical change. Widespread use of tracers in this capacity became possible with the development of, first, the rectilinear scanner and, later, the Anger or gamma scintillation camera.[95] Both these instruments record the gamma emissions from patients injected with appropriate tracers. The cameras use a scintillation crystal that has the ability to fluoresce on interaction with gamma rays. This flash of light (or fluorescence) is detected by a photomultiplier tube that magnifies and amplifies the signal many times to produce an image. Use of a scintillation crystal for the acquisition of data for image formation has led to the labeling of this technique scintigraphy.

Although many gamma-emitting isotopes have been employed in radionuclide imaging—including iodine (^{131}I), gallium (^{67}Ga), and selenium (^{74}Se)—the most commonly used is technetium 99m (^{99m}Tc). As technetium pertechnetate, technetium 99m will mimic iodine distribution when injected intravenously. Additionally, when it is manipulated chemically and attached to other compounds, it may be used to perform scans of virtually every organ of the body.

A stationary Anger camera or a rectilinear scanner is capable of producing a flat plane image of an area or organ in question. Use of an Anger camera with the capacity to rotate 360 degrees about the patient or specialized ring detectors makes single photon emission computed tomography (SPECT) possible.[8] In this technique multiple detectors or a single moving detector allows acquisition of data from a number of contiguous transaxial slices, similar to computed tomography by x ray. These data may then be used to construct multiplaner images of the area of study.

An even more recent development than SPECT in the field of nuclear medicine is positron emission computed tomography (PET).[8] PET, which is reported to have a sensitivity nearly 100 times that of a gamma camera, relies on positron-emitting radionuclides generated in a cyclotron.[68] As a positron is emitted within tissue, it meets a free electron and mutual annihilation occurs, resulting in the production of two 551 keV photons emitted at 180 degrees to each other. When electronically coupled opposing detectors simultaneously identify this pair of gamma photons, the annihilation event is known to have occurred along the line joining the two detectors. Raw PET scan data consist of a number of these coincidence lines, which are reorganized into projections that identify where activity was concentrated within the patient. The utility of PET is based not only on its sensitivity but also on the fact that the most commonly used radionuclides (^{11}C, ^{13}N, ^{15}O, ^{18}F) are isotopes of elements that occur naturally in organic molecules. Although fluorine does not technically fit into this category, it is a chemical substitute for hydrogen. At the present time the use of PET is somewhat limited because of high cost. PET facilities require more space, electricity, and air conditioning than conventional nuclear medicine clinics do. Additionally, PET requires an on-site cyclotron because of the short half-life of positron emitting radionuclides (the half-life of ^{15}O is 124 seconds).

Scintigraphy is not widely used at present in the diagnosis of oral and maxillofacial disease and injury. Reports* exist, however, of several dental conditions—periodontal and periapical inflammation, periapical cemental dysplasia, chronic focal sclerosing osteomyelitis, condylar hyperplasia, TMJ dysfunction, irritations caused by ill-fitting dentures (Fig. 13-18), trauma, and healing wounds—that have shown increased uptake of isotopes on skeletal images. In some cases positive findings on nuclear medicine scans have been demonstrated before clinical evidence of disease was noted.[83,85]

On the other hand, radionuclide imaging has provided valuable information concerning the functional capacity of the salivary glands in patients who have undergone radiotherapy or are suspected of having either acute or chronic sialadenitis, salivary gland aplasia, or sialolithiasis.[55,89] Nuclear medicine has an absolute indication when the ductal orifice of a major salivary gland cannot be found or cannulated in the course of sialography. Scintigraphy has also been found to be useful in the diagnosis and follow-up of patients with Sjögren's syndrome and other systemic diseases of the salivary glands. However, this imaging technique is of limited use for studies of the morphologic status of salivary glands because it cannot resolve lesions less than 1 cm in diameter. Additionally, differentiation between benign and malignant tumors of the salivary glands is not possible because of the nonspecificity of the technique.

Although radionuclide imaging is noninvasive, the radiation dose to the patient as a result of the intravenous injection of radionuclide-labeled tracers should be considered. It has been reported[55] that the injection of 3.7×10^8 Bq of ^{99m}Tc-pertechnetate delivers a whole body radiation dose of 1 mGy. This quantity is about one third the average annual effective dose resulting from natural radiation. (See Chapter 3.)

---

*References 4, 5, 25, 49, 59.

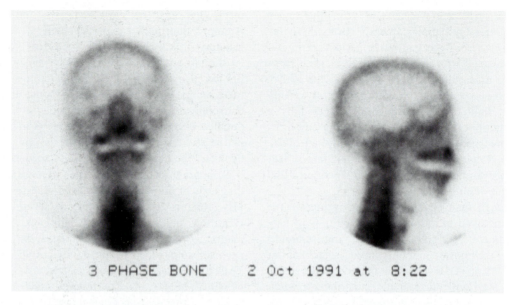

FIG. 13-18. Radionuclide image. The increased uptake of isotope in the region of the maxilla and mandible was attributed to an inflammatory response resulting from poorly fitting complete dentures. (Courtesy Radiology Department, Baylor University Medical Center, Dallas Tex.)

ULTRASOUND

The phenomenon perceived as sound is the result of periodic changes in the pressure of air against the eardrum. The periodicity of these changes lies anywhere between 1500 and 20,000 cycles per second (hertz, Hz). By definition, ultrasound has a periodicity of greater than 20 kHz. Thus it is distinguished from other mechanical waveforms simply by having a vibratory frequency greater than the audible range. Diagnostic ultrasonography (sonography), the clinical application of ultrasound, employs vibratory frequencies in the range of 1 to 20 MHz.[16]

Scanners used for sonography generate electrical impulses that are converted into ultra–high-frequency sound waves by a transducer, which is simply a device that can convert one form of energy into another, in this case electrical energy into sonic energy.[10,97] The most important component of the transducer is a thin piezoelectric crystal or material made up of a great number of dipoles arranged in a geometric pattern. A dipole may be thought of as a distorted molecule that appears to have a positive charge on one end and a negative charge on the other. Currently the most widely used piezoelectric material is lead zirconate titanate (PZT). The electrical impulse generated by the scanner causes the dipoles within the crystal to realign themselves with the electrical field and thus sud-denly change the crystal's thickness. This abrupt change begins a series of vibrations that produce the sound waves that are transmitted into the tissues being examined.

As the ultrasonic beam passes through, or interacts with, tissues of different acoustic impedance, it is attenuated by a combination of absorption, reflection, refraction, and diffusion. Sonic waves that are reflected back (echoes) toward the transducer cause a change in the thickness of the piezoelectric crystal, which in turn produces an electrical signal that is amplified, processed, and ultimately displayed on a monitor. In this system the transducer serves as both a transmitter and a receiver. High-resolution ultrasonography systems operating in the B mode, which produces a picture of a slice of tissue, may achieve an axial (depth) resolution of 0.5 mm or less and a lateral resolution of 1 mm or less. Techniques currently in use permit echoes to be processed at a sufficiently rapid rate to allow for the perception of motion. This is referred to as *real-time imaging*.

In contrast to x-ray imaging, wherein the image is produced by transmitted radiation, in sonography the image is produced by the reflected portion of the beam. The fraction of the beam that is reflected back to the transducer is dependent on the acoustic impedance of the tissue, which is a product of its

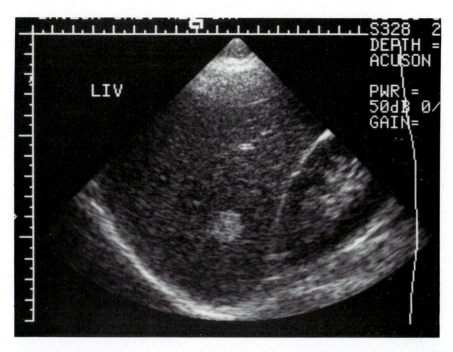

FIG. 13-19. Ultrasound image of the liver. The oval structure in the *right* represents the gallbladder. Note the round radiopacity within the *lower center* of the image. This represents a cavernous hemangioma. (Courtesy Radiology Department, Baylor University Medical Center, Dallas Tex.)

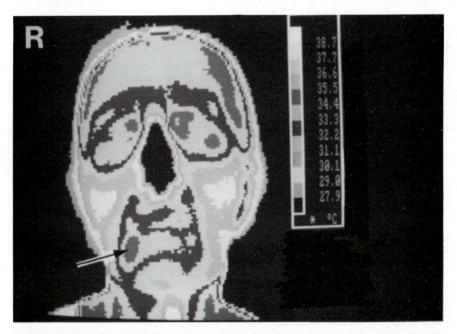

FIG. 13-20. Electronic thermography. Black and white photograph of a multicolored facial thermogram. The *arrow* indicates heat emission over the right mentum. This patient has a deficit of the right inferior alveolar nerve, the result of surgical implant trauma. (Courtesy Dr. Barton M. Gratt, Los Angeles.)

density (and thus the velocity of sound through it) and the beam's angle of incidence. Because of its acoustic impedance a tissue has an internal echo pattern that is characteristic. Consequently, not only can changes in echo patterns delineate different tissues, they may also be correlated with pathologic changes in a tissue. The interpretation of sonograms, then, relies on knowledge of both the physical properties of ultrasound and the anatomy of tissues being scanned (Fig. 13-19).

In the region of the head and neck diagnostic ultrasound has been applied to the evaluation of many structures and conditions: lymph nodes,[14] postsurgical edema and hematoma,[104] and the eye,[105] thyroid gland,[13] and parotid, submandibular, and sublingual salivary glands.[30,106] Additionally, ultrasound has been suggested[88] as a method to demonstrate the thickness of the masticactory mucosa; it thus may prove to be useful for determining the extent of soft tissue displacement under dentures by the forces of occlusion.

ELECTRONIC THERMOGRAPHY

"Thermography" is a term given methods of temperature pattern resolution and analysis. The utility of thermography in diagnosis is based on the fact that disease processes and/or abnormal conditions may result in different temperature patterns because of alterations in blood supply or the presence of inflammation. Sensors used to record temperatures may be small electronic probes called *thermisters* (which are used for point determinations), liquid crystals, or infrared scanners used to record temperatures over wide areas. Infrared scanners appear as small television cameras. When an individual is viewed by such a scanner in a draft-free temperature-controlled environment, the temperature differences recorded are displayed as a color image on a video monitor (Fig. 13-20). Color differences may represent temperature changes as little as 0.1° C. Although the technique is still in the prototype stage for diagnosing disease of the maxillofacial complex, it has been suggested as a useful method for determining a tooth's vitality, evaluating a case of atypical odontalgia, and assessing an internal derangement of the temporomandibular joint.[27-29, 69]

SPECIFIC REFERENCES

1. Aggarwal S, Mukhopadhyay S, Berry M, Bhargava S: Bony ankylosis of the temporomandibular joint: A computed tomography study, *Oral Surg* 69:128-132, 1990.
2. Altman NR, Altman DH, Wolfe SA, Morrison G: Three-dimensional CT reformation in children, *AJR* 146:1261-1267, 1986.
3. Artzy E, Frieder G, Herman GT: The theory, design, implementation and evaluation of a three-dimensional surface detection algorithm, *Comput Graph Image Process* 15:1-24, 1981.
4. Beirne OR, Leake DL: Technetium 99m pyrophosphate uptake in a case of unilateral condylar hyperplasia, *J Oral Surg* 38:385-386, 1980.
5. Bellizzi R, Krakow AM, Drobotij E, Keller D: A serendipitous discovery of ocult pathosis following a technetium 99m diphosphonate bone scan, *J Endod* 7:36-39, 1981.
6. Benson BW, Frederiksen NL: Effect of slit collimation on image contrast, *J Dent Res* (In press, 1993.)
7. Benz C, Mouyen F: Evaluation of the new Radio-VisioGraphy system image quality, *Oral Surg* 72:627-631, 1991.
8. Bernier DR, Christian PE, Langan JK, Wells LD: *Nuclear medicine technology and techniques*, ed 2, St Louis, 1989, Mosby.
9. Brennan RP, Krestin GP, Hauser M, Fuchs WA: Plastic model construction from CT data, *Radiology* 185 (suppl):369, 1992.
10. Buddemeyer EU: The physics of diagnostic ultrasound, *Radiol Clin North Am* 13:391-402, 1975.
11. Bushong SC: *Magnetic resonance imaging. Physical and biological principles,* St Louis, 1988, Mosby.
12. Bushong SC: *Radiologic science for technologists: physics, biology, and protection*, ed 4, St Louis, 1988, Mosby.
13. Butch RJ, Simeone JF, Mueller PR: Thyroid and parathyroid ultrasonography, *Radiol Clin North Am* 23:57-71, 1985.
14. Chodosh PL, Silbey R, Oen KT: Diagnostic use of ultrasound in diseases of the head and neck, *Laryngoscope* 90:814-821, 1980.
15. Christiansen EL, Thompson JR, Zimmerman G, et al: Computed tomography of condylar and articular disk positions within the temporomandibular joint, *Oral Surg* 64:757-767, 1987.
16. Curry TS, Dowdey JE, Murry RC: *Christensen's Physics of diagnostic radiology,* ed 4, Philadelphia, 1990, Lea & Febiger.
17. DelBalso AM, Werning JT: The role of computed tomography in the evaluation of cemento-osseous lesions, *Oral Surg* 62:354-357, 1986.
18. Doi K, Rossmann K, Duda EE: Application of longitudinal magnification effect to magnification stereoscopic angiography: a new method of cerebral angiography, *Radiology* 124:395-401, 1977.
19. Dolowy WC, Lind JC: Stereoscopic dental radiography: a practical dental office procedure (technical tip), *Oral Surg* 68:367, 1989.
20. Engelke W, de Valk S, Ruttimann U: The diagnostic value of subtraction radiography in the assessment of granular hydroxylapatite implants, *Oral Surg* 69:636-641, 1990.
21. Fuchs H, Kedem ZM, Uselton: Optimal surface reconstruction from planar contours, *Commun ACM* 20:693-702, 1977.
22. Fugita M, Kodera Y, Ogawa M, et al: Digital image processing of dentomaxillofacial radiographs, *Oral Surg* 64:485-493, 1987.
23. Fugita M, Kodera Y, Ogawa M, et al: Digital image processing of periapical radiographs, *Oral Surg* 65:490-494, 1988.

24. Furkart AJ, Dove SB, McDavid WD, et al: Direct digital radiography for the detection of periodontal bone lesions, *Oral Surg* 74:650-652, 1992.

25. Garcia DA, Tow DE, Sullivan TM, et al: The appearances of common dental diseases on radionuclide bone images of the jaws, *J Dent Res* 58:1040-1046, 1979.

26. Gibbs SJ: Comparative imaging of the jaws, *Curr Sci* 2:55-63, 1992.

27. Gratt BM, Pullinger A, Sickles EA, Lee JJ: Electronic thermography of normal facial structures: a pilot study, *Oral Surg* 68:346-351, 1989.

28. Gratt BM, Sickles EA, Grall-Radford SB, Solberg WK: Electronic thermography in the diagnosis of atypical odontalgia: a pilot study, *Oral Surg* 68:472-481, 1989.

29. Gratt BM, Sickles EA, Ross JB: Electronic thermography in the assessment of internal derangement of the temporomandibular joint, *Oral Surg* 71:364-370, 1991.

30. Gritzmann N: Sonography of the salivary glands, *AJR* 153:161-166, 1989.

31. Gröndahl HG, Gröndahl K, Webber RL: A digital subtraction technique for dental radiography, *Oral Surg* 55:96-102, 1983.

32. Halse A, White SC, Espelid I, Tveit AB: Visualization of stannous fluoride treatment of carious lesions by subtraction radiography, *Oral Surg* 69:378-381, 1990.

33. Hansson LG, Eriksson L, Westesson PL: Magnetic resonance evaluation after temporomandibular joint diskectomy, *Oral Surg* 74:801-810, 1992.

34. Haug RH, Lieberman JM, Picard U, et al: Use of three-dimensional computerized tomography in the diagnosis of an obstructed coronoid process, *Oral Surg* 68:793-796, 1989.

35. Heffez L, Mafee MF, Langer B: Double contrast arthrography of the temporomandibular joint: role of direct sagittal CT imaging, *Oral Surg* 65:511-514, 1988.

36. Heffez L, Mafee MF, Vaiana J: The role of magnetic resonance imaging in the diagnosis and management of ameloblastoma, *Oral Surg* 65:2-12, 1988.

37. Hemmy DC, Tessier PL: CT of dry skulls with craniofacial deformities: Accuracy of three-dimensional reconstruction, *Radiology* 157:113-116, 1985.

38. Herman GT, Coin CG: The use of three-dimensional computer display in the study of disk disease, *J Comput Assist Tomogr* 4:564-567, 1980.

39. Herman GT, Liu KH: Display of three-dimensional information in computed tomography, *J Comput Assist Tomogr* 1:155-160, 1977.

40. Herman GT, Liu HK: Three-dimensional display of human organs from computed tomograms, *Comput Graph Image Process* 9:1-21, 1979.

41. Hildebolt CF, Vannier MW, Pilgram TK, Shrout MK: Quantitative evaluation of digital dental radiograph imaging systems, *Oral Surg* 70:661-668, 1990.

42. Hounsfield GN: Computerized transverse axial scanning (tomography). I. Description of the system, *Br J Radiol* 46:1016-1022, 1973.

43. Kaplan AS, Assael LA: *Temporomandibular disorders: diagnosis and treatment,* Philadelphia, 1991, WB Saunders.

44. Kashima I, Kanno M, Higashi T, Takano M: Computed panoramic tomography with scanning laser-stimulated luminescence, *Oral Surg* 60:448-453, 1985.

45. Kashima I, Tajima K, Nishimura K, et al: Diagnostic imaging of diseases affecting the mandible with the use of computed panoramic radiography, *Oral Surg* 70:110-116, 1990.

46. Kassebaum DK, McDavid WD, Dove SB, Waggener RG: Spatial resolution requirements for digitizing dental radiographs, *Oral Surg* 67:760-769, 1989.

47. Katagiri S, Yoshie H, Hara K, et al: Application of computed tomography for diagnosis of alveolar bony defects, *Oral Surg* 64:361-366, 1987.

48. Katzberg RW: Temporomandibular joint imaging, *Radiology* 170:297-307, 1989.

49. Kircos LT, Ortendahl DA, Hattner RS, et al: Emission imaging of patients with craniomandibular dysfunction, *Oral Surg* 65:249-254, 1988.

50. Kraut RA: Utilization of 3D/Dental software for precise implant site selection: clinical reports, *Implant Dentistry* 1:134-139, 1992.

51. Lam EWN, Hannam AG, Wood WW, et al: Imaging orofacial tissues by magnetic resonance, *Oral Surg* 68:2-8, 1989.

52. Lambert PM: Three-dimensional computed tomography and anatomic replicas in surgical treatment planning, *Oral Surg* 68:782-786, 1989.

53. Larheim TA, Smith H, Aspestrand F: Rheumatic disease of temporomandibular joint with development of anterior disk displacement as revealed by magnetic resonance imaging: a case report, *Oral Surg* 71:246-249, 1991.

54. Ludlow JB, Soltmann R, Tyndall D, Grady JJ: Digitally subtracted linear tomograms: three techniques for measuring condylar displacement, *Oral Surg* 72:614-620, 1991.

55. Luyk NJ, Doyle T, Ferguson MM: Recent trends in imaging the salivary glands, *Dentomaxillofac Radiol* 20:3-10, 1991.

56. Marsh JL, Vannier MW: The "third" dimension in craniofacial surgery, *Plast Reconstr Surg* 71:759-767, 1983.

57. Marsh JL, Vannier MW: Surface imaging from computerized tomographic scans, *Surgery* 94:159-165, 1983.

58. Matteson SR, Bechtold W, Phillips C, Staab EV: A method for three-dimensional image reformation for quantitative cephalometric analysis, *J Oral Maxillofac Surg* 47:1053-1061, 1989.

59. Matteson SR, Staab EV, Fine JT: Bone-scan appearance of benign oral pathologic conditions, *J Oral Surg* 38:759-763, 1980.

60. McDavid WD, Dove SB, Welander U, Tronje G: Direct digital extraoral radiography of the head and neck with a solid-state linear x-ray detector, *Oral Surg* 74:811-817, 1992.

61. McDavid WD, Dove SB, Welander U, Tronje G: Electronic system for digital acquisition of rotational panoramic radiographs, *Oral Surg* 71:499-502, 1991.

62. McEnergy KW, Wilson AJ, Murphy WA, Marushack MM: Spiral CT imaging of the musculoskeletal system, *Radiology* 185(suppl):367, 1992.

63. Molteni R: Visualix, a new system for direct dental x-ray imaging: a preliminary report, *Dentomaxillofac Radiol* 21:222-223, 1992.

64. Mouyen F, Benz C, Sonnabend E, Lodter JP: Presentation and physical evaluation of RadioVisioGraphy, *Oral Surg* 68:238-242, 1989.

65. Nelvig P, Wing K, Welander U: Sens-A-Ray: a new system for direct digital intraoral radiography, *Oral Surg* 74:818-823, 1992.

66. Ohki M, Okano T, Yamada N: A contrast-correction method for digital subtraction radiography, *J Periodontol Res* 23:277-280, 1988.

67. Okano T, Mera T, Ohki M, et al: Digital subtraction of radiograph in evaluating alveolar bone changes after initial periodontal therapy, *Oral Surg* 69:258-262, 1990.

68. Ott RJ: Nuclear medicine in the 1990s: a quantitative physiologic approach, *Br J Radiol* 62:421-432, 1989.

69. Pogrel MA, Yen CK, Taylor RC: Studies in tooth crown temperature gradients with the use of infrared thermography, *Oral Surg* 67:583-587, 1989.

70. Putnins E, Lavelle CLB, Holthuis A: Detection of three-walled infrabony defects by subtraction radiography, *Oral Surg* 65:102-108, 1988.

71. Reddy MS, Bruch JM, Jeffcoat MK, Williams RC: Contrast enhancement as an aid to interpretation in digital subtraction radiography, *Oral Surg* 71:763-769, 1991.

72. Redington RW, Berninger WH: Medical imaging systems, *Physics Today* 34:36-44, 1981.

73. Roberts D, Pettigrew J, Udupa J, Ram C: Three-dimensional imaging and display of the temporomandibular joint, *Oral Surg* 58:461-474, 1984.

74. Rothman SLG, Chaftez N, Rhodes ML, Schwartz MS: CT in the preoperative assessment of the mandible and maxilla for endosseous implant surgery, *Radiology* 168:171-175, 1988.

75. Rudolph DJ, White SC, Mankovich NJ: Influence of geometric distortion and exposure parameters on sensitivity of digital subtraction radiography, *Oral Surg* 64:631-637, 1987.

76. Ruttimann UE, Webber RL, Schmidt E: A robust digital method for film contrast correction in subtraction radiography, *J Periodontol Res* 21:486-495, 1986.

77. Schwarz MS, Rothman SLG, Chafetz N, Rhodes M: Computed tomography in dental implantation surgery, *Dent Clin North Am* 33:555-597, 1989.

78. Schwarz MS, Rothman SLG, Rhodes ML, Chafetz N: Computed tomography. I. Preoperative assessment of the mandible for endosseous implant surgery, *Int J Oral Implantol* 2:137-141, 1987.

79. Schwarz MS, Rothman SLG, Rhodes ML, Chafetz N: Computed tomography. II. Preoperative assessment of the maxilla for endosseous implant surgery, *Int J Oral Implantol* 2:143-148, 1987.

80. Schwimmer AM, Roth SE, Morrison SN: The use of computerized tomography in the diagnosis and management of temporal and infratemporal space abscesses, *Oral Surg* 66:17-20, 1988.

81. Smith JP, Barrow JW: Reformatted CT imaging for implant planning, *Oral Maxillofac Surg Clin North Am* 3:805-825, 1991.

82. Southard TE, Harris EF, Walter RG: Image enhancement of the mandibular condyle through digital subtraction, *Oral Surg* 64:645-647, 1987.

83. Strittmatter EJ, Keller DL, LaBounty GL, et al: The relationship between radionuclide bone scans and dental examinations, *Oral Surg* 68:576-581, 1989.

84. Takahashi M, Ozawa Y: Stereoscopic magnification angiography using a twin focal-spot x-ray tube, *Radiology* 142:791-792, 1982.

85. Telfer N, Abelson SH, Witmer RR: Role of bone imaging in the diagnosis of active root canal infection: case report, *J Endod* 6:570-572, 1980.

86. Totty WG, Vannier MW: Complex musculoskeletal anatomy: Analysis using three dimensional surface reconstruction, *Radiology* 150:173-177, 1984.

87. Tyndall DA, Phillips C, Malone-Trahey A, Renner J: Validity of digital subtraction of transcranial plain films in quantification of positional changes of the mandibular condyle, *Oral Surg* 71:748-755, 1991.

88. Uchida H, Kobayashi K, Nagao M: Measurement *in vivo* of masticatory mucosal thickness with 20 MHz B-mode ultrasonic diagnostic equipment, *J Dent Res* 68:95-100, 1989.

89. van den Akker HP: Diagnostic imaging in salivary gland disease, *Oral Surg* 66:625-637, 1988.

90. van der Stelt PF: Improved diagnosis with digital radiography, *Curr Sci* 2:1-6, 1992.

91. van der Stelt PF, Ruttiman UE, Webber RL: Determination of projections for subtraction radiography based on image similarity measurements, *Dentomaxillofac Radiol* 18:113-117, 1989.

92. Vannier MW, Gado MH, Marsh JL: Three-dimensional display of intracranial soft-tissue structures, *AJNR* 4:520-521, 1983.

93. Vannier MW, Hildebolt CF, Marsh JL, et al: Craniosynostosis: diagnostic value of three-dimensional CT reconstruction, *Radiology* 173:669-673, 1989.

94. Vannier MW, Marsh JL, Warren JO: Three-dimensional CT reconstruction images for craniofacial surgical planning and evaluation, *Radiology* 150:179-184, 1984.

95. Verdon TA: *Nuclear medicine for the general physician,* Littleton Mass, 1980, PSG Publishing.

96. Walker A, Horner K, Czajka J, et al: Quantitative assessment of a new dental imaging system, *Br J Radiol* 64:529-536, 1991.

97. Walter JP: Physics of high-resolution ultrasound: practical aspects, *Radiol Clin North Am* 23:3-11, 1985.

98. Webber RL, Ruttimann UE, Heaven TJ: Calibration errors in digital subtraction radiography, *J Periodontol Res* 25:268-275, 1990.

99. Webber RL, Tzukert TA, Ruttimann U: The effects of beam hardening on digital subtraction radiography, *J Periodontol Res* 24:53-58, 1989.

100. Welander U, Nelvig P, Tronje G, et al: Basic technical properties of a system for direct acquisition of digital intraoral radiographs, *Dentomaxillofac Radiol* 21:222, 1992.

101. Wenzel A, Halse A: Digital subtraction radiography after stannous fluoride treatment for occlusal caries diagnosis, *Oral Surg* 74:824-828, 1992.

102. Wenzel A, Hintze H, Mikkelsen L, Mouyen F: Radiographic detection of occlusal caries in noncavitated teeth: a comparison of conventional film radiographs, digitized film radiographs, and RadioVisioGraphy, *Oral Surg* 72:621-626, 1991.

103. Westesson P, Cohen JM, Tallents RH: Magnetic resonance imaging of temporomandibular joint after surgical treatment of internal derangement, *Oral Surg* 71:407-411, 1991.

104. Wilson IR, Crocker EF: An introduction to ultrasonography in oral surgery, *Oral Surg* 59:236-241, 1985.

105. Wilson IR, Crocker EF, McKellar G, Rengaswamy V: An evaluation of the clinical applications of diagnostic ultrasonography in oral surgery, *Oral Surg* 67:242-248, 1989.

106. Wittich GR, Scheible WF, Hajek PC: Ultrasonography of the salivary glands, *Radiol Clin North Am* 23:29-37, 1985.

107. Worthington C, Peters TM, Ethier R, et al: Stereoscopic digital subtraction angiography in neuroradiologic assessment, *AJNR* 6:802-808, 1985.

14

ALLAN G. FARMAN, CHRISTOFFEL J. NORTJÉ, and ROBERT E. WOOD

Principles of Image Interpretation

SYSTEMATIC APPROACH

Radiographs and other diagnostic images form only a part of the diagnostic process. Although it is useful to develop one's ability to perceive features within isolated radiographs, the interpretation of these features is rarely pathognomonic. Furthermore, it is ethically unsound, from a radiation health and safety point of view, to make radiographs without following selection criteria. For these reasons a thorough case history and clinical examination should precede selection of the radiographic procedures for every patient. Laboratory tests may also be required as part of the diagnostic process.

Case history

Enough emphasis can hardly be placed on the necessity of a thorough case history. It is important to approach history taking, like radiologic interpretation, in a rational and systematic way. Besides such demographic details as the patient's name, address, age, and gender, this should include the patient's chief complaint (if any), a history of the present condition, the patient's past medical and dental history, and a brief note on the direction in which the investigation is headed. The precise technique for history taking is beyond the scope of this book, but the history should be as thorough as possible. If recorded in this manner, it becomes an invaluable record to refer to when evaluating the clinical, radiologic, histologic, and other laboratory test evidence.

Clinical examination

Radiographs should not be obtained before performing a thorough clinical examination and recording the findings in detail on the patient's chart. A clinical examination helps the clinician select the radiographic projections most likely to provide useful information for an evaluation (and eventual diagnosis) of the patient's condition. The examination need not be restricted to the area of chief complaint, however. It can include a thorough extraoral and intraoral inspection. A clinical evaluation is still essential even when the patient is asymptomatic and is merely requesting a periodic dental review. The decision concerning which radiographs are needed will vary for different patients depending on such clinical findings as oral health status, presence or absence of teeth, and dental alignment. Adjustments in radiographic technique may be necessary to compensate for anatomic variations (e.g., a torus, shallow palate, or ankyloglossia). It is the responsibility of the clinician to select and prescribe the appropriate radiographs to assist in the determination of oral and maxillofacial health status of the individual patient. This responsibility must not be delegated.

Existing diagnostic radiographs

An effective means of reducing the patient's unnecessary exposure to ionizing radiation is to avoid redundancy by not exposing radiographs that are already available. If the patient is not certain which views have already been made, it is the dentist's responsibility to obtain this information from earlier providers.

Previous radiographs are still of value even when they are too old to replace new exposures. A comparison of old radiographs with new images allows one to evaluate changes over a specific time interval. This information on the progression of a radiologic feature can be of great value in helping to differentiate between disease entities and between normal and disease states. It also provides a dynamic assessment of the rate of development of such common chronic dental diseases as caries and periodontitis.

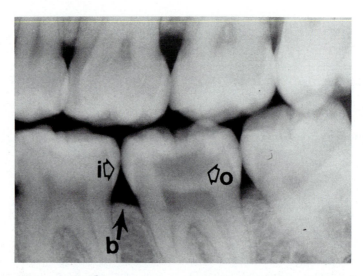

FIG. 14-1. Bitewing radiograph showing interproximal *(i)* and occlusal *(o)* dental caries. The level of the supporting bone is also clearly demonstrated *(b)*.

Image selection

Professional judgment should be used to determine the type, frequency, and extent of each radiographic examination.[1] As noted above, this requires a complete patient history, a thorough clinical examination, and the acquisition of information from existing radiographs.

Symptomatic patients. For patients having signs or symptoms of disease, all radiographs necessary, in the judgment of the dentist, to evaluate the patient's condition should be made. Failure to obtain them constitutes negligence and a failure to provide the appropriate standard of care. If a patient refuses to have radiographs made, the clinician would be wise to document this fact and not proceed with treatment.

The type of radiograph to be made depends on the site and dimensions of the probable lesion and on clinical practicality. For the more common dental conditions intraoral periapical and bitewing films provide the best resolution and coverage of the area of interest (Fig. 14-1). When the patient is unable to open his or her mouth because of trismus, extraoral alternatives to intraoral radiographs must be sought. Such alternatives include a panoramic radiograph or a lateral oblique projection of the jaw. These views are also valuable when the lesion extends beyond the dimensions of standard intraoral films (Fig. 14-2). Special series of radiographs are often used to examine traumatic injuries, progressive dysfunction of the temporomandibular joint, dental malocclusion requiring orthodontic evaluation, syndromes of the head and neck, and multifocal or systemic diseases.

Asymptomatic patients. For patients in need of a regular dental checkup and who are asymptomatic, the selection of radiographs still rests largely on professional judgment. In these patients the principal reason for obtaining a radiograph is to detect incipient proximal dental caries and to evaluate clinically detectable periodontitis. Guidelines to the selection of radiographic examinations for such patients have been developed by the Center for Devices and Radiological Health of the Food and Drug Administration[2] and are described in Chapter 4. Professional judgment is important in this activity. Radiographs should not be made merely as a routine or for administrative purposes.

Initial examination of images

Newly obtained radiographs are evaluated for proper exposure, positioning, and processing. They should have adequate density to illustrate the specific structures under consideration. Different densities are acceptable in certain circumstances but unacceptable in others. Adequate contrast will also depend on the individual clinical situation. For example, a long scale of contrast is desirable for evaluation of periodontal disease. Exposure and processing techniques influence density and con-

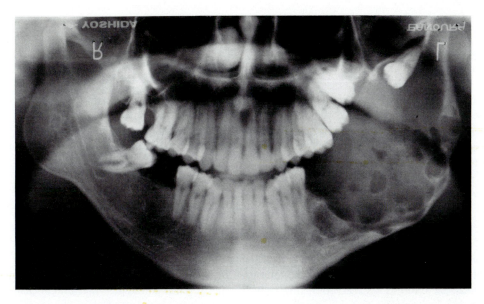

FIG. 14-2. Ameloblastoma of the left mandibular ramus. This lesion was positioned beyond the area of coverage of intraoral radiographs. A panoramic radiograph provides the best initial study in this case.

trast and may be altered to improve these properties (see Chapter 5). Radiographs that are technically inferior should not be used for patient care.

The final questions to be asked are whether these radiographs show the examiner the structures of interest and, if not, what further ones are needed. Since radiographs are generally two-dimensional representations of three-dimensional objects, a single exposure is often inadequate to determine the interpretation in an optimum manner. For pathologic lesions it is often necessary to obtain a minimum of two radiographs at right angles to one another. On occasion, the patient may need to be referred for more advanced imaging modalities (e.g., CT or MRI). (See Chapter 13.)

Viewing environment

The proper environment should be available for reading radiographs. It should have low ambient lighting and freedom from distraction. The darker the ambient lighting, the better able one will be to detect fine details that might go unnoticed in normal room lighting. Such viewing conditions are present in most medical facilities; however, the dentist often views radiographs only at chairside, with normal lighting and with all the distractions of the clinical atmosphere. One should get into the habit of evaluating radiographs under appropriate viewing conditions and away from distractions of the clinic.

The viewing area should have a viewbox of sufficient size, with bright and even illumination, and be in a comfortable position for use by the operator. A bright light or dense-spot viewer is indispensable for viewing dark portions of radiographs. Magnifying glasses should be available to allow the examiner to focus on areas of the film that are of importance. Opaque masks should also be available to block out extraneous light from the viewbox since it is difficult for the observer's eyes to accommodate the range of light intensities both transmitted through the radiographs and coming directly from the viewbox.

It is a good habit for the dentist to view all patients' radiographs at a time when there are no other distractions, perhaps at the beginning of the day before patients arrive or at the end of the day when they have departed. Improved interpretation and treatment planning are certainly worth the extra effort.

Observation and interpretation

Identification. All radiographs must be marked with the patient's name, any extra details that will help discriminate between patients having the same name (e.g., date of birth, social security number, hospital number, or address), and the date of exposure. This information should be checked carefully before writing a report. The legal and medical literature abounds with cases in which this simple precaution was not taken. It is best not to rely on unlabeled radiographs when making a diagnosis.

Localization. Localizing a radiograph should be a simple matter if the dentist has performed the imaging procedure; however, this is not always the case. It may be necessary to orient radiographs taken by other clinicians. This can be done by calling on one's knowledge of normal anatomic landmarks or by relying on special markers to distinguish between right and left sides of the patient. Metallic markers are generally used for extraoral radiographs. For intraoral radiographs there is no room for metallic markers to distinguish between the right and left sides. In this case the manufacturers of the x-ray film place an embossed dot whose convexity is directed toward the source of the radiation during exposure. Correct orientation of films must be assured, because confusing right and left could lead to inappropriate treatment of the patient and would be impossible to defend against in a court of law.

Evaluation sequence. The evaluation sequence begins with history taking, clinical examination of the patient, and selection of appropriate tests (including radiographs). The radiographs are examined under suitable viewing conditions, and observations listed before any significance is attached to them or a determination made of the likely nature of any disease process. In this way a radiologic differential interpretation will be based on the radiologic features alone. Then the radiologic features are correlated with the patient's clinical information, history, and results of other tests (including histologic information) to formulate a working diagnosis. Radiologic interpretation is only one factor in the ultimate diagnosis; it is an "interpretation," not the diagnosis. Additional special tests, possibly including further diagnostic imaging, may be needed before a definitive diagnosis is reached, a treatment plan formulated, or the necessary treatment performed. Table 14-1 summarizes this sequence.

Normal versus abnormal. After assuring the identity of the patient whose images are to be evaluated and assessing image quality and orientation, one needs to determine whether the radiologic features are normal. Such a determination requires a thorough knowledge of normal anatomy and of the factors involved in the production of radiographs. Remember: normal is a range; it is relative rather than specific. Consequently, it must be ascertained which observations are outside the normal range and which require further investigation or treat-

TABLE 14-1. The diagnostic sequence

- History taking and clinical examination
- Radiograph selection and quality assessment
- Radiographic examination
- Radiologic evaluation
- Attach significance and hypothesize likely disease nature
- Formulate differential interpretation
- Integrate patient history with clinical and other findings
- Formulate working diagnosis
- Consider additional tests
- Formulate definitive diagnosis and treatment plan
- Perform necessary treatment

ment. As a generalization, relative bilateral symmetry tends to suggest that one is dealing with a normal structure; and lack of change in the features between radiographs taken at distant time intervals tends to support a conservative approach.

Listing of observations. Observations should be listed in a systematic manner. When viewing a radiograph for the purposes of interpretation it is important to examine all parts of the radiograph. Because radiographs are usually made to evaluate clinical impressions, it is all too easy to examine a few parts of the image and neglect the majority. Often when an abnormality is discovered, the observer will not complete the examination of the remainder of the radiograph, and thereby neglects potentially important observations. Hence, on locating an abnormality, it is wise to ignore it for a time and to carry on with the complete evaluation of the radiograph, keeping in mind the thought of finding a second or even a third area of interest. One can use a system of analysis to ensure examination of all parts of the radiograph, but it takes discipline, and each practitioner should develop a personal method for assuring evaluation of all the information present. A systematic approach for evaluating panoramic radiographs is presented in Chapter 12. A similar approach is necessary for viewing a full-mouth series of periapical and bitewing radiographs:

1. To mask out extraneous light, mount radiographs in an opaque mount. It is usual to view the films with the embossed dot convexities facing the observer, so the patient's right side is on your left, as if you were looking at the patient. Before progressing, check the embossed dots and the normal anatomic details to assure that the films are correctly mounted.

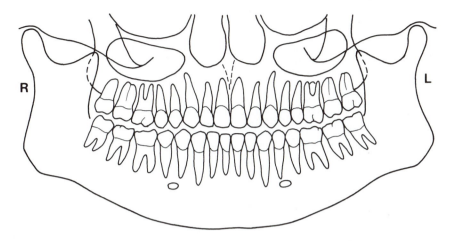

FIG. 14-3. Standard diagram for recording radiologic findings. This one is for panoramic and intraoral radiographs, but a similar arrangement can be used for other projections. In the form of rubber stamps these diagrams can be placed anywhere in the patient's notes.

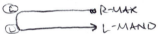

Failure to do so could lead to misdiagnosis and inappropriate treatment for the patient. Also be sure to check the patient's name and the date of the radiographs to assure proper labeling.

2. Begin by viewing the posterior bitewing radiographs starting with the right maxillary teeth and continuing across the maxilla. Then proceed to view the mandibular teeth from the left side to the right. Evaluate the posterior teeth for primary or recurrent dental caries, paying special attention to the enamel surfaces just below the interproximal contact points. When in doubt, refer to the adjacent periapical views for additional information. Be sure to view the surfaces of every tooth.

3. Evaluate the anterior periapical radiographs for primary or recurrent dental caries.

4. Check for the periodontal margin level of all interproximal alveolar crests in a systematic manner, starting with the right maxillary molars and working your way around the arches to the left maxilla, then from the left mandible and working around to the right. Also chart the presence of dental calculus.

5. Evaluate the pulp chamber and periodontal ligament space of each tooth in turn, starting with the right maxilla and progressing around the arches tooth by tooth.

6. Evaluate the bone around the teeth, noting the overall density and extent of trabeculation. Note also normal anatomic bony landmarks, including but not limited to both maxillary sinuses, the outlines of the nasal passages, the anterior nasal spine, the nasopalatine canal and fossa, each mental foramen, and the mandibular canals.

For a lesion to be demonstrated radiologically, there should be a substantive change in the tissues. This change may be in the general architecture or in radiodensity of the involved tissues.

A comprehensive description of each significant lesion should be entered in the patient's clinical notes—including the lesion's site, size, shape, symmetry, borders, and content and its associations. In the ensuing discussion these descriptors will be applied to lesions affecting bone, but they can also be extended to include the dental structures and surrounding soft tissues.

Site. Designate the position of the lesion carefully, preferably using standard diagrams in addition to narrative form (Fig. 14-3). The epicenter of the lesion may help in determining its origin. For instance, lesions arising in the body of the mandible above the mandibular canal are more likely to be odontogenic than are those arising below the canal. Determine also whether the lesion is solitary or multiple, and whether it affects one bone or several (i.e., is multifocal). This will help in differentiating between local and systemic disease.

Size. Indicate the size of the lesion (in millimeters) as measured on the radiographs. Lesion size is an important factor in potential treatment planning and certainly is an important measure in judging change with time. A ruler is an important

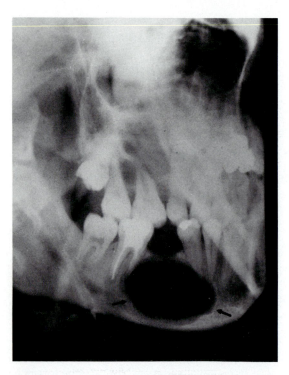

FIG. 14-4. Lesions involving both bone and soft tissues that have a "brandy glass" configuration probably arose in bone. This was a residual radicular cyst. (Lateral-oblique projection.)

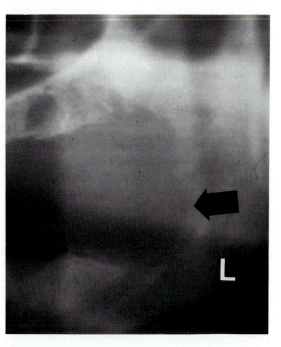

FIG. 14-5. Squamous cell carcinoma arising in the soft tissues of the floor of the mouth. A saucerized appearance tends to indicate that the lesion originated in soft tissues. This cropped panoramic radiograph shows extensive destruction of the ramus and body of the mandible extending from the third molar region.

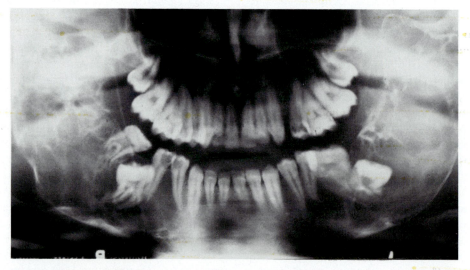

FIG. 14-6. Bilateral symmetry is a feature that suggests either a variant of the normal range or an inherited condition. Symmetry of mandibular lesions is the common feature in the dominantly inherited condition cherubism (seen on this panoramic radiograph).

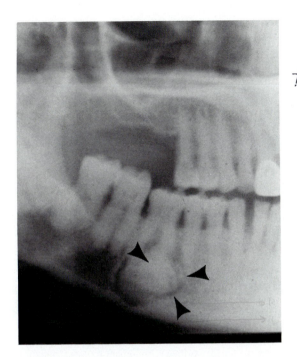

FIG. 14-7. "Encapsulated" benign lesion. Note its radiolucent halo, separating the well-corticated outline from the lesion. This condition proved to be a cementoblastoma.

instrument to keep at the side of the viewbox. A radiographic projection is subject to some shape and size distortion, generally magnification.

Shape. Describe the shape of the lesion from at least two perspectives, using radiographs taken at right angles wherever possible. The shape often provides clues as to origin. For example, a "brandy glass" appearance tends to indicate a lesion that begins within bone and secondarily extends to soft tissues (Fig. 14-4). On the other hand, a saucerized appearance suggests a lesion originating within the soft tissues and secondarily involving bone (Fig. 14-5). Usually, lesions grow in the direction of least resistance, and this will be reflected in their shape.

Symmetry. Asymmetry is more worrisome than symmetry. Bilateral symmetry usually means that a condition is either a variant of normal or inherited (Fig. 14-6).

Borders. There are several factors to consider relating to the border, or outline, of a lesion in bone. First, for a lesion to be detected radiographically, there must be significant alteration of its architecture resulting from the resorption or deposition of bone. Early stages of disease processes may be too subtle to be detected radiographically,

as in the case of an initial carious lesion of enamel where the loss of hydroxyapatite is insufficient to cause a perceptible change in radiodensity. Second, the border of a lesion is perhaps its most significant feature, since the active process in any lesion tends to be at the periphery. Just as the histopathologist gains the best information about a lesion from biopsy specimens taken at the growing edge of the lesion (where abnormal meets normal), so the diagnostic radiologist can obtain a great deal of information from interpretation of the radiologic outline of a lesion.

The border may be well-defined, moderately defined, poorly defined, or undefined. With the exception of inflammatory lesions, benign conditions tend to be either well defined (as in the case of cysts and tumors, Fig. 14-4) or ill defined (as in the case of developmental conditions like late fibrous dysplasia). With the latter it is the structural architecture that changes. The degree of border cortication will vary depending on the type of lesion. Lesions that are poorly defined tend also to be poorly corticated. A radiolucent zone within a well-corticated well-demarcated border suggests encapsulation of the lesion—a feature most consistent with benign processes (Fig. 14-7).

When there is a detectable border, this can be further subtyped. We have already seen the sharp sclerotic margin of benign cysts and neoplasms (Figs. 14-4 and 14-7). Some, usually more aggressive, benign lesions such as ameloblastomas and odontogenic keratocysts tend to have a crenated or multiocular rather than a unilocular outline (Figs. 14-2 and 14-8). The term "infiltrative" (i.e., bays within bays) suggests malignancy whereas a ragged "moth-eaten" (or "worm-eaten") border can occur in both severe inflammatory conditions and malignant neoplasia (Fig. 14-9). Well-defined "punched-out" lesions with noncorticated margins typically occur in the histiocytoses and in myeloma (Fig. 14-10).

Contents. Lesions may be entirely radiolucent, homogeneously radiopaque, or mixed radiolucent and radiopaque. One should, however, be careful when applying these terms. Remember: the terms "radiolucent" and "radiopaque" are relative depending on the density and thickness of adjacent structures and the radiographic technique used. Also a lesion that appears as a radiolucency or a mixed radiolucency and radiopacity by a particular technique may appear as a homogeneous radiolucency by another (Figs. 14-11 and 14-12). If the bulk of the tissue being examined is not considered,

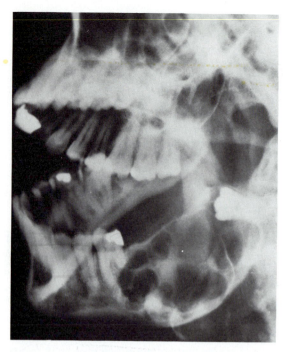

FIG. 14-8. Multiocular radiolucent outlines are often found in more locally aggressive benign cysts and neoplasms of the jaws. (Lateral-oblique projection.)

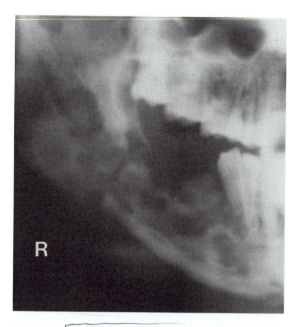

FIG. 14-9. Poorly defined lesion with a moth-eaten appearance in this primary malignancy of the mandible. The lesion was a leiomyosarcoma (shown on a cropped panoramic radiograph).

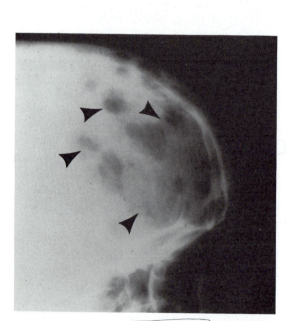

FIG. 14-10. "Punched-out" lesions of multiple myeloma (shown on a cropped lateral projection of the skull.)

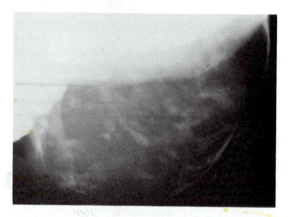

FIG. 14-11. In this projection the cementifying fibroma is seen as a mixed radiolucency and radiopacity.

comparisons of radiodensity are fraught with error.

Another facet to consider is the pathogenesis of the radiologic features. Most lesions start out radiolucent; some progress to become mixed radiolucent and radiopaque, others to become homogeneously radiopaque. The actual appearance of a lesion can vary with the stage of pathogenesis. For example, periapical cemental dysplasia starts as multiple radiolucencies that progressively calcify to become radiopaque (Figs. 14-13 and 14-14).

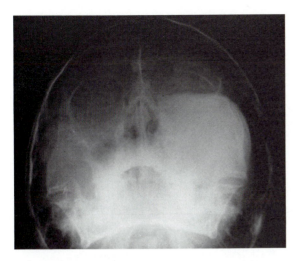

FIG. 14-12. On this Waters view of the sinus the lesion appears as a homogeneous radiopacity. On a lateral view the beam would pass through a much greater bulk of tumor tissue; hence its increased attenuation.

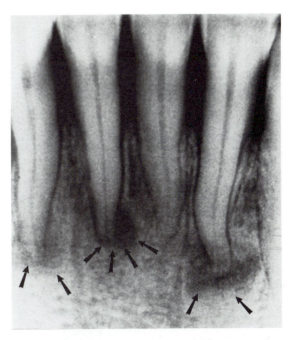

FIG. 14-13. The early lesions of periapical cemental dysplasia are radiolucent.

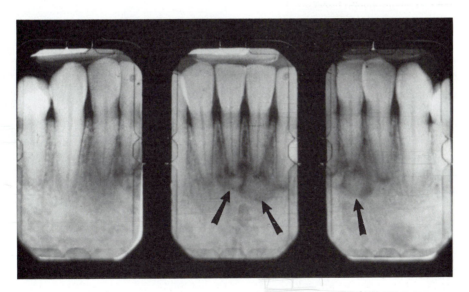

FIG. 14-14. The late lesions of periapical cemental dysplasia are radiopaque.

Essentially, a radiolucent lesion suggests that there has been lysis of normal bone. The development of a calcified product within a lesion results in varying degrees of radiopacity depending on the nature of the calcified material (e.g., cementum vs dentin vs enamel), the degree of calcification, the size of the lesion, and the distribution of the calcified product (Fig. 14-15). Foreign bodies can be much more opaque than calcified products manufactured by the body. They are usually easy to identify (Fig. 14-16).

Another consideration concerning content is the size and distribution of trabeculations, both at the affected site and throughout the jaws. The normal trabecular pattern is usually coarser and more angular, with relatively larger marrow spaces in the

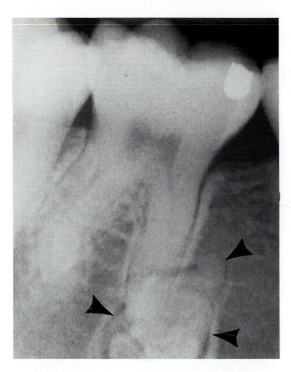

FIG. 14-15. Odontoma. Note that the calcified component has the same opacity as adjacent teeth.

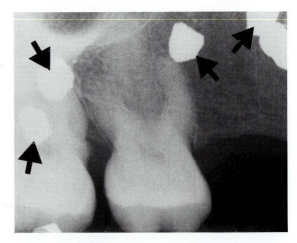

FIG. 14-16. Metallic foreign bodies.

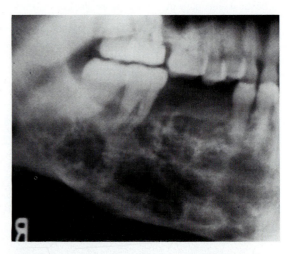

FIG. 14-17. "Honeycomb" angular trabeculations in odontogenic myxoma. (Cropped panoramic radiograph.)

mandible than in the maxilla. The normal pattern tends to be for more dense bone in blacks than in whites; however, there is a wide range of normal. Particularly thin trabeculation and rarefied bone patterns of the jaws can usually be associated with such systemic conditions as hyperparathyroidism, early stages of Paget's disease of bone (osteoporosis circumscripta), and osteoporosis. Unusually dense generalized trabeculations occur in osteopetrosis and a number of other less frequently encountered conditions.

Trabecular patterns within a discrete lesion may be in the form of multiple septa, creating varying degrees of multilocularity. Lucent lesions presenting as a single discrete cavity are termed "unilocular." When septa divide the cavity into two or more segments, the lesion is "multilocular." The term "soap bubble" describes multilocular lesions when such septa are few and the locules are relatively round and large. This type of trabeculation commonly develops in ameloblastomas, central giant cell granulomas, and odontogenic keratocysts (Fig. 14-8). Narrower "honeycomb" separations with angular interstices typically occur in odontogenic myxomas, and intraosseous hemangiomas (Fig. 14-17).

Some lesions show particular trabecular patterns that help in the diagnosis. The "hair on end" appearance of trabeculations in the skull is typical of the hemolytic beta thalassemia and sickle cell anemia (Fig. 14-18). The coarse trabeculation leaves space for hematopoietic marrow to persist. An irregular "sunburst" appearance of trabeculations within a destructive and productive lesion is a typical feature of osteogenic sarcoma (Fig. 14-19), in which the structure of new bone is completely unrelated to the stress-bearing requirements of the bone. Dense patches of sclerotic bone can form in response to a local inflammatory stimulus, as in condensing osteitis (Fig. 14-20), and can be more widespread as the "cotton ball" appearance in late

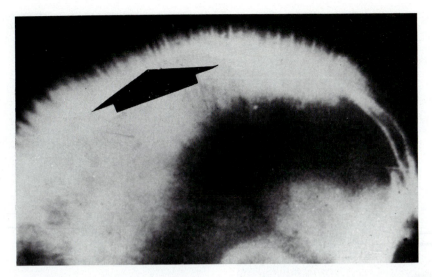

FIG. 14-18. "Hair-on-end" appearance typical of the hemolytic anemias. (Cropped lateral skull radiograph.)

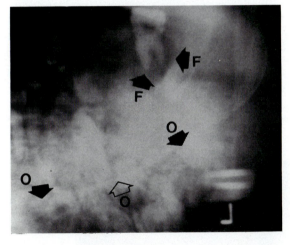

FIG. 14-19. "Sunburst" appearance typical of osteogenic sarcoma. (Cropped panoramic radiograph.) Note the "floating" mandibular third molar tooth *(F)*. The original lower border of the mandible is denoted by *O*.

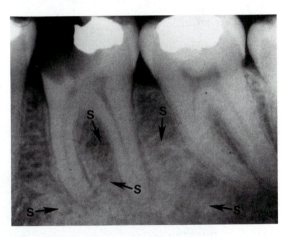

FIG. 14-20. Sclerotic bone in condensing osteitis *(S)*. (Periapical radiograph.)

stages of Paget's disease of bone or in florid osseous dysplasia (Fig. 14-21). In late stages of fibrous dysplasia the bone trabeculations are fine but dense. This results in an "orange peel" appearance on intraoral radiographs (Fig. 14-22). Because the resolution of extraoral radiographs is lower than that of intraoral radiographs, lesions that are "orange peel" on the latter appear "ground glass" ("frosted glass") on the former (Fig. 14-23).

Associations. The effects of a lesion on structures in the jaws (e.g., teeth, mandibular canal,

maxillary sinuses) can be useful aids to interpretation. One of the major divisions can be "tooth associated" versus lesions "definitely not tooth associated." Odontogenic conditions tend to appear in the dental arches. Lesions surrounding, or enveloping, the crown of an unerupted tooth may have developed from the reduced enamel epithelium (e.g., a dentigerous cyst) or have invaded the dental follicle space (e.g., an envelopmental odontogenic keratocyst). Lesions associated with a radiolucent widening of the apical periodontal liga-

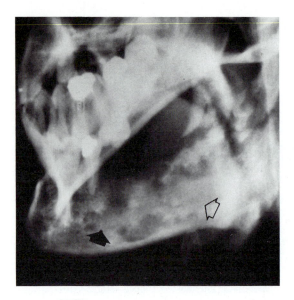

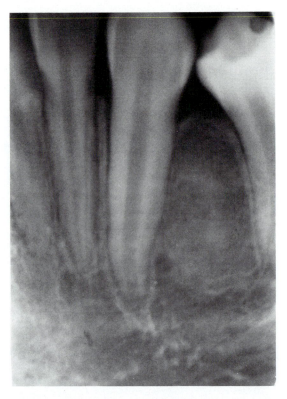

FIG. 14-21. Sclerotic bone in florid osseous dysplasia. (Lateral-oblique projection.)

FIG. 14-22. "Orange peel" appearance in fibrous dysplasia between canine and premolar. (Periapical radiograph.)

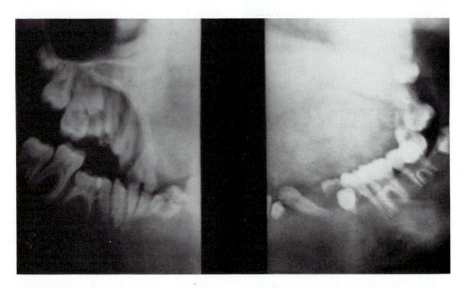

FIG. 14-23. "Ground glass" appearance in fibrous dysplasia. (Detail from a split-image panoramic radiograph.)

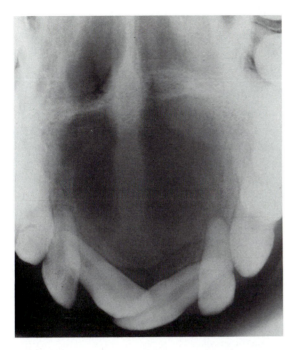

FIG. 14-24. Nasopalatine duct cyst displacing subjacent teeth. (Topographic occlusal radiograph.)

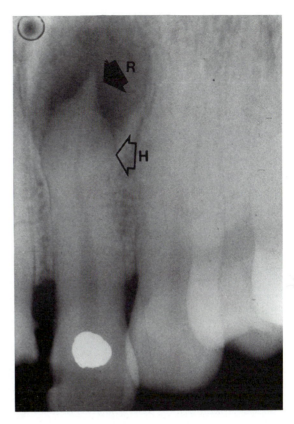

FIG. 14-25. Root resorption *(R)* and hypercementosis *(H)* due to a local inflammatory process.

ment space are most frequently of dental origin following an insult to the pulp of the affected tooth.

Lesions may have one of three effects on the associated structures: displacement, resorption or no effect.[3] Assessing these changes aids in determining the nature of the disease process. As a rough generalization, the less-aggressive benign cysts and tumors tend to displace adjacent structures (Fig. 14-24), locally aggressive benign lesions tend to infiltrate the jaws without much effect on the involved structures, and malignancies and severe infections tend to cause erosion or resorption of structures (Figs. 14-5 and 14-25). Keep in mind that this is a generalization; lesions developing from reduced enamel epithelium (e.g., dentigerous cysts) may be benign but also cause extensive resorption of the roots of adjacent teeth.[4]

Attaching significance to the observations

It is obvious from the above that certain features are highly suggestive, or even pathognomonic, of a particular disease process; however, most radiologic features are contributory rather than diagnostic pieces of evidence. The combination of radiologic features provides a direction for further inquiry. These features can also be used with artificial-intelligence computer programs to produce a list of possible diagnoses based on interpretation

of their various characteristics and other requested information. Whether or not one employs computer-aided diagnosis, it is important to correlate the radiologic features with other diagnostic information to determine a working diagnosis, what further tests will be necessary to formulate the definitive diagnosis, and whether biopsy of the lesion is indicated.

For dentists, skill and success in radiologic diagnosis are dependent on a comprehension of the broad spectrum of disease (Table 14-2) that may be encountered in oral and perioral structures. Although the history and clinical manifestations can provide persuasive evidence of a condition's existence, the radiographic examination usually furnishes significant new information. Except for limited situations such as proximal dental caries, however, diagnosis and treatment should not be based solely on radiographic evidence. When the general nature of a disease is recognized and coupled with basic pathologic changes seen on the radiograph (Table 14-3), a differential diagnosis can be composed; but the list of probable lesions

TABLE 14-2. Broad classification of disease

Normal
Abnormal
  Developmental
    Congenital
    Hereditary
  Acquired
    Inflammatory
    Traumatic
    Cystic
    Benign neoplasia
    Malignant neoplasia
      Primary
      Secondary
    Fibro-osseous
    Metabolic or systemic

must also be qualified by an appreciation of the wide ranges of morphology that are consistent with *normal* as well as the relative incidences of the various entities.

Radiologic differential interpretation

Ideally, one should read radiographs while being blind to the other information that will eventually contribute to the diagnosis. In this way an unbiased list of possibilities, based solely on the radiologic observations, can be made. This is an interpretation rather than a diagnosis. Then the differential radiologic interpretations can be integrated with other available information to form a working diagnosis. If the radiographs are observed by an individual

TABLE 14-3. Radiographic patterns of jaw lesions

Density	Radiolucent, mixed opacity, or radiopaque
Number of lesions	Solitary or multiple
Borders of lesion	Well defined or poorly defined
Shape of lesion	Unilocular, multilocular, or not loculated
Association with teeth	Tooth associated or tooth independent
Adjacent structures	Displaced, eroded, or unaffected

Radiolucent lesions

Unilocular with well-defined borders
  Cyst
  Early periapical cemental dysplasia
  Benign tumor
  Dental granuloma
  Submandibular salivary gland defect
Unilocular with poorly defined borders
  Abscess
  Dental granuloma
  Metastasis
  Osteoporotic bone marrow defect
Multilocular with well-defined borders
  Ameloblastoma
  Keratocyst
  Myxoma
  Cherubism
  Early fibrous dysplasia
  Giant cell granuloma
  Hemangioma
  Traumatic bone cyst
  Aneurysmal bone cyst
Multilocular with poorly defined borders
  Osteomyelitis
  Sarcoma
  Early fibrous dysplasia

Radiopaque lesions

Solitary
  Osteosclerosis
  Condensing osteitis
  Cementoblastoma
  Odontoma
  Torus palatinus
  Superimposed sialolith
  Superimposed foreign body
Multiple
  Florid osseous dysplasia
  Paget's disease of bone
  Late fibrous dysplasia
  Superimposed foreign bodies
  Late periapical cemental dysplasia
  Torus mandibularis
  Osteopetrosis

Mixed opacity lesions

Solitary
  Late adenomatoid odontogenic tumor
  Ameloblastic fibro-odontoma
  Osteogenic sarcoma
  Chondrosarcoma
  Cystic odontoma
  Calcifying epithelial odontogenic tumor
  Ossifying or cementifying fibroma
Multiple
  Periapical cemental dysplasia
  Osteoblastic metastases

who has not been biased by the history or clinical examination, there is less likelihood that salient features will be ignored.

Synthesis of diagnostic information (decision making)

The synthesis of diagnostic information requires the addition of radiologic interpretations to other collected data, including clinical observation, history, and any other special tests such as histopathologic evaluation. This synthesis allows for a narrowed group of differential diagnoses—the working diagnoses—from which a protocol for further special tests may be needed to develop the definitive diagnosis. The additional special tests can include further radiographs or other diagnostic images. Remember: Effective and efficient treatment is unlikely without a definitive diagnosis. Radiologic interpretation is but one step in this process.

Treatment

Radiographs are not only used during the diagnostic stages; they sometimes are an integral component of the treatment process. A good dental example is the radiologic evaluation of various stages of endodontic therapy. Furthermore, radiographs are used to check successful healing following endodontic therapy, dental implantation, and certain other oral surgical procedures.

Expert observation versus supervised neglect

When a radiologic abnormality is detected, there are several pertinent questions: Should it be ig-

nored? Should it be observed? Should it be tested further or treated? These are "bottom line" questions that face all practitioners responsible for interpreting radiographs. If one suspects a benign process that does not generally require treatment and the patient is reliable, one can occasionally place the patient under "expert observation" for a short period to assess whether the condition is progressive. If one suspects a benign process that will invariably require treatment, there is no sense in procrastinating. Since the patient is always entitled to be informed, it is much better to formulate a definitive diagnosis without delay. It is unpleasant to have uncertainty about one's health placed on one's mind. Furthermore, since most disease processes are easier to treat and have a better prognosis if treated early, when a condition is likely to be locally aggressive or malignant or to have other systemic consequences, there is no such thing as "expert observation." In such a situation delay always constitutes "supervised neglect."

SPECIFIC REFERENCES

1. American Dental Association, Council on Dental Materials, Instruments, and Equipment. Recommendations in radiographic practices: an update, 1988, *J Am Dent Assoc* 118:115-7, 1989.
2. Center for Devices and Radiological Health. The selection of patients for x-ray examinations, HHS Publ (FDA) 88-8273, 1987.
3. Farman AG, Nortjé CJ, Grotepass FW: Pathological conditions of the mandible: their effect on the radiologic appearance of the inferior dental canal, *Br J Oral Surg* 15:64-72, 1977.
4. Struthers PJ, Shear M: Root resorption produced by enlargement of ameloblastomas and cysts of the jaws, *Int J Oral Surg* 5:128-132, 1976.

15

BARTON M. GRATT

Dental Caries

"Caries," translated from the Latin, means "rot."[30] Dental caries is a common infectious disease affecting 95% of the population.[25] Bacterial microorganisms (e.g., *Streptococcus mutans, Lactobacillus casei,* and *Actinomyces viscosus*) are concentrated on specific tooth sites as an adherent gelatinous mat known as bacterial plaque. Cariogenic plaque may contain more than 2×10^8 bacteria per milligram wet weight. In susceptible individuals bacterial plaque is capable of fermenting sucrose, glucose, and fructose, with a resultant drop in plaque pH. A pH of 5.5 is usually considered[19] to be the critical threshold for demineralization of enamel. Repeated cycles of acid generation can, in time (usually 18 ± 6 months), cause an incipient carious lesion.[2] The initial lesion appears as an opaque white or brown spot beneath the plaque layer. As more intercrystalline voids form, mineral loss continues faster. In time the surface enamel loses hardness, bacteria penetrate into the enamel, and a microscopic cavity develops.[4,19] Without treatment, carious lesions may progress through the enamel, the dentin, and eventually into the pulp and may destroy the entire tooth (Fig. 15-1).

Rationale for the use of intraoral radiographs

Radiography is useful for the detection of dental caries because the carious process causes tooth demineralization. The carious lesion (the demineralized area of the tooth that allows greater passage of x rays) is darker than the unaffected portion (more radiolucent) and may be detected on radiographs.

Intraoral radiography can reveal carious lesions that otherwise might go undetected during a thorough clinical examination. A number of studies*

*References 6, 7, 16, 21, 22, 28, 29, 32.

have shown the value of dental radiographs by repeatedly demonstrating that approximately half of all proximal surface lesions cannot be seen clinically and may be detected only with radiographs. This is especially true for individuals above the age of 12 years.[8] On the other hand, early carious lesions are difficult to detect with radiographs, particularly when they are small and limited to the enamel.[9,18,20,27,34] Therefore both clinical examination and x-ray examination are necessary in the detection of dental caries.

Examinations

Posterior bitewing radiographs are the most useful x-ray projection for detecting caries in the distal third of a canine and the interproximal and occlusal surfaces of premolars and molars. Periapical radiographs are useful primarily for detecting changes in the periapical and interradicular bone. Use of a paralleling technique for obtaining periapical radiographs increases the value of this projection in detecting caries of both anterior and posterior teeth.

Radiographic examination for caries in children should include bitewing films (Fig. 15-2). In children younger than 3 years of age with a small mouth, it may not be possible to use the larger no. 2 size film or even the smaller no. 1 size; however, it is possible to gain the child's cooperation by using a small no. 0 film. As the child grows, he should be able to tolerate a no. 1 size and, by age 6, 7, or 8, should willingly take the no. 2 size film. The larger the film used, the greater will be the chance of projecting the appropriate anatomic structures onto it; and the smaller the film, the less discomfort will be felt and the better the child's acceptance of the procedure.

The most useful adult bitewing examination consists of four no. 2 size films for separate premolar and molar projections.

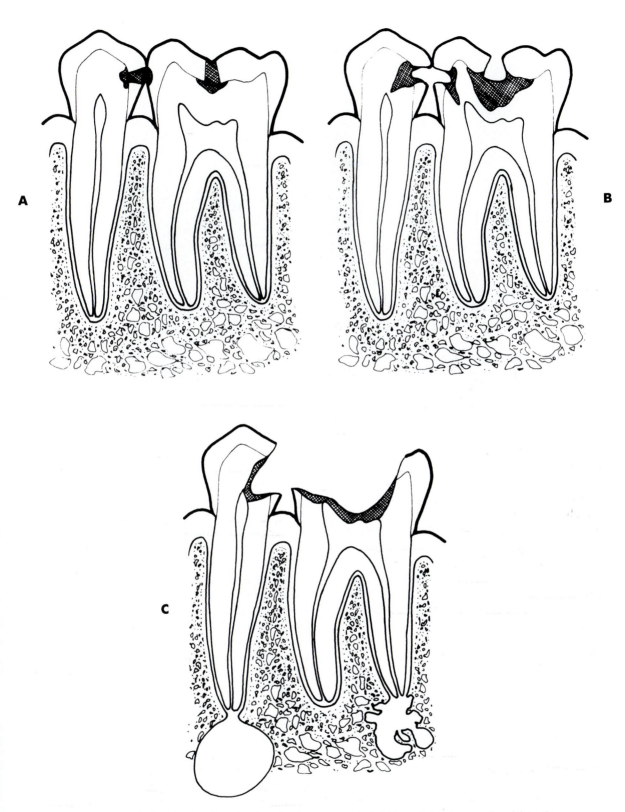

FIG. 15-1. A, Proximal and occlusal caries having penetrated through tooth enamel and into the dentin. **B,** Severe proximal and occlusal caries nearing the pulp chamber of two vital teeth. **C,** Severe proximal and occlusal caries having invaded the pulp chambers results in two nonvital pulps and periapical disease.

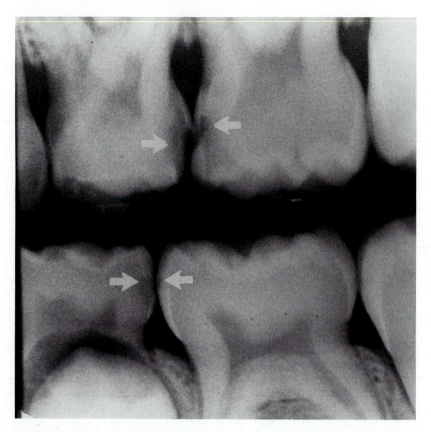

FIG. 15-2. Posterior bitewing radiograph demonstrating both permanent and deciduous teeth. Note the proximal caries *(arrows)*.

Frequency

Radiographs are useful for detecting proximal caries when the teeth are in contact and cannot be directly inspected. The frequency of any radiographic procedure must be decided on the basis of a patient's needs—with factors such as oral hygiene, fluoride exposure, diet, caries history, extent of restorative care, and age considered in determining whether radiography will contribute to the diagnosis.[24] (See Chapter 4.)

RADIOGRAPHIC APPEARANCE OF CARIES

Occlusal caries

New carious lesions in children and adolescents most often occur on the occlusal surfaces of posterior teeth. Bitewing radiographs are useful in detecting them on the occlusal surfaces of premolars and molars. The demineralization process originates in enamel pits and fissures and penetrates to the dentinoenamel junction (DEJ). The carious lesion spreads along the DEJ and is seen as a thin radiolucent line between enamel and dentin. In most cases there is no early radiographic evidence of enamel involvement[17,31] (Fig. 15-3) since the lesion is in a pit or fissure surrounded by dense sound enamel. The enamel obscures the small lesion, which penetrates only a thin layer. Although radiographs may provide the first indication of occlusal caries, a careful clinical examination will reveal most destruction. As the carious process spreads, the thin radiolucent line extends below the enamel and extends pulpally in a spherical pattern (Fig. 15-4). The margin of the expanding radiolucent area between the carious and noncarious dentin is very diffuse. As the lesion spreads through the dentin, it undermines the enamel, and masticatory forces frequently cause cavitation (Fig. 15-5).

Interpretation of incipient occlusal lesions. Radiographs are usually not effective for the detection of an occlusal carious lesion until it reaches the dentin.[17,31] Figure 15-3 shows examples of teeth requiring restorations that exhibit little or no radiographic changes. The only detectable evidence of an early lesion at the occlusal surface

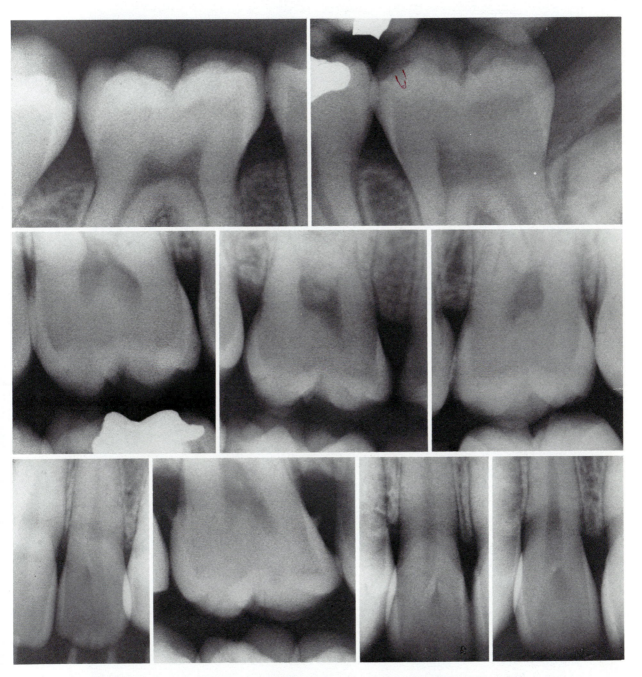

FIG. 15-3. Incipient occlusal caries. Note that these nine radiographic images show little or no changes; yet occlusal caries requiring treatment is present in each case.

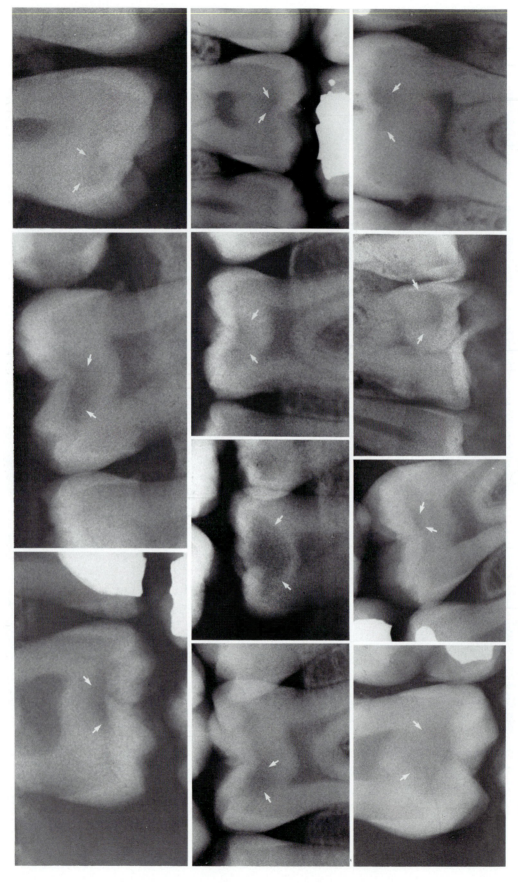

FIG. 15-4. Moderate occlusal caries. Eleven radiographs show a radiolucent zone within dentin, but little or no changes apparent in the overlying enamel.

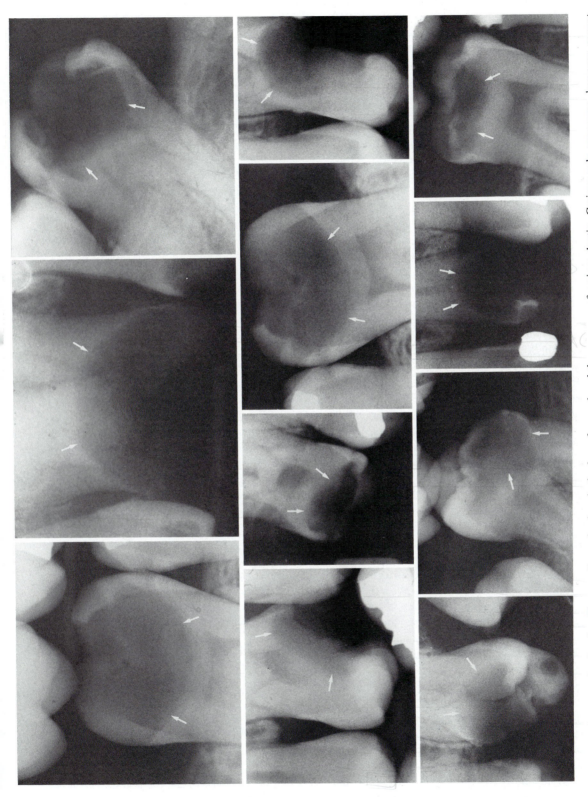

FIG. 15-5. Severe occlusal caries. Eleven radiographs show both a loss of enamel and the presence of carious dentin. Carious pulp exposures, however, cannot be determined by these radiographs. Only with clinical evaluation is it possible to substantiate the extent of a carious process and the accuracy of its x-ray appearance.

may be a fine gray shadow just under the DEJ. A similar but usually less broad shadow, however, is frequently apparent on the images of unaffected teeth below (or above) the occlusal enamel. This line of increased density at the junction represents an optical illusion referred to as a Mach band. The occlusal carious lesion generally starts in the sides of a fissured wall rather than at the base, and it tends to penetrate nearly perpendicularly toward the DEJ.[15] The clinician usually makes the radiographic decision of normal or equivocal for caries and refers to a careful clinical evaluation before deciding to restore the tooth. Visual changes such as chalkiness or yellow, brown, or black discolorations may develop on the occlusal surface of the tooth, although a stained fissure is not a reliable criterion for caries.

Interpretation of moderate occlusal lesions. The moderate occlusal lesion is usually the first to induce specific radiographic changes prompting a definitive decision regarding the presence of caries. The classic radiographic change is a broad-based thin radiolucent zone in the dentin with little or no changes apparent in the enamel. Figure 15-4 shows examples of moderate occlusal caries with minor radiolucent changes. Note carefully the region of dentin next to the DEJ, because if a radiolucent region is present a decision of either equivocal or positive for caries must be considered. When present, another significant manifestation of occlusal caries in the dentin is a band of increased opacity between the lesion and the pulp chamber. This light band, which represents calcification within the primary dentin, is not usually seen with buccal caries. The area must be carefully evaluated clinically before making a treatment decision.

Interpretation of severe occlusal lesions. Severe occlusal lesions are readily observed both clinically and radiographically. They appear as a large hole, or cavity, in the crown of a tooth. Since the underlying dentin is carious and cannot support the enamel, masticatory forces cause a collapse of the occlusal surface. Figure 15-5 shows examples of the radiographic appearance of such severely carious teeth. Pulp exposures cannot be determined by radiographs, however; only clinical evidence can substantiate the radiographic impression.

Radiographic pitfalls in the interpretation of occlusal lesions. There are three common errors made in interpreting occlusal caries[36]: First is the failure to recognize that occlusal caries of enamel will not ordinarily be detectable on radiographs

because of the superimposition of heavy cuspal enamel over the fissured (carious) areas. Second is the carelessness of not observing the rather long thin radiolucency that first appears at the DEJ as a sign of occlusal caries. Third is the confusion shown by many clinicians in distinguishing between occlusal and buccal caries. This occurs when lesions in the buccal grooves of molars are superimposed on the occlusal area and simulate occlusal lesions. A direct clinical inspection of the tooth will eliminate any such confusion.

Proximal caries

Radiographic detection of carious lesions on the proximal surfaces of teeth depends on loss of enough mineral to result in a detectable change in radiographic density. Because the proximal surfaces of posterior teeth are often broad, the loss of small amounts of mineral from incipient lesions or the advancing front of more advanced lesions is often difficult to detect on a radiograph. For this reason, the actual depth of penetration of a carious lesion is deeper than may be detected radiogaphically.[5,13,27,34,37] Approximately 40% demineralization is required for radiographic detection of a lesion.[35,36]

Interpretation of incipient proximal lesions. Interproximally the earliest carious lesions develop slowly, taking 3 to 4 years to become clinically apparent.[1] Clinically the lesions are first seen as having a loss of enamel transparency, resulting in an opaque chalky region ("white spot").[15] These generally occur on the outer surface of the enamel between the contact point and the height of the free

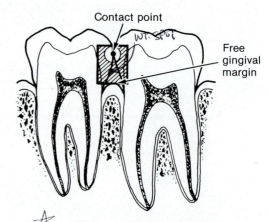

FIG. 15-6. Proximal caries-susceptible zone. This region exists from the contact point down to the height of the free gingival margin. Note that it increases with recession of the alveolar bone and gingival tissues.

gingival margin. Proximally this caries-susceptible zone has a vertical dimension on the radiograph of 1 to 1.5 mm and continues to enlarge with receding of the gingiva[23] (Fig. 15-6). Since caries do not begin below the free margin of the gingiva, recognition of this "zone" minimizes difficulties in differentiating caries from cervical burnout. (See Chapter 8.) The early lesions are radiolucent and do not appear radiographically to penetrate more than half the thickness of the enamel. The general radiographic appearance of an incipient lesion is of a radiolucent "notch" on the outer surface of the tooth (Fig. 15-7). Often, incipient lesions may not DEJ.

be visualized radiographically because of the small volume of tooth mineral lost.

A magnifying glass is very useful for examining the film when evaluating the extent of incipient carious lesions and any of the other fine details that appear on a radiograph. Figure 15-8 is a series of radiographs showing early lesions with and without magnification.

Interpretation of moderate proximal lesions. Moderate proximal lesions are those that involve more than the outer half of the enamel but are not seen radiographically to extend into the DEJ. These lesions generally have one of three

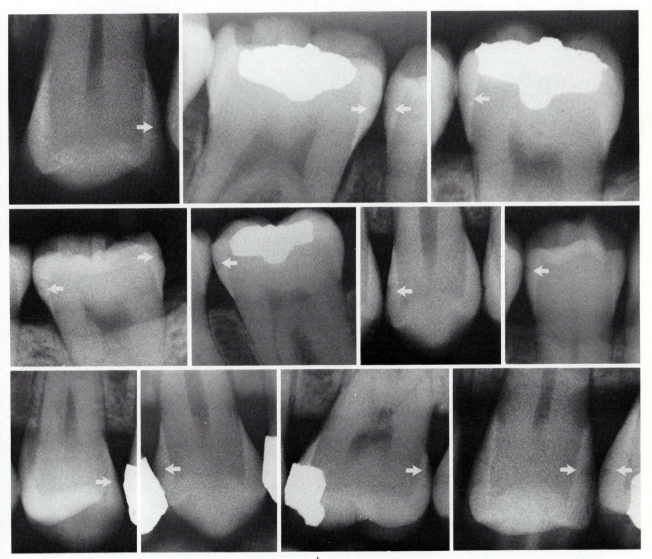

FIG. 15-7 "Notched" incipient proximal enamel caries. (*Arrows* indicate the areas showing demineralization.) Note the shape, size, and location of these 14 early lesions.

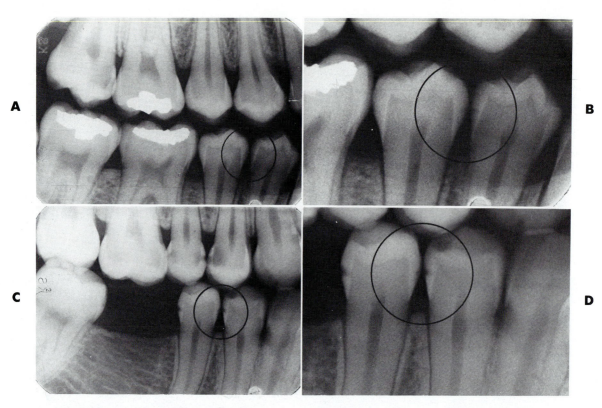

FIG. 15-8. A, A magnifying glass is important for examining the extent of dental caries. **A** and **C** are without magnification, **B** and **D** with magnification.

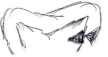

radiographic appearances: first, and most common (67%), is a triangle with its broad base at the surface of the tooth; second, and less common (16%), is a diffuse radiolucent image; and third (17%), is a combination of these two types.[36] The larger the radiolucent area is, the larger will be the lesion found on clinical examinations.[35] Figure 15-9 is a series of radiographs showing moderate proximal carious lesions.

Interpretation of advanced proximal lesions. Advanced carious lesions are those that have invaded the DEJ. The description of an advanced lesion classically includes a radiolucent penetration through the enamel. The configuration is usually triangular, but it may be diffuse or a combination of triangular and diffuse. In addition, there is spreading of the demineralization process at the DEJ, undermining the enamel and subsequently extending into the dentin. This forms a second triangular radiolucent image in the dentin with its base at the DEJ and its apex directed toward the pulp cavity. Figure 15-10 presents examples of advanced lesions that can be seen radiographically not to have spread through more than half the thickness of the dentin. Occasionally, lesions that have penetrated into the dentin will appear not to have penetrated from the enamel.

Interpretation of severe proximal lesions. A severe carious lesion is one that radiographically penetrates through more than half the dentin and is approaching the pulp chamber. Examination of the image usually reveals a narrow path of destruction through the enamel, an expanded radiolucency at the DEJ (forming the base of its triangular shape), and the extent of lesional development toward the pulp chamber. The lesion may or may not appear to involve the pulp. An important point to stress is that it is not possible to identify pulp exposures by radiographs alone. The relationship of caries to the pulp is important, and certain information may be gained from a radiograph, but care must be taken not to place too great a reliance on the film. Because a radiograph is a two-dimensional image on which all parts of the tooth are projected, the full extent of the carious process may not be revealed. A lesion far removed from the pulp chamber may be superimposed on it.[26] Only by clinical appraisal can the impression conveyed by

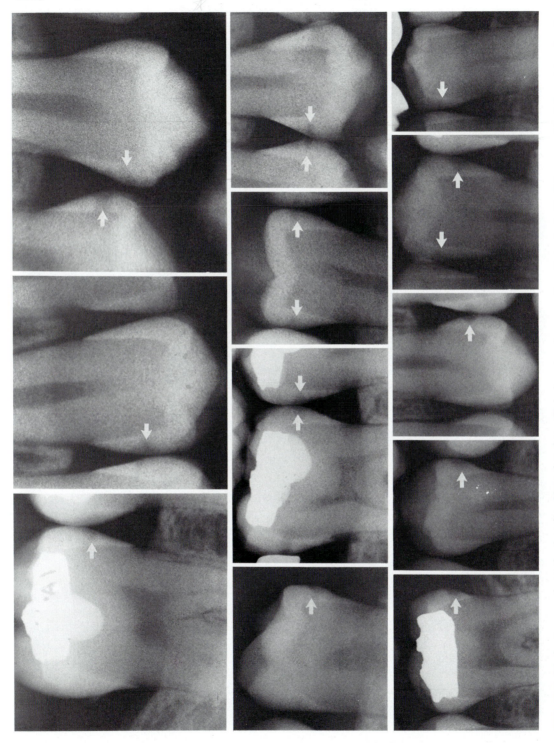

FIG. 15-9. Moderate enamel proximal caries. Note that these 17 lesions involve more than the outer half of the enamel but do not involve the dentinoenamel junction (DEJ) to a radiographically detectable extent.

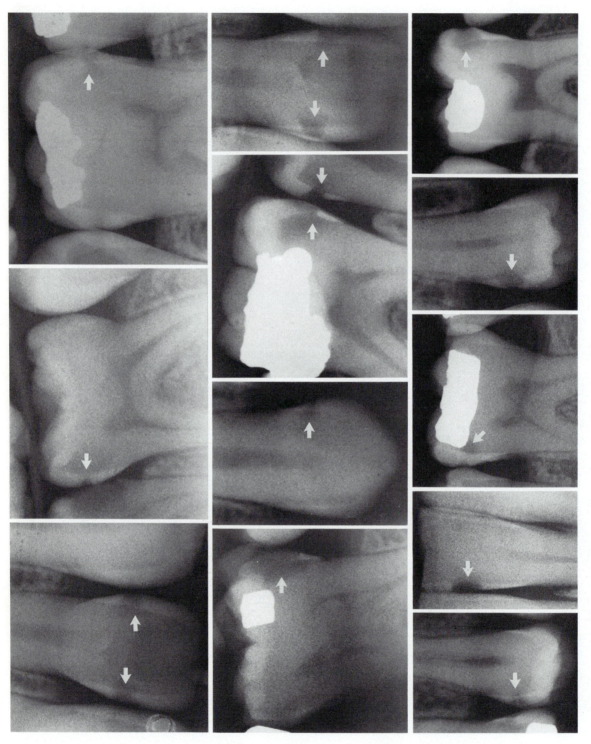

FIG. 15-10. Advanced proximal caries. Note the size, shape, and location of these 15 lesions and the radiographic changes (increased radiolucency) of both enamel and dentin.

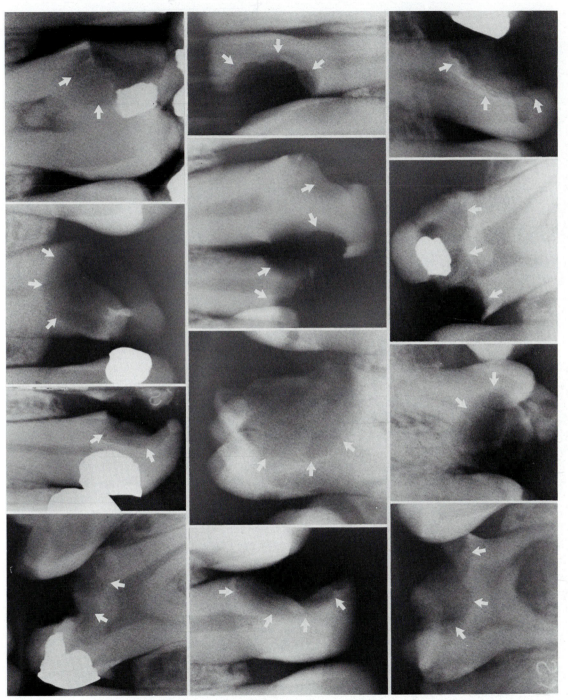

FIG. 15-11. Severe proximal caries. Note in these 13 examples the loss of enamel structure. Only an approximation of the degree of dentinal involvement toward the pulp can be made.

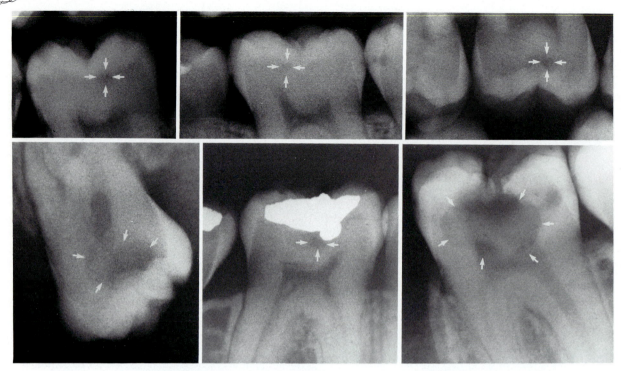

FIG. 15-12. Facial, buccal, and lingual caries. Note in these six examples the uniform enamel surrounding each radiolucent lesion. Clinical observation is the definitive method for making treatment decisions.

the x-ray interpretation be substantiated.

Severe interproximal lesions with much dentinal destruction also will undermine the enamel. Subsequently forces of mastication will cause the undermined enamel to collapse, leaving a very large cavity, or hole, in the tooth. Figure 15-11 shows examples of severe proximal dental caries.

Radiographic pitfalls in the interpretation of proximal caries. Accurate radiographic detection of proximal surface caries is challenging. One must differentiate cervical burnout from proximal caries. Also various dental anomalies such as hypoplastic pits or concavities produced by wear on the proximal surfaces can mimic caries on sound surfaces. Accordingly, the clinician must diagnose proximal caries cautiously and with the benefit of a careful clinical and radiographic examination.

Facial, buccal, and lingual caries

Facial, buccal, and lingual carious lesions occur in enamel pits and fissures of teeth. When small, these radiolucencies are usually round; as they enlarge, they become elliptic or semilunar in shape. They demonstrate sharp well-defined borders between the intact and demineralized (radiolucent) enamel.

It is difficult to differentiate between buccal and lingual caries on a radiograph. When viewing buccal, lingual, or palatal caries, the clinician should look for a uniform noncarious region of enamel surrounding the apparent radiolucency. This well-defined circular area represents parallel noncarious enamel rods surrounding the buccal or palatal decay. It is necessary to examine more than one view of the area because a margin of a buccal or lingual lesion may be superimposed on the DEJ and suggest occlusal caries. Also a buccal or lingual lesion at or near the mesial or distal line angle of the tooth may project onto a proximal surface and appear as a proximal lesion. Occlusal caries, however, will ordinarily be more extensive than lingual or buccal caries and its outline not as well defined (Fig. 15-12). Clinical evaluation and probing of buccal or lingual caries are usually straightforward and the definitive method of diagnosis.

Root surface caries

Root surface caries (also called *cemental caries*) involves both cementum and dentin. Its prevalence is approximately 40% to 70% in an aged population.[33] The tooth surfaces most frequently affected are, in order, buccal, lingual, and proximal.[15] The exposed cementum is relatively soft and usually only 20 to 50 μm thick near the cementoenamel junction, so it rapidly degrades by attrition, abrasion, and erosion. Consequently, root caries is a lesion of dentin associated with gingival recession.[23] The carious process is a scooping out that results in a radiographic appearance usually described as ill defined, saucerlike, and radiolucent. If the peripheral surface area is small, the appearance of the carious lesion will be more "notched" than saucerlike. Root surface caries does not involve enamel except by extension into the dentin immediately under the enamel along the DEJ. In such cases fracturing of the unsupported enamel frequently occurs. Figure 15-13 shows examples of typical root surface dental caries.

Pitfalls in the interpretation of root surface caries. Intact root surfaces may appear to be carious as a result of the phenomenon called *cervical burnout* (Fig. 8-2). The true carious lesion may be distinguished from the intact surface primarily by the absence of an image of the root edge and by the appearance of a diffuse rounded inner border where the tooth substance has been lost.[2] Clinical evaluation and probing of root surface caries are the definitive method of diagnosis.

Recurrent caries

Recurrent caries is that occurring immediately next to a restoration. It may result from poor adaptation of a restoration, which allows for marginal leakage, or it may be due to inadequate extension of a restoration. In addition, caries may remain if there has not been complete excavation of the original lesion, which later may appear as residual or recurrent caries. Approximately 16% of restored tooth surfaces have recurrent caries.[11] It is important to treat these lesions without delay because they are a frequent cause of pulp necrosis.[19]

The radiographic appearance of recurrent caries depends on the amount of decalcification present and whether a restoration is obscuring the lesion. It is common for radiopaque restorations to hide small and large regions of demineralized (radiolucent) dentin. In this case its discovery and conformation are dependent on careful clinical examination. Recurrent lesions at the mesiogingival, distogingival, and occlusal margins are most frequently discovered radiographically. In contrast, there may be considerable destruction about the margins of buccal, facial, and lingual restorations before it becomes apparent radiographically.[35,36] Figure 15-14 demonstrates several examples of recurrent dental caries as seen on the mesial, distal,

and occlusal borders of amalgam, gold, and composite dental restorations.

Restorative and base materials

Restorative materials vary in their radiographic appearance depending on thickness, density, atomic number, and the photon energy used to make the radiographic projection. Some can be confused with caries. Older calcium hydroxide preparations without barium, lead, or zinc (added to lend radiopacity) appear radiolucent and may resemble recurrent caries. Despite the calcium present, the relatively large proportion of low–atomic number material in calcium hydroxide causes its radiodensity to approximate that of a carious lesion. Composite, plastic, or silicate restorations also may simulate caries (Fig. 15-15). It is often possible, however, to identify and differentiate these radiolucent materials from caries by their well-defined and smooth classic outline. Again, although the radiographic interpretation may be equivocal for recurrent caries it is possible to make treatment decision on the basis of dental history and a careful clinical examination.

Rampant caries

Rampant caries usually occurs in children with poor dietary habits, who generally demonstrate extensive interproximal and smooth surface caries. This condition, however, is becoming increasingly rare because of the extensive availability of water fluoridation[14] and the more widespread and enlightened practices of good nutrition and oral hygiene. Radiographs (Fig. 15-16) demonstrate severe (advanced) carious lesions, especially of the mandibular anterior teeth. Treatment requires extensive dental care and education of the child's parents.

Radiation caries

Patients who have received therapeutic radiation to the head and neck may suffer a loss of salivary gland function, leading to xerostomia (or dry mouth). Untreated, this induces rampant destruction of the teeth, termed "radiation caries." (See Chapter 2.) Typically the destruction begins at the cervical region and may aggressively encircle the tooth, causing the entire crown to be lost, with only root fragments remaining in the jaws. The radiographic appearance of radiation caries is characteristic[26]: dark radiolucent shadows appearing at the necks of teeth, most obvious on the mesial and distal aspects. Variations in the depth of destruction may be present, but generally there is uniformity within a given region of the mouth.

Text continued on p. 325.

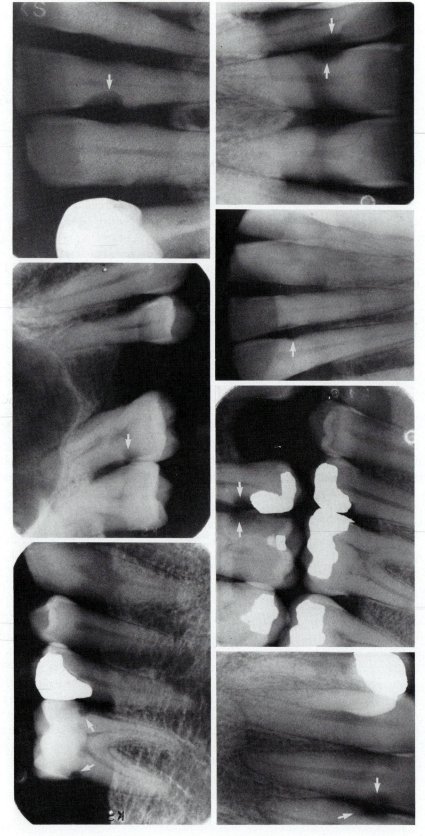

FIG. 15-13. Root surface (cementum) caries. Note the radiographic appearance of these 11 ill-defined saucer-shaped defects on the mesial or distal portion of the root exposed as a result of gingival recession.

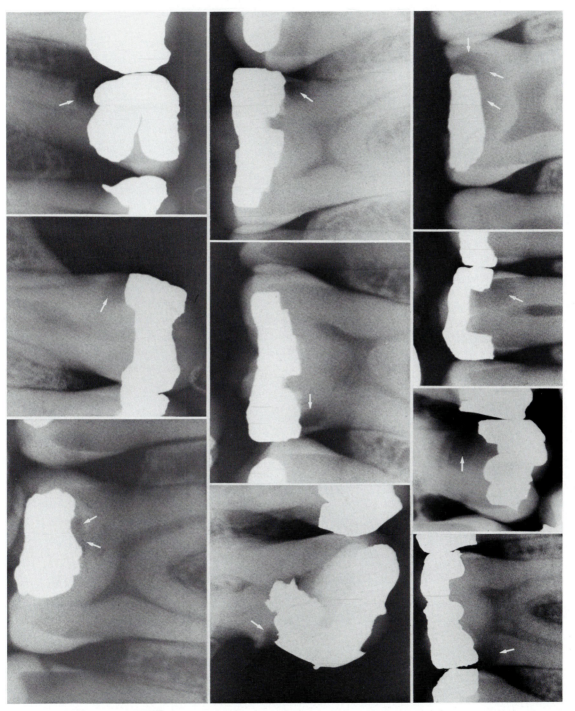

FIG. 15-14. Recurrent caries. Note carefully the increased radiolucency at the margins of existing restorations in these 10 examples.

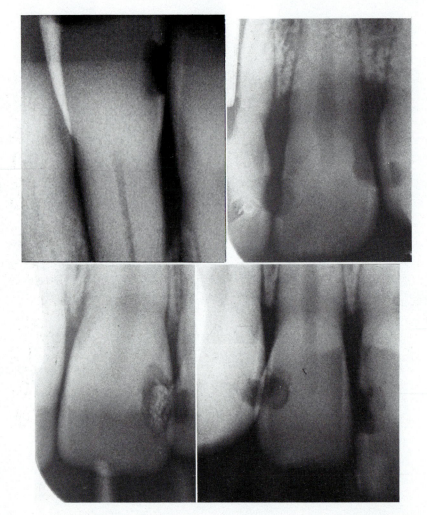

FIG. 15-15. Restorative materials resembling radiolucent dental caries. Note the smooth classic outlines of these radiolucent areas, which are actually prepared cavity preparations.

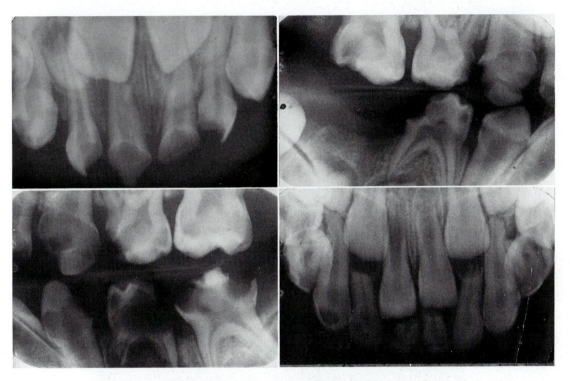

FIG. 15-16. Rampant (advanced) caries. These four examples were found in young children. (Courtesy Dr. Raphael Yeung, Alhambra Calif.)

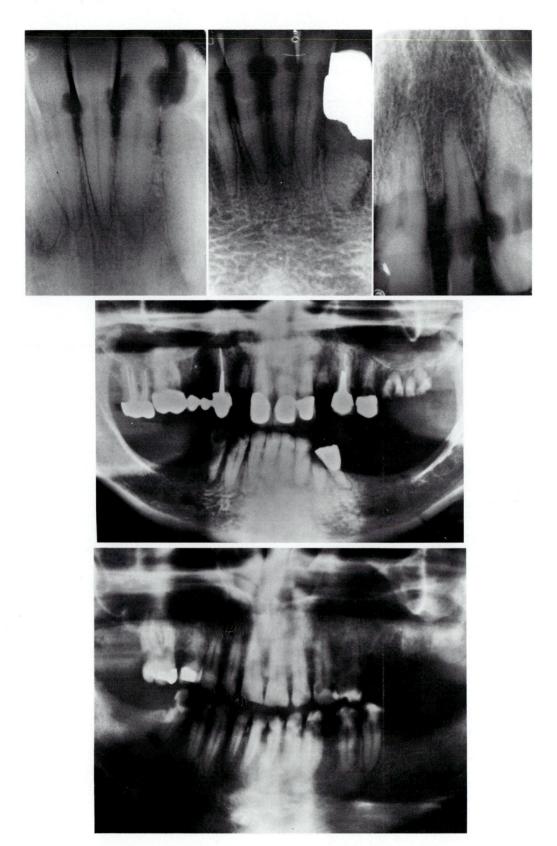

FIG. 15-17. Radiation caries. In these five postirradiation patients there was a loss or decrease of salivary gland function (xerostomia).

Figure 15-17 shows examples of radiation caries in patients wtih xerostomia following therapeutic radiation for cancer of the head and neck. Use of topical fluorides, remineralizing solutions, and meticulous oral hygiene can markedly reduce the radiation damage to teeth resulting from xerostomia.

TREATMENT CONSIDERATIONS

The treatment of severe and even moderate dental caries requires removal of the lesion and restoration of the tooth to form and function. Incipient (or early) dental caries, however, may require only preventive and/or remineralization treatment. Since dental caries is a daily ongoing dynamic process that is reversible in the earliest stages, many of the lesions detected radiographically impose the obligation of deciding whether treatment should be by restoration or by preventive and/or remineralization methods. The consensus seems to be that when the surface of a lesion is no longer intact, meaning that cavitation has occurred, a restoration is required. Remineralization techniques will be ineffective when a radiograph of the carious lesion indicates it has progressed into dentin and cavitation is certain.[12] When the radiograph shows a lesion limited to enamel, the current view[3,27] is that the probability of cavitation is low and the prospect of arresting or reversing the decay process good. If subsequent radiographic examinations show no change in these incipient lesions, then the preventive or remineralization methods can be considered to have been proper and effective.

SPECIFIC REFERENCES

1. Backer Dirks O: Longitudinal dental caries study in children 9-15 years of age, *Arch Oral Biol* 6:94-108, 1961.
2. Berry H: Cervical burnout and mach band: two shadows of doubt in radiologic interpretation of carious lesions, *J Am Dent Assoc* 106:622-625, 1983.
3. Bille J, Thylstrup A: Radiographic diagnosis and clinical tissue changes in relation to treatment of proximal carious lesions, *Caries Res* 16:1-6, 1982.
4. Brudevald F: A study of the phosphate solubility of the human enamel surface, *J Dent Res* 27:320-329, 1948.
5. Buchholz R: Histologic-radiographic relation of proximal surface carious lesions, *J Prevent Dent* 4:23-24, 1977.
6. Cheyne VD, Home EV: The value of the roentgenograph in the detection of carious lesions, *J Dent Res* 27:58-67, 1948.
7. Delabarre FA: Preschool age dentistry, *J Am Dent Assoc* 20:124-128, 1933.
8. de Vries HCB, Ruiken HMHM, König KG, van't Hof MA: Radiographic versus clinical diagnosis of proximal carious lesions, *Caries Res* 24:364-370, 1990.
9. Douglass CW, Valachovic RW, Wijesinha A, et al: Clinical efficacy of dental radiography in the detection of dental caries and periodontal diseases, *Oral Surg* 62:330-339, 1986.
10. Edward S, Fjellstrom A, Henrikson C, Nord C: A comparative study of clinical and roentgenological recording of proximal caries in primary molars of preschool children, *Odontol Rev* 24:317-324, 1973.
11. Goldberg J, Tanzer J, Munster E: Cross-sectional clinical evaluation of recurrent enamel caries, restoration of marginal integrity and oral hygiene status, *J Am Dent Assoc* 102:(4):635-641, 1981.
12. Gröndahl HJ, Hollender L: The value of the radiographic examination in caries diagnosis. In Thylstrup A, Fejerskov O (eds): *Textbook of cariology*, Copenhagen, 1986, Munksgaard.
13. Gwinnett A: A comparison of proximal carious lesions as seen by a clinical radiograph, contact microradiography, and light microscopy, *J Am Dent Assoc* 83:1078-1080, 1971.
14. Interim report of the American Dental Association's Special Committee on the Future of Dentistry: Issue papers on dental research, manpower, education, practice, and public and professional concerns, *J Am Dent Assoc* September 1982.
15. Katz RV: Assessing root caries in populations: the evolution of the root caries index, *J Publ Health Dent* 40:7-16, 1980.
16. Kidd EAM, Pitts NB: A reappraisal of the value of the bitewing radiograph in the diagnosis of posterior proximal caries, *Br Dent J* 1689:195-200, 1990.
17. King N, Shaw L: Value of bitewing radiographs in detection of occlusal caries, *Community Dent Oral Epidemiol* 7:218-221, 1979.
18. Lundeen RC, McDavid WD, Barnwell GM: Proximal surface caries detection with direct-exposure and rare earth screen/film imaging, *Oral Surg* 734-745, 1988.
19. Mandel ID: Dental caries, *Am Sci* 67:680-688, 1979.
20. Mileman PA, van der Weele LT: Accuracy in radiographic diagnosis: Dutch practitioners and dental caries, *J Dent* 18:130-136, 1990.
21. Muhler J: The ability of different clinical examination techniques to diagnose caries prevalence, *J Dent Child* 30:3-8, 1963.
22. Murray J, Shaw L: Errors in diagnosis of approximal caries on bitewing radiographs, *Community Dent Oral Epidemiol* 3:276-282, 1975.
23. Newbrun E: *Cariology,* ed 3, Baltimore, 1989, Williams & Wilkins, pp 13-375.
24. Radiation exposure in pediatric dentistry. Conference proceedings, *Pediatr Dent* 3 (spec issue 2):461-463, 1981.
25. Schachtele CF: Dental caries. In Schuster GS (ed): *Oral microbiology and infectious disease,* student ed 2, Baltimore, 1983, Williams & Wilkins.
26. Shafer WG, Hine MK, Levy BM: *A textbook of oral pathology,* ed 4, Philadelphia, 1983, WB Saunders, pp 406-478.
27. Silverstone L: Relationship of the macroscopic, histological, and radiographic appearance of interproximal lesions in human teeth: in vitro study using artificial caries technique, *Pediatr Dent* 3(Spec Issue 2):414-422, 1981.
28. Smith RK: The x-ray: An essential to diagnosis and prognosis of the child patient, *J Am Dent Assoc* 29:796-804, 1942.
29. Sognnaes RJ: The importance of a detailed clinical examination of carious lesions, *J Dent Res* 19:(1):11-15, 1940.

30. Spouge JD: *Oral pathology,* St Louis, 1973, Mosby, pp 3-40.
31. Stephens R, Kogon S, Reid J: A comparison of Panorex and intraoral surveys for routine dental radiography, *J Can Dent Assoc* 43:382-386, 1977.
32. Trithart A, Donnelly C: A comparative study of proximal cavities found by clinical and roentgenographic examinations, *J Am Dent Assoc* 40:33-37, 1950.
33. Vehkalahti M, Rajala M, Tuominen K, et al: Prevalence of root caries in the adult Finnish population, *Community Dent Oral Epidemiol* 11:188-190, 1983.
34. White S, Hollender L, Gratt B: Comparison of xeroradiographs and film for detection of proximal surface caries, *J Am Dent Assoc* 108:755-759, 1984.
35. Worth HW: *Principles and practice of oral radiologic interpretation,* Chicago, 1963, Year Book Medical Publishers, pp 150-154.
36. Wuehrmann AH: Roentgenographic interpretation of dental caries, *Prac Dent Monogr,* pp 3-46, September 1959.
37. Zamir T, Fisher D, Fishel D, Sharav Y: A longitudinal radiographic study of the rate of spread of human approximal dental caries, *Arch Oral Biol* 21:523-526, 1976.

SELECTED REFERENCES

Eastman Kodak, Dept 840 B: *Kodak dental x-ray products: intraoral radiography,* Rochester NY, 1976, Eastman Kodak.
Gibilisco JA: *Stafne's Oral radiographic diagnosis,* ed 5, Philadelphia, 1985, WB Saunders, pp 74-77.
Leijon G, Marken KE: Roentgenologic diagnosis of approximal caries, *Acta Odontol Scand* 26:35-61, 1968.
Mandel ID: Histological, histochemical and other aspects of caries initiation, *J Am Dent Assoc* 51:432-442, 1955.
Rowe NH (ed): *Incipient caries of enamel,* Ann Arbor, November 11-12, 1977, The University of Michigan School of Dentistry and The Dental Research Institute.
Wuehrmann AH, Manson-Hing LR: *Dental radiology,* ed 5, St Louis, 1981, Mosby, pp 305-320.

16

Periodontal Diseases

Several distinct yet related disorders of the periodontium are collectively known as periodontal disease. The most common of these are gingivitis and periodontitis. *Gingivitis* is a sequela of infection. It is limited to the marginal gingiva and is usually seen as a common nonspecific form. *Periodontitis* is also the result of infection, but it differs from gingivitis in that there is also a loss of alveolar bone. The various types of periodontal disease are caused by different specific infections that are classified according to their distinctive clinical manifestations.[35] There are localized and generalized forms of prepubertal periodontitis (patients 1 to 12 years of age), general and localized forms of juvenile periodontitis (13 to 20 years), a rapidly progressing periodontitis, and generalized or localized forms of adult periodontitis (usually after 30 years).[34,47] These various periodontal diseases share the fact that they are of infectious origin and result in deleterious changes to the supporting tissues of the dentition. They differ with respect to cause, pathogenesis, progression, natural history, and response to treatment.[32]

Recent epidemiologic studies[33] suggest that approximately half of the population is completely free of any form of inflammatory periodontal disease and probably less than 20% of American adults have active periodontitis. A recent cross-sectional survey of 15,132 employed adults in the United States[4] found that 14% had pockets 4 mm or greater. The prevalence of attachment loss of 3 mm or more was 44%, and the extent of these findings increased with age. The prevalence of juvenile periodontitis is less than 1%.[29] It also seems that the prevalence of gingivitis in the United States is declining, apparently because of the extensive use of fluoride and antibiotics. In addition, there is increasing evidence[32] that patients will demonstrate periods in which the rate of periodontal destruction lessens or even ceases. Rather than progressing smoothly from mild to moderate to severe, adult periodontitis is being recognized as having quite variable progression. There are periods of loss of attachment followed by periods (often years) of no appreciable change. As the size of the elderly population increases, and with increased retention of their teeth as a result of improved preventive and restorative measures, it may be that the prevalence of periodontal disease will increase in the future.[19] The development of improved treatment methods, however, may well modify this picture.

The causes of periodontal disease are multifactorial—involving the interplay of various host and environmental factors. Smokers are more prone to periodontal disease,[2,3] as are persons of increased age and those with poor education, neglected dental care, previous periodontal destruction, and diabetes.[11] Plaque-forming bacteria play an intimate role in the initiation and progression of periodontal destruction. They colonize the root surface, spread into the region between the root and the gingival margin, and stimulate a chronic inflammatory response. This results in pocket formation, subsequent apical migration of the epithelial attachment, and loss of bone. The immune system plays a primarily protective role. Bacterial antigens stimulate antibody responses that promote destruction and elimination of the bacteria. Bacteria also serve as potent mitogens of B cells, stimulating broad immunoglobulin production. The roles of neutrophilic granulocytes and monocytes are important in causing bacterial destruction and thus preventing periodontitis. Many patients with periodontitis are found to have functional defects in these cells.[35] The immune system may, however, contribute to destruction of the periodontium by the release of lymphokines (e.g., osteoclast activation factor and lymphotoxin).[32]

The clinical manifestation of the presence of bacteria and the host response is an inflammatory reaction in the periodontium. Gingivitis is the most common first clinical sign, although some forms of periodontitis may be seen without gingivitis. Progression of these diseases leads to pocket formation, the universal manifestation of all periodontal disease. Other clinical signs include bleeding, purulent exudate, edema, resorption of the alveolar crest, and tooth mobility. In most cases of adult periodontitis the disease is episodic, characterized by alternating periods of inflammation and quiescence. Exacerbations of this disease probably begin with infection, antibody production, and clearance of the specific species of pathogen. Then there is a quiescent period, followed by reinfection by an unrelated species. This cycle of disease activity may repeat.[36] Other factors, such as occlusal trauma, will influence the progression of the disease. The relative duration of the destructive and quiescent phases depends on the form of periodontitis, nature of the bacterial pathogens, and host response. Host factors such as the presence of systemic disease, age, immune system status, and stress will influence the course of the disease. There may even be spontaneous remission of the destructive process. The disease is usually painless, and most patients are unaware of its presence. Various forms of therapy—including oral hygiene, scaling, and surgical treatment—are effective.

Contributions of radiographs

Radiographs play an integral role in the assessment of periodontal disease.[37,41] They are often valuable in assessing:

The amount of bone present
  Condition of the alveolar crests
  Bone loss in the furcation areas
  Width of the periodontal ligament space
Local initiating factors that cause or intensify periodontal disease
  Calculus
  Poorly contoured or overextended restorations
Root length and morphology and the crown-to-root ratio
Anatomic considerations
  Position of the maxillary sinus in relation to a periodontal deformity
  Missing, supernumerary, or impacted teeth
Pathologic considerations
  Caries
  Periapical lesions
  Root resorptions

Radiographs also provide a permanent record of the condition of the bone throughout the course of the disease.

In recent years computers and image-processing techniques have been used to enhance radiographs for the improved detection of alveolar bone loss associated with periodontal disease. The most widely used of these techniques has been subtraction radiography. (See Chapter 13.) The advantage of this method is that it allows better detection of small amounts of bone loss between radiographs made at different times than may be achieved by visual inspection.[20] It is difficult to use, however, since the images must be made using the same orientation of the x-ray machine, bone, and film at each examination, which is quite difficult to accomplish in general practice.

It is important to emphasize that the clinical and radiographic examinations are complementary. The clinical examination should include periodontal probing, a gingival index, mobility charting, and an evaluation of the amount of attached gingiva.[42] Features that are not well delineated by the radiograph are most apparent clinically, and those that the radiograph best demonstrates are difficult to identify and evaluate clinically. Radiographs are an adjunct to the diagnostic process. Although a radiograph will demonstrate advanced periodontal lesions well, other equally important changes in the periodontium may not be seen radiographically. Accordingly, a complete diagnosis of periodontal disease requires insight from a clinical examination of the patient combined with radiographic evidence.[16]

Limitations of radiographs

The primary limitation of radiographs in evaluating periodontal disease is the inability of a viewer to perceive bony defects that are overlapped by existing bony walls. This is primarily because the radiograph provides a restricted (two-dimensional) representation of the (three-dimensional) situation.[13] There is often failure to image buccal and lingual bone levels. Furthermore, the earliest (incipient) mild destructive lesions in bone do not cause sufficient alterations in density to be detectable.[1] Also, the density of the root superimposed on the image of the defect tends to obscure the bone height. Radiographs will tend to show less severe destruction than is present. In addition, radiographs do not demonstrate the soft tissue to hard tissue relationships. Thus, although they play an invaluable role in treatment planning, their use must be supplemented by careful clinical examination. It is important to emphasize that radiographs will not identify a successfully managed case as opposed to an untreated one.[37] Nevertheless, in spite of the limitations detailed above, radiographs made with standardized techniques have proved useful in evaluating bone changes over relatively long periods of observation.

TECHNICAL PROCEDURES

The usefulness of radiographs in evaluating periodontal disease is dependent on the technical quality of the image.

Film placement

Interproximal (bitewing) and periapical radiographs are useful for evaluating the periodontium. The film is placed parallel with the long axis of the teeth, or as near to this ideal position as the size and structure of the mouth permit. This will ensure that the images of the teeth on the radiograph are not distorted and bear the same relationship to their supporting structures as they normally do. Typically the bone level is lower on interproximal films. Interproximal films more accurately record the distance between the cementoenamel junction (CEJ) and the crest of the interseptal alveolar bone. They do not have the restrictions imposed by anatomy in the posterior maxilla, which tend to produce image foreshortening. There are significant differences between the appearance of bone levels recorded by the interproximal and periapical paralleling techniques. Of the periapical radiographic examinations, the paralleling technique produces images with less distortion than occurs with the bisecting-angle technique (Chapter 6). Because the assesssment and comparisons of bone height during the course of disease and treatment are only relative, however, the primary consideration must be not which technique to use but to consistently use images produced by a single technique for all comparisons.[40]

In recent years some periodontists[8] have recommended the use of vertical interproximal radiographs for patients with periodontal disease. This method uses seven no. 2 films as vertical interproximal radiographs to cover the molar, premolar, canine, and midline regions. It is best to expose these projections in a standardized and reproducible fashion to facilitate comparison of radiographs exposed at different times. For periapical radiographs it is usually necessary to place the film some distance from the teeth to achieve a parallel relationship. To compensate for this increased object-to-film distance, and to minimize the distortion it would introduce, it is advisable that the target-to-film distance be increased to at least 16 inches. This will minimize shape distortion and maximize image sharpness (see Chapter 6). One of the commercially available film holders can be used to facilitate placement and retention of the properly aligned film. Panoramic radiographs are not recommended for evaluation of periodontal disease.[38] When images from this technique were compared with those from a long cone paralleling technique,[15] there was a tendency to underestimate minor marginal bone destruction and overestimate major destruction.

Angle of projection

After the film is placed in optimum relation to the teeth, the x-ray beam is directed so the best undistorted images of the teeth and periodontal tissues will project onto the film. The vertical angulation should be such that the beam is perpendicular to the long axis of the tooth and the plane of the film,[23] with the horizontal angulation tangential to the interproximal surfaces at the contact points (surfaces) of the teeth.

The images of teeth cast at the optimum angle of projection will show properly proportioned anatomic features (e.g., correct crown-to-root ratios), and the CEJ and crest of the interseptal alveolar bone at their actual relative levels. If a radiograph meets the following criteria, there is some assurance that the teeth will be depicted in their correct relative positions in the alveolar process with (1) the interproximal spaces between tooth roots not overlapped, (2) the proximal contacts between crowns not overlapped, and (3) overlap of the buccal and lingual cusps of molars.

Film exposure and processing

For radiography of the alveolar bone it is desirable to use a beam energy of 80 kVp or more.[23,37] This increased penetration provides better visualization of the extent of bony detail and tooth roots. Films that are slightly light are more useful for examining cortical margins of bone. A properly collimated beam will reduce scattered radiation and improve image definition.

Proper darkroom techniques, such as protection of the opened film from extraneous light, maintenance of active (fresh) solutions at the recommended temperature, and complete development of the film, will assure that the maximum amount of information on the film is perceived.

Special considerations and techniques

The dentist must determine the optimum frequency of radiographic examination for patients with periodontal disease. Certainly radiographs of all diseased areas must be available at the beginning of periodontal therapy to allow treatment planning and serve as a baseline for later comparisons. The extent of continued disease activity should dictate the frequency of subsequent radiographic examinations.

Some clinicians have found it useful to superimpose fine wire grids when exposing radiographs to aid measurement of relative bone height. Typically the grids form 1 mm squares, which apppear as fine radiopaque lines on the resultant radiograph, that allow quantitative measurement of the position of the alveolar bone with respect to the dentition. This procedure is particularly useful in evaluating osseous changes on radiographs made at different times with a reproducible positioning technique.

NORMAL ANATOMY

The normal alveolar bone supporting the dentition has a characteristic radiographic appearance. A thin layer of opaque cortical bone often covers the alveolar crest. The height of the crest lies at a level approximately 1 to 1.5 mm below the level of the CEJs of adjacent teeth. Between posterior teeth the alveolar crest will also be parallel with a line connecting adjacent CEJs (Fig. 16-1). Between anterior teeth the alveolar crest is usually pointed and has a dense cortex (Fig. 16-2). As between the posterior teeth, the alveolar crest between anterior teeth will lie within 1 to 1.5 mm of a line connecting the adjacent CEJs.

The alveolar crest is continuous with the lamina dura of adjacent teeth. In the absence of disease, this bony junction between the alveolar crest and the lamina dura of posterior teeth will form a sharp angle next to the tooth root. There may be a slight widening of the periodontal ligament space around the cervical portion of the tooth root. In this situation, if the lamina dura still forms a sharp well-defined angle with the alveolar crest, it represents a variant of normal and is not an indication of disease. There is wide variability in the density of alveolar crests, with no clear correlation between the density of the crestal lamina dura and periodontal status.[14,28]

Gingivitis is an inflammatory condition of the gingiva resulting from the presence of a bacterial plaque. In this early condition the destruction has not spread to the underlying bone. When only gingivitis is present, the radiographic appearance of the bone will be normal, because by definition gingivitis shows no radiographic evidence of bone loss.

EARLY PERIODONTITIS

The early lesions of adult periodontitis present as areas of localized erosion of the alveolar bone crest (Fig. 16-3). In the anterior regions there will be blunting of the alveolar crests. In the posterior regions there may also be a loss of the normally

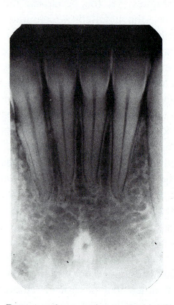

FIG. 16-2. Between the anterior teeth the alveolar crest will normally be pointed and well corticated, coming to within 1 to 1.5 mm of the adjacent cementoenamel junctions.

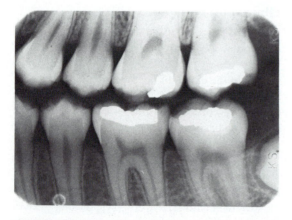

FIG. 16-1. The normal alveolar crest lies 1 to 1.5 mm below the adjacent cementoenamel junctions and forms a sharp angle with the lamina dura of the adjacent tooth.

sharp angle between the lamina dura and the alveolar crest. In the presence of early periodontal disease, this angle may lose its normal cortical surface (margin) and appear rounded off with an irregular and diffuse border. If only slight radiographic changes are apparent, the disease process may not be of recent onset. This is because significant loss of attachment must be present for 6 to 8 months before there is radiographic evidence of bone loss.[12] Also variations in the x-ray beam's angle of projection can cause a slight change in the apparent height of the alveolar bone. Early lesions progress episodically, with some remaining quiescent for years. The presence of a slight lesion does not necessarily mean that it will later become more severely involved.[33]

MODERATE PERIODONTITIS

If the lesions of adult periodontitis progress, the destruction of alveolar bone extends beyond early changes in the alveolar crest and may induce a variety of defects. The buccal or lingual cortical plate may resorb, or there may be defects of bone between the buccal and lingual plates. The pattern of bone loss may show on radiographs as generalized horizontal erosion or as localized vertical (angular) defects. There may be clinical evidence of tooth mobility. It is important to restate that the radiograph is valuable in showing areas of residual bone but the complete extent of bone loss will not necessarily be evident on the radiograph.

Horizontal bone loss

Horizontal bone loss is a term used to describe the radiographic appearance of loss in height of the alveolar bone; the crest is still horizontal, that is, parallel with the occlusal plane. Localized horizontal bone loss is limited to a few teeth whereas generalized loss involves a quadrant or more. Horizontal bone loss may also be mild, moderate, or severe depending on its extent. In horizontal bone loss the buccal and lingual cortical plates and the intervening interdental bone have been resorbed (Fig. 16-4). The extent of bone loss evident at a single examination does not indicate the current activity of the disease. For example, a patient who previously had generalized periodontal disease that resulted in moderate horizontal bone loss may have undergone successful periodontal therapy, with elimination of all pockets and inflammation. Such

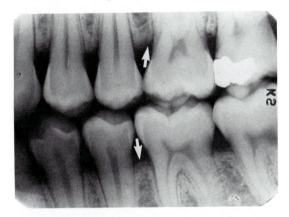

FIG. 16-3. Initial periodontal disease is seen as a loss of cortical density *(arrows)* and a rounding of the junction between the alveolar crest and lamina dura.

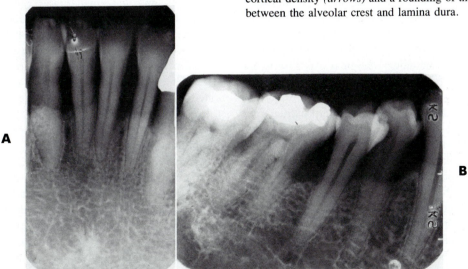

FIG. 16-4. Horizontal bone loss is seen in the anterior, **A,** and posterior, **B,** regions as a loss of the buccal and lingual cortical plates and interdental alveolar bone.

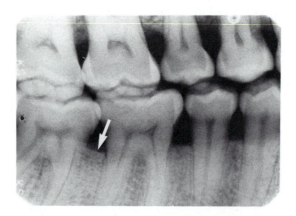

FIG. 16-5. An interproximal crater, seen through a defect between the buccal and lingual cortical plates, shows as a radiolucency below the level of the crestal edges *(arrow)*.

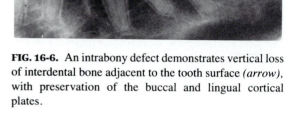

FIG. 16-6. An intrabony defect demonstrates vertical loss of interdental bone adjacent to the tooth surface *(arrow)*, with preservation of the buccal and lingual cortical plates.

a patient will show a moderate degree of horizontal bone loss but the condition will be stable. The return of a relatively dense alveolar cortex suggests the absence of periodontal disease.

Osseous defects

The term *osseous defects* describes the types of vertical (angular) bony lesions that are localized to one or two teeth. (An individual may, however, have multiple osseous defects.) These defects typically display an oblique angulation to the alveolar bone in the area of involved teeth.

The four most common types of osseous defects are interproximal crater, proximal intrabony defect, interproximal hemisepta, and inconsistent bony margins. Often these lesions are difficult or impossible to recognize on a radiograph because one or both of the cortical bony plates remain superimposed with the defect. Surgical exposure is the best means of determining the true bony architecture.

Interproximal crater. The interproximal crater is the most common type of bone deformity associated with moderate periodontal disease.[37] It is a troughlike depression that occurs in the crests of the interproximal septal bone between adjacent teeth. It has two side walls, composed of the buccal and lingual cortical plates, and two additional walls created by the roots of adjacent teeth (Fig. 16-5).

The coronal limits of the buccal and lingual walls will usually be radiographically apparent. The image of the wall projected more coronally will show reduced density compared to the image of the apical wall superimposed on it. If the crestal edges of the

two walls are exactly superimposed, the troughlike interproximal crater may appear as an irregular linear area of reduced density between adjacent teeth. Craters detectable radiographically are 1 mm or more deep. The apical margin of the defect is typically ill defined. As a result the relatively radiolucent image of the crater will gradually blend with the normal bone apical to it. In the mandible the external oblique ridge may obscure interproximal craters involving the third molars.

Proximal intrabony defect. The proximal intrabony defect is a three-walled vertical deformity within bone. It extends apically along the root from the alveolar crest, surrounded by three walls: a hemisepta and the lingual and buccal cortical plates. The hemisepta is interdental septal bone that remains on the root of the uninvolved adjacent tooth after destruction of either the distal or the mesial portion of the septum. Proximal intrabony defects may result from occlusal trauma complicated by inflammation and are more common on the distal surface of teeth, where they usually occur in association with loss of attachment, increased tooth mobility, and open contacts.[31]

Radiographically the intrabony defect is generally V shaped and sharply outlined. It lies immediately next to the root surface of the affected tooth. The adjacent bone has a normal radiographic appearance (Fig. 16-6). A crestal lamina often appears coronal to the defect and represents the coronal limits of the highest remaining buccal or lingual wall. Visualization of the depth of the pockets may be aided by inserting a gutta-percha point. The point will follow the defect and appear on the

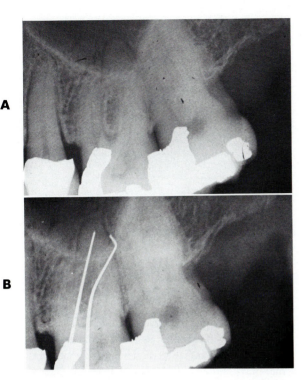

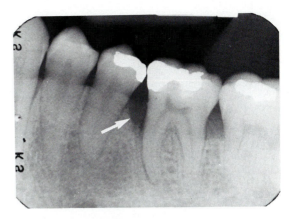

FIG. 16-8. An interproximal hemiseptum *(arrow)* has one side wall remaining and one wall lost.

FIG. 16-7. Gutta-percha may be used to visualize the depth of intrabony defects. **A** fails to show the osseous defect without the use of the gutta-percha points. **B** reveals an osseous defect extending to the region of apex. (Courtesy Dr. H. Takei, Los Angeles, Calif.)

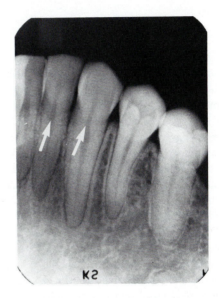

FIG. 16-9. Inconsistent bony margins are seen as irregular coronal edges of the buccal or lingual cortical plates superimposed over an image of the tooth roots *(arrows).*

radiograph because gutta-percha is relatively inflexible and radiopaque (Fig. 16-7).

Interproximal hemisepta. Hemiseptal defects (one or two wall) form when only a mesial or distal portion of the interproximal bony septum is resorbed (as in the proximal intrabony defect). Also the interproximal hemiseptum must have one or both of the cortical plates (side walls) missing to be distinguishable from an intrabony defect. These lesions extend more frequently onto the buccal surfaces of teeth.

The radiographic image of a one-wall interproximal hemiseptum (with both buccal and lingual walls resorbed) is similar to that of a proximal intrabony defect. The image of the side walls, however, will not be superimposed on that of the defect. As a consequence the defect next to a hemiseptum is better demarcated from the adjacent normal bone than is the intrabony defect. Sometimes it will appear to have a well-corticated margin; and even where the margin extends over the root of an affected tooth, it may be very distinct. This condition probably results from arrested disease in which

there has been time for a cortical margin to reform. Two-walled defects (one side wall remaining) next to hemisepta are usually indistinguishable from a proximal intrabony defect (Fig. 16-8).

Inconsistent bony margins. An inconsistent bony margin is the result of uneven resorption of the alveolar cortical plate on the lingual or vestibular surface, with the result that the crest of the margin is irregular (Fig. 16-9). Marginal inconsistencies occur only where the marginal bone is thin and completely removed by the inflammatory process. These defects apparently form quite rapidly and then can remain constant for relatively long periods.

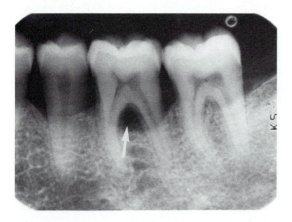

FIG. 16-10. Advanced destruction of the periodontal bone has led to destruction of both cortical plates and interradicular bone in the furcation region of the first molar *(arrow)*.

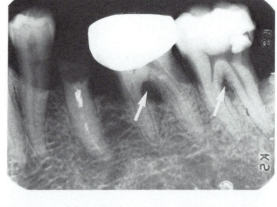

FIG. 16-11. Advanced destruction of the cortical plates without complete destruction of interradicular bone in the furcation region is revealed as a reduction in normal bone density in this region *(arrows)*.

ADVANCED PERIODONTITIS

In advanced adult periodontitis the bone loss is so extensive that the remaining teeth show excessive mobility and drifting and are in jeopardy of being lost because of inadequate support. There may be extensive horizontal bone loss or extensive osseous defects. As with moderate bone loss, the lesions seen at surgery will usually be more extensive than is suggested by the radiographs alone.

Osseous deformities in the furcations of multirooted teeth

Progressive periodontal disease and its associated bone loss may invade the furcations of multirooted teeth. As bone resorption extends down the side of a multirooted tooth, eliminating the marginal cortical bone over the root, it can reach the level of the furcation and beyond. Thickening of the periodontal ligament space at the apex of the interradicular bony crest is strong evidence that the furcation is being invaded by the periodontal disease process. If there is sufficient bone loss on the lingual and buccal aspects of a mandibular molar furcation, the radiolucent image of the lesion will be sharply outlined between the roots (Fig. 16-10). The bony defect may involve either the buccal or the lingual cortical plate and extend under the roof of the furcation. In such a case, where it does not extend through to the other cortical plate, it will appear more irregular than, and of increased radiolucency compared to, the adjacent normal bone (Fig. 16-11). Radiographs will not reveal whether the septal bone has been lost from the buccal or the lingual cortical plate.

Furcation defects involve maxillary molars about three times as frequently as mandibular molars.[43] The loss of interradicular bone in the furcation of a maxillary molar may originate from the buccal, mesial, or distal surface of the tooth. The most common avenue for furcation involvement of the maxillary permanent first molar is from the mesial side. The image of furcation involvement is not as sharply defined around maxillary first molars as around mandibular molars, however, because the palatal root is superimposed on the defect. Mesial or distal furcation involvement of the maxillary molars is also not usually apparent on periapical radiographs because of the superimposition of one or both cortical plates.

With mandibular molars the trabecular pattern of cancellous bone within the furcation will be faintly apparent on the film. If the crestal bone is above or below the furcation but the disease process has not invaded the interradicular bone, the image of the crestal bone and that of the periodontal ligament space about the septal bone will appear normal. In the mandible the external oblique ridge may mask furcation involvement of the third molars. Convergent roots may also obscure furcation defects in maxillary and mandibular second and third molars.

Alveolar dehiscence

Alveolar dehiscence results when the marginal bone dips apically and exposes a length of root surface.[24] The defect may be wide and irregular and extend as far as the apex of the affected tooth. It occurs on either the lingual or the vestibular side

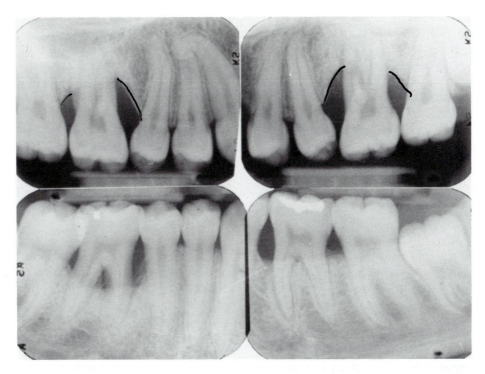

FIG. 16-12. Typical vertical bone loss in juvenile periodontitis. Note how it is localized to the region of the first molars. (Courtesy Dr. T.D. Charbeneau, Dallas.)

of the root. A dehiscence is usually not seen well on radiographs. Under optimum conditions it will appear as a faint radiopaque line (representing its apical extension). Also, on the portion of the root image covered by bone, a faintly recognizable trabecular pattern will be discernible.

Periodontal abscess

A periodontal abscess is a rapidly progressing destructive lesion that usually originates in a deep soft tissue pocket. It occurs when the coronal portion of the pocket becomes occluded or when foreign material becomes lodged between a tooth and the gingiva. Clinically there will often be pain and swelling in the region. If the lesion persists, a generalized radiolucency can form. After treatment there may be regeneration of some of the lost bone.

JUVENILE PERIODONTITIS

Juvenile periodontitis is an aggressive but uncommon form of periodontal disease found in children and young adults. It has a familial distribution that is most likely an X-linked dominant trait; but because it is an infectious disease, this probably represents a genetic transmission of susceptibility.[36] Both localized and generalized forms occur. The localized form results in severe and rapid loss of alveolar bone. The radiographic appearance of the bone loss is typically vertical[44] (Fig. 16-12) and confined to the region of the first molars and incisors.[18] The amount of bony destruction at these sites is more exaggerated than can be attributed to the relatively small amounts of local irritants (e.g., subgingival calculus) identifiable.[26] Maxillary teeth are slightly more frequently involved than mandibular teeth, and there is strong left-right symmetry. The disease usually begins in the early teens and is more common in women. Most (75% to 90%) affected individuals have an inherited defect of neutrophil chemotactic function.[6,35] "This deficiency affects the ability of the polymorphonuclear leukocytes to phagocytose and to degranulate and may consequently impair the host defense and mediate the rapid progress of the juvenile periodontitis lesions."[27]

The generalized form involves most of the dentition. It generally has a later onset, usually between the ages of 20 and 30 years. Also, besides the first molars and incisors, it involves the canines, premolars, and second molars. Whether the generalized form of juvenile periodontitis is an outgrowth of the localized form or a separate disease is not clear. Since it begins at a later age, some maintain that the generalized form started as the localized juvenile form and, left untreated, spread.[18] Others,[34] however, believe it is a separate entity and have named it *rapidly progressive periodontitis*. As with the localized form, gross deposits of subgingival calculus are uncommon. The generalized form of juvenile periodontitis also displays the rapid and typically angular loss of alveolar bone that may progress to tooth loss. As with the localized form, there is usually a defect in neutrophil production and in some cases monocyte chemotaxis.

In spite of the rather unusual nature of this disease, it responds to total plaque control, just as does the advanced adult periodontitis.[27] Treatment often consists of scaling, curettage, and antibiotics.

DENTAL CONDITIONS ASSOCIATED WITH THE PERIODONTAL DISEASES

Various changes in the dentition and its supporting structures that are frequently associated with periodontal disease include overhanging and faulty restorations, occlusal trauma, tooth mobility, open contacts, and local irritations. These conditions are usually apparent on radiographs.

Occlusal trauma

Traumatic occlusion does not cause gingivitis or periodontitis, affect the epithelial attachment, or lead to pocket formation. It does, however, cause some traumatic lesions, which generally develop in response to occlusal pressures that are greater than the physiologic tolerances of the tooth's supporting tissues. These lesions occur as a result of malfunction. In addition to clinical symptoms such as increased mobility, wear facets, unusual response to percussion, and a history of contributing habit(s), there may be radiographic evidence suggesting increased tooth mobility[45]—widening of the periodontal ligament (PDL) space, decreased definition of the lamina dura, bone loss, and altered trabeculation. Other radiographic signs of traumatic occlusion include hypercementosis and root fractures.[23]

Tooth mobility

Widening of the PDL space suggests tooth mobility resulting from occlusal trauma. If the affected tooth has a single root, the socket may develop an hourglass shape. If it is a multirooted tooth, it may show widening of the PDL space at the apices and in the region of the furcation. These changes result when the tooth moves about an axis of rotation at some midpoint on the roots. The widened PDL is due to resorption of both the root and the alveolar bone (lamina dura). In addition, the radiographic image of the lamina dura may appear broad and hazy and of increased density (osteosclerosis). In some cases, if the trauma is extensive, there may not be any apparent lamina dura in evidence. In the case of multirooted teeth the interradicular bone may be blunt, especially if the trauma has moved the tooth buccally and lingually.

Open contacts

When the mesial and distal surfaces of adjacent teeth are not touching, the patient has an open contact. This condition is potentially dangerous to the periodontium because of the potential to trap food debris in the region. Trapped food particles may damage the soft tissue and induce an inflammatory response (leading to periodontal disease). Areas with open contacts and early periodontal disease show more bone loss than areas of closed contacts do.[21] Similar problems may follow when there is a discrepancy in height of two adjacent marginal ridges. These conditions are both examples of the importance of proper tooth alignment for the prevention of periodontal disease.

Local irritating factors

Local irritating factors may cause or aggravate periodontal defects. The presence of calculus deposits will prevent effective cleansing of a sulcus and lead to the progression of periodontal disease. Similarly, defective restorations with overhanging or poorly contoured margins can lead to the accumulation of bacterial deposits and periodontal disease (Fig. 16-13). Radiographs will often reveal these conditions. Occasionally crowns have insufficient contour and fail to protect the gingiva. Gingivitis and periodontitis may then result from trauma to the tissues. Prior surgical removal of an impacted third molar has been shown to be associated with a higher incidence of plaque, gingivitis, and pockets on the distal surface of the second molar than on other surfaces of the first and second molars.[22]

EVALUATION OF PERIODONTAL THERAPY

Radiographs may show signs of successful treatment of periodontal disease. The relatively radio-

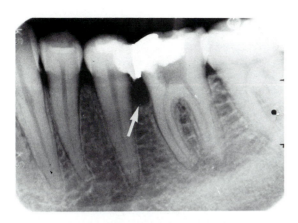

FIG. 16-13. Overhanging amalgam restorations have resulted in the loss of alveolar bone *(arrow)*.

lucent margins of bone that were undergoing active resorption before treatment may become more sclerotic (radiopaque) after successful therapy. In other cases, however, the radiographic appearance of the alveolar process may not change after successful periodontal treatment. The enlarged marrow spaces are reduced and the bone becomes more dense, creating the illusion of vertical bone growth (bone regeneration after therapy). Other changes may not be seen. For instance, radiographs will not disclose the therapeutic elimination of (radiolucent) soft tissue periodontal pockets unless there has been an alteration in the appearance of the alveolar process.

Radiographs made with poor technique may not accurately demonstrate the condition of bone after treatment. Even though periodontal therapy does not restore marginal bone or bone in the furcation region, alterations in beam orientation may give the false impression that such additive changes have taken place. The effect of exposure and processing must also be critically controlled and evaluated when assessing the result of treatment. Too high an x-ray exposure and too long a developing time will create the impression of destroyed bone as a result of alveolar crest burnout. If followed (posttreatment) by too low an exposure and too short a developing time, the denser-appearing image may suggest vertical bone growth.

The clinical *crown-to-tooth ratio* is a useful criterion not only for determining the nature of the restorative treatment to be performed on a tooth but also for deciding what the prognosis of an individual tooth will be. It is a measure of the tooth's bony support, relating the proportion of tooth length that is beyond the level of bone (clinical

crown) to that supported by the lowest level of bone (bony investment). Teeth have an unfavorable crown-to-root ratio when the length of the tooth out of bone exceeds the length of root supported by bone.

SYSTEMIC DISEASE AND THEIR EFFECT ON PERIODONTAL DISEASE

Although systemic diseases do not cause periodontal disease, they do influence its course by interfering with the natural defenses against irritants or by limiting the capacity of the individual to effect repair. Although any systemic disease may have some influence on other body systems, only a few appear to influence the periodontium and periodontal treatment: diabetes mellitus, hematologic disorders (monocytic and less often myelogenous leukemia, neutropenia, hemophilia, abnormal bleeding, nonhemophilic polycythemia vera), genetic and hereditary disturbances (e.g., hyperkeratosis palmoplantaris,[10] Down's syndrome,[5] hypophosphatemia, Chediak-Higashi syndrome),[25] hormonal changes (puberty, pregnancy, menopause), and stress.[7]

AIDS

There has been an increase in frequency and severity of periodontal disease in patients with AIDS.[46] The disease process in these individuals is characterized by a rapid progression that leads to bone sequestration and loss of multiple teeth. Patient does not respond to standard periodontal therapy.

Diabetes mellitus

Diabetes mellitus is the most prevalent and most important systemic disease that will influence the onset and course of periodontal disease. Uncontrolled, it may result in protein breakdown, degenerative vascular changes, lowered resistance to infection, and increased severity of infections.[13] Consequently patients with diabetes are more disposed to develop periodontal disease than those with normal glucose metabolism.[9,30] It is also true that patients with uncontrolled diabetes and periodontal disease show more severe and rapid alveolar bone resorption and are more prone to the development of periodontal abscesses. There is, however, nothing especially destructive about their periodontal disease, in contrast to that afflicting persons without diabetes. In those with controlled diabetes periodontal pathosis responds normally to traditional treatment.[37]

Hyperkeratosis palmoplantaris

Hyperkeratosis palmoplantaris (Papillon-Lefèvre syndrome) is a rare heritable condition (autosomal dominant) manifested by hyperkeratosis of the palms and soles. There is also extensive, mostly prepubertal, destruction of the periodontal bone, usually manifested as extensive generalized horizontal bone loss. The condition may result in loss of the entire primary dentition by the age of 5 years and loss of the secondary dentition before age 20.[39]

SPECIFIC REFERENCES

1. Ainamo J, Tammisalo EH: Comparison of radiographic and clinical signs of early periodontal disease, *Scand J Dent Res* 81:548-552, 1973.

2. Beck JD, Koch GG, Rozier RG, Tudor GE: Prevalence and risk indicators for periodontal attachment loss in a population of older community-dwelling blacks and whites, *J Periodontol* 61:521-528, 1990.

3. Bergström J, Eliason S, Preber H: Cigarette smoking and periodontal bone loss, *J Periodontol* 62:242-246, 1991.

4. Brown LJ, Oliver RC, Löe H: Evaluating the periodontal status of US employed adults, *J Am Dent Assoc* 121:226-232, 1990.

5. Cutress TW: Periodontal disease and oral hygiene in trisomy 21, *Arch Oral Biol* 16:1345-1355, 1971.

6. Davies R, Smith R, Porter S: Destructive forms of periodontal disease in adolescents and young adults, *Br Dent J* 158:429-436, 1985.

7. DeMarco TJ: Periodontal emotional stress syndrome, *J Periodontol* 47:67-68, 1976.

8. Duckworth J, Judy P, Goodson J, Socransky S: A method for the geometric and densitometric standardization of intraoral radiographs, *J Periodontol* 54:435-440, 1983.

9. Emrich LJ, Shlossman M, Genco RJ: Periodontal disease in non–insulin-dependent diabetes mellitus, *J Periodontol* 62:123-130, 1991.

10. Farzim I, Edalat M: Periodontosis with hyperkeratosis palmaris and plantaris (the Papillon-Lefèvre syndrome): a case report, *J Periodontol* 45:316-318, 1974.

11. Fox CH: New considerations in the prevalance of periodontal disease, *Curr Opin Dent* 2:5-11, 1992.

12. Goodson JM, Haffajee AD, Socransky SS: The relationship between attachment level loss and alveolar bone loss, *J Clin Periodontol* 11:348-359, 1984.

13. Grant D, Stern IB, Everett FG: *Periodontics: in the tradition of Orban and Gottlieb,* ed 5, St Louis, 1979, Mosby.

14. Greenstein G, Polson A, Iker H, Meitner S: Association between crestal lamina dura and periodontal status, *J Periodontol* 52:362-366, 1981.

15. Gröndahl HG, Gröndahl K: Subtraction radiography for the diagnosis of periodontal bone lesions, *Oral Surg* 55:208-213, 1983.

16. Gröndahl K, Gröndahl HG, Webber RL: Influence of variations in projection geometry on the detectability of periodontal bone lesions: a comparison between subtraction radiography and conventional radiographic technique, *J Clin Periodontol* 11:411-420, 1984.

17. Gröndahl HG, Johnson E, Lindahl B: Diagnosis of marginal bone destruction with orthopantomography and intraoral radiographs, *Tandlak Tidskr* 64:439-446, 1971.

18. Hormand J, Frandsen A: Juvenile periodontitis: localization of bone loss in relation to age, sex, and teeth, *J Clin Periodontol* 6:407-416, 1979.

19. Interim report of the American Dental Association, Special Committee on the Future of Dentistry: *Issue papers on dental research, manpower, education, practice, and public and professional concerns,* Chicago, 1982, American Dental Association.

20. Jeffcoat MK: Diagnosing periodontal disease: new tools to solve an old problem, *J Am Dent Assoc* 122:55-59, 1991.

21. Koral SM, Howell TH, Jeffcoat MK: Alveolar bone loss due to open interproximal contacts in periodontal disease, *J Periodontol* 52:477-550, 1981.

22. Kugelberg CF, Ahlstrom U, Ericson S, Hugoson A: Periodontal healing after impacted lower third molar surgery: a retrospective study, *Int J Oral Surg* 14(1):29-40, 1985.

23. Lang NP, Hill RW: Radiographs in periodontics, *J Clin Periodontol* 4:16-28, 1977.

24. Larato DC: Alveolar plate fenestrations and dehiscences, *Oral Surg* 29:816-819, 1970.

25. Lavine WS, Page RC, Padgett GA: Host response in chronic periodontal disease. V. The dental and periodontal status of mink and mice affected by Chediak-Higaski syndrome, *J Periodontol* 47:621-635, 1976.

26. Liljenberg B, Lindhe J: Juvenile periodontitis: some microbiological, histopathological, and clinical characteristics, *J Clin Periodontol* 7:48-61, 1980.

27. Liljenberg B, Lindhe J: Treatment of localized juvenile periodontitis: results after 5 years, *J Clin Periodontol* 11:399-410, 1984.

28. Mann J, Pettigrew J, Beideman R et al: Investigation of the relationship between clinically detected loss of attachment and radiographic changes in early periodontal disease, *J Clin Periodontol* 12:247-253, 1985.

29. Melvin WL, Sandifer JB, Gray JL: The prevalence and sex ratio of juvenile periodontitis in a young racially mixed population, *J Periodontol* 62:330-334, 1991.

30. Nelson RG, Shlossman M, Budding LM et al: Periodontal diseases and NIDDM in Pima Indians, *Diabetes Care* 13:836-840, 1990.

31. Nielsen IM, Glavind L, Karring T: Interproximal periodontal intrabony defects: prevalence, localization, and etiological factors, *J Clin Periodontol* 7(3):187-198, 1980.

32. Page RC: Periodontal research: implications of the future of academic dentistry, *J Dent Educ* 47:226-231, 1983.

33. Page RC: Oral health status in the United States: prevalence of inflammatory periodontal disease, *J Dent Educ* 49:354-363, 1985.

34. Page RC, Altman LC, Ebersole JL et al: Rapidly progressive periodontitis: a distinct clinical condition, *J Periodontol* 54:197-209, 1983.

35. Page RC, Schroeder HE: *Periodontitis in man and other animals,* Basel, 1982, S Karger.

36. Page RC, Vandesteen GE, Ebersole JL et al: Clinical and laboratory studies of a family with a high prevalence of juvenile periodontitis, *J Periodontol* 56:602-610, 1985.

37. Prichard JF: *Advanced periodontal disease: surgical and prosthetic management,* ed 2, Philadelphia, 1972, WB Saunders.

38. Prichard JF: The roentgenographic depiction of periodontal disease, *J Am Soc Periodontol* 3(2):44-50, 1973.

39. Rateitschak-Pluss EM, Schroeder HE: History of periodontitis in a child with Papillon-Lefèvre syndrome, *J Periodontol* 55:35-46, 1984.

40. Reed B, Polson A: Relationships between bitewing and periapical radiographs in assessing crestal alveolar bone levels, *J Periodontol* 55:22-27, 1984.

41. Robinson PJ: Diagnostic yield criteria and the use of radiological examination in periodontics. Presented at NCHCT technology assessment forum on dental radiology, Arlington Va, 1981.

42. Robinson PJ, Vitek RM: Periodontal examination, *Dent Clin North Am* 24:597-611, 1980.

43. Ross IF, Thompson RH: Furcation involvement in maxillary and mandibular molars, *J Periodontol* 51:450-454, 1980.

44. Sugarman MM, Sugarman EF: Precocious periodontitis: a clinical entity and a treatment responsibility, *J Periodontol* 48:397-409, 1977.

45. Wank GS, Kroll YJ: Occlusal trauma: an evaluation of its relationship to periodontal prostheses, *Dent Clin North Am* 25:511-532, 1981.

46. Winkler JR, Graffi M, Murray PA: Clinical description and etiology of HIV-associated periodontal disease. In Robinson PB and Greenspan JS: Prospectus on Oral Manifestations of AIDS. Littleton MA, 1988, PSG Publishing Co. Inc.

47. World workshop in clinical periodontics: report of section on periodontal diagnosis and diagnostic aids, Princeton NJ, 1989.

17

Dental Anomalies

Dental anomalies generally reflect either a change in the number of teeth or a change in their shape. Changes in shape may involve the enamel or dentin. Given the complexities and interactions involved in tooth development, from initiation at about the sixth week in utero to eruption, the number of anomalies described should come as a surprise; the surprise is that the number is not greater. Most of the defects considered in this chapter are inherited. In all cases radiographs play an important role in identifying the nature or severity of the condition.

SUPERNUMERARY TEETH

Supernumerary teeth (also known as *hyperdontia*) are those found in addition to the normal complement. They occur in 1% to 4% of the population.[11,62] Although they may develop in both dentitions, they are more frequent in the permanent.[10] Their form may vary from normal to conical. Some are just masses of dental tissue without recognizable tooth form. They usually do not erupt but are discovered radiographically. Although their

cause is unknown, the tendency is familial. Most cases are polygenetic and represent initial spontaneous gene mutations. When an increased number of teeth are a component of a syndrome, it is inherited as an autosomal dominant trait.[32] When the anomaly is restricted to supernumerary teeth only, it is inherited as an autosomal recessive trait.[24]

The supernumerary teeth that occur between the maxillary central incisors are *mesiodens* (Fig. 17-1); those occurring in the molar area are *paramolar* teeth (Fig. 17-2); and, more specifically, those that erupt distal to the third molar are *distodens* or *distomolar* teeth (Fig. 17-3). Also supernumerary teeth that erupt ectopically either buccally or lingually to the normal arch are *peridens*.

Clinical features. Supernumerary teeth may occur anywhere in either jaw. Single teeth are most common in the anterior maxilla and in the maxillary molar region. Multiple teeth not associated with syndromes occur most frequently in the premolar regions, usually in the mandible (Fig. 17-4).[11,62] The mandibular counterpart of the mesiodens is

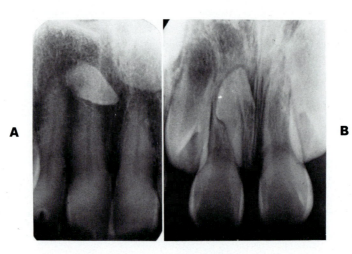

FIG. 17-1. Mesiodens is a supernumerary tooth in the midline of the maxilla. **A,** In the region of the maxillary central incisor apex. **B,** Inverted and lying just lateral to the intermaxillary suture.

rare. Supernumerary teeth occur twice as often in males[23] and have a greater incidence in Asians and Native Americans than in whites.[24]

Supernumerary teeth may cause impaction or delay the eruption of normal members of the dentition (Fig. 17-5). Although a patient may appear clinically to be missing teeth, an appropriate radiographic examination will occasionally reveal a supernumerary tooth interfering with normal tooth eruption. When supernumerary teeth erupt, they usually lie outside the normal arch because of space restriction.[6] Because multiple supernumerary teeth occur with increased frequency in a number of syndromes, the recognition of this trait should alert the clinician to the possibility of other, more serious, physical disabilities.

Radiographic features. Radiographs may reveal supernumerary teeth in the deciduous dentition (Fig. 17-6) after 3 or 4 years of age, when the deciduous teeth have formed. In the permanent dentition they may be detected after 9 to 12 years. There is no difficulty in recognizing the presence of more than the usual number of teeth. Their radiographic image will be characteristic. Since most supernumerary teeth remain unerupted, and many also interfere with the eruption of members of the normal dentition, radiographic examination may be required to rule out missing teeth. Besides the periapical intraoral examination, occlusal radiographs will aid in determining the location and number of unerupted supernumerary teeth.

Differential diagnosis. The recognition of supernumerary teeth and follicles, both clinically and radiographically, is usually straightforward.

Management. The management of supernumerary teeth depends on their potential effect on

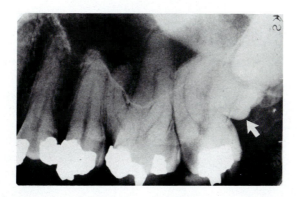

FIG. 17-2. A paramolar *(arrow)* blocking the path of eruption of the third molar.

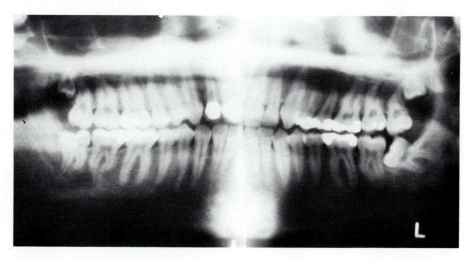

FIG. 17-3. Distomolars or fourth molars may be seen in both maxillary quadrants. Note also the coincidental mucous retention cysts in both maxillary antra.

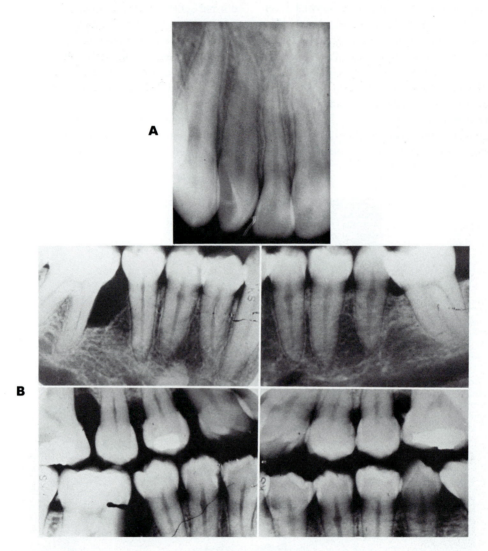

FIG. 17-4. Supernumerary lateral incisors, **A,** and premolars, **B,** may also be seen. Note the presence of four mandibular left premolars.

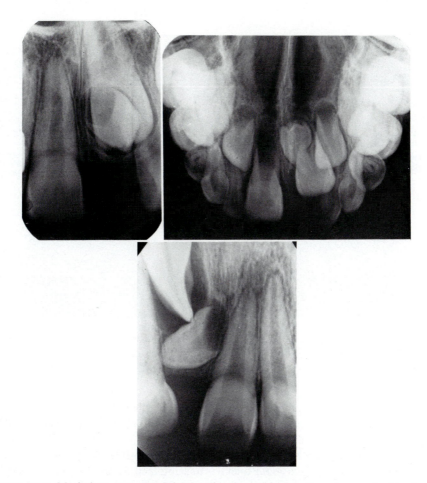

FIG. 17-5. Mesiodens may retard the eruption or cause impaction of permanent teeth.

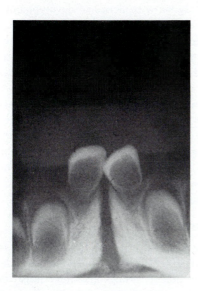

FIG. 17-6. Supernumerary primary central incisors that erupted soon after birth. Note the open mandibular suture, normal for an infant.

the developing normal dentition, on their position and number, and on the complications that may result from surgical intervention. If they erupt, they can cause malalignment of the normal members of the dentition. Those that remain in the jaws may cause root resorption or interfere with the normal eruption sequence. Follicles of unerupted supernumerary teeth occasionally develop into dentigerous cysts.

DEVELOPMENTALLY MISSING TEETH

The expression of developmentally missing teeth may range from the absence of one or a few teeth (hypodontia), to the absence of numerous teeth (oligodontia), to the failure of all teeth to develop (anodontia). Although missing primary teeth are relatively uncommon, when there is one missing it is usually a maxillary incisor.[6] Hypodontia in the permanent dentition, excluding third molars, is found in 3% to 10% of the population.[1,26] Anodontia is uncommon.[6] The most commonly missing

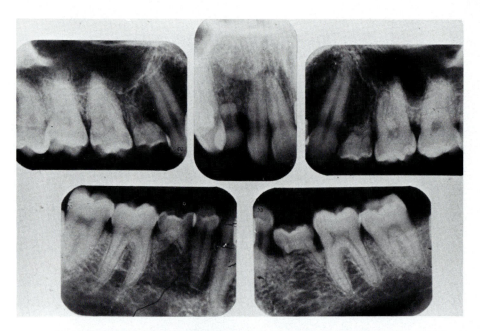

FIG. 17-7. Developmental absence of all maxillary premolars and both mandibular second premolars. Note the retention of the maxillary primary canine as a result of posterior position of maxillary permanent canine.

teeth are third molars, second premolars (Fig. 17-7), and maxillary lateral[29] and mandibular central incisors. The absence may be either unilateral or bilateral. There is a tendency for children who have developmentally missing teeth to have more than one missing and for more than one morphologic group (incisors, premolars, molars) to be involved.[7] Anodontia or oligodontia frequently occurs in patients with ectodermal dysplasia*[14] (Fig. 17-8). Developmentally missing teeth may also be the result of numerous independent pathologic mechanisms that can affect the orderly formation of the dental lamina—including the orofaciodigital syndrome,[9] failure of a tooth germ to develop at the optimum time, lack of necessary space imposed by a maldeveloped jaw,[40] and a genetically determined disproportion between tooth mass and jaw size.[13]

Clinical features. In the more common cases of hypodontia, a tooth or a morphologic group of teeth will be absent from the dentition. The patient will not describe previous extractions, and the radiographic examination does not reveal unerupted teeth. Hypodontia is more frequently found in Asian and Native Americans than in white populations.[35]

Radiographic features. The recognition of missing teeth is not difficult, although it is well to consider the marked variability in development of teeth. Some teeth may be developmentally delayed by a number of years after the established time and others may show evidence of development as late as a year after the contralateral tooth.

Differential diagnosis. A tooth may be considered to be developmentally missing when it cannot be discerned clinically or radiographically and there is no history of its extraction.

Management. Missing teeth, abnormal occlusion, or altered facial appearance may cause some patients psychologic distress. If the extent of hypodontia is mild, the associated changes may likewise be slight and manageable by orthodontics. In more severe cases restorative or prosthetic procedures can be undertaken.

TOOTH SIZE

There is a positive correlation between tooth size (mesiodistal diameter × buccolingual diameter) and body height.[8] Males also have larger primary and permanent teeth than females. Beyond these normal variations, however, individuals may occasionally develop unusually large or small teeth.

---

*Ectodermal dysplasia is a syndrome characterized by malformation of one or more ectodermal structures. Often patients with this condition show abnormalities of the skin, nails, hair, eyes or teeth.

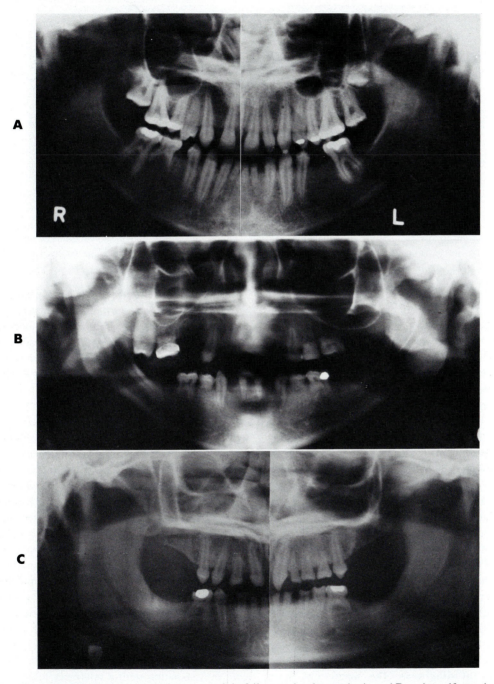

FIG. 17-8. Ectodermal dysplasia may result in failure to develop teeth, **A,** and **B,** or in malformation of the teeth, **C.**

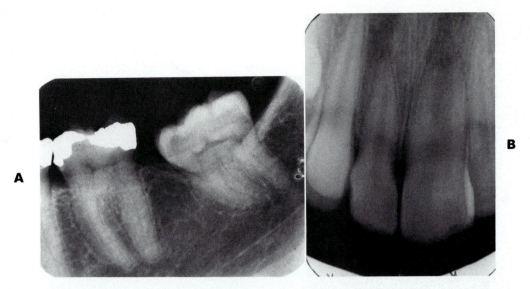

FIG. 17-9. Macrodontia is a condition that results in an enlarged tooth. **A,** The macrodont molar shows an increased mesiodistal dimension. **B,** The macrodont central incisor shows enlargement of both its mesiodistal and its longitudinal dimension. (**A** courtesy Dr. B. Gratt, Los Angeles.)

Macrodontia

In macrodontia the teeth are larger than normal. When the teeth are of normal size but occur in smaller than normal jaws, the condition is relative macrodontia. Macrodontia may rarely affect the entire dentition, but more commonly it involves a group of teeth, individual contralateral teeth, or a single tooth (Fig. 17-9). A unilaterally macrodont tooth may be difficult to differentiate from fusion of a normal and a supernumerary tooth or partial twinning (gemination) of a normal tooth. Localized true macrodontia can occur at times in hemihypertrophy of the face[42] and with angioma of the jaw.[16] True generalized macrodontia may occur with pituitary giantism.[29] The cause of macrodontia is unknown, but there is probably a genetic component.

Clinical features. The large size of the teeth is apparent on clinical examination. There may be crowding, malocclusion, and impaction.

Radiographic features. Radiographs reveal the increased size of both erupted and unerupted macrodont teeth. The crowding may cause impaction of other teeth.

Differential diagnosis. The macrodont may appear so characteristic that its identity is not in doubt, or it may resemble gemination or fusion. Because the management of a macrodont tooth, a partially geminated tooth, or a fusion between normal and supernumerary teeth is the same, the distinction among the three conditions does not influence patient care.

Management. In most cases macrodontia does not require treatment. Orthodontic treatment may be necessary, however, if there is malocclusion. Extraction may be necessary for an impacted macrodont, and the same guidelines should be followed as govern the removal of any impacted tooth.

Microdontia

In microdontia the involved teeth are smaller than normal. As with macrodontia, microdontia may involve all the teeth or be limited to a single tooth or groups of teeth. Relative microdontia can also occur. In this condition normal-sized teeth develop in an individual with large jaws. Microdont molars may have altered shape—from five to four cusps in the case of mandibular molars, and from four to three in the case of upper molars (Fig. 17-10). Microdont lateral incisors are also smaller and peg shaped (Fig. 17-11). Generalized microdontia is extremely rare,[33] although it does occur in some patients with pituitary dwarfism.[42] Supernumerary teeth are frequently microdont. Also the lateral incisors and third molars, which often are developmentally missing, may be small. Microdontia occurs in association with a relatively large number of syndromes (e.g., congenital heart disease, and progeria).

Clinical features. The involved teeth are noticeably small and may have altered morphology.

Radiographic features. Radiographs will permit evaluation of the size and shape of both erupted and unerupted microdonts.

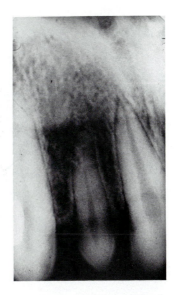

FIG. 17-11. Microdontia of the maxillary lateral incisor results in a characteristic peg-shaped deformity.

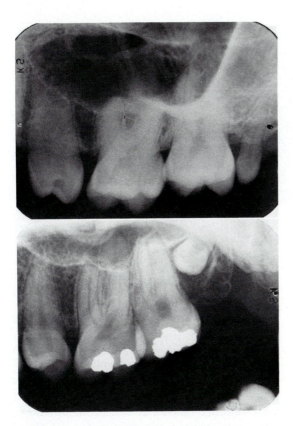

FIG. 17-10. Microndontia of the maxillary third molars, showing reduction in both the size and the number of cusps.

Differential diagnosis. The recognition of small teeth indicates the diagnosis. The number and distribution of microdonts may also suggest consideration of syndromes.

Management. The only treatment that may be in order is restorative dentistry.

TRANSPOSITION

Transposition is the condition in which two teeth have exchanged position.

Clinical features. The most frequently transposed teeth are the permanent canine and first premolar (more often than the lateral incisor).[39] Second premolars infrequently lie between first and second molars. The transposition of central and lateral incisors is rare. Apparently transposition in the primary dentition has not been reported.[29] It can occur with hypodontia, supernumerary teeth, or the persistence of a deciduous predecessor.

Radiographic features. Radiographs reveal transposition when the teeth are not in their usual sequence in the dental arch (Fig. 17-12).

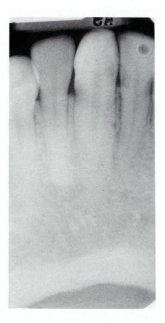

FIG. 17-12. Mandibular canine transposed with the lateral incisor. (Courtesy Dr. N.L. Frederiksen, Dallas.)

Differential diagnosis. Transposed teeth are usually easily recognized.

Management. Transposed teeth are frequently altered prosthetically to improve function and esthetics.

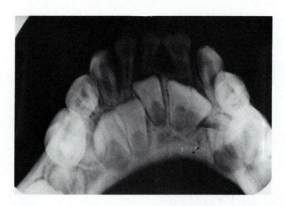

FIG. 17-13. Fusion of the central and lateral incisors in both the primary and the permanent dentition. Note the reduction in number of dental structures and the increased width of the fused tooth mass.

FUSION

Fusion of teeth (known as *synodontia*) results from the combining of adjacent tooth germs, resulting in union of the developing teeth. Some authors believe that fusion results when two tooth germs develop so close together that as they grow they contact and fuse before calcification. Others contend that a physical force or pressure generated during development causes contact of adjacent tooth buds. The genetic basis for the anomaly is probably autosomal dominant with reduced penetrance.[6] Fusion may be total or partial depending on the stage of odontogenesis and the proximity of the developing teeth. The result can vary, from a single tooth of about normal size to a tooth of nearly twice normal size. There may be a bifid crown or two recognizable teeth joined by dentin or enamel. The sex ratio is 1 to 1, and the incidence is higher in Asians and Native Americans than in whites or blacks.[18]

Clinical features. Fusion usually causes a reduced number of teeth in the arch. It occurs in deciduous and permanent dentitions, although it is more common between deciduous teeth. When a deciduous canine and lateral incisor fuse, the corresponding permanent lateral incisor is often absent.[12] Fusion is more common in anterior teeth of both the permanent and deciduous dentition (Fig. 17-13). The crowns of fused teeth usually appear to be large and single, or there may be an incisocervical groove of varying depth or a bifid crown.[45]

Radiographic features. Radiographs disclose the unusual shape or size of the entire tooth. The true nature and extent of the union will frequently be more evident on the radiograph than can be determined by clinical examination. Fused teeth may show an unusual configuration of the pulp chamber, root canal, or crown.

Differential diagnosis. The differential diagnosis for fused teeth includes gemination and macrodontia. Such comparison is of greater academic interest than practical importance because the treatment objective of both is esthetic improvement. Since fusion can take place between a normal and a supernumerary tooth, it may often be difficult to differentiate fusion from gemination.

Management. The management of a case of fusion will depend on which teeth are involved, the degree of fusion, and the morphologic result. If the affected teeth are deciduous, they may be retained as they are. If the clinician contemplates extraction, it is important first to determine whether the succedaneous teeth are present. In the case of fused secondary teeth, the fused crowns may be reshaped with a restoration that mimics two independent crowns. The morphology of fused teeth should be evaluated radiographically, however, before they are reshaped. Endodontic therapy may become necessary and perhaps be difficult or impossible if the root canals are of unusual shape. There is also always the option, and this is generally the most prudent, to leave the teeth as they are.

CONCRESCENCE

Concrescence occurs when the roots of two or more teeth are united by cementum. It may involve either primary or secondary teeth. Although its cause is unknown, many authorities suspect that space restriction during development, local trauma, excessive occlusal force, or local infection after development plays an important role. If the con-

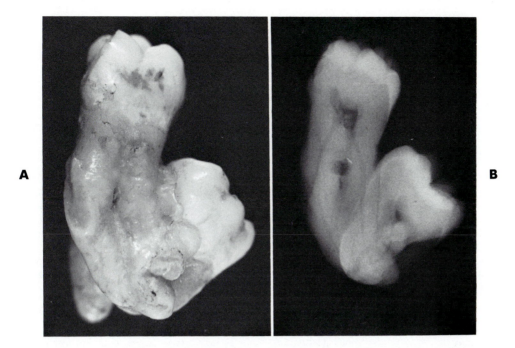

FIG. 17-14. A, Concrescence occurs when two teeth are joined by a mass of cementum. **B,** Extraction of one tooth may result in the unintended removal of the second, because cementum is often not well visualized radiographically. (Courtesy Dr. R. Kienholz, Dallas.)

dition occurs during development, it is called *true* concrescence; if later, it is *acquired* concresence.

Clinical features. Maxillary molars are the teeth most frequently involved, especially a third molar and a supernumerary tooth. Involved teeth may fail to erupt or may erupt incompletely. The sexes are equally affected.[20]

Radiographic features. A radiographic examination may not always distinguish between concrescence and teeth that are in close contact or are simply superimposed (Fig. 17-14). When the condition is suspected on a radiograph and extraction of one of the teeth is being considered, additional projections at different angles may be obtained to delineate the condition better.

Differential diagnosis. It will usually be impossible to determine radiographically with certainty whether the teeth whose root images are superimposed are actually joined. If the roots are joined, it may not be possible to tell whether the union is by cementum or by dentin (fusion).

Management. Concrescence affects treatment only when the decision is made to remove one or both of the involved teeth. This condition will surely complicate the extraction. The clinician should warn the patient that an effort to remove one may result in the unintended and simultaneous removal of the other.

GEMINATION

Gemination (twinning) is a rare anomaly that arises when the tooth bud of a single tooth attempts to divide. The result may be an invagination of the crown, with partial division, or in rare cases complete division throughout the crown and root, producing identical structures.[6] Complete twinning results in a normal tooth plus a supernumerary tooth in the arch. Its cause is unknown, but there is some evidence that it is familial.[48]

Clinical features. Gemination more frequently affects the primary teeth, but it may occur in both dentitions, usually in the incisor region.[19] It can be detected clinically after the anomalous tooth erupts. The occurrence in males and females is about equal.[19] The enamel or dentin of geminated teeth may be hypoplastic or hypocalcified.

Radiographic features. Radiographs reveal the altered shape of the geminated tooth's hard tissue and pulp chamber. Radiopaque enamel outlines the clefts in the crowns and invaginations and thus accentuates them. The pulp chamber is usually single and enlarged and may be partially divided (Fig. 17-15). In the rare case of premolar gemination the tooth image suggests a molar with an enlarged crown and two roots. Its position in the arch will prompt its identity.

Differential diagnosis. The differential diag-

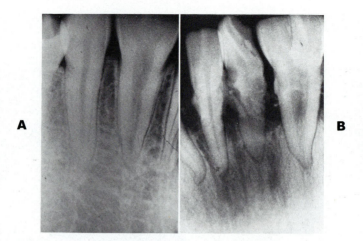

FIG. 17-15. A, Gemination of a mandibular lateral incisor showing bifurcation of the crown with a single enlarged pulp chamber. **B,** Gemination of a mandibular central incisor, with two crowns and a common root.

nosis of gemination includes fusion. If the malformed tooth is counted as one, individuals with gemination will have a normal tooth count whereas those with fusion will be missing a tooth.

Gemination, however, may be difficult to distinguish from fusion if the fusion is between a normal and a supernumerary tooth. In this case there will be a normal number of teeth in the affected area. Because the distinction is not important to the formulation of a treatment plan, the following guideline should be used: In vague situations a tooth structure with two separate root canals and with either one root or two roots is the result of fusion. Alternatively, an enlarged tooth with a bifid crown containing an enlarged and possibly partially divided pulp chamber is the result of gemination.

Management. A geminated tooth in the anterior region may compromise arch esthetics. Areas of hypoplasia and invagination lines or areas of coronal separation represent caries-susceptible sites that may in time result in pulpal infection. Affected teeth can cause malocclusion and lead to periodontal disease. Consequently the affected tooth may be removed (especially if it is decidious), the crown(s) may be restored or reshaped, or the tooth may be left untreated and periodically examined to preclude the development of complications. Before treatment is initiated on primary teeth, the status of the succedaneous teeth and configuration of their root canals should be determined radiographically.

TAURODONTISM

Taurodont teeth have longitudinally enlarged pulp chambers. The crown is of normal shape and size, but the body is elongated and the roots are short. The pulp chamber extends from a normal position in the crown throughout the length of the extended body, leading to an increased distance between the cementoenamel junction and the furcation.

Taurodontism may occur in either the permanent or the primary dentition (or both). Although some evidence of the trait can be seen in any tooth, it is usually fully expressed in the molars and less often in the premolars.[2] Single or multiple teeth may show taurodont features, unilaterally or bilaterally and in any combination of teeth or quadrants.

Clinical features. Since the body and roots of taurodont teeth lie below the alveolar margin, the distinguishing features of these teeth are not recognizable clinically.

Radiographic features. The distinctive morphology of taurodont teeth is quite apparent on radiographs. The peculiar feature is an extension of the rectangular pulp chamber into the elongated body of the tooth (Fig. 17-16). The shortened roots and root canals are a function of the long body and normal length of the tooth. The size of the crown is normal.

Differential diagnosis. The image of the taurodont tooth is characteristic and easily recognized radiographically. The inexperienced clinician may

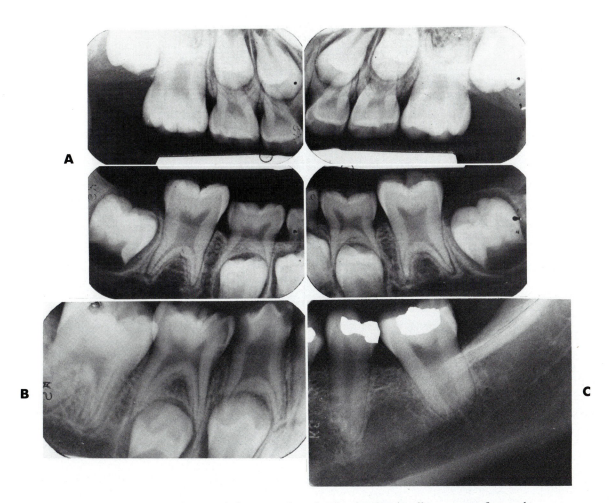

FIG. 17-16. Taurondontia, revealed as an enlarged pulp chamber in all permanent first molars, **A,** in a primary first molar, **B,** and in a permanent first molar, **C.**

identify a developing mandibular molar as a tau-rodont tooth, but attention to the wide apical foramina, incompletely formed roots, and dental papillae will correct this misimpression.

Management. Taurodont teeth do not require treatment.

DILACERATION

Dilaceration is a disturbance in tooth formation that produces a sharp bend or curve in the tooth. One of the oldest concepts is that it is probably the result of mechanical trauma to the calcified portion of a partially formed tooth. It is more likely, however, a true developmental anomaly with trauma not a factor.[40] The angular distortion may occur anywhere in the crown or root. Some of the angles that develop are so acute that the tooth will not erupt. The condition occurs most often in perma-

nent maxillary premolars. One or more teeth may be affected.

Clinical features. Most cases of radicular dilaceration are not recognized clinically. If the dilaceration is so pronounced that the tooth does not erupt, the only clinical indication of the defect will be a missing tooth. If the defect is in the crown of an erupted tooth, it may be readily recognized as an angular distortion (Fig. 17-17).

Radiographic features. Radiographs provide the best means of detecting a radicular dilaceration. If the roots bend mesially or distally, the condition is clearly apparent on a periapical radiograph (Fig. 17-18). When the roots are bent buccally (labially) or lingually, the central ray will be passing approximately parallel with the deflected portion of the root. The dilacerated portion will then appear at the apical end of the unaltered root as a rounded

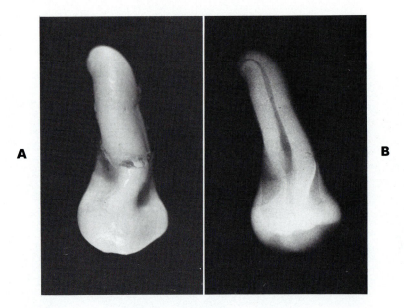

FIG. 17-17. A, Dilaceration of the crown may be readily recognized clinically. **B,** Radiograph of this specimen. (Courtesy Dr. R. Kienholz, Dallas.)

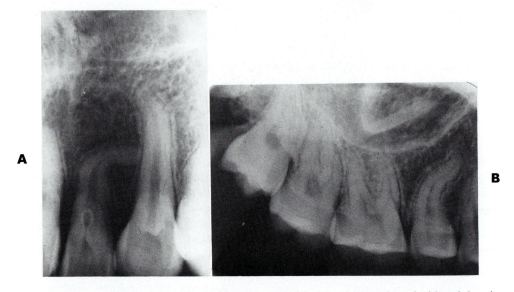

FIG. 17-18. Dilaceration of the root of a maxillary lateral incisor, **A** (note the coincidental dens in dente), and a maxillary second premolar, **B.**

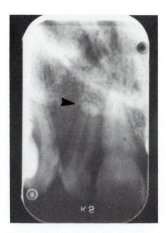

FIG. 17-19. Dilacerated root. The apical portion of the root is bent buccally or lingually into the plane of the central ray. Note the halo in the apical region, produced by the periodontal ligament space *(arrow)*.

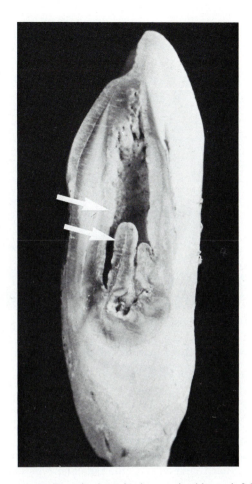

FIG. 17-20. Dens in dente is characterized by an infolding of enamel into the tooth. This sectioned canine with a dens in dente shows enamel *(arrows)* folded into the tooth's interior.

opaque area with a dark shadow in its central region cast by the apical foramen and root canal. The PDL space around this dilacerated portion may be seen as a radiolucent halo (Fig. 17-19). In some cases, especially in the maxilla, the geometry of the projections may preclude the recognition of a dilaceration.

Differential diagnosis. Occasionally dilacerated roots will be difficult to differentiate from fused roots, condensing osteitis, or periapical idiopathic osteosclerosis. They can usually be identified, however, by obtaining radiographs exposed from different angles.

Management. The dilacerated root generally does not require treatment, because it provides adequate support. If it must be extracted for some other reason, its removal can be complicated, especially if the surgeon is not prepared with a preoperative radiograph. In contrast, dilacerated crowns are frequently restored with a crown—the aim being to improve esthetics and function and to preclude dental caries and periodontal disease.

DENS IN DENTE

Dens in dente (also known as *dens invaginatus*) results from an infolding of the outer enamel surface of a tooth into the interior. This can occur in either the crown or the root during tooth development and may involve the pulp chamber or root canal, resulting in deformity of either the crown or the root. These anomalies are seen most often in tooth crowns, and in most instances at the site

of an anatomically defined pit. Coronal invaginations usually originate from an anomalous infolding of the enamel organ into the dental papilla. In a mature tooth the result is a fold of hard tissue within the tooth characterized by enamel lining the fold and coating the peripheral dentin (Fig. 17-20). Dens in dente occurs most frequently in the permanent maxillary lateral incisors, followed (much less frequently) by occurence in the maxillary central incisors, premolars, and canines, and less often in the posterior teeth.[15] Invagination is rare in the crowns of mandibular teeth and in deciduous teeth.[29] It occurs symmetrically in about half the cases. Concomitant involvement of the central and lateral incisors is also observed.

When dens in dente involves a root (radicular dens invaginatus), it appears to be the result of an invagination of Hertwig's epithelial root sheath.

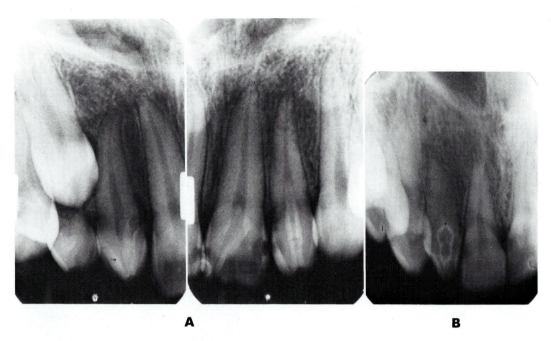

A   **B**

FIG. 17-21. Dens in dente is seen radiographically as a radiopaque infolding of enamel into the tooth's pulp chamber. **A,** Involvement of both maxillary lateral incisors. **B,** Altered coronal morphology.

This results in an accentuation of the normal longitudinal root groove.[44] In contrast to the coronal type (lined with enamel) the radicular-type defect is lined with cementum. If the invagination retracts and is cut off, it leaves a longitudinal structure of cementum, bone, and remnants of periodontal ligament within the pulp canal. These often extend for most of the root length.[36] In other cases the root sheath may bud off a sacklike invagination that produces a circumscribed cementum defect in the root.[27] Mandibular first premolars and second molars are especially prone to develop the radicular variety of this invagination anomaly.[27]

There seems to be little difference in the frequency of occurrence among whites and Asian peoples. If all grades of expression of invagination, mild to severe, are included, the condition will be found in approximately 5% of these two racial groups.[29] The condition appears to be rare in blacks.[15] There is no sexual predilection. Although no specific mode of inheritance seems to fit all the data, there does seem to be a high degree of inheritability.[6]

Clinical features. The clinical appearance of the affected tooth may suggest dens in dente. With this condition the lingual marginal ridges or cingula are prominent. Also the pit in the cingulum is par-

ticularly broad and deep, especially when these features occur in the lateral incisor. In most cases, however, the dens in dente is not large and there are no clinically apparent changes in crown morphology.

The clinical importance of dens invaginatus results from the risk of pulpal disease. Although enamel lines the coronal defect, it is frequently thin, often of poor quality, and even missing in some areas. Furthermore, the cavity is usually separated from the pulp chamber by a relatively thin wall and opens into the oral environment through a narrow constriction. Consequently it offers conditions favorable for the development of caries. Such carious lesions are difficult to detect clinically and will rapidly involve the pulp. In addition, sometimes fine canals extend between the invagination and the pulp chamber, causing pulpal disease even in the absence of caries.

Radiographic features. Most cases of dens in dente are discovered radiographically. The infolding of the enamel lining the cavity is recognized by its greater radiodensity (Fig. 17-21). Less frequently the radicular invaginations will appear as poorly defined, slightly radiolucent, structures running longitudinally within the root. The defects, especially the coronal variety, may vary in size and

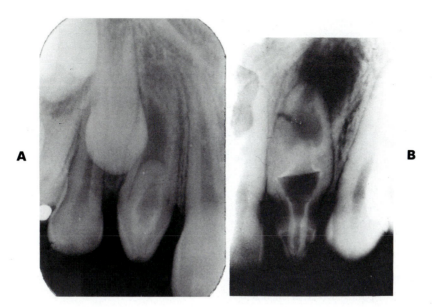

FIG. 17-22. Severe malformation of dens in dente may produce open apices, **A,** and often periapical lesions, **B.**

shape from small and superficial to large and deep. If a coronal invagination is extensive, the crown is almost invariably malformed; and when the crown is malformed, the apical foramen is usually wide (Fig. 17-22). All these features are apparent on radiographs even before the tooth erupts.

Differential diagnosis. The appearance and usual occurrence in incisors are so characteristic that, once recognized, there is little probability that the anomaly will be confused with another condition.

Management. Although it is important to evaluate every case individually, the placement of a prophylactic restoration in the defect is typically the treatment of choice and should assure a normal life span for the tooth. Failure to treat the tooth may result in its premature loss or the requirement for root canal therapy.

DENS EVAGINATUS

In contrast to the dens in dente, dens evaginatus is the result of an outfolding of the enamel organ. The result is an enamel-covered tubercle, usually in or near the middle of the occlusal surface of a premolar or occasionally a molar (Fig. 17-23). Canines are rarely affected. Dens evaginatus may occur bilaterally and usually in the mandible.[61] The tubercle often has a dentin core, and a pulp horn frequently extends into the evagination.[28] Fracture or indiscriminate surgical removal may precipitate a pulpal infection. Its frequency of occurrence is highest in Asians and lower in whites.[47] Although its mode of transmission is unknown, dens evaginatus is a heritable trait, as evidenced by its almost exclusive occurrence in patients with Down's syndrome.

Clinical features. Clinically dens evaginatus appears as a tubercle of enamel on the occlusal surface of the affected tooth. There is a polyplike protuberance in the central groove or lingual ridge of a buccal cusp.

Radiographic features. The radiographic image shows an extension of a dentin tubercle on the occlusal surface. The dentin core is usually covered with opaque enamel. A fine pulp horn may extend into the tubercle. If the tubercle has been worn to the point of pulpal exposure or has fractured, pulpal necrosis may result. This will be indicated by a periapical radiolucency.

Differential diagnosis. The clinical and radiographic appearance of dens evaginatus is so characteristic that it is unlikely to be confused with another entity.

Management. If the tubercle causes any occlusal interference or shows evidence of marked abrasion, it should probably be removed under aseptic conditions and the pulp capped, if necessary. Such a precaution may preclude pulpal exposure and infection as the result of accidental fracture or advanced abrasion.

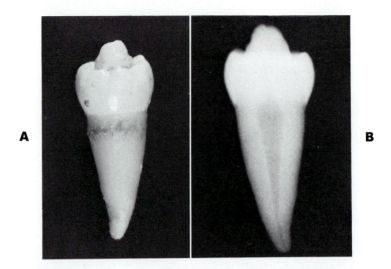

FIG. 17-23. A, Dens evaginatus, seen as a tubercle on the mandibular premolar. **B,** Radiograph of the specimen. (Courtesy Dr. R. Kienholz, Dallas.)

AMELOGENESIS IMPERFECTA

Amelogenesis imperfecta is a developmental disturbance that interferes with normal enamel formation. It leads to marked changes in the enamel of all or nearly all the teeth in both dentitions. Most forms are autosomal dominant or recessive, but two types are X linked.[5,57] It is not related to any time or period of enamel development or any clinically demonstrable alteration (disease or dietary abnormality) in other tisuses. The enamel may lack the normal prismatic structure, being laminated throughout its thickness or at the periphery. As a result these teeth are more resistant to decay.[49] The dentin and root form are usually normal.[59] Eruption of the affected teeth is often delayed, and there is a tendency for impaction. Although at least 14 variants of the condition have been described, there are four general types that have characteristic clinical or radiographic appearances[57]: a hypoplastic type, a hypomaturation variety, a hypocalcified type, and a hypomaturation-hypocalcified type associated with taurodontism.

Clinical features

Hypoplasia. As a result of some defect in ameloblasts, the enamel of the affected teeth fails to develop to its normal thickness.[54] It is so thin that the dentin shows through and imparts a yellowish brown color to the tooth. In the various hypoplastic forms the enamel may be pitted, rough, or smooth and glossy. The crowns of the teeth may not have the usual contour of enamel but rather appear squarish. The reduced enamel thickness also causes the teeth to be undersized, with lack of contact between adjacent teeth (Fig. 17-24). The occlusal surfaces of the posterior teeth are relatively flat with low cusps. This is a result of the attrition of cusp tips that were initially low and not fully formed. There may be an anterior open bite.

Hypomaturation. In the hypomaturation form of amelogenesis imperfecta the enamel has a normal thickness but a mottled appearance. It is softer than normal and may crack off the crown. Its color may range from clear to cloudy white, yellow, or brown. In one form of hypomaturation the teeth appear to be snow capped (with white opaque enamel).

Hypocalcification. Hypocalcification of teeth is more common than the hypoplastic variety of amelogenesis imperfecta.[29] The crowns of the teeth are normal in size and shape when they erupt because the enamel is of regular thickness (Fig. 17-25). Because the enamel is poorly mineralized, however, it starts to fracture away shortly after it comes into function. This creates defects that are clinically recognizable. The soft enamel abrades rapidly and the softer dentin also wears down rapidly, resulting in a grossly worn tooth, sometimes to the level of the gingiva. An explorer point under pressure can penetrate the soft enamel. Yet caries in these worn teeth is unusual. The hypocalcified enamel has increased permeability and becomes stained and darkened. The teeth of a young person with generalized hypomineralization of the enamel are frequently dark brown from food stains.

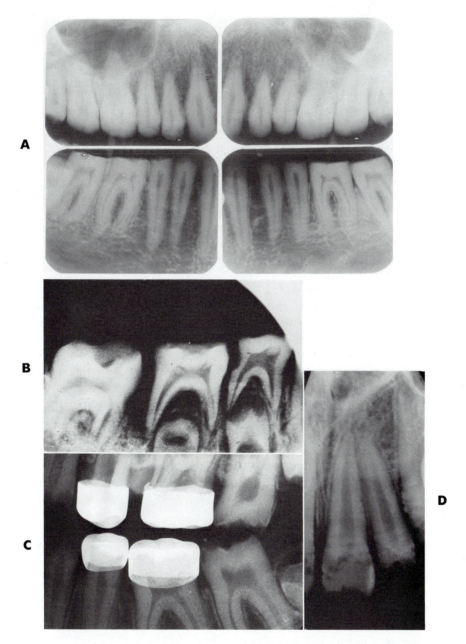

FIG. 17-24. A, Amelogenesis imperfecta (generalized hypoplastic form (is recognized by the complete absence of enamel. **B,** Primary and permanent dentition with amelogenesis imperfecta. **C** and **D,** Severe mottling of the enamel surface.

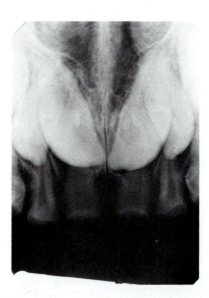

FIG. 17-25. Amelogenesis imperfecta (generalized hypomineralized form). Note the reduced enamel density and the rapid abrasion of the crowns of the primary teeth.

Radiographic features. Identification of amelogenesis imperfecta is primarily made by clinical examination. Although there are radiographic manifestations of this condition, they primarily substantiate the clinical impression.

The radiographic signs of the hypoplastic amelogenesis imperfecta include a squarish shape of the crown, a relatively thin opaque layer of enamel, and low or absent cusps. The density of the enamel is normal. Pitted enamel will appear as sharply localized areas of mottled density, quite different from the image cast by a tooth that is normal in shape and density. The hypomaturation form demonstrates a normal thickness of the enamel, but its density is the same as that of dentin. In the hypocalcified forms the enamel thickness is normal but its density is even less than that of dentin. With advanced abrasion, obliteration of the pulp chambers may complicate recognition of the radiographic picture.

Differential diagnosis. If there is advanced abrasion and secondary dentin obliterates the pulp chambers, the radiographic picture of the amelogenesis imperfecta appears similar to that of dentinogenesis imperfecta. However, the presence of bulbous crowns and narrow roots, the relatively normal density of any remaining enamel, and the obliteration of pulp chambers and root canals, in the absence of marked attrition, should distinguish dentinogenesis imperfecta (see below) from amelogenesis imperfecta.

Management. Appropriate treatment for amelogenesis imperfecta is restoration of the esthetics and function of the affected teeth.

DENTINOGENESIS IMPERFECTA

Dentinogenesis imperfecta (also called *hereditary opalescent dentin**) is a developmental disturbance primarily of the dentin. Enamel may be thinner than normal in this condition. Dentinogenesis imperfecta is an autosomal dominant disturbance of high penetrance and occurs with equal frequency in both sexes.[52,54] Both the deciduous and the permanent dentition may show this defect. It usually affects whites.[51]

There are two types of dentinogenesis imperfecta.[57] Type I is associated with osteogenesis imperfecta.† The tooth roots and pulp chambers are generally small and underdeveloped. It affects the primary dentition more severely than the permanent teeth. Type II lesions are similar to Type I lesions but affect only the dentin without any skeletal defects. The expression of Type II lesions is variable, and occasionally individuals will show enlarged pulp chambers in the primary teeth.

Clinical features. The appearance of the teeth with dentinogenesis imperfecta is characteristic. They show a high degree of amberlike translucency and a variety of colors from yellow to blue gray. The colors change according to whether the teeth are observed by transmitted light or reflected light.[51] The enamel easily fractures from the teeth and the crowns wear readily. In adults they may frequently wear down to the gingiva. The exposed dentin becomes stained. The color of the abraded teeth may change to dark brown or even black.

---

*Although the terms "dentinogenesis imperfecta" and "hereditary opalescent dentin" have been used interchangeably for more than 40 years, there is evidence[56] that suggests they are two distinct entities. Dentinogenesis imperfecta is the dental defect that accompanies osteogenesis imperfecta whereas hereditary opalescent dentin is an isolated defect.[57] Because these conditions share common clinical, radiographic, and dental features, we refer to the defect for convenience as dentinogenesis imperfecta, which is the term that most dentists associate with this condition.

†Osteogenesis imperfecta is a hereditary disorder characterized by osseous fractures. It is usually transmitted as an autosomal dominant trait. Patients may have blue sclerae, wormian bones, skeletal deformities, and progressive osteopenia. In addition to dentinogenesis imperfecta, oral findings may include class III malocclusions and an increased incidence of impacted first and second molars.[41] The pathogenesis is believed to be in some cases an inborn error of collagen metabolism.[30]

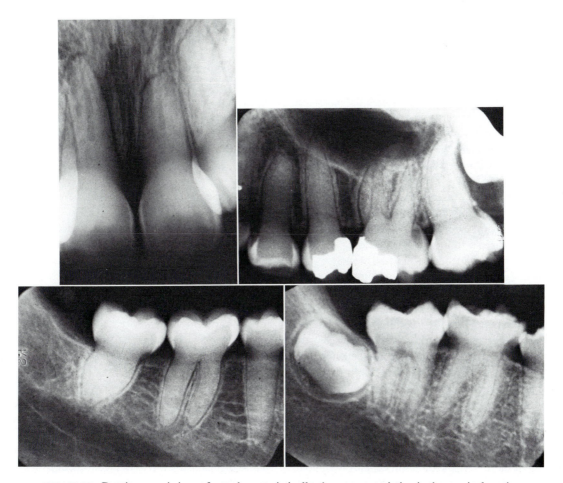

FIG. 17-26. Dentinogenesis imperfecta characteristically shows a constriction in the cervical portion of the root, a bulbous crown, short roots, and a reduced size of the pulp chamber and root canals.

Some patients will demonstrate an anterior open bite.

Radiographic features. The images of the crowns in patients with dentinogenesis imperfecta are usually of normal size, but a constriction of the cervical portion of the tooth gives them a bulbous appearance. Radiographs may reveal slight to marked attrition of the occlusal surface. The roots are usually short and slender. Types I and II show partial or complete obliteration of the pulp chambers. The root canals may be absent or threadlike (Fig. 17-26). Occasional periapical radiolucencies are seen in association with sound teeth without evidence of pulpal involvement. These lesions do not occur as frequently as in dentin dysplasia. The architecture of the bone in the maxilla and mandible is normal.

Differential diagnosis. See under the differential diagnosis of dentin dysplasia (below).

Management. Crowning affected teeth is usu-

ally unsuccessful unless they have good root support. The teeth should not be extracted from patients 5 to 15 years of age. It is generally preferred to place full overdentures over the teeth to prevent alveolar resorption. In adults extraction of the teeth and their replacement can be recommended. Alveolectomy may be required in these latter cases.[56]

DENTIN DYSPLASIA

Dentin dysplasia is an autosomal dominant trait that resembles opalescent dentin. It is rarer than dentinogenesis imperfecta (1:100,000 compared to 1:8,000).[53,56] Two types have been described[43,57]: Type I (radicular) and Type II (coronal) dentin dysplasia. In Type I disease the most marked alterations are found in the appearance of the roots. In Type II disease changes in the crown are most clearly seen in the altered shape of the pulp chambers.

Clinical features. Clinically, teeth with dentin dysplasia have characteristic features:

In the radicular pattern (Type I) there will be mostly normal color and shape in both dentitions. Occasionally a slight bluish brown translucency is apparent.[58] The teeth in patients with the Type I defect are often malaligned in the arch, and the patient may describe drifting and state that the teeth exfoliate with little or no trauma.

In the coronal pattern (Type II) the crowns of primary teeth appear to be of the same color, size, and contour as those in dentinogenesis imperfecta. The permanent teeth will be normal in these respects. Apparently there are no other distinctive clinical features, although some authors[55] contend that the primary teeth, in keeping with their appearance, rapidly abrade; nevertheless, others[34] have not found evidence of unusual wear.

Radiographic features. The radiographic images of radicular and coronal dentin dysplasia demonstrate the appropriateness of the names.

In Type I the roots of all teeth, primary and permanent, are either short or abnormally shaped (Fig. 17-27). The roots of primary teeth may be only spicules. The pulp chambers and root canals completely fill in before eruption. The extent of obliteration of the pulp chambers and canals is variable.[25] In addition, about 20% of teeth with Type I disease have periapical radiolucencies, which are described[25] as either cysts or granulomas. Association of these periapical radiolucencies with noncarious teeth is an important feature for recognition of this particular entity.[37]

The changes most apparent in coronal dentin dysplasia (Type II) are obliteration of the pulp chamber and reduced root canals that occur after eruption (at least by 5 or 6 years).[2] These changes are not seen before eruption. As the chambers of the molars are being filled with hypertrophic dentin, the pulp chambers may become flame shaped. Occasionally the anterior teeth and premolars develop a pulp chamber that is thistle-tube in shape because of its extension into the root. The roots of the coronal variety are normal in shape and proportions.

Differential diagnosis. The differential diagnosis for dentin dysplasia may include only one other entity, dentinogenesis imperfecta. Because these two conditions seem to form a continuum, their differentiation may be difficult at first. Both entities can have altered color and occluded pulp chambers. In Type II dentin dysplasia, however, the pulp chambers do not fill in before eruption. Also finding a thistle-tube–shaped pulp chamber in a single-rooted tooth strengthens the probability

of dentin dysplasia. In addition, crown size can help distinguish between the two: the teeth in dentinogenesis imperfecta have typical bell-shaped crowns with a constriction in the cervical region whereas the crowns in dentin dysplasia are usually of normal shape, size, and proportions. If the roots are short and narrow, the condition is likely to be dentinogenesis imperfecta. On the other hand, normal-appearing roots or practically no roots at all should suggest dentin dysplasia. Periapical rarefactions in association with noncarious teeth are strong presumptive evidence that the condition is dentin dysplasia.

Management. Teeth with Type I dentin dysplasia have such poor root support that prosthetic replacement is about the only course practical. On the other hand, teeth that are of normal shape, size, and support (Type II) can be crowned if they seem to be rapidly abrading. At the same time the esthetics of discolored anterior teeth can be improved by crowning or by restoring the surfaces.

REGIONAL ODONTODYSPLASIA

Regional odontodysplasia (also known as *odontogenesis imperfecta*) is a relatively rare condition in which both enamel and dentin are hypoplastic and hypocalcified. The result is localized arrest in tooth development. Typically regional odontodysplasia affects only a few adjacent teeth in a quadrant. They may be either primary or permanent teeth. If the primary teeth are affected, their successors will usually be involved. Central incisors are most often affected, with lateral incisors and canines also occasionally showing the defect (most often in the maxilla). Eruption of the defective teeth is often delayed. Although there are many theories as to the etiology of this condition, its cause is unknown.[4]

Clinical features. Teeth affected with regional odontodysplasia are small and mottled brown as a result of staining of the hypocalcified hypoplastic enamel. They are especially susceptible to caries, are brittle, and are subject to fracture and the pulpal infection resulting from either. In severe cases they may not erupt.

Radiographic features. The radiographic images of teeth with regional odontodysplasia have a ghostlike appearance. The pulp chambers are large and the root canals wide because the hypoplastic dentin is thin, just serving to outline the image of the root (Fig. 17-28). The poorly outlined roots are short. The enamel is, likewise, thin and less dense than usual, sometimes so thin and poorly

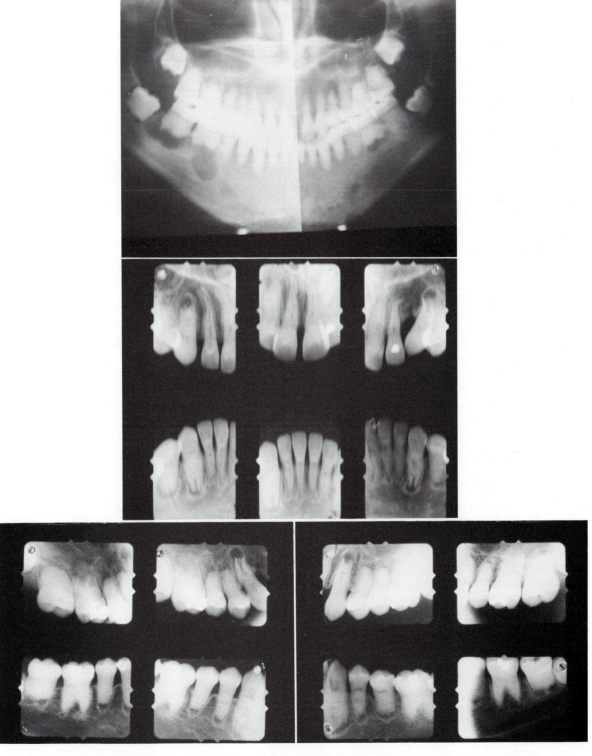

FIG. 17-27. Dentin dysplasia, Type I (radicular), showing the short and poorly developed roots, the obliterated pulp chambers and root canals, and the pathognomonic radiolucencies associated with noncarious teeth (panoramic and periapical radiographs). (Courtesy Dr. Ralph Nothhelfer, Detroit.)

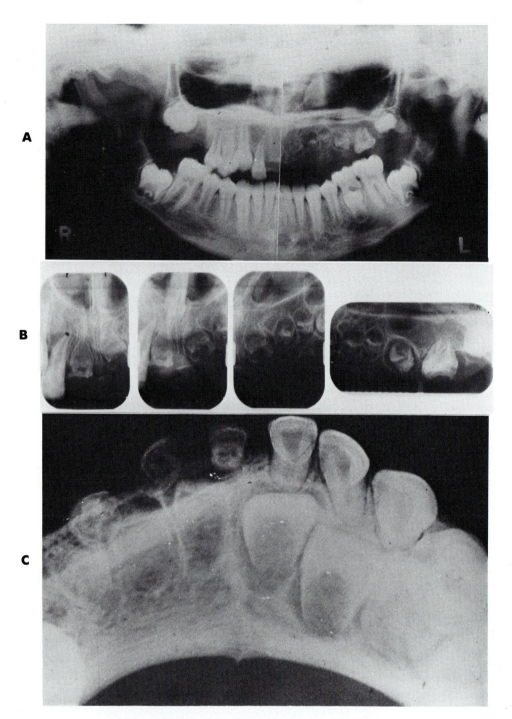

FIG. 17-28. Odontodysplasia revealing poor mineralization of both the enamel and the dentin. **A** and **B,** Note the involvement of the left maxilla. **C,** There is involvement also of the primary and secondary dentitions.

d f   *l d*

mineralized that it may not be evident on the radiograph. The tooth is little more than a thin shell of hypoplastic enamel and dentin. Teeth that do not erupt are so hypomineralized and hypoplastic that they appear to be resorbing.

Differential diagnosis. The malformed teeth[2] occasionally seen in one of the expressions of dentinogenesis imperfecta may occasionally be confused with those in regional odontodysplasia. The fact that the dentinogenesis imperfecta trait usually carries a history of familial involvement, however, in contrast to odontodysplasia (which is not hereditary), is an important distinguishing feature. Also the enamel in regional odontodysplasia is obviously hypoplastic, which is not the case in dentinogenesis imperfecta. Finally, only a few teeth of either dentition in an isolated segment of the arch will be affected in regional odontodysplasia, whereas the type of dentinogenesis imperfecta that resembles regional odontodysplasia involves all primary teeth.

Management. With the advent of newer restorative materials it is recommended to retain and restore the affected teeth as much as possible. Unerupted teeth should be retained during the period of skeletal growth. Severely damaged permanent teeth that become pulpally involved may require removal and replacement.

ENAMEL PEARL

The enamel pearl (also known as an *enamel drop, enamel nodule,* or *enameloma*) is a small globule of enamel 1 to 3 mm in diameter that occurs on the roots of molars (Fig. 17-29). It is found in about 3% of the population,[21] probably formed by Hertwig's epithelial root sheath before the epithelium loses its enamel-forming potential. Enamel pearls generally develop at the trifurcation of a maxillary molar (usually third molar) or the bifurcation of a mandibular molar. Some lie at or just apical to the cementoenamel junction. Those that form on the maxillary molars are usually at the mesial or distal aspect, in contrast to those on the mandibular molars, which are most often buccal or lingual. Usually only one pearl develops, but occasionally there will be more. Enamel pearls may have a core of dentin and rarely a pulp horn extending from the chamber of the host tooth. Their presence is of limited clinical importance, although they may promote periodontal pocket development and subsequent periodontal disease.[60]

Clinical features. Most enamel pearls form below the crest of the gingiva and are not detected during a clinical examination. There are usually no clinical symptoms associated with their presence although they may predispose to periodontal pocket formation.

Radiographic features. The enamel pearl will appear smooth, round, and comparable in radiodensity to the enamel over the crown. When projected over the crown of the tooth, it may be obscured or mistaken for a pulp stone. If it is at the cementoenamel junction, its image may be confused with that of calculus.[42]

Differential diagnosis. It is possible to mistake an enamel pearl for an isolated piece of calculus or a pulp stone. The differentiation between a pulp stone and an enamel pearl can be made by increasing the angle of projection to interpose the image of some root between the pulp chamber and the enamel pearl. If the opacity is calculus, it will usually be clinically detectable.

Management. As a rule the recognition that an opacity superimposed on the tooth is an enamel pearl will preclude the necessity for treatment. The clinician can remove the mass if its location at the cementoenamel junction predisposes to periodontal disease. The possibility must always be considered that it may contain a pulp horn.

TALON CUSP

The talon cusp is an anomalous hyperplasia of the cingulum of a maxillary or mandibular incisor. It results in the formation of a supernumerary cusp. When viewed from its incisal edge an incisor bearing the cusp is T shaped.[29] Normal enamel covers the cusp and fuses with the lingual aspect of the tooth. There may be developmental grooves that become caries-susceptible areas. The cusp may or may not contain an extension (horn) of the pulp.

Clinical features. The talon cusp is infrequently encountered. It may be found in either sex and on both primary and permanent incisors,[22] It varies in size from that of a prominent cingulum to that of a cusplike structure extending to the level of the incisal edge. There does not appear to be a racial association. Although it usually occurs as an isolated entity, its incidence has been reported to be increased in teeth related to cleft palate[17] and in association with other anomalies.[22]

Radiographic features. The image of a talon cusp is usually superimposed radiographically on that of the incisor on which it occurs (Fig. 17-30). Its outline is smooth, and a layer of normal-appearing enamel is generally distinguishable. The radiograph may not reveal a pulp horn. The cusp

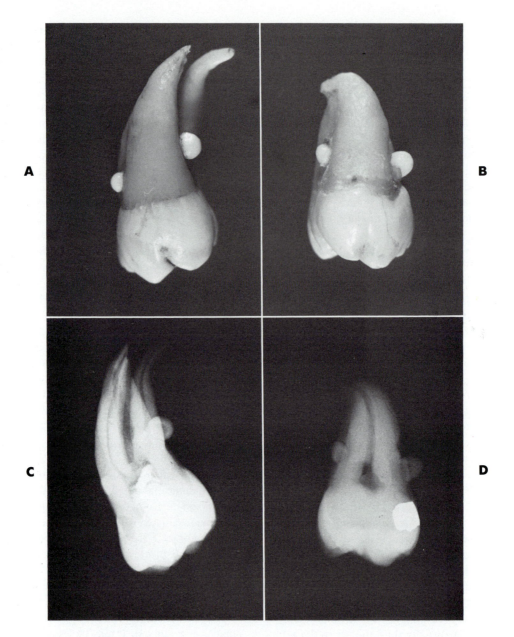

FIG. 17-29. **A** and **B,** Enamel pearls are small outgrowths of enamel and dentin seen in the furcation area of a tooth. **C** and **D,** Radiographs of these teeth. (**A** to **D** courtesy Dr. R. Kienholz, Dallas.)

is often apparent radiographically before eruption and may suggest the presence of a supernumerary tooth. Another radiograph obtained with a different horizontal angulation may be needed to rule out this possibility.

Differential diagnosis. The appearance of a talon cusp is quite distinctive, and an awareness of this entity usually assures its recognition. Although it may not be radiographically distinguishable from a supernumerary tooth, the tube-shift

technique can demonstrate its close association with the tooth.

Management. If developmental grooves are present where the cusp fuses with the lingual surface of the incisor, a prophylactic restoration may be in order, depending on the individual's oral hygiene. If the cusp is large, it may pose an esthetic or occlusal problem. Slowly removing the cusp may remedy this situation by permitting the formation of secondary dentin and preventing expo-

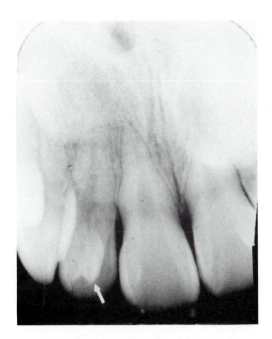

FIG. 17-30. Maxillary lateral incisor bearing a talon cusp (*arrow*). Note that the tooth also has two enamel invaginations. (Courtesy Dr. R.A. Cederberg, Dallas.)

sure of a pulp horn. Mechanical exposure of such a pulpal extension will require endodontic treatment.

TURNER'S HYPOPLASIA

"Turner's hypoplasia" (also known as *Turner's tooth*) is a term used to describe a permanent tooth with a local hypoplastic defect in its crown. This defect may have been caused by the extension of a periapical infection from its deciduous predecessor or by mechanical trauma transmitted through the deciduous tooth. If the trauma (whether infectious or mechanical) takes place while the crown is forming, it may adversely affect the ameloblasts of the developing tooth and result in some degree of enamel hypoplasia or hypomineralization.

Clinical features. Turner's hypoplasia most often affects the mandibular premolars,[42] generally because of the relative susceptibility of the deciduous molars to caries, their proximity to the developing premolars, and their relative time of mineralization. The severity of the defect depends on the severity of the infection or mechanical trauma and on the stage of development of the permanent tooth.[50] It may disturb matrix formation or calcification, in which case the result will vary from a

hypoplastic defect to a hypomineralized spot in the enamel. The hypomineralized area may become stained, and the tooth will usually show a brownish spot on the crown. If the insult is severe enough to cause hypoplasia, the morphology of the crown may show pitting or a more pronounced defect. The hypoplastic defect may contain cementum, which may also be stained a yellowish brown.

Radiographic features. The enamel irregularities associated with Turner's hypoplasia that alter the normal contours of the affected tooth will be apparent on a radiograph (Fig. 17-31). A stained hypomineralized spot will not be apparent because the difference in its relative radiodensity is probably not detectable by routine radiographic techniques. Also the hypomineralized areas may become remineralized by continued contact with saliva.

Differential diagnosis. An image of a single tooth (usually a premolar or a maxillary incisor) with a deformed crown or a defect in a portion of the crown is characteristic of Turner's hypoplasia. A carious lesion on an otherwise normal tooth will not cause the malformation seen in a Turner's tooth.

Management. If the radiograph of a tooth affected by Turner's hypoplasia shows that the tooth has good root support, the esthetics and function of the deformed crown can be restored.

CONGENITAL SYPHILIS

About 30% of people with congenital syphilis develop dental hypoplasia that involves the permanent incisors and first molars.[38] Development of primary teeth is seldom disturbed. The affected incisors are called *Hutchinson's teeth,* and the molars *mulberry molars.* The changes characteristic of the condition seem to result from a direct infection of the developing tooth, because the spirochete of syphilis has been identified in the tooth germ.[3]

Clinical features. The affected incisor has a characteristic screwdriver-shaped crown, with the mesial and distal surfaces tapering from the middle of the crown to the incisal edge (Fig. 17-32). The effect is that the edge may be no wider than the cervical area of the tooth. The incisal edge is also frequently notched. Although maxillary central incisors usually demonstrate these syphilitic changes, the maxillary lateral and mandibular central incisors may also be involved.

As with incisor crowns, the crowns of affected first molars are quite characteristic, being usually

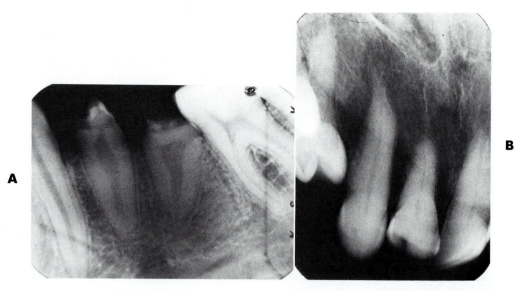

FIG. 17-31. A, Turner's hypoplasia, demonstrated as an extensive malformation and hypomineralization of the crowns of both premolars. **B,** Defect in the incisal edge of the lateral incisor, with rotation of the central incisor following trauma to the primary dentition. (**B** courtesy Dr. William Brown, Dallas.)

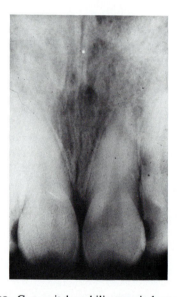

FIG. 17-32. Congenital syphilis may induce a developmental malformation of the maxillary central incisors characterized by tapering of the mesial and distal surfaces toward the incisal edge with notching of the incisal edge.

smaller than normal and maybe even smaller than second molar crowns.[53] The most distinctive feature is the constricted occlusal third of the crown, with the occlusal surface no wider than the cervical portion of the tooth. The cusps of these molars are also reduced in size and poorly formed. The enamel over the occlusal surface is hypoplastic, unevenly formed in irregular globules, like the surface of a mulberry. Some patients with congenital syphilis will have a defect that resembles a hypoplastic type of amelogenesis imperfecta.[46] Not all patients with Hutchinson's incisors or mulberry molars will have congenital syphilis, however, and some who do will not have the dental changes.[42]

Radiographic features. The characteristic shapes of the affected incisor and molar crowns can be identified on radiographs. Because the crowns of these teeth form at about 1 year of age, radiographs may reveal the dental features of congenital syphilis 4 to 5 years before the teeth erupt.

Differential diagnosis. Because the shape and size of Hutchinson's teeth and mulberry molars are so characteristic, there is little chance of confusion with other dental abnormalities. When the hypoplasia is not characteristic, other lesions exist that are indicative of the condition, especially when a number occur in concert.[42]

Management. Hutchinson's teeth and mulberry molars often do not require dental treatment. Esthetic restorations may be used to correct the hypoplastic defects as indicated clinically.

SPECIFIC REFERENCES

1. al-Emran S: Prevalence of hypodontia and developmental malformation of permanent teeth in Saudi Arabian school children, *Br J Orthod* 17(2):115-118, 1990.
2. Bixler D: Heritable disorders effecting dentin. In Steward RE, Prescott GA (eds): *Oral facial genetics,* St Louis, 1976, Mosby.
3. Bradlaw RV: Dental stigmata of prenatal syphilis, *Oral Surg* 6:147-158, 1953.
4. Crawford PJ, Aldred MJ: Regional odontodysplasia: a bibliography *J Oral Pathol Med* 18(5):251-263, 1989.
5. Crawford PJ, Aldred MJ: X-linked amelogenesis imperfecta: presentation of two kindreds and a review of the literature, *Oral Surg* 73(4):449-455, 1992.
6. Dixon GH, Stewart RE: Genetic aspects of anomalous tooth development. In Steward RE, Prescott GH (eds): *Oral facial genetics,* St Louis, 1976, Mosby.
7. Garn SM, Lewis AB: The relationship between third molar agenesis and reduction in tooth number, *Angle Orthod* 32:14-18, 1962.
8. Garn SM, Lewis AB, Kerewsky BS: The magnitude and implications of the relationship between tooth size and body size, *Arch Oral Biol* 13:129-131, 1968.
9. Gorlin RJ: Orofaciodigital syndrome. In Bergsma D (ed): *Birth defects compendium,* ed 2, New York, 1979, Alan R Liss.
10. Grahnen H, Lindahl B: Supernumerary teeth in the permanent dentition: a frequency study, *Odontol Rev* 12:290-294, 1961.
11. Grimanis GA, Kyriakides AT, Spyropoulos ND: A survey on supernumerary molars, *Quintess Int* 22(12):989-995, 1991.
12. Hagman FT: Anomalies of form and number, fused primary teeth, a correlation of the dentitions, *J Dent Child* 55(5):359-361, 1988.
13. Keene HJ: The relationship between third molar agenesis and the morphologic variability of the molar teeth, *Angle Orthod* 35:289-298, 1965.
14. Levin LS: Dental and oral abnormalities in selected ectodermal dysplasia syndromes, *Birth Defects* 24(2):205-227, 1988.
15. McCarter TJ: Dens in dente. In Bergsma, D (ed): *Birth defects compendium,* ed 2, New York, 1979, Alan R Liss.
16. Meskin LH: Macrodontia: In Bergsma D (ed): *Birth defects compendium,* ed 2, New York, 1979, Alan R Liss.
17. Meskin LH, Gorlin RJ: Agenesis and peg-shaped permanent lateral incisors, *J Dent Res* 42:1476-1479, 1963.
18. Messer LB, Cline JT: Fused teeth. In Bergsma D (ed): *Birth defects compendium,* ed 2, New York, 1979, Alan R Liss.
19. Messer LB, Cline JT, Walker PO: Geminated teeth. In Bergsma D (ed): *Birth defects compendium,* ed 2, New York, 1979, Alan R Liss.
20. Messer LB, McKibben DH: Concrescence of tooth roots. In Bergsma D (ed): *Birth defects compendium,* ed 2, New York, 1979, Alan R Liss.
21. Moskow BS, Canut PM: Studies on root enamel. II. Enamel pearls: a review of their morphology, localization, nomenclature, occurrence, classification, histogenesis, and incidence, *J Clin Periodontol* 17(5):275-281, 1990.
22. Natkin E, Pitts DL, Worthington P: A case of talon cusp associated with other odontogenic abnormalities, *J Endod* 9:491-495, 1983.
23. Niswander JD: Effects of hereditary and environment on development of the dentition, *J Dent Res* 42:1288-1296, 1963.
24. Niswander JD, Suyaku C: Congenital anomalies in Japanese children, *Am J Phys Anthropol* 21:569-574, 1963.
25. O Carroll MK, Duncan WK, Perkins TM: Dentin dysplasia: review of the literature and a proposed subclassification based on radiographic findings, *Oral Surg* 72(1):119-125, 1991.
26. O'Dowling IB, McNamara TG: Congenital absence of permanent teeth among Irish school-children, *J Ir Dent Assoc* 36(4):136-138, 1990.
27. Oehlers FAC: The radicular variety of dens invaginatus, *Oral Surg* 11:1251-1260, 1958.
28. Oehlers FA, Lee KW, Lee EC: Dens evaginatus (evaginated odontome), *Dent Pract* 17:239-244, 1967.
29. Pindborg JJ: *Pathology of the dental hard tissues,* Philadelphia, 1970, WB Saunders.
30. Prockop DJ, Kirvirikko KI, Tuderman L, Guzman NA: The biosynthesis of collagen and its disorders. I and II, *N Engl J Med* 301:13-23, 77-85, 1979.
31. Putkonen P: Dental changes in congenital syphilis, *Acta Dermatol Venereol* 42:44-62, 1962.
32. Rao SR: Supernumerary teeth. In Bergsma D (ed): *Birth defects compendium,* ed 2, New York, 1979, Alan R Liss.
33. Rao SR, Witkop CJ: Microdontia. In Bergsma D (ed): *Birth defects compendium,* ed 2, New York, 1979, Alan R Liss.
34. Richardson AS, Fantin TD: Occlusal anomalous dysplasia of dentin: report of a case, *J Can Dent Assoc* 36:189-191, 1970.
35. Rosengweig K, Gabarski D: Numerical aberration in the permanent teeth of grade school children in Jerusalem, *Am J Phys Anthropol* 23:277-284, 1965.
36. Rushton MA: A collection of dilated composite odontomes, *Br Dent* 63:65-68, 1937.
37. Rushton MA: A case report of dentinal dysplasia. *Guys Hosp Rep* 89:369-373, 1939.
38. Sarnat BG, Shaw NG: Dental development in congenital syphilis, *Am J Orthod* 29:270-284, 1943.
39. Schacter H: A treated case of transposed upper canine, *Dent Res* 71:105-108, 1951.
40. Schulze C: Developmental abnormalities of the teeth and jaws. In Gorlin RJ, Goldman HM (eds): *Thoma's Oral pathology,* ed 6, St Louis, 1970, Mosby, vol 1.
41. Schwartz S, Tsipouras P: Oral findings in osteogenesis imperfecta, *Oral Surg* 57:161-167, 1984.
42. Shafer WG, Hine MK, Levy BM: *Oral pathology,* ed 4, Philadelphia, 1983, WB Saunders.
43. Shields EP, Bixler D, El-Kafraevy AM: A proposed classification for heritable human dentin defects with a description of a new entity, *Arch Oral Biol* 18:543-553, 1973.
44. Soames JV, Kuyebi TA: A radicular dens invaginatus, *Br Dent J* 152:308-309, 1982.
45. Sperber GH: Genetic mechanisms and anomalies in odontogenesis, *J Can Dent Assoc* 33:433-442, 1967.
46. Stafne EC, Gibilisco JA: *Oral roentgenographic diagnosis,* ed 4, Philadelphia, 1975, WB Saunders.
47. Sykaras SN: Occlusal anomalous tubercle on premolars of a Greek girl, *Oral Surg* 38:88-91, 1974.
48. Tannenbaum KA, Alling EE: Anomalous tooth development: case report of germination and twinning, *Oral Surg* 16:883-887, 1963.

49. Toller PA: A clinical report of six cases of amelogenesis imperfecta, *Oral Surg* 12:325-333, 1959.

50. Via WF Jr: Enamel defects induced by trauma during tooth formation, *Oral Surg* 25:49-54, 1968.

51. Winter GB: Hereditary and idiopathic anomalies of tooth number, structure, and form, *Dent Clin North Am* 13:355-373, 1969.

52. Witkop CJ Jr: Hereditary defects in enamel and dentin. Proceedings of the First International Congress on Human Genetics, *Acta Genet Stat Med* 7:236-239, 1957.

53. Witkop CJ Jr: Hereditary defects of dentin, *Dent Clin North Am* 19:25-45, 1975.

54. Witkop CJ Jr: Amelogenesis imperfecta. In Bergsma D (ed): editor: *Birth defects compendium,* ed 2, New York, 1979, Alan R Liss.

55. Witkop CJ Jr: Dentin dysplasia, coronal. In Bergsma D (ed): *Birth defects compendium,* ed 2, New York, 1979, Alan R Liss.

56. Witkop CJ Jr: Dentinogenesis imperfecta. In Bergsma D (ed): *Birth defects compendium,* ed 2, New York, 1979, Alan R Liss.

57. Witkop CJ Jr: Amelogenesis imperfecta, dentinogenesis imperfecta and dentin dysplasia revisited: problems in classification, *J Oral Pathol* 17(9-10):547-553, 1988.

58. Witkop CJ Jr, Rao S: Inherited defects in tooth structure. In Bergsma D (ed): *Birth defects.* XI. *Orofacial structures,* Baltimore, 1971, Williams & Wilkins, vol 7, no 7.

59. Witkop CJ Jr, Saulk JJ: Heritable defects of enamel. In Stewart RE, Prescott GA (eds): *Oral facial genetics,* St Louis, 1976, Mosby.

60. Worth HM: *Principles and practice of oral radiologic interpretation,* Chicago, 1963, Year Book Medical Publishers.

61. Yip WW: The prevalence of dens evaginatus, *Oral Surg* 38:80-87, 1974.

62. Yusof WZ: Non-syndrome multiple supernumerary teeth: literature review, *J Can Dent Assoc* 56:147-149, 1990.

18

Regressive Changes of the Dentition

A number of acquired degenerative changes affect the dentition. Such changes may be of no clinical significance or may compromise the involved teeth so severely that they are lost if the precipitating cause is not identified and eliminated. This chapter describes the more common and important of these degenerative changes.

ATTRITION

Attrition is the physiologic wearing away of the dentition resulting from occlusal contacts between the teeth during chewing. It occurs on the incisal, occlusal, and interproximal surfaces. Interproximal wear causes the contact points to become flattened into interproximal surfaces. Attrition may play important physiologic roles. It helps maintain an advantageous crown-to-root ratio by reducing the coronal height when there is a loss of alveolar bone from periodontal disease. It also gains intercoronal space (possibly as much as 1 cm) around the arch, which facilitates third molar eruption.[17] Attrition occurs in over 90% of young adults and is generally more severe in men than women.[23] Its extent depends on the abrasiveness of the diet,[22] salivary factors,[26] mineralization of the teeth,[20] occupations such as farming (e.g., excessive grit in the air can enter the oral cavity),[11] and emotional tension.[23] Physiologic attrition is a component of the aging process. When the loss of dental tissue becomes excessive, however, as from bruxism, the attrition becomes pathologic.

Clinical features. The clinically observable wear caused by attrition develops in a predictable progressive pattern. Wear facets first appear on cusps and marginal oblique and transverse ridges. The incisal edges of the maxillary and mandibular incisors, in turn, start to show evidence of broadening. The wear facets on the occlusal surfaces of molars become more pronounced, with the lingual cusps of maxillary teeth and the buccal cusps of

mandibular posteriors showing the most wear. When the dentin is exposed, it usually becomes stained and the color contrast between stained dentin and enamel highlights the areas of attrition. The incisal edges of mandibular incisors tend to become pitted because the dentin wears more rapidly than its surrounding enamel. In the case of pathologic attrition the patterns of wear are generally not as uniformly progressive as those described for physiologic attrition. The wear facets develop at a higher rate, and the areas of distribution are different. It is important to emphasize, however, that "physiologic attrition" is a relative term and its clinical manifestations will vary with the customs (dietary and otherwise) of the population in question.

Radiographic features. The radiographic appearance of attrition is a smooth wearing of the incisal and occlusal surfaces of the involved teeth. There is a shortened image of the crown with absence of opaque enamel on the involved surfaces (Fig. 18-1). Often a number of adjacent teeth in each arch will show this wear pattern. Sclerosis of the pulp chambers and canals may occur since attrition stimulates the deposition of secondary dentin. This narrows or obliterates the pulp canals and chambers. There is also frequently a simultaneous loss of alveolar bone, and even some widening of the periodontal ligament space or hypercementosis.

Differential diagnosis. Recognition of physiologic attrition is usually not difficult given the characteristic history, location, and extent of wear. The general pattern is predictable and familiar.

Management. Physiologic attrition does not require treatment. On the contrary, it may likely mitigate periodontal disease by eliminating cuspal interference (producing a free-sliding occlusion) and reducing lateral stresses on the periodontium. It may also minimize caries by modifying or eliminating the susceptible pits and fissures.

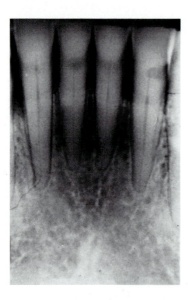

FIG. 18-1. Attrition is the physiologic wearing away of tooth structure during mastication. Note the wearing of incisal edges of these lower incisors plus the secondary pulpal sclerosis.

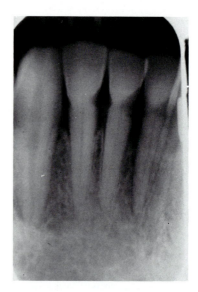

FIG. 18-2. Abrasion of the cervical portion of these teeth is evident from excessive (and improper) use of dental floss. Note the pulpal sclerosis.

ABRASION

Abrasion is the nonphysiologic wearing away of teeth by contact with foreign substances. It results from friction induced by habits or occupational hazards. A clinical examination will usually readily reveal it. Although there are many causes, two occur with moderate frequency and can usually be eliminated[6,15]: that from improper tooth brushing and that from dental floss. Other causes include pipe smoking,[1] opening hair pins with the teeth, improper use of toothpicks, and cutting thread with the teeth.[1]

Toothbrush injury

Clinical features. Toothbrush abrasion is probably the most frequently observed type and is usually the result of improper technique, most frequently a back-and-forth movement of the brush with heavy pressure. This causes the bristles to assume a wedge-shaped arrangement between the crowns and the gingiva. The brushing wears a V-shaped groove into the cervical area of the tooth, usually involving enamel and the softer root surface. Abraded teeth may become sensitive as the dentin is exposed. The abraded areas are usually most severe at the cementoenamel junction on the labiobuccal surfaces of maxillary premolars, canines, and incisors, in about that order.[20] The enamel generally limits the coronal extension of

abrasion. The lesions are more common and more pronounced on the left side for a right-handed person, and vice versa.[8] The deposition of secondary dentin opposite the abraded areas usually keeps pace with the destruction at the surface, so pulpal exposure is rarely a complication.

Radiographic features. The radiographic appearance of toothbrush abrasion is radiolucent defects at the cervical level of teeth. These defects have well-defined semilunar shapes with borders of increasing density. The pulp chambers of the more seriously involved teeth are frequently partially or completely sclerosed. The most common location of this injury is in the premolar areas usually in the upper arch.

Dental floss injury

Clinical features. Excessive and improper use of dental floss, particularly in conjunction with a toothpaste, may result in abrasion of the dentition[15] (Fig. 18-2). The most frequent site is the cervical portion of the proximal surfaces just above the gingiva.

Radiographic features. The radiographic appearance of dental floss abrasion is narrow semilunar grooves, in the interproximal surfaces of buccal teeth near the cervical area. Most often the grooves on the distal surfaces of the teeth are deeper than those on the mesial surfaces, probably because it is easier to exert more pressure in a forward direction by pulling than by pushing the floss backward into the mouth.

Differential diagnosis. Dental floss abrasion is readily identified by its clinical and radiographic appearance. Its location will provide some evidence as to the nature of the cause. This can be verified by the patient history.

Management. The primary treatment recommended for abrasion is elimination of the causative agents or habits. Extensively abraded areas can be restored, but this may involve removing a considerable amount of tooth substance. Restoration of the defect will probably not add to the support of the tooth but will improve esthetic appearance and reduce the susceptibility of the area to caries.

EROSION

Erosion of teeth results from a chemical action not involving bacteria. Although in many cases the cause is not apparent, in others it is obviously the contact of acid with teeth. The source of the acid may be (1) chronic vomiting or acid reflux from gastrointestinal disorders[11] or (2) the diet when the individual consumes large amounts of acidic foods, citrus fruits, or carbonated beverages.[30] Some occupations involve contact with acids that can induce dental erosion. The location of the erosion, the pattern of eroded areas, and the appearance of the lesion will usually provide a clue as to the origin of the decalcifying agent. Regurgitated acids attack lingual surfaces; dietary acids primarily demineralize labial surfaces. All surfaces are affected by industrial dental erosion.[5]

Clinical features. Dental erosion is usually found on incisors, often involving multiple teeth. The lesions are generally smooth glistening depressions in the enamel surface, frequently near the gingiva. Erosion may result in so much loss of enamel that a pink spot shows through the remaining enamel.

Radiographic features. Areas of erosion appear as radiolucent defects on the crown. Their margins may be either well-defined or diffuse. A clinical examination will usually resolve any questionable lesions.

Differential diagnosis. The diagnosis of erosion is based on the recognition of dished-out or V-shaped defects in the buccal and labial enamel and dentinal surfaces. The margins of a restoration may project above the remaining tooth surface.[22] The edges of lesions caused by erosion are usually more rounded off than those caused by abrasion.[11]

Management. As with abrasion, erosion is managed with identification and removal of the causative agent. If the cause is chronic vomiting from a psychologic disorder, then a daily fluoride rinse should be prescribed during counseling therapy.[11] If the cause is unknown, management depends solely on restoration of the defect. This will prevent additional damage, possible pulp exposure, and objectionable esthetic appearance.

RESORPTION

Resorption is classified as internal or external on the basis of the origin of the odontoclastic cells. External resorption originates outside the tooth and periodontal ligament whereas internal resorption begins internally from cells of the pulp. These two types produce changes that are radiographically distinct. The most appropriate treatment depends on their proper identification. The resorption discussed here is not that associated with the normal loss of deciduous teeth but that observed when the teeth have been subjected to unusual stimuli. Although the cause of many resorptive lesions is unknown, there is at least presumptive evidence that some lesions are the sequelae of chronic infection (inflammation),[21,32] excessive pressure and function,[4,19] or factors associated with local tumors and cysts.[7,24]

Internal resorption

Internal resorption is a condition starting in the pulp. The pulp chamber or root canal, or both, expand by resorbing the surrounding dentin. This condition may be transient and self-limiting or progressive. Although the cause of internal resorption is unknown, there is speculation that whatever the precipitating factor, it produces a vascular change in the pulp that involves an inflammation and the formation of granulation tissue. There is an accompanying metaplasia of normal connective tissue and macrophages to form osteoclast-like giant multinucleated odontoclasts. These lie in lacunae that scallop the resorbing wall of the pulp chamber or canal. Internal resorption has been reported to be initiated by acute trauma to the tooth,[25] direct and indirect pulp capping, pulpotomy,[3] enamel invagination,[12] and pulp polyps.[1]

Clinical features. Internal resorption may affect any tooth in either the primary or the secondary dentition. It occurs most frequently in permanent teeth, usually in central incisors and first and second molars,[1] beginning during the fourth and fifth decades and generally in men.[9] When the lesion is in the crown, it may expand until the crown shows a dark shadow. If the expanding pulp perforates the dentin and involves the enamel, it may appear as a pink spot; and if the condition is not intercepted, it may perforate the crown, with hemorrhagic tissue projecting from the perforation, and lead to infectious pulpitis. When the lesion occurs in the root of a tooth, it is for the most part clinically silent. If the resorption is extensive, it may weaken the tooth and result in a fracture. It is also possible that the pulp may expand into the periodontal ligament and communicate with a deep periodontal pocket or the gingival sulcus, also leading to a pulpal infection. Internal resorption may cease enlarging at any time.

Radiographic features. Because internal resorption does not usually cause any subjective symptoms, early lesions are detected only radiographically. The lesion is radiolucent and round, oval, or elongated within the root. It causes a widening of the pulp chamber or canal (Fig. 18-3). It is characteristically homogeneous without bony trabeculation or pulp stones. The outline is sharply defined and smooth or slightly scalloped. In some cases virtually the whole pulp may enlarge within a tooth, although more commonly the lesion remains localized.

Differential diagnosis. The most common lesions to be confused with internal root resorption are dental caries on the buccal or lingual surface of a tooth and external root resorption. *Carious lesions* have more diffuse margins than lesions caused by internal root resorption. Clinical inspection will quickly reveal caries on the buccal or lingual surface of a tooth. The walls of the pulp canal or chamber are superimposed with the margins of the lesion. For the distinguishing contrasts between internal and external resorption, see the differential diagnosis section under external resorption (p. 374).

Management. The treatment for internal resorption depends on the tooth's condition. If the process has not led to a serious weakening defect in the structure, filling the root canal will halt the resorption. If the expanding pulp has not structurally compromised the tooth but a perforation of the root has occurred, the perforated surface can be surgically exposed and retrofilled. If the tooth has been badly excavated and weakened by the resorption, extraction may be the only alternative.

External resorption

External resorption begins on the surface of the root and is quite variable in appearance. It may appear at the apex or on the lateral root surface. Lesions on the lateral surface generally begin on a broad front or in a relatively small area of the root. The latter can invade cementum and dentin and produce an expanding excavated defect in the dentin. One form of external resorption, called *invasive* or *cervical resorption,* originates in the cervical area of a tooth.[2] Although it usually involves only one tooth, external resorption may occur in several. There are numerous causes—localized infection, reimplanted teeth, tumors and cysts, excessive mechanical (orthodontic) and occlusal forces, and impacted teeth. In many lesions the cause is unknown.

External resorption is slightly more prevalent in mandibular teeth than in maxillary teeth and involves primarily the central incisors, canines, and premolars.[31] Idiopathic root resorption is common. One study of 18- to 25-year-old men and women[14] found that all patients exhibited some degree of external root resorption in four or more teeth.

Clinical features. External resorption is usually not recognized, since there are often no characteristic signs or symptoms. Even when there is considerable loss of tooth structure, the tooth in question will frequently be firm and immobile in the dental arch. In advanced cases there may be some nonspecific pain or fracture of the resorbed root.[9]

Radiographic features. External root resorption usually involves the apices of teeth but on occasion will involve the lateral surfaces. When the lesion begins at the apex, it generally causes a smooth resorption of the tooth structure as it progresses occlusally (Fig. 18-4). Almost always the bone and lamina dura will follow the resorbing root and present a normal appearance around this shortened structure. External root resorption may, however, be caused by a periapical abscess or granuloma. In this case the lamina dura will be absent around the apex. Because the root canal is fully formed before the initiation of external root resorption, the lateral walls of the canal at the edge of the lesion will seem to be straight and not convergent near the apex, as with normal fully formed teeth.

Occasionally external root resorption involves the lateral aspects of roots (Fig. 18-5). Such lesions tend to be irregular, may involve one side more than the other, and occur in any tooth. A common cause of external resorption on the side of a root is the presence of an unerupted adjacent tooth. Examples of such include resorption of the distal aspect of the roots of an upper second molar by the

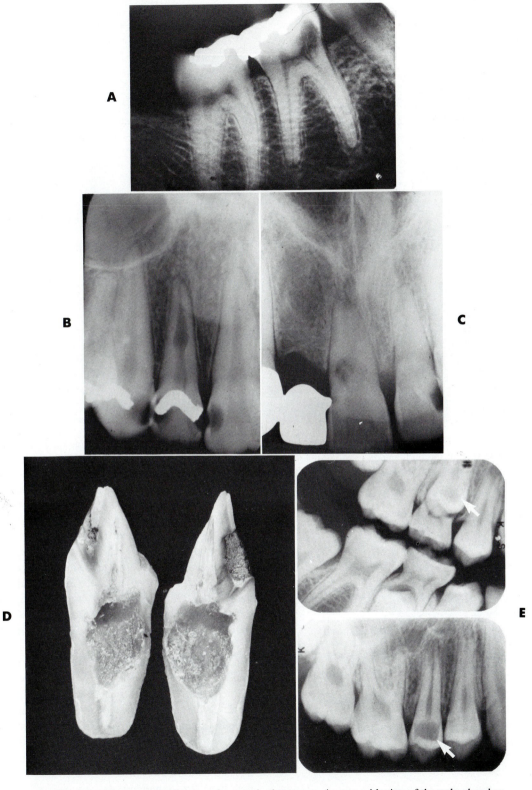

FIG. 18-3. Internal root resorption may be seen in the crown, **A,** as a widening of the pulp chamber or in the root, **B** and **C,** as widening of the pulp canal. In a sectioned incisor (after crown reduction), **D,** note the large area of internal root resorption. Internal resorption can also be seen in the crown of a second premolar, **E,** before eruption. (**D** courtesy Dr. R. Kienholz, Dallas.)

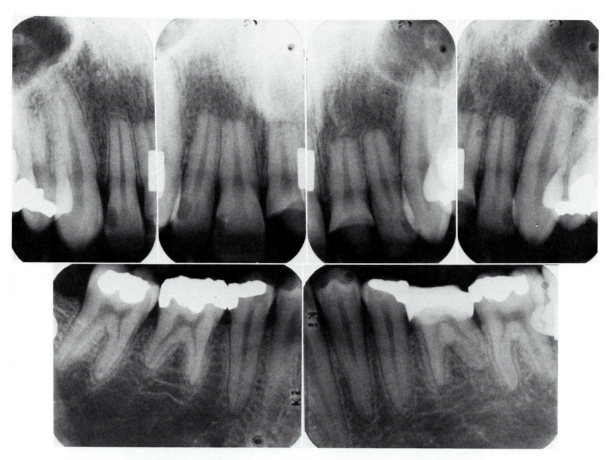

FIG. 18-4. External root resorption results in a loss of tooth structure from the apex. Note the wide openings of the pulp canals. The lamina dura is intact adjacent to the remaining tooth.

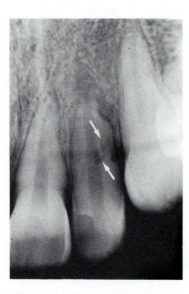

FIG. 18-5. External root resorption. Note the irregular radiolucent defects *(arrows)* associated wtih resorption on the buccal or palatal surface as well as at the apex.

crown of the adjacent third molar and resorption of the root of a permanent central or lateral incisor, or both, by an unerupted maxillary canine.

External resorption of an entire tooth can occur when the tooth is unerupted and completely embedded in bone (Fig. 18-6), usually in the maxilla and usually involving the maxillary canine or third molar.[29] In such instances the entire tooth, including the root and crown, may undergo resorption.

Differential diagnosis. External root resorption on the apex or lateral surface of a root is radiographically self-evident. When the lesion lies on the buccal or lingual surface of a root and above the level of the adjacent bone, the differential diagnosis includes caries (p. 318) and internal resorption. Internal resorption characteristically appears as an expansion of the pulp chamber or canal. Careful examination of the pulpal walls will show that they are expanded. In the case of external resorption the image of the normal intact pulp chamber or canal may be traced through the radio-

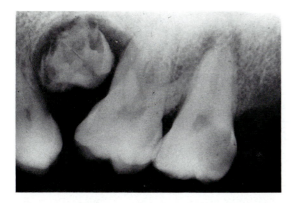

FIG. 18-6. External root resorption of an unerupted tooth, showing loss of enamel and dentin.

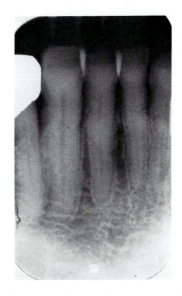

FIG. 18-7. Secondary dentin formation may cause apparent obliteration of the pulp canal and chamber.

lucent area of external resorption. Also projections made at different angles can be compared. The location of the radiolucency caused by external root resorption will move with respect to the pulp canal while the image of internal resoprtion maintains fixed to the canal. A tooth with a necrotic pulp and a rarefying lesion in bone found at the opening of a lateral canal may also cause a lesion that appears like external root resorption.[27] Successful endodontic therapy will resolve this lesion.

Management. When the cause of external root resorption is known, the treatment is usually to remove the etiologic factors. This may mean cessation of excessive mechanical forces, removal of an adjacent impacted tooth, or eradication of a cyst, tumor, or source of inflammation. If it is necessary to endodontically treat a tooth that has external resorption at the apex, apicoectomy may be necessary to remove the portion of root and soft tissue that cannot be adequately instrumented and filled. If the area of resorption is broad and on an accessible surface of the root, curettement and restoring the resorbed area will usually stop the process.

SECONDARY DENTIN

Secondary dentin is that deposited in the pulp chamber after the formation of primary dentin has been completed. The process is a normal consequence of aging and results from such stimuli as chewing or slight trauma. Secondary dentin also develops following chronic trauma from such pathologic conditions as moderately progressive caries, fracture of the crown, erosion, attrition, abrasion, or a dental restorative procedure. This specific stimulus promotes a more rapid and localized coronal response than that seen as a result of normal aging. The term "tertiary dentin" has been suggested[13] to identify dentin specifically initiated by stimuli other than the normal aging response and normal biologic function.

Clinical features. The response of odontoblasts in producing secondary dentin reduces the sensitivity of teeth to stimuli from the external environment. In elderly individuals with extensive secondary dentin formation this reduced sensitivity may be especially pronounced. Similarly, the formation of an additional layer of dentin between the pulp and a region of insult will reduce the sensitivity often experienced by individuals with recent dental restorations or coronal fractures.

Radiographic features. Radiographically, secondary dentin is indistinguishable from primary dentin. It presents as a reduction in size of the normal pulp chamber and canals (Fig. 18-7). When secondary dentin formation results from the normal aging process, the result is a generalized reduction in pulp chamber and canal size. Often there remains only a thin narrow pulp chamber and canal. The pulp horns usually disappear relatively early, followed by a reduction in size of the pulp chamber and narrowing of the canals. When more specific stimuli initiate secondary dentin formation, it begins in the region adjacent to the source of stimuli. Although formation of secondary dentin may continue until the pulp appears to be completely obliterated, histologic studies show that even in these severe cases a small thread of viable pulp material will still remain.

Differential diagnosis. Secondary dentin is readily recognized by the reduction in size of the pulp chamber that takes place, which is a reduction in most of its dimensions. This is contrasts with the reduction in size that accompanies the formation of a pulp stone. The pulp stone (see below) simply occupies some pulp chamber or canal space, but its round to oval shape (conforming to the chamber) will be apparent and the stone recognized.

Management. Secondary dentin per se does not require treatment. The precipitating cause is removed if possible and the tooth restored when appropriate. If the insult is likely to cause eventual pulpal death of the affected tooth, it is wise to anticipate this problem. It may be necessary to perform endodontic therapy before the chamber and canal become so obliterated as to complicate or preclude future treatment.

PULP STONES

Pulp stones are foci of calcification in the dental pulp. They are probably apparent microscopically in more than half the teeth from young people and in almost all from people older than 50 years of age.[16] Although most are microscopic, they vary in size, with some as large as 2 or 3 mm in diameter almost filling the pulp chamber. Only these larger concretions are radiographically apparent. Although the larger masses represent but 15% to 25% of pulpal calcification,[16] they are a common radiographic finding and may appear in a single or several teeth. Their cause is unknown, and no firm evidence exists that they are associated with any systemic or pulpal disturbance.[16]

Clinical features. Pulp stones are not clinically discernible. They develop in normal pulps and do not cause any alteration in tooth morphology. Whereas they occur in all tooth types, they are most common in molars.

Radiographic features. The radiographic appearance of pulp stones is quite variable; they may be seen as radiopaque structures within pulp chambers or root canals or extending from the pulp chamber into the root canals (Fig. 18-8). There is no uniform shape or number. They may be round or oval; and some, occupying most of the pulp chamber, will conform to its shape. Also they may occur as a single dense mass or as several small opacities. Their outline, likewise, varies from sharply defined to a more diffuse margin.

Differential diagnosis. Although pulp stones are variable in size and form, their recognition is not difficult. They require little more than an appreciation of what they are and a recognition of their innocence.

Management. Because they do not cause symptoms and are not detrimental, pulp stones do not require treatment.

PULPAL SCLEROSIS

Pulpal sclerosis is another form of calcification in the pulp chamber and canals of teeth. In contrast to pulp stones, pulpal sclerosis is a diffuse process. Its specific cause is unknown, although its appearance correlates strongly with age. About 66% of all teeth in individuals between the ages of 10 and 20 years, and 90% of all teeth in individuals between the ages of 50 and 70 years,[10] showed histologic evidence of pulpal sclerosis. Histologically the pattern of calcification is amorphous and unorganized, being evident as linear strands or columns of calcified material paralleling blood vessels and nerves in the pulp.

Clinical features. Pulpal sclerosis is a clinically silent process without clinical manifestation. It is an incidental finding of no clinical significance. As with pulp stones, its only importance may be that it can cause difficulty in the performance of endodontic therapy when such a procedure is indicated for other reasons.

Radiographic features. Early pulpal sclerosis, a degenerative process that precedes the formation of pulp stones, is not radiographically demonstrable.[10] Diffuse pulpal sclerosis produces a generalized calcification throughout large areas of the pulp chamber and pulp canals (Fig. 18-9).

Differential diagnosis. Pulpal sclerosis has such a characteristic radiographic appearance that it is unlikely to be confused with other conditions.

Management. Pulpal sclerosis does not require treatment.

HYPERCEMENTOSIS

Hypercementosis is a regressive change in teeth manifested by the excessive deposition of cementum on roots. In most cases its cause is unknown. Occasionally it will appear on a supraerupted tooth following the loss of an antagonist. Under these circumstances cementum production usually occurs around the apex of the tooth that serves to maintain the normal root length.[28] Another cause of hypercementosis is inflammation, usually resulting from periapical infection. In this condition cementum is deposited on the root surface at some

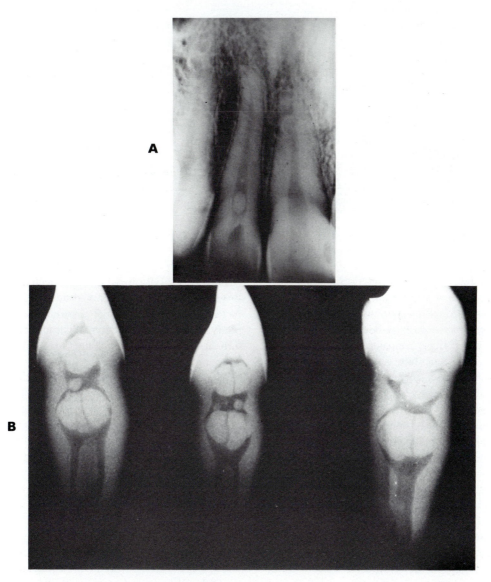

FIG. 18-8. Pulp stones may be found as isolated calcifications in the pulp, **A,** or may cause deformation of pulp chamber and canals, **B.**

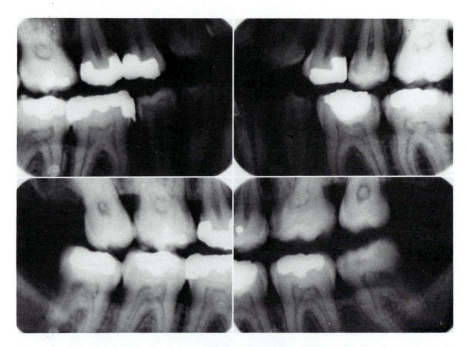

FIG. 18-9. Pulpal sclerosis is seen as diffuse calcification of the pulp chamber and canals.

distance from the apex. Its function is apparently to serve as a barrier to inflammatory products as they diffuse through the periapical tissues. Occasionally hypercementosis will be associated with teeth that are in hyperocclusion or that have been fractured. The cementum is related to the repair process. Other cases of hypercementosis have no obvious cause. Finally, hypercementosis occurs in patients with Paget's disease of bone (p. 525). In such instances it may be localized or generalized and associated with the loss of lamina dura and other bony changes characteristic of Paget's disease. Hypercementosis can also occur with hyperpituitarism (gigantism and acromegaly).[28]

Clinical features. Hypercementosis does not cause any clinical signs or symptoms. Its presence per se is not of clincial significance. If possible, its cause should be determined so appropriate therapy can be instituted to remove existing deleterious factors.

Radiographic features. Hypercementosis is evident radiographically as an excessive buildup of cementum around all or part of a root (Fig. 18-10). It is most evident at the apical end and is usually seen as a mildly irregular accumulation of cementum. This cementum is slightly more radiolucent than dentin. The lamina dura will follow the outline of the cementum and show a normal periodontal ligament space.

Differential diagnosis. There is little difficulty in recognizing the thickening and blunting of affected roots caused by the accumulation of relatively radiolucent cementum. The excess cementum usually does not obscure the outline of the dentinocemental juction.

Management. Hypercementosis itself requires no treatment. When possible, however, the circumstances responsible for it should be identified in case they can or should be treated. Perhaps the primary significance of hypercementosis relates to the difficulty that the root configuration can pose if extraction is indicated.

BONE RESORPTION

Resorption of the alveolar bone will occur following loss of the dentition. Apparently it results from a loss of the occlusal forces transmitted through the teeth by way of the collagen fibers of the PDL. Without such stress on the bone, it resorbs as a form of disuse atrophy.

Clinical features. The region of alveolar bone resorption may be limited to one or two teeth, or it may be large involving all regions of both jaws. Clinically the loss of supporting alveolar bone causes a depression between remaining teeth in the more limited cases and a generalized loss in height and width of the alveolar bone when a large region is involved.

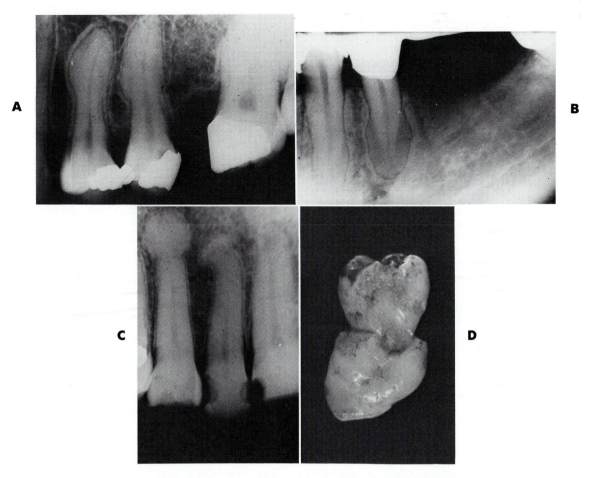

FIG. 18-10. A to **C,** Hypercementosis is evident as a buildup of cementum around the roots of teeth. Note the continuity of the lamina dura and the normal periodontal ligament space. **D,** Extracted molar, showing extensive hypercementosis. (**D** courtesy Dr. R. Kienholz, Dallas.)

Radiographic features. Where one or a few teeth are missing, the bone slopes away from the remaining teeth. If a large region is involved, there will be a generalized loss of alveolar bone. The trabecular pattern in the remaining bone may be either normal or somewhat less dense than normal. In the latter case localized osteoporotic changes in the alveolar bone will take place. The trabeculae will be thinner and the narrow spaces somewhat larger than in the tooth-bearing regions. In the absence of disease, however, the cortical outline of the bone will be intact. In the maxilla the loss of cortical bone may be so severe that there is only a paper-thin shelf of residual bone separating the maxillary sinus from the oral cavity. The cortical outline may even show defects where areas of the bony floor appear to be completely missing. In the mandible, severe loss of the alveolar bone may cause the mental foramen to lie on the superior surface of the remaining body. Indeed, in some cases the resorption exposes the superior portion of the inferior alveolar dental canal.

Differential diagnosis. The clinical and radiographic appearance of disuse atrophy of the alveolar bone is so distinctive and the associated circumstances so predictable that it is likely to be properly recognized.

Management. The alveolar bone loss per se is usually not treated. If an implant is planned for this area, a surgical effort may be made to restore the alveolar ridge if the resorption has been extensive.

SPECIFIC REFERENCES

1. Baden E: Environmental pathology of the teeth. In Gorlin RJ, Goodman HM (eds): *Thoma's Oral pathology,* ed 6, St Louis, 1970, Mosby, vol 1.
2. Bakland LK: Root resorption, *Dent Clin North Am* 36(2):491-507, 1992.
3. Bennett TG, Paleway SA: Internal resorption, post-pulpotomy type, *Oral Surg* 17:228-234, 1964.

4. Bhaskar SN, Orban B: Experimental occlusal trauma, *J periodontol* 26:270-284, 1955.

5. Bruggen ten Cate JH: Dental erosion in industry, *Br J Industr Med* 25:249-266, 1968.

6. Bull WH, Callender RM, Pugh BR, Wood GD: The abrasion and cleaning properties of dentifrices, *Br Dent J* 125:331-337, 1968.

7. Davidoff SM, Damowa N: Histologic changes in structure of teeth situated in regions of benign and malignant tumors, *Dent Abst* 3:148, 1958.

8. Erwin JC, Buchner CM: Prevalence of tooth root exposure and abrasion among dental patients, *Dent Items Interest* 66:760-769, 1944.

9. Goldman HM: Spontaneous intermittent resorption of teeth, *J Am Dent Assoc* 49:522-532, 1954.

10. Hill TJ: Pathology of the dental pulp, *J Am Dent Assoc* 21:820-844, 1934.

11. Johnson GK, Sivers JE: Attrition, abrasion, and erosion: diagnosis and therapy, *Clin Prev Dent* 9(5):12-16, 1987.

12. Kramer IRH: The pathology of pulp death in noncarious maxillary incisors with minor palatal invaginations, *Proc R Soc Med* 46:503-506, 1953.

13. Kuttler, Y: Classification of dentin into primary, secondary and tertiary, *Oral Surg* 12:966-1001, 1959.

14. Massler M, Perreault JG: Root resorption in the permanent teeth of young adults, *J Dent Child* 21:158-164, 1954.

15. Mitchell DF, Standish SM, Fast TB: *Oral diagnosis/oral medicine,* Philadelphia, 1978, Lea & Febiger.

16. Moss-Salentijn L, Hendricks-Klyvert M: Calcified structures in human dental pulps, *J Endod* 14(4):184-189, 1988.

17. Murphy TR: Reduction of the dental arch by approximal attrition: quantitative assessment, *Br Den J* 116:483-488, 1964.

18. Nadler SC: Bruxism, a classification. Critical review, *J Am Dent Assoc* 54:615-622, 1957.

19. Phillips JR: Apical root resorption under orthodontic therapy, *Angle Orthod* 20:1-22, 1955.

20. Pindborg JJ: *Pathology of the dental hard tissues,* Philadelphia, 1970, WB Saunders.

21. Reichborn-Kjennerud I: Dentoalveolar resorption in periodontal disorders. In Sognnaes RF (ed): *Mechanisms of hard tissue destruction,* Washington DC, 1963, American Association for the Advancement of Science.

22. Russell MD: The distinction between physiological and pathological attrition: a review, *J Ir Dent Assoc* 33(1):23-31, 1987.

23. Seligman DA, Pullinger AG, Solberg WK: The prevalence of dental attrition and its association with factors of age, gender, occlusion, and TMJ symptomatology, *J Dent Res* 67(10):1323-1333, 1988.

24. Shafer WG, Hine MK, Levy BM: *Oral pathology,* ed 4, Philadelphia, 1983, WB Saunders.

25. Simpson HE: Internal resorption, *J Can Dent Assoc* 30:355-359, 1964.

26. Sognnaes RF: Dental and hard tissue destruction with special reference to idiopathic erosions. In Sognnaes RF (ed): *Mechanism of hard tissue destruction,* Washington DC, 1963, American Association for the Advancement of Science.

27. Solomon CS, Notaro PJ, Kellert M: External root resorption: fact or fancy, *J Endod* 15(5):219-223, 1989.

28. Sponge JD: *Oral pathology,* St Louis, 1973, Mosby.

29. Stafne EC, Austin LT: Resorption of embedded teeth, *J Am Dent Assoc* 32:1003-1009, 1945.

30. Stafne EC, Lovestedt SA: Dissolution of tooth substance by lemon juice, acid beverages, and acid from some other sources, *J Am Dent Assoc* 34:586-592, 1949.

31. Stafne EC, Slocumb CH: Idiopathic resorption of teeth, *Am J Orthod* 30:41-49, 1944.

32. Tronstad L: Root resorption: etiology, terminology, and clincial manifestations, *Endod Dent Traumatol* 4:241-252, 1988.

19

Infection and Inflammation of the Jaws and Facial Bones

Infections and inflammations of the jaws and facial bones occur fairly often and develop from a variety of causes. Infection is the most common source of inflammatory disease of the pulp resulting from caries and leading to pulp death.[12] The inflammatory agents from the pulp gain access to the periapical connective tissue of the jaws by way of the root canals of involved teeth. Although infections at the apices of teeth usually remain localized in this region, they may occasionally extend beyond the periapical region into bone and produce an osteomyelitis. Tooth extraction wounds are the second most common source of bony infections, despite the fact that they are responsible for considerably fewer inflammatory episodes in the facial bones than pulpal infections are. Other sources of infection are from some types of periodontal disease, compound fractures, and rarely a hematogenous-carried microorganism. When the infection extends into the soft tissues of the face or neck, it may cause a cellulitis that may impair breathing. Rarely the infection may spread to the cavernous sinus and cause a life-threatening cavernous sinus thrombosis.

PERIAPICAL INFECTIONS

The infectious products from a necrotic pulp may be released from the tooth into the oral cavity or into the periapical tissues. If an infected tooth drains only into the oral cavity, it will remain asymptomatic and cause no detectable pathologic response in bone. If, however, the infectious agents or their degradation products from the infected pulp reach the periapical connective tissue, a lesion in the bone may form. The severity of the reaction they elicit will depend on their nature and amount and on the resistance of the host. If they reach the periapical tissues in such small amounts that they are effectively neutralized by the defenses of the

host, no clinical symptoms or radiographic changes will develop. Consequently, the only evidence of this balance between the virulence of an infection and the resistance of the host will be some clinical indication of pulpal injury. In such cases the crown may be discolored or missing or it may have deep caries or a large restoration near the pulp (Fig. 19-1). Alternatively, when the source of the inflammatory degradation products overcomes the host's defenses, a lesion will develop within the bone at the apex of the tooth. The nature and radiographic appearance of these bony lesions are the subject of this chapter.

The inflammatory reaction in the periapical tissues following pulpal necrosis may be acute, leading to an acute periapical abscess, or chronic, leading to a periapical granuloma or radicular cyst.

Acute periapical abscess

An acute periapical abscess starts to develop when the inflammatory degradation products from

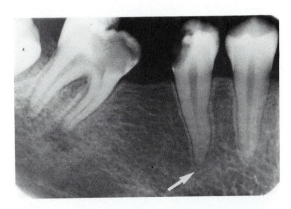

FIG. 19-1. A deep carious lesion in this second premolar has resulted in pulpal damage, but without evidence of changes in the lamina dura or periapical bone (*arrow*). Note the loss of lamina dura and periapical bone around the apex of the mesial root of the second molar.

an infected pulp penetrate the apical PDL in sufficient quantity to provoke the host's defense and initiate an inflammation. The result will be a minimum inflammatory reaction, mostly edema, localized in the apical PDL. If the exudate from the diseased pulp continues to pass into the periapical tissues or is somewhat more irritating, tissue death with pus formation may develop. (The acute periapical abscess is also called an *acute dental* or *dentoalveolar abscess*.) The acute periapical abscess may progress to a chronic form. (See below.)

Clinical features. With an acute periapical abscess, the pulp is nonvital and inflammation is restricted to the PDL. Pain may develop spontaneously and is usually throbbing. There will be evidence of deep caries, a large restoration, or trauma to the tooth. The tooth is not sensitive to hot, cold, sweet, or sour foods because the pulp is necrotic. The tooth elevates in its socket because of edema and is sensitive to pressure and percussion. Regional lymphadenitis and fever are absent.

Radiographic features. The initial, radiographically apparent, change of an acute periapical abscess is widening of the PDL space. The widening is caused by edema with accumulation of inflammatory exudate in the connective tissue of the apical periodontal ligament. Because of the rapidity of lesional development, the bone remains intact.

Management. The primary objective of treating an acute periapical abscess is to establish drainage. Usually this requires opening the pulp chamber or extraction of the tooth. If a periapical abscess is untreated, it may extend into the surrounding tissues as a cellulitis or osteomyelitis or cause a

bacteremia. The abscess may develop a fistula to the oral mucosa or skin.

Chronic inflammation of the periapical region

A chronic inflammation of the periapical tissues may be either a sequela of an acute episode or, more frequently, a low-grade reaction to a pulpal infection or to inflammatory products of relatively long duration and low virulence. The radiographic appearances of the chronic periapical inflammatory conditions described below are often similar and go by the general term "periapical rarefying osteitis." This is a radiographic term and does not imply a specific diagnosis.

Chronic periapical abscess

A chronic periapical abscess occasionally develops from an acute periapical abscess, or it may develop without an acute stage. If the infection in a root canal is of low virulence and the resistance of the host is high, a critically balanced equilibrium between disease and defense may be maintained for years. The response to this low-grade insult may be confined to the region of the PDL. (The chronic periapical abscess is also called a *chronic dental* or *dentoalveolar abscess*.)

Clinical features. Patients with a chronic periapical abscess describe only minimum intermittent discomfort. The patient reports that the tooth has been in need of restoration for a long period but has rarely had pain or swelling in the area. Clinically there will typically be a moderate to large carious lesion. The pus from the lesion may drain through a sinus tract to the oral mucosa or skin.

Radiographic features. The radiographic appearance of a chronic periapical abscess at the apex of a tooth is quite variable. Initially the only radiographic sign may be a widened PDL space. In other cases there may be a radiolucent lesion with ill-defined borders that is indistinguishable from a periapical granuloma or radicular cyst. Surrounding the radiolucent space may be a band of radiopaque sclerotic (dense, thick) trabeculae of variable width. This bone represents an additional response to the irritants that have passed through the PDL but are of such low intensity as to do not much more than stimulate bone production (Fig. 19-2). The sclerotic response is a mark of chronicity.[17]

Periapical granuloma

The periapical granuloma is the most common lesion found at the apex of a nonvital tooth. It

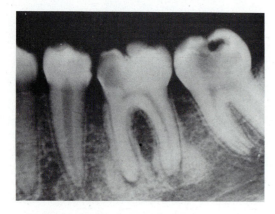

FIG. 19-2. A chronic periapical abscess with areas of surrounding condensing osteitis.

develops in response to an intense or prolonged irritation from an infected root canal. The irritation produces a lesion that extends beyond the PDL. The periapical granuloma may develop from either an acute or a chronic periapical abscess or may result directly from pulpal necrosis without abscess formation. The expanding inflammation and increased vascular pressure cause resorption of bone in the area. Eventually granulation tissue replaces the necrotic soft tissue and bone.

Clinical features. Usually there are not any direct clinical symptoms associated with a periapical granuloma. The tooth is nonvital, may be darker in color, and is not sensitive to percussion. Typically it will have a deep carious lesion or restoration. Because the size of a periapical granuloma is self-limiting, there is seldom any swelling or expansion of the overlying cortical bone.

Radiographic features. Radiographically the periapical region of an affected tooth is radiolucent with loss of the lamina dura (Fig. 19-3). The radiolucency may vary in extent but will rarely, if ever, become large enough to cause expansion of the cortical plates. A radiolucency greater than 2 cm in diameter is most likely to have evolved into a radicular cyst from a periapical granuloma.[24] (See Chapter 21.) The border of the radiolucent lesions may vary from a well-defined sclerotic band to a diffuse region that blends into the adjacent bone. Often the border is well defined but not corticated. Usually the radiographic image of the affected tooth will show a deep carious lesion or restoration suggesting pulpal infection.

Condensing osteitis

If the exudate from an infected pulp is of low toxicity and long-standing, the resulting mild ir-

ritation may lead to a circumscribed proliferation of the periapical bone. This opaque lesion is called *condensing* (or *sclerosing*) *osteitis* or *focal sclerosing osteomyelitis*.[21] This sclerosis in the periapical region is accomplished by the deposition of new bone along existing trabeculae, which increases their size and constricts the marrow spaces. Condensing osteitis occurs most frequently in the mandible, around teeth with a periapical granuloma or radicular cyst, root canal treatment, or restorations.[14] This osseous reaction to inflammation is necessarily observed at the apices of either nonvital teeth or teeth with a pulp in the process of degeneration. (The latter may give a positive response to pulpal vitality tests.)

On radiographs the condensing osteitis may be of variable size and extent, with margins ranging from well-defined to diffuse (Fig. 19-4). The margins of thickened trabeculae are diffuse and blend gradually into the trabeculae of surrounding normal bone. Individual segments of the outline of a single sclerotic lesion may show all these variations. If the lesion represents resolution of an acute periapical abscess, the thickened PDL space may persist and be apparent on radiographs within the image of the sclerotic reaction. Following endodontic therapy, there is usually regression of the condensing osteitis.[4]

Differential diagnosis. The first step in identifying a periapical radiolucency as a *periapical granuloma or radicular cyst* is to establish whether

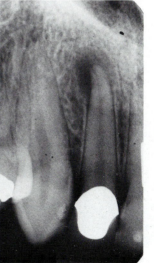
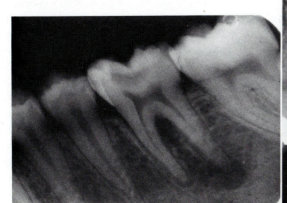

FIG. 19-3. Periapical granuloma. Note the loss of lamina dura and the periapical radiolucency associated with the deep occlusal lesion at the apex of **A,** a mandibular first molar and **B,** a restored maxillary lateral incisor.

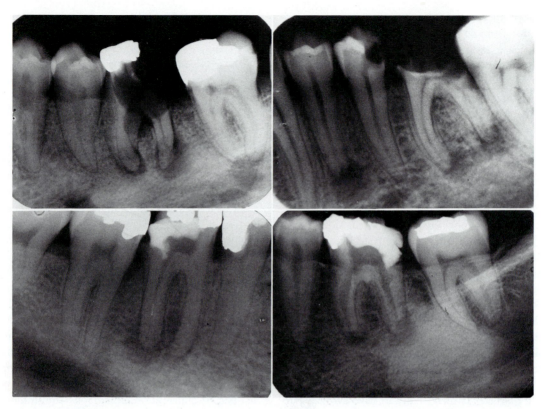

FIG. 19-4. Condensing osteitis, showing the formation of sclerotic bone around periapical granulomas.

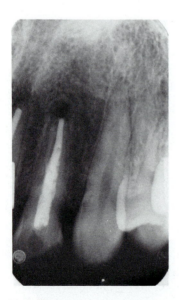

FIG. 19-5. Radiolucent periapical scar or surgical defect with a hyperostotic border around the radiolucent scar tissue.

the involved tooth is vital or nonvital. If it is vital, the possibility of a periapical granuloma or radicular cyst is eliminated. Periapical cemental dysplasia or other benign fibroosseous lesions should be considered. If, however, the tooth has a root canal filling, the radiolucency may represent a periapical scar or surgical defect (Fig. 19-5). If there are no associated symptoms or evidence that the lesion is increasing in size, the diagnosis of periapical scar or surgical defect is appropriate. A patient history of prior surgery or radiographic evidence of modification of the root apex confirms the diagnosis of a surgical defect. Also the surgical defect will probably be more radiolucent than the periapical scar because one or both cortical plates in the area may be missing. Accordingly, the occurrence of a radiolucency at the apex of a nonvital untreated tooth is convincing evidence of a granuloma or radicular cyst because these two diseases account for 90% of all pathologic periapical radiolucencies.

Condensing osteitis may be confused with such periapical radiopacities as osteosclerosis, periapical cemental dysplasia, hypercementosis, and some projected radiopacities. *Hypercementosis* appears

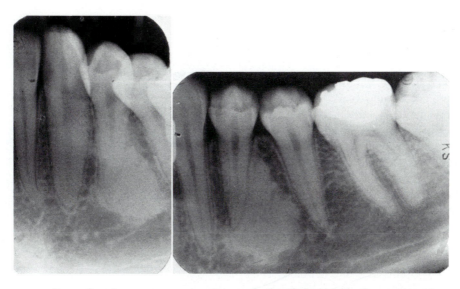

FIG. 19-6. Osteosclerosis seen as an opaque mass of sclerotic bone without any apparent cause.

to be an integral part of a malformed root, lying within the intact lamina dura and PDL space; thus it can usually be distinguished from condensing osteitis. In contrast, the radiographic image of condensing osteitis is outside the lamina dura and periodontal ligament. Furthermore, the teeth involved with hypercementosis are vital (in the absence of other disease). Maturing lesions of *periapical cemental dysplasia* may also be differentiated from condensing osteitis because they occur in association with vital teeth and do not have a trabecular pattern. In addition, a radiolucent border of varying thickness separates the lesions of periapical cemental dysplasia from the surrounding normal bone. Condensing osteitis is not so sharply delineated from the adjacent normal bone. Distinguishing condensing osteitis from *osteosclerosis* when the radiopaque lesion occurs in an edentulous area is a matter of conjecture; however, if the sclerotic area lies near the area of a root tip or nonvital tooth, whether present or missing, condensing osteitis is a reasonable conclusion.

Radicular cyst

The radicular cyst (also known as *periapical cyst* or *dental cyst*) is the next stage, following granuloma, in the sequence of diseases in the periapical tissues that are chronically irritated by exudates from an infected root canal. Proliferation of epithelial rests within the granuloma initiates development of the radicular cyst. When the masses of proliferating epithelium reach a critical size, the central cells degenerate and liquefy. This series of

events leads to the formation of a cyst: a liquid-filled cavity lined with epithelium in the periapical region of a tooth with an infected root canal. Depending on the study, about 17% to 54% of periapical lesions around nonvital teeth are cysts, with the remainder being granulomas.[19] The clinical and radiographic features, differential diagnosis, and management of this lesion are considered in Chapter 20.

Osteosclerosis

Although osteosclerosis does not appear to be the sequela of an infectious process, its radiographic appearance so closely resembles that of condensing osteitis that its consideration in this discussion is appropriate. Osteosclerotic areas that do not seem to be associated with infection are frequently observed on radiographs of the jaws. Some of these lesions do indeed appear to be part of the reparative process, and others a compensatory response to abnormal stress, but the cause is usually obscure.

Clinical features. There are no clinical symptoms to suggest the presence of this entity.

Radiographic features. Areas of exceptionally dense bone are relatively common on radiographs of the jaws of individuals over 20,[5] usually appearing as solitary but maybe also as multiple and bilateral radiodensities. They vary in size from 2 or 3 mm to 1 or 2 cm in diameter and in shape from round to irregular (Fig. 19-6). Their borders may vary from a well-defined outline to an indistinct and ragged blending with the adjacent normal bone. The density of the sclerotic areas, likewise, is variable and may range from a vague thickening of trabeculae in the area, to a ground-glass appearance, to a dense homogeneous mass. Although most of these areas occur near the apices of normal mandibular premolars and molars, any vital tooth may be involved.[5] The osteosclerotic areas also occur in areas of the jaws removed from teeth, in the alveolar process, between the roots of teeth, and about the roots of teeth subjected to unusual masticatory stresses, heavy occlusal forces, or forces applied in abnormal directions.

Occasionally after extraction of a tooth, the socket will heal with sclerotic bone. In such cases of *socket sclerosis,* the new bone forms first on the borders of the socket and progresses inward. When healing is almost complete, a thin radiolucent line remains in the middle, running the length of the socket, and may resemble a root canal. At this stage the sclerosis is so dense that a trabecular pattern is not radiographically apparent. The sclerotic alveolus may thus resemble a root that was not removed when the tooth was extracted. Although close examination of radiographs may reveal the persistence of a lamina dura, the absence of a PDL space provides the clue for the recognition of socket sclerosis (Fig. 19-7).

Differential diagnosis. A differential diagnosis of sclerotic areas that develop at the apices of teeth should include osteosclerosis, condensing osteitis, mature lesions of periapical cemental dysplasia, hypercementosis, and other fibroosseous lesions.

The primary distinguishing feature between osteosclerosis and *condensing osteitis* at the apex of a tooth is that osteosclerosis is associated with a vital tooth whereas condensing osteitis occurs when there is a significant indication of intraosseous infection from a tooth with an infected or nonvital pulp. Although the calcified lesions of *periapical cemental dysplasia* or other fibroosseous lesions develop at the apex of a tooth with a healthy pulp, they differ from osteosclerosis by having a peripheral radiolucent zone and a well-defined border. The border of osteosclerosis will be diffuse and continuous with the adjacent normal bone, not separated from it by an intervening radiolucent structure. The radiolucent PDL space at the periphery of the affected root separates hypercementosis from the adjacent normal bone. The characteristic bulbous shape it imparts to the root apex usually identifies hypercementosis.

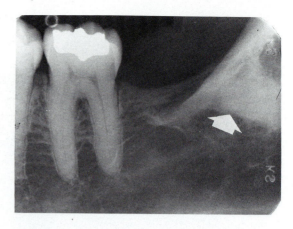

FIG. 19-7. Socket sclerosis *(arrow)* evident as dense sclerotic bone in the site of a previous extraction.

A number of radiopaque entities that occur in jaws (e.g., retained roots, mature odontomas, and unerupted teeth) have distinctive and recognizable shapes and densities and should be readily distinguishable from areas of osteosclerosis not contacting teeth. Similarly, exostoses, tori, and peripheral osteomas should not be mistaken for osteosclerosis, because they will be palpable and recognized during the clinical examination.

Diffuse sclerosing osteomyelitis is much larger than osteosclerosis, which is generally less than 1 cm in diameter. The mild bone infection is also accompanied by the symptoms of chronic infection, and radiographically the sclerotic areas that occur with sclerosing osteomyelitis may be intermingled with radiolucent zones. The usual mixed radiolucent-radiopaque appearance of *osteoblastic malignancy* in the jaw differentiates it from the solely radiopaque osteosclerosis. Also the symptoms and other clinical findings of malignancy help to distinguish these tumors from the symptomless lesions of osteosclerosis.

OSTEOMYELITIS

Osteomyelitis is an inflammation of the bone marrow that produces clinically apparent pus and secondarily affects the calcified component. It usually results from an odontogenic infection in a root canal, from an infection through the PDL space, or from an extraction wound.[18] Other predisposing causes are trauma resulting in a fracture or metastasis from a remote area of infection. When a pyogenic infection spreads into the bone marrow of a healthy individual, it is effectively walled off and

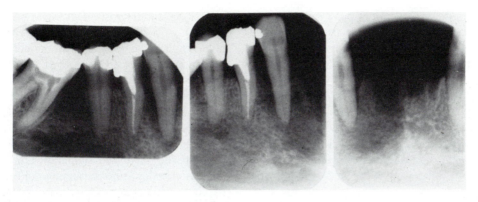

FIG. 19-8. Acute osteomyelitis, with initial blurring of the bony trabeculae near the canine forward to the midline of the mandible. (Courtesy Dr. L. Hollender, Seattle.)

localized by the host's defensive response. If a concomitant disease lowers the host's resistance, however, or rarely, if the infectious agent is especially virulent, the infection may spread through the medullary spaces of the bone. Predisposing conditions that may be present when osteomyelitis develops are malnutrition, diabetes, leukemia, and various anemias as well as conditions that are characterized by the formation of avascular bone that precludes an effective defensive response—including osteopetrosis, Paget's disease, florid osseous dysplasia, post-irradiation states, and fluorosis.[11] Patients with a history of alcoholism also constitute a high-risk group for osteomyelitis.[3]

Osteomyelitis occurs more often in men and more frequently in the mandible (predominantly in the premolar-molar areas), and the incidence slowly increases after the age of 20 years. The mandible's predisposition toward infection compared to the maxilla's results from a combination of factors. Because of the dense mandibular cortical plates of bone, especially in the posterior region, it takes longer for a sinus to form and for pus to be released. Consequently, the infection remains contained within the cortical plates and spreads within the spongiosa. Also the bone surrounding the sockets of mandibular posterior teeth is more dense, which makes the teeth more difficult to extract. As a result, the removal of posterior mandibular teeth causes more damage to the bone and there is a greater probability that portions of infected teeth will be left in the sockets. There is also the important consideration that the mandible is much less vascularized than the maxilla.[21]

Osteomyelitis may be acute or chronic, differing in onset, symptoms, and course. Pain is a characteristic feature and can vary from mild to severe. Other features usually present are swelling, fever, general malaise, and intermittent purulent discharge.

Acute osteomyelitis

Acute osteomyelitis develops in a matter of days and does not show any early radiographic changes. Most commonly it arises from a periapical abscess.

Clinical features. The local signs and symptoms are severe pain, regional lymphadenopathy, and soreness of the involved teeth, which are also loose. If infection involves the mandibular canal, a paresthesia or anesthesia of the lip is common. There is no swelling or redness until later when the infection has penetrated the cortex and involved the periosteum. The white blood count and temperature will be elevated.[18] There may also be reflex spasms of the muscles attached to the involved area of bone.

Radiographic features. Initially there are no radiographic manifestations of acute osteomyelitis. About 10 days following its appearance, however, the trabeculae are decreased in density and their outlines become blurred or fuzzy (Fig. 19-8). Subsequently, solitary or multiple small radiolucent areas appear on the radiograph representing enlarged trabecular spaces caused by foci of necrosis and frank bone destruction.[20]

Acute subperiosteal osteomyelitis

In some cases (e.g., a mandibular periapical abscess that develops close to and rapidly ruptures the cortex) exudate invades the subperiosteal space and elevates the periosteum as pus pools below it, stripping more and more of the periosteum. The pressure of the exudate on the cortex produces a local necrosis, causing resorption of the cortical plate, and interrupts the blood supply to the cortex. The result is an acute subperiosteal osteomyelitis. Eventually the pus ruptures intraorally or extraorally through multiple sinuses.[11]

Clinical features. As pus starts to pool beneath the periosteum, the patient is in severe pain (with intraoral or extraoral swelling and redness) and regional lymphadenitis develops. The involved teeth are only mildly sensitive to percussion. When the intraoral and extraoral sinus tracts develop and start discharging pus, there is an easing of symptoms.[10]

Radiographic features. An occlusal radiograph of the area will show erosion of the cortex but not extensive involvement of the adjacent cancellous bone. On a lateral radiograph, however, the image of a moth-eaten cortex superimposed on the jaw will be hard to distinguish from an intermedullary osteomyelitis.[10]

Chronic osteomyelitis

Following an acute phase, osteomyelitis may subside and the infection evolve into a prolonged chronic course. If the virulence of the infectious agent is low or the resistance of the host especially effective, however, a chronic osteomyelitis may develop without the initial acute stage. Its clinical features are similar to those of an acute infection but the symptoms are milder, bone destruction is slower, and the patient is in less pain. Sinus tracts develop intermittently and then cease draining and close.

Chronic osteomyelitis is a persistent abscess of bone characterized by inflammatory processes, including necrosis of mineralized and marrow tissues, suppuration, resorption, sclerosis, and hyperplasia. In any specific lesion certain of these reactions may predominate. Accordingly, it is common to describe lesions in terms of the feature that is most prominent. A persistent lesion confined largely to bone is a chronic osteomyelitis. A lesion that extends to the periosteum and then dissects laterally may cause a subperiosteal osteomyelitis. Similar lesions in children or young adults may lead to elevation of the periosteum and the deposition of new bone, resulting in an osteomyelitis with proliferative periostitis. Lesions that extend into the facial tissues may cause a cellulitis. Other forms of osteomyelitis may be focal or produce a diffuse chronic sclerosis. The *focal* type of chronic sclerosing osteomyelitis is the localized osteoblastic reaction in the periapical region that is initiated by dental infection and is described above as *condensing osteitis*.

Chronic osteomyelitis is usually localized to the bone around one or a few teeth. It persists because the infected necrotic area is effectively isolated from the host's defensive reactions. As in the acute form, tissue death and suppuration predominate; but this infection is milder and more localized than its acute counterpart. Chronic lesions within the bone may be single or multiple, and the process may persist for a variable period (up to many years) with intermittent exacerbations.

Clinical features. Local tenderness and swelling develop over the bone in the affected area. There is mild leukocytosis with low-grade fever, and a regional lymphadenopathy will be present. Intraoral or extraoral sinuses intermittently develop and drain a small amount of pus and then close. The symptoms then moderate, and the patient becomes more comfortable. The most frequent site is the body of the mandible, and some patients develop pathologic fractures.[2]

Radiographic features. The radiographic picture is one of single or multiple radiolucencies of variable size with irregular outlines and poorly defined borders. As the infection progresses, the affected bone becomes moth-eaten in appearance as the radiolucent areas enlarge, remain irregular in outline, and are separated by islands of normal-appearing bone (Fig. 19-9). Segments of the necrotic bone become detached, and irregular calcified areas separated from the remaining bone may be distinguishable as *sequestra*.

On radiographs the sequestra are usually more dense and better defined, with a sharper outline than the surrounding vital bone. Their increased density is the result of sclerosis induced before the bone became necrotic. Also the inflammatory reaction probably stimulates the demineralization of vital bone surrounding the sequestra, thereby enhancing the contrast. The smaller sequestra may become less dense as they are slowly dissolved by the lytic action of the purulent fluid surrounding them.

Suppuration may perforate the cortical bone, periosteum, and overlying skin or mucosa, forming a fistulous tract to the surface. This tract will show on the radiograph as a radiolucent band traversing the body of the jaw and penetrating the cortical plate (Fig. 19-10).

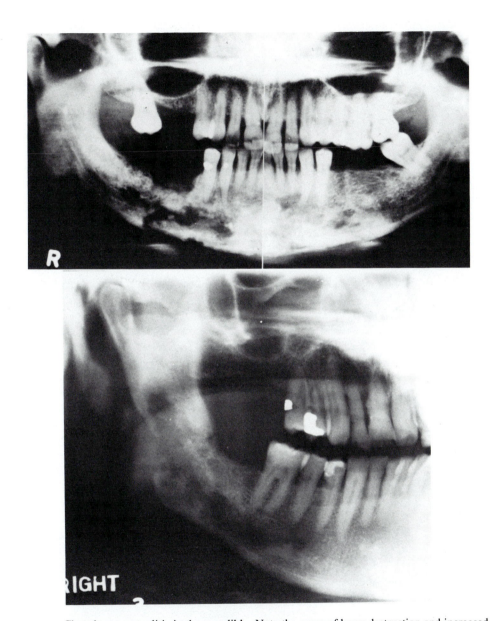

FIG. 19-9. Chronic osteomyelitis in the mandible. Note the areas of bony destruction and increased density, the small bony islands with irregular and ill-defined margins, and the irregular cortex along the borders.   *Continued.*

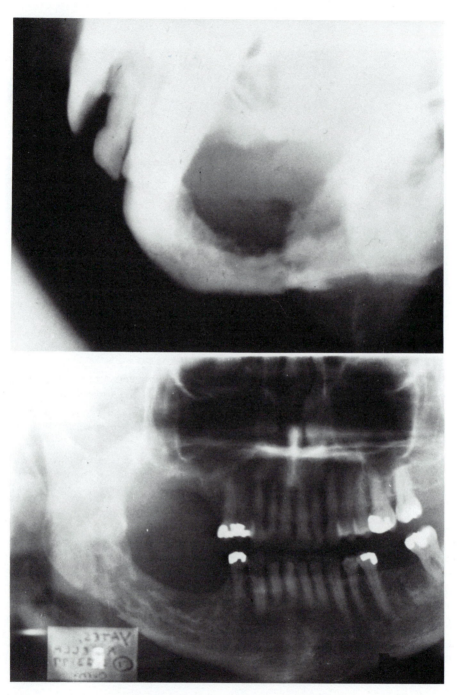

FIG. 19-9, cont'd. For legend see page 389.

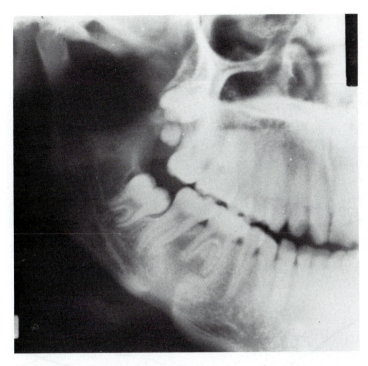

FIG. 19-10. A fistulous tract extending inferiorly from the apex of the first molar to the inferior cortex of the mandible. Note the incidental paramolar blocking the path of eruption of the maxillary third molar.

Diffuse sclerosing osteomyelitis

In the *diffuse* type of sclerosing osteomyelitis (DSO) there is a low-grade infection of the bone. In contrast to tissue death and pus formation, which are characteristic of the chronic osteomyelitis, reactive proliferation of the bone is the primary response in DSO.[6] The diffuse type may occur at any age, but it is observed most often in older age groups. Because the host seems unable to control the subvirulent infection completely, it frequently involves relatively large segments of the jaw, so large that it is not feasible to treat it surgically. The lesion occurs primarily in the mandible, but the maxilla, femur, tibia, and elbow may be involved.[8] There is also evidence[23] that DSO may result from a chronic tendoperiostitis because of muscle overuse.

Clinical features. Symptoms of DSO are usually mild or absent, except that the jaw may enlarge slightly on the affected side from the subperiosteal deposition of bone. During the periods of enlargement, patients may complain of pain and tenderness. The pain persists for a few weeks, with quiet periods of months to years.[7] DSO affects patients of any age, females more often than males.[1] Approximately half the patients show elevated erythrocyte sedimentation rates and fever. Most improve with long-term antibiotic therapy. Treatment by decortication is also effective in relieving pain and increasing the interval between periods of pain.[7]

Radiographic features. The early radiographic changes associated with DSO resemble those of osteomyelitis and include ill-defined osteolytic and osteosclerotic zones. As the lesions progress, they become more sclerotic and there is an increase in the size of the involved part (Fig. 19-11). Typically the margins are ill defined. Occasionally, small lucent areas will appear in association with painful periods. Usually DSO involves a large portion of the mandible, but it usually does not cross the midline. Shortening of tooth roots may occur in affected areas.[9] Scintigraphic examination of DSO has shown consistent uptake of ^{99m}Tc-polyphosphate or ^{99m}Tc-diphosphonate in diseased areas, suggesting active bone deposition.[9] The areas of radiographic change generally correlate with areas of isotope uptake, and scintigraphy displays a more distinctly outlined lesion.

Differential diagnosis. A mixed radiolucent-radiopaque lesion with ill-defined borders should be regarded with suspicion. As in osteomyelitis,

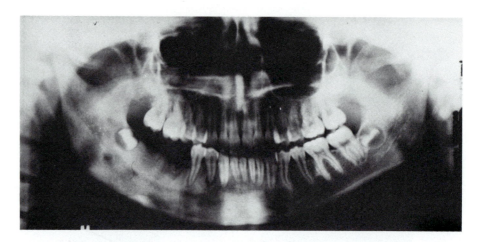

FIG. 19-11. Diffuse sclerosing osteomyelitis. Note the widespread sclerosis of the right mandible from the midline posteriorly. There is also a slight enlargement of the bone. Some radiolucent areas may be identified. (Courtesy Dr. L. Hollender, Seattle.)

malignancies (e.g., osteosarcoma, metastatic osteoblastic carcinoma, and chondrosarcoma) may appear as radiolucent-radiopaque lesions. In addition, none of these lesions, including osteomyelitis, has a radiographic appearance that is uniquely characteristic. Even though symptoms of infection accompany a radiolucent-radiopaque image, the lesion cannot be identified solely as an infection, because osteomyelitis or secondary infection may complicate the tumors. In formulating a differential diagnosis, however, one would favor osteomyelitis over tumors merely on the basis of its greater frequency. Also, a malignant tumor would not likely become infected until it was quite large and, even then, would be assigned a relatively low priority in the differential diagnosis.

Intermediate-stage *Paget's disease of bone* also is characterized by radiopaque areas within a generalized radiolucency. Paget's, however, can usually be distinguished from osteomyelitis since it generally affects multiple bones and there is complete involvement of the individual bones. There is also, however, a predisposition for osteomyelitis to develop in the dense avascular bone affected by Paget's disease, which can complicate recognition of the latter by superimposing the symptoms of infection. Conversely, a patient with an established diagnosis of Paget's and symptoms of infection reinforces the impression of concurrent osteomyelitis. Finally, the presence of uncontrolled systemic disease that reduces host resistance strengthens the impression of osteomyelitis when the characteristic radiographic image is present.

The occurrence of a large osteolytic lesion in the jaw—possibly accompanied by local pain, swelling, and tenderness—also suggests *eosinophilic granuloma*. This would have to be distinguished from osteomyelitis by biopsy. Usually the margins of eosinophilic granuloma are better defined than for osteomyelitis. They also show no evidence of bony sclerosis.

Chronic subperiosteal osteomyelitis

In acute subperiosteal osteomyelitis, pus from an adjacent periapical abscess pools beneath the periosteum and causes necrosis of the compact bone. As soon as drainage for the pus is established through intraoral or extraoral sinuses, the chronic phase of the infection begins. When the pooling pus elevates a region of the periosteum, the cortex becomes deprived of its blood supply. As a result, multiple small necrotic sequestra form in a portion of the cortical plate. The area of affected cortex may be relatively large. The spongiosa below the plate is only slightly involved, if at all. The sequestra, which act as foreign bodies and perpetuate the suppurative process, eventually discharge through the multiple sinuses that usually form. After their discharge, healing of the infection occurs relatively rapidly if the precipitating odontogenic infection has been controlled.

Clinical features. In the chronic stage of subperiosteal osteomyelitis there will be only slight pain and some regional lymphadenitis. The swelling will be confined to the sulcus. In addition, there will be multiple draining sinuses in the area.

Radiographic features. Lateral radiographs will show the moth-eaten appearance of an intra-

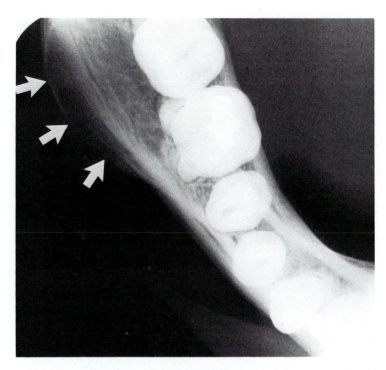

FIG. 19-12. Proliferative periostitis *(arrows)* lateral to an erupting second molar with clinical pericoronitis.

medullary osteomyelitis. In an occlusal projection the cortical sequestration will appear as multiple small radiopaque flakes. Although the lesion is mainly confined to the cortex, some mottling of the adjacent trabecular bone will usually be apparent.

Proliferative periostitis

Proliferative periostitis (also called *Garré's osteomyelitis*) is a rare nonsuppurative type of osteomyelitis. It occurs as a hard bony swelling at the periphery of the jaw (a reactive periostitis) induced by mild infection below the periosteum from the cancellous portion of the jaw that penetrates the cortex. Although periapical infection is the most frequent cause, Garré's is occasionally associated with a pericoronitis. The lesion is rare because its development depends on the occurrence of a set of critically integrated conditions: a chronic infection in an individual, usually a young person with a periosteum capable of vigorous osteoblastic activity, and an equilibrium between the virulence of the infection and the resistance of the host.

Clinical features. The most frequent site of the hard nontender swelling of proliferative periostitis is the inferior border of the mandible below the first molar. Medial and lateral expansion may also

occur. Proliferative periostitis occurs more frequently in females, almost exclusively in the mandible, and usually in persons younger than 30 years of age. The mass may vary in size from 1 to 2 cm to involve the entire length of the mandible on the affected side. The cortex may become 2 to 3 cm thick. Although pain is not a prominent feature of this condition, there may initially be some from the precipitating odontogenic infection. It develops before enlargement of the jaw becomes clinically apparent. Also the lesion may be secondarily infected and cause considerable discomfort.

Radiographic features. Radiographs of a patient with an early lesion of proliferative periostitis show the shadow of a thin convex shell of bone outside the cortex. There are no trabecular shadows in the radiolucent space between the shell and the cortex (Fig. 19-12). As the infection persists, the cortex thickens and becomes laminated, with alternating radiolucent-radiopaque layers (the onionskin appearance) (Fig. 19-13). The adjacent cancellous bone may remain normal in appearance, become sclerotic, or show areas of osteolytic change within the sclerosed spongiosa. After removal of the irritation, the cortical bone may remodel to a normal appearance.

Differential diagnosis. A number of bony con-

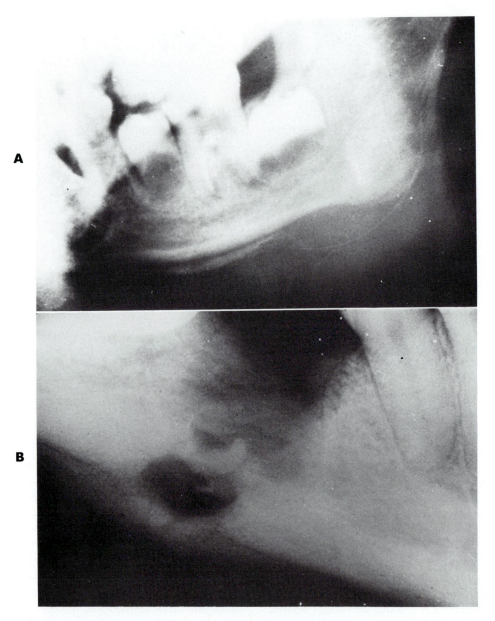

FIG. 19-13. Proliferative periostitis, demonstrating the deposition of bone inferior to the first molar region. **A,** Minimal intramedullary bone changes. **B,** Considerable lateral bony sclerosis and loss of bone after the offending tooth was removed.

ditions that cause expansion of the jaws are necessarily included in the differential diagnosis of proliferative periostitis: Ewing's sarcoma, infantile cortical hyperostosis (Caffey's disease), fibrous dysplasia, osteosarcoma, exostoses, tori, and peripheral osteomas.

Ewing's sarcoma may resemble proliferative periostitis in that one of its manifestations is swelling of the involved bones as a result of the formation of layers of subperiosteal bone with an on-

ionskin appearance. Both conditions also occur in young individuals. The bony enlargement caused by sarcoma, however, develops much more rapidly. In addition, the tumor frequently produces osteophytes with sunray appearance. Although Ewing's sarcoma may cause some sclerosis of the spongiosa, it is generally more osteolytic than the bone infection. Also, in contrast to proliferative periostitis, the sarcoma produces facial neuralgia and lip paresthesia as frequent complications.

The radiographic pictures of *Caffey's disease* (also known as *infantile cortical hyperostosis*) and proliferative periostitis may be quite similar in that the bone produced in both entities is deposited in layers parallel with the cortex (onionskin appearance). Although the lesions of Caffey's disease may clinically somewhat resemble the swellings of the lower jaw seen in proliferative periostitis, they usually develop at the angle or in the ramus of the mandible and their onset becomes apparent at an earlier age, in most cases before 2 years. In contrast, proliferative periostitis usually occurs in the posterior tooth-bearing areas of the mandibular body and at a considerably later age. These lesions develop from a periapical infection after the teeth have erupted. In addition, whereas proliferative periostitis is unlikely to develop in more than one location, cortical hyperostosis is likely to involve other bones besides the mandible (especially the clavicle).

An expansion of the jaw as a result of *fibrous dysplasia* may suggest proliferative periostitis in size and shape and would have its onset in children or young adults. Unlike proliferative periostitis, however, fibrous dysplasia is not associated with a dental infection and is more likely in the maxilla. The radiographic pictures of the two entities also provide some reasonably definitive contrasts. The expanding lesion of proliferative periostitis is primarily a thickened cortex, whereas the cortex in fibrous dysplasia is thinned or completely replaced by altered bony tissue extending to the limit of the bone. Likewise, the density of a fibrous dysplastic lesion is usually more uniform than that in proliferative periostitis (which is more mottled, with alternating areas of sclerosis and osteolysis). Also the characteristic ground-glass appearance of fibrous dysplasia usually involves the entire thickness of the affected bone.

Osteosarcoma may produce a bony hard mass on the jaw like the one with proliferative periostitis. Although some overlap may occur at the upper limits of the age groups for proliferative periostitis and osteosarcoma, the irregular mixed-density bone formed by the tumors suggests a malignancy and is dissimilar to the linear array of bone deposited in the periostitis.

The hard nodular or pedunculated growth of such entities as *peripheral osteomas, tori,* and *exostoses* that occur on the mandibular body should be clinically distinguishable from the smoothly contoured swelling observed in proliferative periostitis. Radiographically they appear as dense uniformly radiopaque masses on the jaw or protruding from the cortex, depending on the angle of projection.

Specific chronic infections of the jaws

A number of agents that produce the so-called granulomatous inflammations occasionally lead to chronic osteomyelitis of the jaw. Unlike the pyogenic agents, however, these do not provoke tissue damage by the direct action of toxins; rather, their pathologic effect is the result of cell-mediated hypersensitivity. Some of the bacterial and mycotic agents that produce these chronic processes of bone are the ones responsible for tuberculosis, syphilis, brucellosis, actinomycosis, blastomycosis, and coccidioidomycosis; but, from the standpoint of radiographic diagnosis, there is nothing characteristic about the appearance of the bony changes induced by any of these entities: they are all radiographically indistinguishable from the chronic bone infections caused by the pyogenic microorganisms. The recognition of these diseases depends on their systemic symptoms or on immunologic evidence. Their lesions are rare in the jaw bones and usually are not apparent until the general symptoms and indicators develop. Primary lesions of these entities are unusual in the jaws.

Osteoradionecrosis

Following exposure to intense irradiation (between 40 and 80 Gy), bone undergoes a marked decrease in vascularity.[15] This results in a chronic hypoxia in the irradiated bone and a loss of cellularity. Such bone has poor defensive powers and is especially susceptible to traumatic injury and direct infection from extraction wounds, infected pulps, severe periodontitis, or dentures. The bony changes are irreversible, and an increased potential for infection persists for years.[12] Osteoradionecrosis develops when such compromised bone becomes infected from an oral wound, accounting for perhaps half of all cases of osteomyelitis.

Although this pathologic process may develop in any irradiated bone, jaws show a high predisposition, probably because of the higher incidence of infection and trauma to which they are subjected. Osteoradionecrosis occurs more often in the mandible than in the maxilla, primarily because of the anatomic differences between them (especially the more abundant blood supply of the maxilla). Also the mandible is more often therapeutically exposed than the maxilla.[21] The higher incidence in men probably results from their increased incidence of oral carcinomas.

The lesions that develop in such altered bone are similar to those of chronic osteomyelitis.[11] They probably differ only in that the typical inflammatory response is decreased or absent as a result of the reduced vascular bed. Because of the lowered resistance, there is minimum localization of the infection and the spread, though slow, is relatively diffuse, with late sequestration.

Clinical features. There will be signs of inflammation, with swelling and drainage, and the patient will usually have intense pain. This pain may be present long before other clinical or radiographic signs are evident. Even when a lesion involves the teeth, they frequently give positive vitality test results.

Radiographic features. The radiographic appearance of an osteoradionecrosis will be areas of increased radiodensity interspersed with osteolytic (radiolucent) regions and the appearance of late-forming (radiopaque) sequestra (Fig. 19-9). In this regard osteoradionecrosis tends to resemble osteomyelitis. Whereas the osteoradionecrosis may be confined to a limited area, it will usually be more widespread than a chronic osteomyelitis.[2] Furthermore, although distinguishing the two may not always be possible radiographically or clinically,[20] when there is a history of therapeutic radiation to the jaw area, it should establish the nature of the lesion.

Pericoronal infections

Pericoronitis is an infection of the soft tissue surrounding the crown of a partially erupted tooth. At this stage of eruption, with a cusp tip or part of the crown projecting through the gingiva, the follicular space is open to infection by contamination from the oral cavity.[18] Pericoronal infections are fairly common. Those that involve teeth that erupt rapidly and completely are of mild intensity and short duration, because the follicle is eliminated once the tooth has erupted.[12] It is quite common, however, for third molars, especially in the mandible, to develop in such a position that they do not erupt completely. They usually remain in this position until treated. Consequently, pericoronitis is most frequent around third molars that are partially encapsulated by soft or hard tissue.[13]

Clinical features. Pericoronitis involving a third molar will show all the features of inflammation in the soft tissues over and around an impacted crown: pain, redness, and swelling. Occasionally it will lead to cellulitis, muscular trismus, dysphagia, regional lymphadenitis, or a submaxillary or pharyngeal abscess.[16] The inflammation often causes the operculum (a covering of soft tissue) to enlarge to such an extent that it becomes traumatized by the opposing tooth during chewing, a condition that also contributes to the patient's discomfort and perpetuation of the inflammation.[16]

Radiographic features. Pericoronal infections of relatively short duration or involving only a few episodes usually do not cause defects in the bone that are radiographically apparent, even when symptoms are severe. Also the margins of follicles are normally so variable that it is frequently difficult to identify abnormal features.[22] Repeatedly infected follicles, however, may develop chronic pericoronal abscesses that involve the bony crypt and cause changes in the follicular margins. A radiograph will show the defect in bone, usually in the retromolar region, but the defect may be located at the distal or mesial aspect of the tooth. It often appears as a steplike distortion of the crypt wall distal to the crown. The existing follicular margin generally shows some sclerosing osteitis and thickening of the wall of the crypt, indicating a chronic low-grade infection. The inflammatory process may even partially resorb the roots of the adjacent tooth.

Folliculitis

The follicles of developing succedaneous teeth may become infected when their primary predecessors develop chronic periapical abscesses. The abscesses necessarily surround or are next to the follicles of the developing permanent tooth. If the infection causes damage to the ameloblasts of the developing tooth, hypoplastic defects in the enamel will result. The entire enamel surface, or only a portion of it, may be affected. When these isolated teeth erupt, showing the hypoplastic defects not shared by the contralateral tooth, they are called *Turner's teeth*. (See Chapter 17.)

The crowns of mandibular premolars are the teeth most frequently affected[16]; however, on the basis of (1) the number of permanent tooth follicles observed on radiographs of children that appear to be involved by periapical infections of deciduous teeth and (2) the low incidence of Turner's teeth, it must be assumed that many of these follicles either are not infected or are infected but without injurious sequelae. If the infection extends to the developing end of the permanent tooth, it may kill the pulp of the unerupted tooth and terminate further development. The incompletely formed tooth will usually continue to erupt and may be shed shortly after eruption, although it may on occasion be retained.[22]

Clinical features. There is frequently a red and tender swelling of the mucosa in the vestibule next to the infected tooth. The swelling will subside and be replaced by a parulis, which will usually open opposite the primary tooth. There will also be a regional lymphadenitis, and the patient may have a slight fever.

Radiographic features. In some cases of folliculitis, the cortical border surrounding the developing permanent tooth is destroyed and the tooth follicle appears to be infected. Often, however, the radiographic picture of folliculitis is less well defined. It may not show the rather sharp delineation of an infectious process that is observed when a similar lesion affects a permanent tooth.

SPECIFIC REFERENCES

1. Alling C, Martinez M: Comment on reactive hyperplasia of bone, *Oral Surg* 40:445-447, 1975.
2. Calhoun KH, Shapiro RD, Stiernberg CM, et al: Osteomyelitis of the mandible, *Arch Otolaryngol Head Neck Surg* 114(10):1157-1162, 1988.
3. Davies HT, Carr RJ: Osteomyelitis of the mandible: a complication of routine dental extractions in alcoholics, *Br J Oral Maxillofac Surg* 28(3):185-188, 1990.
4. Eliasson S, Halvarsson C, Ljuugheiner C: Periapical condensing osteitis and endodontic treatment, *Oral Surg* 57:195-199, 1984.
5. Farman AG, Joubert JJ, and Nortjé CJ: Focal osteosclerosis and apical periodontal pathosis in European and Cape Colored dental outpatients, *Int J Oral Surg* 7:549-557, 1978.
6. Jacobsson S, Heyden G: Chronic sclerosing osteomyelitis of the mandible, *Oral Surg* 43:357-364, 1977.
7. Jacobsson S, Hollen O, Hollender L, et al: Fibro-osseous lesion of the mandible mimicking chronic osteomyelitis, *Oral Surg* 40:433-444, 1975.
8. Jacobsson S, Hollender L: Treatment and prognosis of diffuse sclerosing osteomyelitis (DSO) of the mandible, *Oral Surg* 49:7-14, 1980.
9. Jacobsson S, Hollender L, Lindberg S, Larsson A: Chronic sclerosing osteomyelitis of the mandible: scintigraphic and radiographic findings, *Oral Surg* 45:167-174, 1978.
10. Killey HC, Kay TW: Subperiosteal osteomyelitis, *Br Dent J* 118:294-298, 1965.
11. Killey HC, Kay TW: Inflammatory diseases of the jaw bones. In Gorlin RJ, Goldman HM [eds]: *Thoma's Oral Pathology,* ed 6, St Louis, 1970, Mosby.
12. Killey HC, Seward GR, Kay TW: *An outline of oral surgery. I,* Bristol U.K., 1975, John Wright & Sons.
13. Leone SA, Edenfield MJ, Cohen ME: Correlation of acute pericoronitis and the position of the mandibular third molar, *Oral Surg* 62(3):245-250, 1986.
14. Marmary Y, Kutiner GA: Radiographic survey of periapical jawbone lesions, *Oral Surg* 61(4):405-408, 1986.
15. Marx RE: Osteoradionecrosis: a new concept of its pathophysiology, *J Oral Maxillofac Surg* 41:283-288, 1983.
16. Ruben MP, Goldman HM, Schulman SM: Diseases of the periodontium. In Gorlin RJ, Goldman HM [eds]: *Thoma's Oral Pathology,* ed 6, St Louis, 1970, Mosby.
17. Schulze C: Developmental abnormalities of the teeth and jaws. In Gorlin RJ, Goldman HM [eds]: *Thoma's Oral Pathology,* ed 6, St Louis, 1970, Mosby.
18. Shafer WG, Hine MK, Levy BM: *A textbook of oral pathology,* ed 4, Philadelphia, 1983, WB Saunders.
19. Stockdale CR, Chandler NP: The nature of the periapical lesion: a review of 1108 cases, *J Dent* 16(3):123-129, 1988.
20. Waldron CA: Local diseases of the jaws. In Tiecke RW [ed]: *Oral Pathology,* New York, 1965, McGraw-Hill.
21. Wood NK, Goaz PW: *Differential diagnosis of oral lesions,* ed 4, St Louis, 1991, Mosby.
22. Worth HM: *Principles and practice of oral radiologic interpretation,* Chicago, 1963, Year Book Medical Publishers.
23. van Merkesteyn JPR, Groot RH, Bras J, et al: Diffuse sclerosing osteomyelitis of the mandible: a new concept of its etiology, *Oral Surg* 70:414-419, 1990.
24. Zain RB, Roswati N, Ismail K: Radiographic evaluation of lesion sizes of histologically diagnosed periapical cysts and granulomas, *Ann Dent* 48(2):3-5, 1989.

20

Cysts of the Jaws

A cyst is a pathologic space filled with fluid, lined by epithelium, and surrounded by a definite connective tissue wall. The cystic fluid either is secreted by the cells lining the cavity or derives from the tissue fluid. It may be clear or turbid, colorless or discolored, thin and watery or thick and cheesy. It may contain crystals of cholesterol. (A space filled with pus or blood is not customarily included in this definition.) Cysts are more common in the jaws than in any other bone, because most begin in the numerous rests of odontogenic epithelium that remain after tooth formation. Cysts are second only to granulomas as the most common pathologic radiolucency of the jaws.

Oral cysts usually arise in bone (centrally), although occasionally they will develop in the soft tissues. (This chapter discusses central cysts.) Typically, oral cysts in bone grow slowly and, apparently in response to hydrostatic pressure. Their general radiographic appearance is a radiolucent area, often with a hyperostotic (well-corticated) border. Large cysts will expand bone cortical plates, but the bony margins usually remain intact.

Most jaw cysts (90%) are odontogenic (i.e., they arise in a cellular component of the enamel organ). Odontogenic cysts are thus in some way associated with teeth. Nonodontogenic cysts arise from epithelial rests in lines of fusion between embryologic processes or from remnants of embryologic oral or perioral structures. The development of a cyst may be stimulated by inflammatory, developmental, traumatic, or neoplastic causes. Despite their specific etiology, most cysts display similar behavior. Even though the dentist may be unable to reach a conclusion as to the exact nature of a cyst, treatment is often the same. On rare occasion, malignant tumors may develop in cysts. Consequently, it is imperative that each smooth-walled radiolucent lesion with or without a radiopaque cortex be thoroughly evaluated and treated.

ODONTOGENIC CYSTS
Radicular cyst

The radicular cyst (also known as a *periapical cyst, apical periodontal cyst,* or *dental cyst*) is the most common of oral cysts. It represents a step in the progressive inflammatory events associated with bacterial invasion, death, and degradation of the dental pulp. It is the next step following the formation of a dental granuloma, developing at the apex of a tooth with a nonvital pulp. It may occasionally originate on the mesial or distal surface of a tooth root, at the opening of an accessory canal, but infrequently arises in a deep periodontal pocket.

Clinical features. A radicular cyst typically develops at the apex of a *nonvital tooth*. The tooth will often have a deep carious lesion, large restoration, or endodontic filling. The patient may be young or old, male or female, and usually will have no discomfort at the site of the lesion. The tooth is not sensitive to percussion. Radicular cysts are most frequently (60%) found in the maxilla,[43] especially around incisors and canines. They tend to remain small but occasionally will cause a painless bony expansion. Such expansion, usually just labial or buccal in the mandible, may be either buccal or palatal in the maxilla.[43] It may be bony hard if the cortex is intact, crepitant as the bone thins, or rubbery and fluctuant if the bone is destroyed. There may be a history of trauma to the affected tooth.

Radiographic features. The typical radiographic appearance of a radicular cyst is a radiolucent rounded or pear-shaped unilocular lesion less than 1 cm in diameter. The tooth typically will have a large carious lesion, restoration, or endodontic filling (Fig. 20-1). The borders of the lesion are generally well defined and may or may not be corticated. When a border is corticated, the radiopaque image will be continuous with the lam-

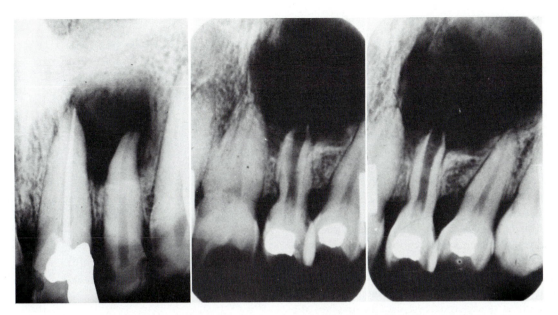

FIG. 20-1. Radicular cysts. Note that they appear as a periapical radiolucency with fairly well-defined margins.

ina dura around the associated root. Radicular cysts are radiographically indistinguishable from dental granulomas; however, although both may have well-defined outlines, the cyst is more apt to have a thin hyperostotic (radiopaque) border than the granuloma.[50] In addition, as the lesion increases in size, the probability that it is a cyst also increases. Virtually all lesions greater than 2 cm in diameter are cysts. Radicular cysts in the posterior maxilla may expand into the sinus and elevate its floor, presenting a halo appearance above the involved tooth. Root resorption of adjacent teeth often occurs in long-standing cases.

Differential diagnosis. The differential diagnosis for a reasonably well-defined radiolucency at the apex of a nonvital tooth includes *periapical granuloma, radicular cyst, periapical scar,* and *surgical defect.* There is only about a 10% probability that the lesion will be one of the latter two lesions listed. A history of apicoectomy or location of the lesion at the apex of an endodontically treated tooth will identify this group. Of the two remaining possibilities, the granuloma is more probable, having the higher incidence.[47] The larger the lesion, however, the greater is the probability of its being a radicular cyst. A history of recurrent episodes of pain and swelling suggests granuloma or infected cyst.

Management. The radicular cyst is usually treated by excision through either extraction and

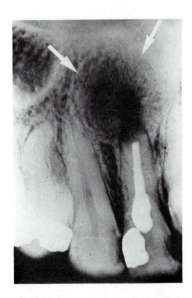

FIG. 20-2. Radicular cyst healing after endodontic treatment. *Arrows* show the original outline of the cyst.

curettage or endodontic therapy and apical surgery. The periapical area of an endodontically treated tooth should be radiographically examined periodically to assure normal healing (Fig. 20-2). If the cyst is large, it may be treated by marsupialization. Recurrence is unlikely if it has been removed completely.

Dentigerous cyst

A dentigerous cyst (also called *follicular cyst*) forms around the crown of an unerupted developing tooth. It begins when fluid accumulates in the layers of reduced enamel epithelium or between the epithelium and crown of an unerupted tooth. It is the second most common of all the oral cysts and the most common pericoronal radiolucency. Some 4% of individuals with at least one unerupted tooth will have a dentigerous cyst. Dentigerous cysts around supernumerary teeth constitute about 5% of all such cysts, and most develop[30] around a mesiodens in the anterior maxilla.

Clinical features. The usual patient with a dentigerous cyst is an adolescent or young adult with unerupted teeth. Most of these cysts form around the crown of a mandibular third molar or maxillary canine, the teeth that are most commonly impacted. In adults a dentigerous cyst usually involves the third molar. Clinical examination will reveal a missing tooth or teeth and possibly a hard swelling around the developing cyst, occasionally resulting in facial asymmetry. Dentigerous cysts grow slowly. The patient typically has no pain or discomfort, although there may be paresthesia on the affected side.

The most important feature of the dentigerous cyst is its potential to expand. It may vary greatly in size, from little more than the diameter of the involved crown to an expansion that causes progressive but painless enlargement of the jaw and facial asymmetry. Teeth next to the developing cyst, as well as the involved tooth, may be severely displaced or resorbed. Although most dentigerous cysts are solitary, bilateral cysts are found in association with the *basal cell nevus syndrome and cleidocranial dysplasia.*[20]

When a dentigerous cyst involves deciduous or permanent teeth that are about to erupt, it may or may not cause fluctuant bulging of the alveolar surface. Occasionally it will contain blood (the blue-domed cyst). The lesions are called *eruption cysts* because of their timing with erupting teeth. In contrast to the usual dentigerous cyst, the eruption cyst associated with a permanent succedaneous tooth may cause pressure on the unprotected pulp of its resorbing predecessor and be extremely painful.

Radiographic features. The usual dentigerous cyst presents as a well-defined radiolucent lesion around the crown of an unerupted third molar or maxillary canine. It has a hyperostotic (well-corticated) border, is unilocular, and includes the

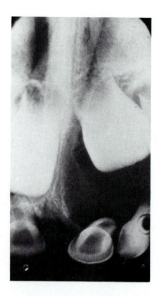

FIG. 20-3. An eruption cyst involving the permanent maxillary central incisor.

crown but usually not the root of the involved tooth. The tooth may be displaced from its usual location. The size of the normal follicular space is 2 to 3 mm. When the follicular space exceeds 5 mm, a dentigerous cyst is likely. Dentigerous cysts may grow to 2 or 3 cm in diameter or even larger. Eruption cysts have the same appearance as dentigerous cysts, except that they develop around the crowns of erupting teeth (Fig. 20-3).

A dentigerous cyst most often envelops the crown symmetrically (Fig. 20-4), but it may expand laterally from the crown. It may displace the associated tooth in any direction and to any position—for instance, a mandibular molar to the inferior border of the jaw or up into the ramus (Fig. 20-5)—and it may extend even into the coronoid process or condyle, at the same time expanding the lateral walls in these areas. A dentigerous cyst can displace a maxillary canine (Fig. 20-6) into the maxillary sinus, next to the nasal fossa, or even to the floor of the orbit.[43] Remember: although a dentigerous cyst develops around the crown, the roots of the tooth are usually in bone outside the lesion.

Differential diagnosis. The appearance of a pericoronal radiolucency suggests the following possible interpretations: *dentigerous cyst, ameloblastoma, calcifying odontogenic cyst, adenomatoid odontogenic tumor,* or *ameloblastic fibroma.* Dentigerous cysts have a much higher incidence than any of these lesions. Furthermore, the ame-

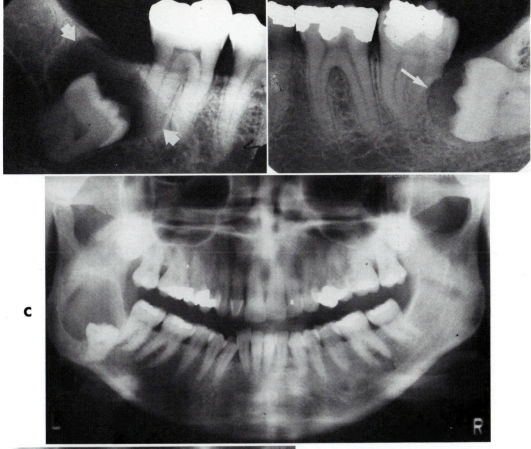

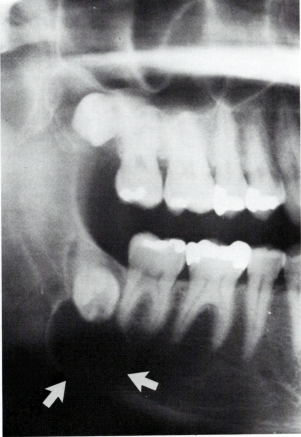

FIG. 20-4. Dentigerous cysts: **A,** surrounding the crown of a third molar *(arrows);* **B,** adjacent to the crown of another third molar *(arrow),* causing resorption of the distal root of the second molar; **C,** involving the ramus of the mandible; **D,** expanding laterally from an unerupted third molar *(arrows).*

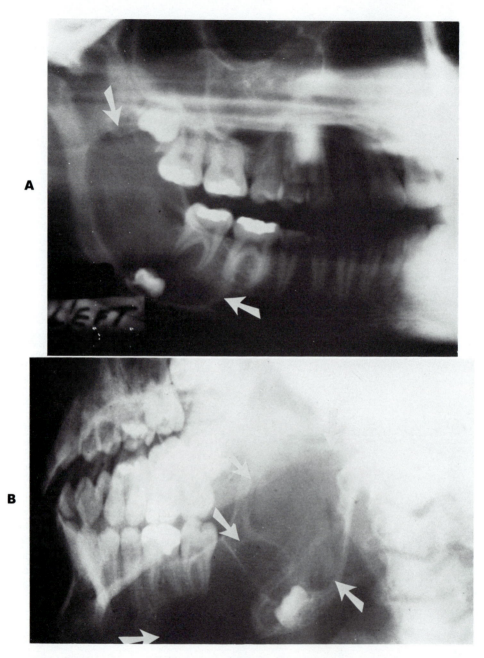

FIG. 20-5. Dentigerous cysts displacing third molar crowns. *Arrows* show the extent of the lesion: **A** and **B,** toward the inferior border of the mandible as well as into the ramus; **C,** toward the coronoid process.

C

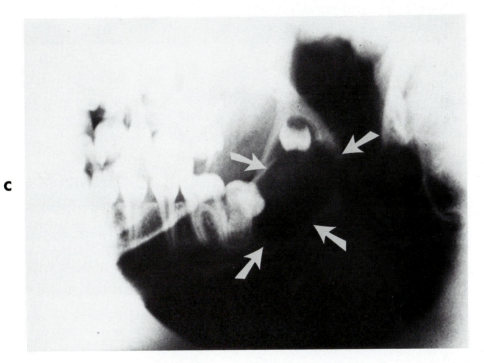

FIG. 20-5, contd. C, For legend see opposite page.

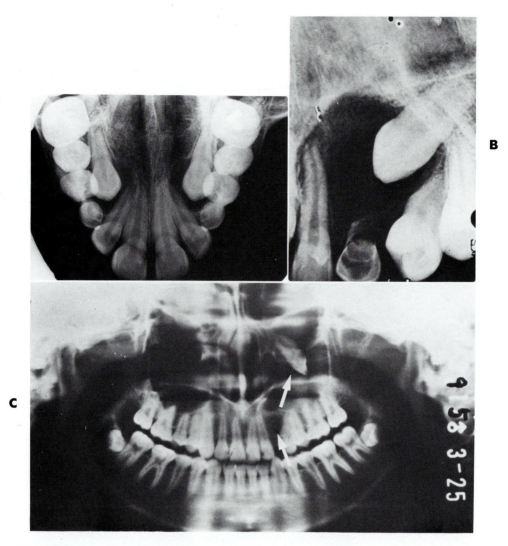

FIG. 20-6. Dentigerous cysts involving the maxillary canines. **A,** Causing displacement toward the midline; **B,** impeding eruption; **C,** causing displacement between the lateral incisor and premolar.

loblastoma and ameloblastic fibroma may be multilocular and not associated with the crown of an unerupted tooth. Also an ameloblastic fibroma associated with an unerupted tooth is likely to grow laterally away from the crown whereas a dentigerous cyst is likely to envelop the crown symmetrically. The calcifying odontogenic cyst and the adenomatoid odontogenic tumor are both rare. The former is usually in the premolar-molar region of the mandible, whereas 75% of the latter occur in the incisor to premolar region of the maxilla. They may contain radiopaque foci within the lesion. Occasionally a radicular cyst at the apex of a primary tooth will surround the crown of the permanent tooth developing apical to

it, giving the false impression that a dentigerous cyst is involving the permanent tooth.[56] The presence of deep caries in a primary tooth suggests residual cyst. The primary tooth will also test nonvital.

Management. Dentigerous cysts are treated by surgical removal of the tooth and cyst lining. Large destructive cysts may be treated by marsupialization. Untreated cysts can destroy bone, and the epithelial lining may be transformed into an ameloblastoma or, rarely, a carcinoma.[32]

Residual cyst

A residual cyst may develop following partial removal of a radicular, lateral, or dentigerous cyst.

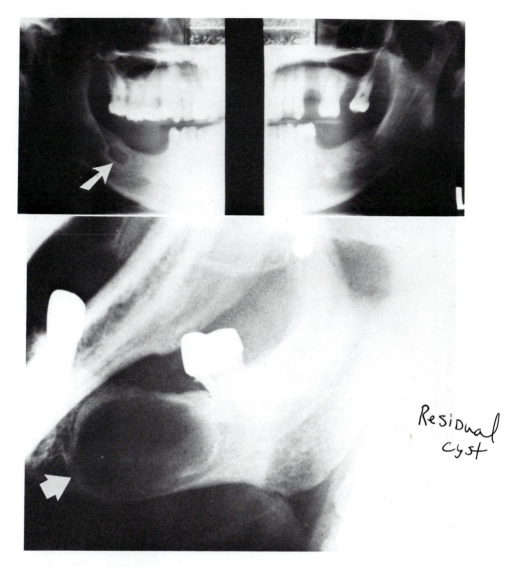

Residual
Cyst

FIG. 20-7. Residual cysts in the posterior regions. *Arrows* identify the lesions.

It may also form after the removal or exfoliation of a tooth, as a result of the cystic degeneration of granulomatous material remaining after a tooth and the associated granuloma are removed, or from residual odontogenic epithelial rests in remnants of the PDL of a lost tooth. About 10% of odontogenic cysts are the residual type, most residual radicular cysts.[25]

Clinical features. The residual cyst typically occurs in middle-aged or older men who have had one or more teeth extracted. It is somewhat more common in the maxilla and is usually asymptomatic and discovered on radiographic examination of an edentulous area. The lesion seldom produces expansion of the cortical plates and, when aspirated, produces an amber colored cystic fluid.

Radiographic features. A residual cyst is typically radiolucent with smooth, round, corticated borders (Fig. 20-7). A thin radiopaque margin is common, although infected cysts will not have such well-defined margins. The lesion is usually 5 mm or less in diameter, infrequently becoming large enough to cause jaw expansion. A preextraction radiograph of the area in question may show a tooth with evidence of deep caries or a fracture adequate for pulpal involvement and an associated radiolucent lesion.

Differential diagnosis. Although any solitary cystlike radiolucency not necessarily contracting teeth should be considered in the differential diagnosis of a residual cyst, the following are most appropriate: *odontogenic keratocyst* and *traumatic* *bone cyst*. A residual cyst requires a history of extraction. If the lesion is below the mandibular canal in the third molar region, a developmental salivary gland defect should be considered.

Management. Depending on the size of the lesion and the patient's health, a residual cyst should be enucleated. When the surgical procedure must be as atraumatic as possible, marsupialization or decompression may be used. Removal of these cysts is important, because of the risk of pathologic fracture and the rare chance of its developing into a carcinoma.[40]

Odontogenic keratocyst

The odontogenic keratocyst (OKC) arises from dental lamina and comprises 5% to 17% of all cysts in the jaws.[28] It is exceptional in that it has the highest recurrence rate of any odontogenic cyst (10% to 60%).[28] It is also unusual in that it often contains a viscous or cheesy material derived from the epithelial lining. Whereas the epithelial lining of many types of odontogenic cysts show evidence of keratinization, the histologic structure of the epithelial lining of an OKC has a thin connective tissue wall and a thin squamous-type epithelial lining (4 to 8 cells thick) that is keratinized, either parakeratinized (87%) or orthokeratinized* (13%),[58] and without rete pegs. The basal layer is of either columnar or cuboidal epithelium; and if prickle cells are present, they are frequently vacuolated.[51] In some cases budlike proliferations from the basal layer into the adjacent connective tissue wall, or the proliferation of odontogenic epithelial islands present in the wall, will give rise to satellite microcysts.[9] A role for these in the high recurrence rate of keratocysts is supported by some authors,[17] but others[53] maintain that there is no correlation. When multiple OKCs are found (4% to 5% of the cases), they may constitute part of the basal cell nevus syndrome (p. 411).

Clinical features. An odontogenic keratocyst can appear in a young child or an aged adult. Most lesions occur during the second and third decades, the mean age being about 30 years,[11,28] and men are somewhat more commonly affected.[11,26] Lesions usually develop in the mandible (75% to 80%),[36,46] with about 40% in the third molar–ramus

region.[26,53] Cortical expansion is a common initial finding. An OKC will often develop in connection with an impacted tooth and is usually symptomless; but as with any other bony lesion, there may be pain and infection. Aspiration produces thick, yellow, cheesy material (keratin). Again, remember: these lesions have a high recurrence rate.

Radiographic features. An odontogenic keratocyst is frequently indistinguishable radiographically from any other odontogenic cyst. The majority (75%) appear as radiolucencies in the mandible, with more than 90% posterior to the canines[2] and more than 50% at the angle. Many of these latter lesions extend into the ramus.[29] As a class, keratocysts are more likely than other odontogenic cysts to show aggressive growth, with undulating borders and an appearance suggestive of multilocularity. The size of the cysts varies from small to 5 cm or more in diameter, with maxillary lesions usually smaller and rounder than mandibular ones,[29] and the margins are usually hyperostotic. Tooth displacement is common. The majority of these cysts are unilocular with smooth borders[10] (Fig. 20-8), but some may be large with irregular shapes and scalloped borders (Fig. 20-9) and can be misinterpreted as multilocular[44] (Fig. 20-10). Although true multilocular lesions do occur, septa are rarely if ever present. Keratocysts may expand through the buccal and lingual cortical plates of bone and spread into the adjacent soft tissue.[13]

Conventional radiography can clearly demonstrate the unilocular variety of these cysts and generally will indicate bony perforations, but it does not show the extent of a cyst into adjacent soft tissues. Even contrast medium frequently fails to delineate all the spaces of an irregularly shaped lesion. Computed tomography, however, can accurately image the margins of an odontogenic keratocyst, including any bony perforations and extensions into the soft tissue[17] (Fig. 20-11). Proper treatment planning is dependent on such complete preoperative information.

Differential diagnosis. Lesions that have a number of features similar to the odontogenic keratocyst are the *residual cyst, traumatic bone cyst, early ameloblastoma,* and *myxoma*. Absence of a tooth without a history of extraction favors odontogenic keratocyst. Although these lesions cannot be radiographically distinguished with confidence, the probabilities can be estimated on the basis of usual location, age of occurrence, association with neurogenic symptoms, and incidence. OKCs also tend to be more aggressive than their nonkeratocyst

---

*Orthokeratinized cysts seem to have a much lower recurrence rate than parakeratinized cysts do.[53] This lower growth potential is reflected by a more complete maturation of the squamous epithelium as indicated by the absence of nuclei in keratinized cells and also by the presence of a granular layer.

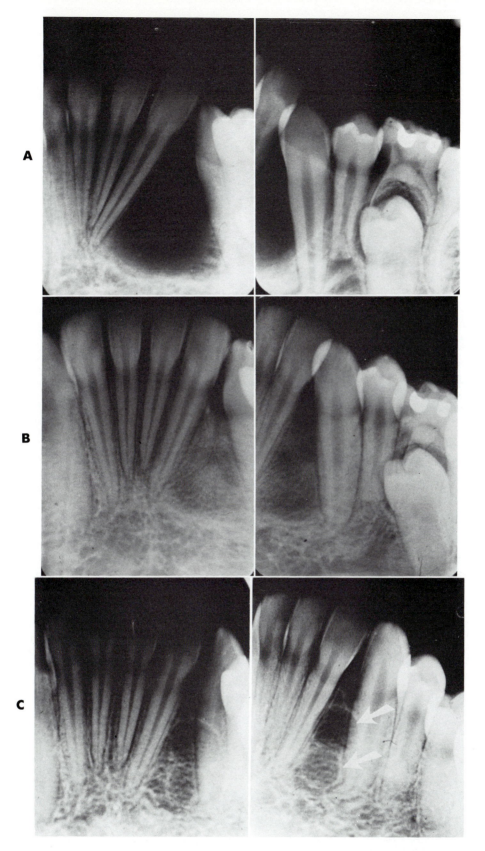

FIG. 20-8. Odontogenic keratocyst between the mandibular left lateral incisor and canine. **A,** Note how it has forced the two roots apart. **B,** After enucleation there is bone filling of the defect. **C,** Unfortunately, the cyst is evident again 3 years later. (**A** to **C** courtesy Dr. L. Hollender, Seattle.)

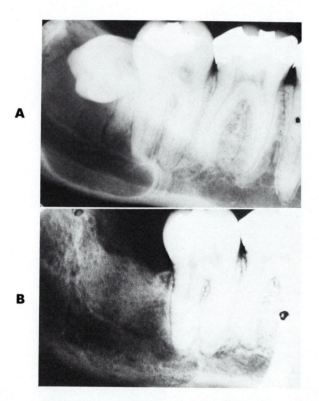

FIG. 20-9. A, Odontogenic keratocyst extending under the second molar before treatment. **B,** After enucleation there is bone filling. (**A** and **B** courtesy Dr. L. Hollender, Seattle.)

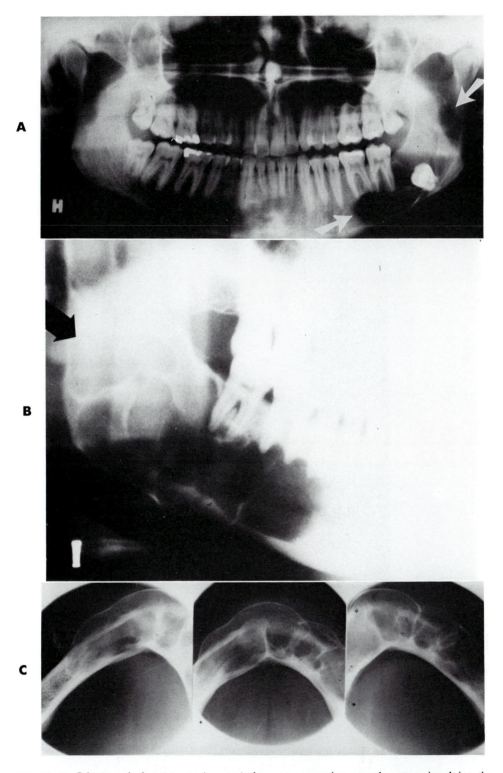

FIG. 20-10. Odontogenic keratocysts *(arrows)* show an aggressive growth pattern involving the body and ramus of the mandible, **A** and **B,** as well as the anterior mandible, **C** and **D.** In **E** the cyst has absorbed most of the ramus and coronoid process and is extending into the midbody of the mandible *(arrows)*. (**A** to **D** courtesy Dr. L. Hollender, Seattle; **E** courtesy Dr. B. Gratt, Los Angeles.) *Continued.*

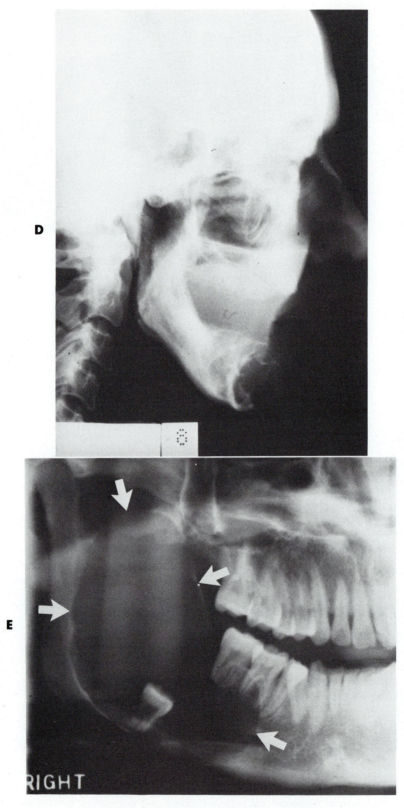

FIG. 20-10, cont'd. For legend see page 409.

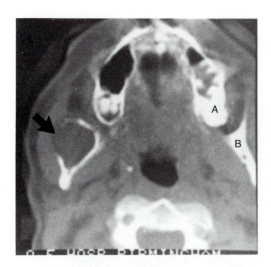

FIG. 20-11. A CT scan at the level of the hard palate illustrates perforation of the cortical plate of the ramus and extension of an odontogenic keratocyst into the masseter muscle *(arrow)*. *A,* Maxillary alveolus; *B,* ramus on the normal side. (From Frame JW, Wake MJC: *Br Dent J* 153:93-96, 1982.)

counterparts. Aspiration produces characteristic semisolid material. Other cystlike radiolucencies that share fewer characteristics and are candidates for lower priorities are the *benign nonodontogenic tumors and completely radiolucent ossifying and cementifying fibromas* (which are uncommon) and the *giant cell granuloma (which is usually multilocular and occurs more anteriorly).*

Management. Cysts are usually treated by surgical removal. If the clinician discovers a yellow, cheesy, granular material in the cyst cavity, more vigorous curettement of the cyst walls should be performed than is the case with a cyst containing typical cyst fluid. Also it is important to make periodic posttreatment clinical and radiographic examinations of the surgical defect to detect any recurrence. Recurrent lesions will usually develop within the first 5 years but may be delayed as long as 10 years. In addition, regular surveillance is prompted by the rare reports[13,31] that keratocysts may transform into ameloblastomas or carcinomas.

Basal cell nevus syndrome

The basal cell nevus syndrome (also known as *nevoid basal cell carcinoma syndrome* and *Gorlin-Goltz syndrome*) includes a number of abnormalities such as multiple nevoid basal cell carcinomas of the skin, bifid ribs, and multiple jaw cysts. It is inherited as an autosomal dominant trait with varying penetrance and expressivity.[21,22] The jaw cysts are odontogenic keratocysts.[14]

Clinical features. The basal cell nevus syndrome starts to appear early in life, usually after the age of 5 and before the age of 30 years, with the development of jaw cysts and skin basal cell carcinomas. The lesions occur as multiple odontogenic keratocysts of the jaws, usually appearing in multiple quadrants. About 1% of patients with this syndrome will have only one odontogenic keratocyst.[11] The skin lesions are small, flattened, and flesh-colored or brownish papules occurring anywhere on the body but especially prominent on the face, neck, and trunk. If these appear early in life during the first decade, additional lesions will usually occur later during the teens and twenties. Occasionally basal cell carcinomas form later in life than the jaw cysts do. The basal cell carcinomas that are part of this syndrome are less aggressive than the solitary basal cell carcinomas that characteristically form later in life.[19] Skeletal anomalies include the bifid rib (most common) and other costal abnormalities such as agenesis, deformity, and synostosis of the ribs, kyphoscoliosis, vertebral fusion, polydactyly, shortening of the metacarpals, temporal and temporoparietal bossing, minor hypertelorism, and mild prognathism.[7] Calcification of the falx cerebri and other parts of the dura occurs early in life, and slight mental retardation is usually apparent. Approximately 4% of these patients will develop a medulloblastoma.[15]

Radiographic findings. The jaw cysts in patients with basal cell nevus syndrome are apparent as multiple cystlike radiolucencies of variable size, from a millimeter to several centimeters in diameter (Fig. 20-12). They occur more frequently in the premolar-molar region of the mandible but may be seen in the third molar area of the maxilla. The radiopaque line of the calcified falx cerebri is also prominent on a posteroanterior skull projection.

Differential diagnosis. The complex of abnormalities that make up the basal cell nevus syndrome constitutes a characteristic pattern of features that should not be difficult to recognize. It is often possible to distinguish the several well-defined radiolucencies of *multiple myeloma, metastatic carcinoma,* and *histiocytosis X* from the jaw cysts of basal cell nevus syndrome because the former usually lack hyperostotic borders characteristic of a cyst. The radiolucent lesions of cherubism are not as well-defined as jaw cysts. Cherubism also produces jaw expansion that is not characteristic of the basal cell nevus syndrome. Dentigerous cysts are unlikely, since it is unusual to find several of them in one patient.

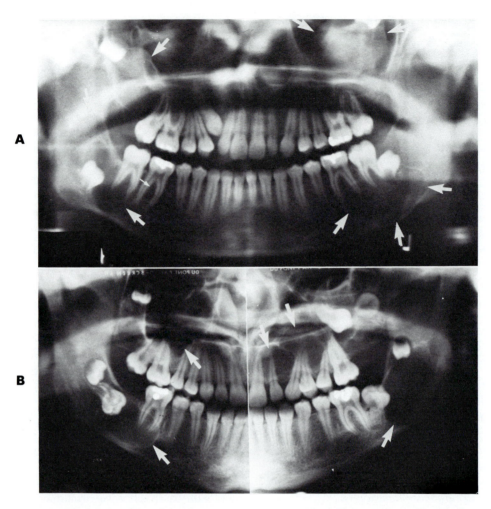

FIG. 20-12. Multiple odontogenic cysts associated with the nevoid basal cell carcinoma syndrome. In **A** the *upper arrows* point to opacified maxillary antra, the *small arrow* to a lesion in the bifurcation of the right mandibular first molar, and the *lower arrows* to lesions involving the roots of the third molars. In **B** cysts are present near the mandibular third molars and in the maxillary incisor region.

Management. Because multiple jaw cysts are so frequently keratocysts, with a high recurrence rate, they require vigorous treatment to ensure complete enucleation. Following their removal, careful periodic reexaminations should be made to detect any recurrence. A basal cell carcinoma may be treated surgically and requires the attention of a physician. The meduloblastoma is life threatening and requires immediate medical care.

Lateral periodontal cyst

The lateral periodontal cyst is similar to the gingival cyst of adults. The names reflect their location. The lateral periodontal cyst arises in periodontium and extends into the interproximal bone between the apex and alveolar crest. The gingival cyst of adults arises as a dome-shaped swelling in the attached gingiva. The clinical appearance and behavior, morpholgic and histochemical features, and site of occurrence of these lesions are so similar that they seem to be intraosseous and extraosseous manifestations of the same condition.[59] Their common physical and histochemical association with clear cells of the dental lamina is also convincing evidence that they are in fact the immediate source of epithelium found in cases of both lateral periodontal and the gingival cysts of adults.[59] In contrast, clear cells do not occur in the walls of radicular or dentigerous cysts.

If a cyst occurs intraosseously, it is a lateral periodontal cyst; but if it appears to be in attached gingiva, it is a gingival cyst of adults. Clinical

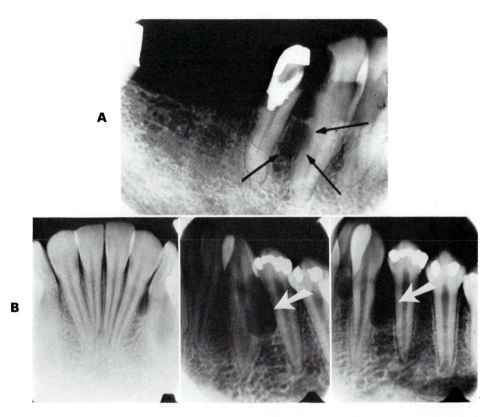

FIG. 20-13. Lateral periodontal cysts in the mandibular premolar region. *Arrows* point to lesions between the canine and first premolar. (**B** courtesy Dr. L. Hollender, Seattle.)

distinction between the two is not always possible, however. Cysts originating in bone may expand, burrow through the bone, and ultimately cause gingival swelling. Similarly, a cyst in the gingiva may expand and create pressure on the bone and cause resorption that extends to the root surface.[34]

Clinical features. The lateral periodontal cyst and gingival cyst of adults are relatively uncommon. Those apparent clinically are customarily identified as gingival cysts of adults. They are usually asymptomatic and appear as dome-shaped fluctuant swellings of the interdental papilla, attached gingiva, or alveolar mucosa. Some clinicians[34] report that they may be emptied with finger pressure. They are covered with normal mucosa and are usually (more than 90%) on the labial or buccal side of the arch (a position corresponding to that of a vestigial structure of the dental lamina).[49] The lesions are usually less than 1 cm in diameter, and 50% to 75% develop in the mandible, mostly between the lateral incisor and first premolar.[5] There does not appear to be any sexual predilection, and the age distribution extends from the second to the ninth decade (mean age about 50 years).[59] Multiple

lesions (botyroid) may also occur.[34,55] The vitality of adjacent teeth is not a factor in their development. Microscopically these cysts seldom show evidence of infection, and their association with accessory root canals is accidental. These observations support the developmental nature of the entities. If they become secondarily infected, they will mimic a lateral periodontal abscess.

Radiographic features. The intrabony periodontal cyst occurs as a well-defined radiolucency, round to ovoid, with a hyperostotic margin (Fig. 20-13). It usually lies somewhere between the cervical margin and the apex of an adjacent root and may or may not be in contact with the root surface.[45] Those primarily confined to the gingiva (gingival cysts of adults) may produce distinct but superficial saucerizations or erosions in the cortical bone that may not be radiographically apparent. If they communicate with the periodontium, a radiographic image is likely.[12,33]

Differential diagnosis. The location and radiographic appearance of a lateral periodontal cyst will cause the following lesions to be included in the differential diagnosis: *lateral periodontal ab-*

scess, lateral dentigerous cyst, radicular cyst at the foramen of a lateral (accessory) pulp canal, residual radicular cyst from primary dentition, and odontogenic keratocyst.[45,57] The multiple (botryoid) cysts with a multilocular appearance resemble a small ameloblastoma.[37,55]

Management. Simple enucleation is the treatment of choice. The cyst does not recur.

Calcifying odontogenic cyst

The calcifying odontogenic cyst (also called a *calcifying epithelial odontogenic cyst* or *Gorlin cyst*) is an uncommon, slow-growing, and completely benign entity. It occupies some position between a cyst and an odontogenic tumor, with the characteristics of a solid neoplasm (epithelial proliferation, tendency for continued growth) and of a cyst.[39] It is not always cystic; and although it resembles an ameloblastoma in some histologic respects, it does not behave like one.[4]

Clinical features. At least three fourths of calcifying odontogenic cysts occur in bone, with a nearly equal distribution between the jaws.[4] Most (75%) occur anterior to the first molar. The youngest patient observed was 1 year old, and the oldest 82 years.[44] The age distribution peaks at 10 to 19 years, and the mean age is 36.[18] There may be a second incidence peak during the seventh decade.[43] These cysts occur more frequently in women before the age of 40 and more frequently in men after age 40. The usual clinical presentation is a slow-growing, painless, nontender swelling of the jaw. Occasionally a patient will complain of pain.[44] In some cases the expanding lesion may destroy the cortical plate, and the cystic mass may be palpable as it extends into the soft tissue. The patient may report a discharge from such advanced lesions.[44] Aspiration often yields a viscous granular yellow fluid.

Radiographic features. The radiographic images of a calcifying odontogenic cyst are quite variable. The central lesion may be radiolucent with a variable margin that is smooth and well defined or irregular and poorly defined. It also may be of variable form, either unilocular or multilocular. Occasionally (20% to 50%) the cyst will be associated with unerupted teeth,[16] and sometimes with a pericoronal radiolucency. The radiolucent area may contain small foci of calcified material that appear as white flecks (Fig. 20-14). In some cases the calcifications will be so small that the lesion looks completely radiolucent. The calcified component may, however, be large and occupy most

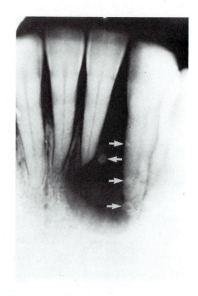

FIG. 20-14. Calcifying odontogenic cyst. Note that it has well-defined borders and multiple small radiopaque masses of calcified material *(arrows)*. There is also evidence of external root resorption on the lateral incisor. (Courtesy Dr. L. Hollender, Seattle.)

of the lesion. This is the only jaw cyst with radiopaque foci.[37] Although unusual, the roots of adjacent teeth may be resorbed. Perforation of the cortical plate can be seen radiographically in enlarging lesions.[39]

Differential diagnosis. The radiographic image of the calcifying odontogenic cyst in its mixed presentation is so variable in form, outline, and radiodensity that a differential diagnosis may well include *partially calcified odontoma, adenomatoid odontogenic tumor, ossifying fibroma, odontogenic fibroma,* and *cementoblastoma.* The less common, completely radiolucent presentation suggests an odontogenic cyst.

Management. Although this cyst does have some neoplastic characteristics, such as a tendency for continued growth, it does not have the invasive growth pattern of the ameloblastoma. The treatment should be enucleation and curettage.[6] Soft tissue lesions are removed by excision.

NONODONTOGENIC EPITHELIUM LINED CYSTS
Nasopalatine canal cyst

The nasopalatine canal conducts the nasopalatine vessels and nerves. It usually contains remnants of the nasopalatine duct, a primitive organ of smell. Occasionally a cyst forms in the nasopalatine canal when embryonic epithelial remnants of the naso-

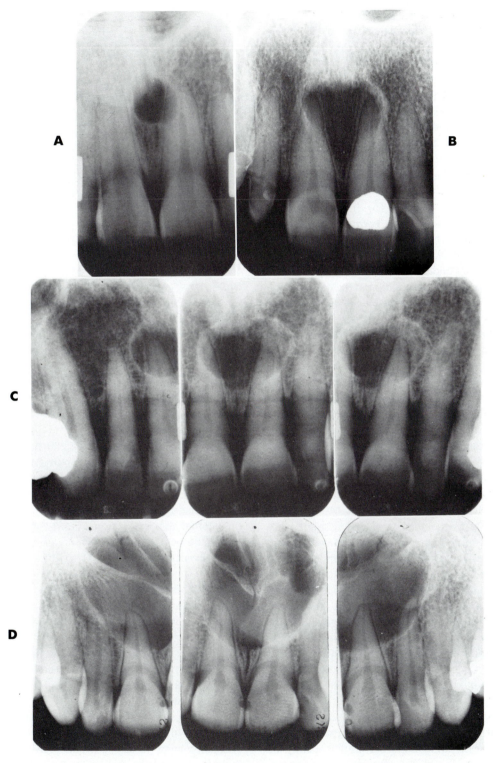

FIG. 20-15. Nasopalatine canal cysts. Note the presence of an intact lamina dura around all the apices. In **A** the lesion is small; in **B** and **C,** medium sized; and in **D,** large.

palatine duct undergo proliferation and cystic degeneration. The nasopalatine canal cyst (nasopalatine duct cyst, incisive canal cyst, or median anterior maxillary cyst) occurs in about 1% of the population and is the most common nonodontogenic cyst in the maxilla. They form in the canal and at the oral terminus in the incisive papilla. Although the soft tissue variety has been called a *cyst of the incisive papilla,* because it originates from the same epithelial remnants as the cyst that forms in the canal, the term "nasopalatine cyst" is preferred for this entity as well.[29]

As the nasopalatine canal cyst enlarges, it may extend posteriorly to involve varying proportions of the hard palate (Fig. 20-15). This condition is frequently called *a median palatal cyst.* It may expand anteriorly between the central incisors, destroying the labial plate of bone and causing the teeth to diverge and a swelling to appear just below the labial frenum. This variation of the nasopalatine duct cyst is frequently called a *median alveolar cyst* (median anterior maxillary cyst). If it occurs at the level of the incisive foramen, it may cause swelling of the incisive papilla and is then called a *nasopalatine cyst.*

Clinical features. The nasopalatine canal cyst accounts for about 10% of jaw cysts.[44] The age distribution is broad, with most cases discovered in the fourth through sixth decades,[1] and the incidence is three times higher in men.[44] The majority are asymptomatic or cause such minor symptoms that they are tolerated for long periods.[24] Consequently, most are detected on radiographs made for other reasons.

The most frequent complaint is a small well-defined swelling just posterior to the palatine papilla. This swelling is usually fluctuant and bluish if the cyst is near the surface. The deeper nasopalatine canal cyst is covered by normal-appearing mucosa unless it is ulcerated from masticatory trauma. If the cyst expands, it may penetrate the labial plate and produce a swelling below the maxillary labial frenum, or to one side (if it is in a branch of the canal), suggesting its origin as associated with the central incisor. The cyst may cause the roots of the central incisors to diverge.[3] The lesion may also bulge into the nasal cavity and distort the nasal septum.[8] Pressure from the cyst on the adjacent nasopalatine nerves that occupy the same canal may cause a burning sensation or numbness over the palatal mucosa. In some cases cystic fluid may drain into the oral cavity through a sinus tract or a remnant of the nasopalatine duct. The

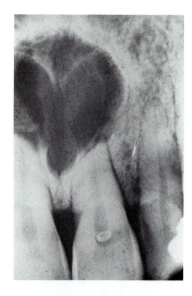

FIG. 20-16. A nasopalatine canal cyst is causing external root resorption of a maxillary central incisor.

patient will usually detect the fluid and report a salty taste.

Radiographic features. The image of a nasopalatine canal cyst is a typical cystlike radiolucency, frequently superimposed on the apices of the central incisors (Fig. 20-15). The image of the radiopaque anterior nasal spine may be superimposed on the dark cystic cavity, giving it a heart shape. The superimposition of the nasal septum over the cystic area may also impart a heart-shaped appearance. If the cyst forms in one of the branches of the canal, its image will deviate to one side of the midline. Divergence of the central incisor roots[3] or external root resorption (Fig. 20-16) will occasionally be apparent.[35]

Differential diagnosis. The differential for a cystlike lesion in the anterior maxillary region should include a large incisive fossa, a radicular cyst or periapical granuloma, a nasopalatine canal cyst, a dentigerous cyst from a mesiodens, and an odontogenic keratocyst.

Although it is not easy to distinguish a *large incisive fossa* from a small cyst, several guides may be useful: Radiolucencies in the midline that are round with well-defined hyperostotic margins most likely are cysts. Oval or irregularly shaped radiolucencies with indistinct outlines probably are an unusually large fossa. Heart-shaped lesions and those that seem to be separating the central incisors are most likely cysts. In addition, a large deep incisive fossa is sharply defined only at its lateral margins but not on its inferior and superior margin,

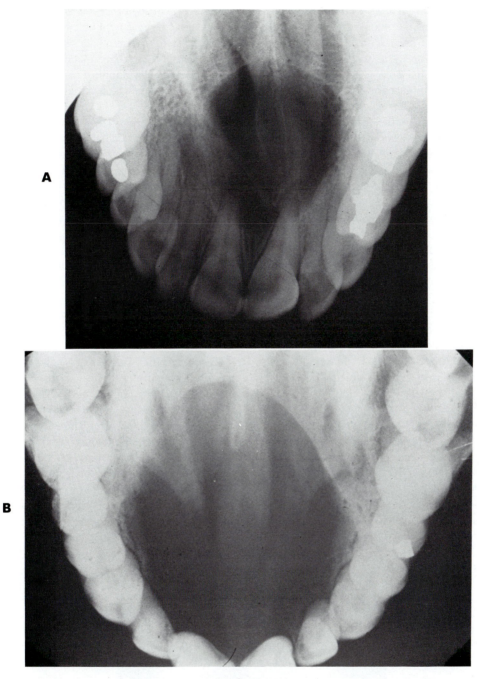

FIG. 20-17. Nasopalatine canal cysts, demonstrating the value of an occlusal radiograph in revealing the size and position of a lesion. **A** is the same patient as in Fig. 20-15, **D.**

in contrast to the cyst, which usually has a well-delineated boundary on all margins. A radiolucency in the area less than 6 mm wide is most likely a normal fossa, in the absence of associated symptoms.[27] Radiolucencies greater than 1 cm in diameter are likely to be cysts. Aspiration will frequently enable the dentist to distinguish between a cyst and an unusually large incisive fossa. Occlusal projections of the area are helpful in recognizing the cyst since it will demonstrate that the radiolucency is lingual to the central incisors (Fig. 20-17). Comparison of a current radiograph with previous films may show whether there has been an increase in size of the questionable area suggesting a cyst.

To distinguish a *radicular cyst* or *periapical granuloma* of one of the maxillary anterior teeth from a *nasopalatine canal cyst,* it is essential to establish the pulp vitality of the incisors and the integrity of the lamina dura. Also the spatial relationship of the radiolucency to the roots of the anterior teeth should be determined by noting whether the location of the lesion changes with respect to the apex in views made at different orientations. (See Chapter 6.) A periapical granuloma or radicular cyst will lie at the apex, whereas a nasopalatine canal cyst usually lies palatal to the teeth.

Although the features of a *dentigerous cyst from a mesiodens* may be quite similar to those of a nasopalatine cyst, the radiographic evidence of association with a supernumerary tooth will establish the true nature of the lesion.

Management. The appropriate treatment for a nasopalatine cyst is enucleation, preferably from the palate to help avoid the nasopalatine nerve.[23] If the cyst is large and there is danger of devitalizing the tooth or creating a nasooral or antrooral fistula, the surgeon may elect to marsupialize the defect.[29]

Nasoalveolar cyst

The nasoalveolar cyst (also called *nasolabial cyst*) is a soft tissue cyst that involves bone only secondarily. Its pathogenesis is unresolved. Some authorities[20,54] maintain that it is a fissural cyst arising from the epithelial rests in fusion lines of the globular, lateral nasal, and maxillary processes, others[51] that there is actually only a merging of the mesenchyme of the processes and not a fusion per se so there can be no epithelial entrapment in the nasooptic furrow. These later authors contend that the location of the nasoalveolar cyst strongly argues in favor of its development from the embryonic nasolacrimal duct, which initially lies on the surface.[38]

Clinical features. This rare lesion produces swelling of the nasolabial fold and in the nose, with flaring of the ale, distortion of the nostrils, and fullness of the upper lip below the nasal vestibule. It may bulge into the floor of the nasal cavity, and cause some obstruction; and if infected, it may drain into the nasal cavity.[48] It generally is unilateral, but bilateral lesions have occurred. Affected patients have a wide range of ages, from 12 to 75 years, with the mean 44 years. The incidence peaks late in the third decade. About 75% of the lesions occur in women. They are fluctuant and may cause pain and difficulty breathing through the nose, although swelling is most often the only complaint.[38]

Radiographic features. Nasoalveolar cysts are primarily soft tissue lesions and may not be apparent on a radiograph. Some are discovered during routine palpation of the nasolabial fold. Occasionally one will cause erosion of the underlying bone (Fig. 20-18), producing an increased radiolucency of the alveolar process beneath the cyst and above the apices of the incisors. Also the usual outline of the inferior border of the nasal fossa may become distorted, resulting in a posterior convexing of this margin.[41] The actual shape and position

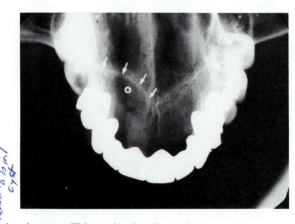

FIG. 20-18. Nasoalveolar cyst. This occlusal radiograph demonstrates pressure erosion of the alveolar bone *(o)* and destruction of the nasal fossa floor *(arrows).* (From Montenegro Chineallato LE, Demante JH: *Oral Surg* 58:729-735, 1984.)

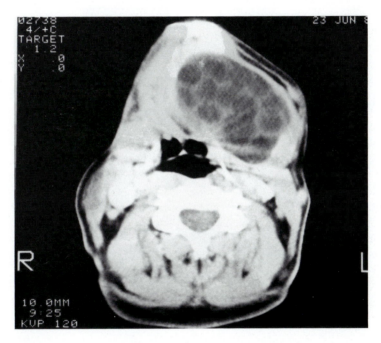

FIG. 20-19. This CT scan of a dermoid cyst illustrates an encapsulated mass on the *left*, with multiple cellular spaces. (From Hunter TB, et al: *Am J Roentgenol* 141:1229-1240, 1983.)

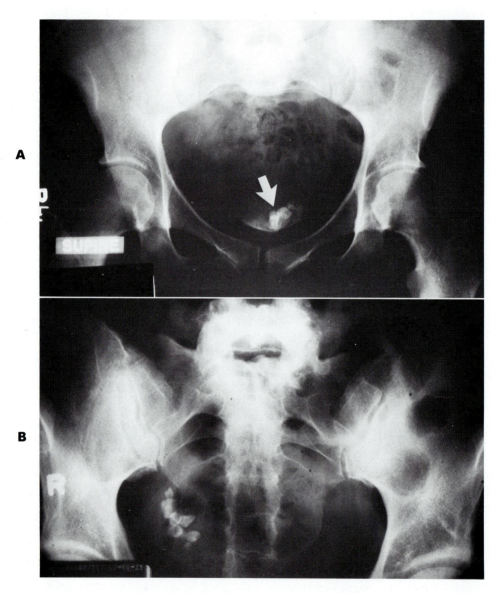

FIG. 20-20. Dermoid cyst containing teeth located, **A,** in the uterus *(arrow)* and **B,** in the ovary. (**A** courtesy Dr. R. Harwood, Los Angeles.)

of the cyst can be demonstrated by aspirating the typical cyst fluid and replacing it with a radiocontrast material.

Differential diagnosis. The swelling caused by an infected nasoalveolar cyst may be mistaken for an *acute dentoalveolar abscess*, especially if it is displaced downward. The adjacent teeth are always vital. It may also resemble a *nasal furuncle* if it pushes upward into the floor of the nasal cavity. A large *mucous extravasation cyst* or a *cystic salivary adenoma* should also be considered in the differential diagnosis of an uninfected nasoalveolar cyst.

Management. The nasoalveolar cyst should be excised using an intraoral approach. There is no tendency to recur.

Dermoid cyst

The dermoid cyst is a rare developmental anomaly that may occur anywhere in the body. About 10% or fewer arise in the head and neck, and only 1% to 2% in the oral cavity. Of those that develop in the oral cavity, about 25% occur in the floor of the mouth and on the tongue. They may be midline or lateral. Clinically, the lateral variety is usually responsible for less swelling than the midline variety.[52] Dermoid cysts are lined with epidermis and cutaneous appendages and filled with keratin or sebaceous material (and rarely with bone, teeth, muscle, or hair, in which case they are properly termed "teratomas").[42]

Clinical features. Dermoid cysts may develop at any time from birth, but they usually become clinically apparent between 12 and 25 years of age, about equally distributed between the sexes.[27] The swelling, which is slow and painless, can be up to several centimeters in diameter and may interfere with breathing, speaking, and eating. Depending on how deep it is in the neck, it can deform the submental area. On palpation these cysts may be fluctuant or doughy according to their contents; and because they usually are in the midline, they do not affect teeth.

Radiographic features. Inasmuch as there are seldom any mineralized structures within a dermoid cyst when it occurs in the oral cavity, it will be radiolucent on conventional radiographs; but a CT projection of the area closely approximates the pathologic description of the lesion (Fig. 20-19). If teeth or bone do form in the cyst, however, their radiopaque images with characteristic shapes and densities will be apparent on the radiograph (Fig. 20-20).

Differential diagnosis. Lesions that are clinically similar to the dermoid cyst are *ranula* (unilateral or bilateral blockage of Wharton's ducts), *thyroglossal duct cyst, cystic hygroma, branchial cleft cyst, cellulitis, tumors* (lipoma and liposarcoma), and *normal fat masses* in the submental area.[27]

Management. Dermoid cysts do not recur after surgical removal.

Former cysts

In recent years it has become clear that various types of cysts have been previously misclassified. These lesions include primordial cysts (now recognized largely to be odontogenic keratocysts), median palatal cysts (now recognized as a variant of the nasopalatine canal cyst), and median mandibular and globulomaxillary cysts (now recognized as being caused by other recognized cysts, mostly odontogenic occurring in the mandibular symphysis and maxillary lateral/canine regions respectively).

REFERENCES

1. Abrams AM, Howell FV, Bullock WK: Nasopalatine cysts, *Oral Surg* 16:306-332, 1963.
2. Ahlfors E, Larsen A, Sjögen S: The odontogenic keratocyst: a benign cystic tumor? *J Oral Maxillofac Surg* 42:10-19, 1984.
3. Allard RHB, Van Der Kwast WAM, Van Der Wall I: Nasopalatine duct cyst, *Int J Oral Surg* 10:447-461, 1981.
4. Altini M, Farman AG: The calcifying odontogenic cyst. eight new cases and a review of the literature, *Oral Surg* 20:751-759, 1975.
5. Angelopoulou E, Angelopoulos AP: Lateral periodontal cyst: review of the literature and report of a case, *J Periodontol* 61(2):126-131, 1990.
6. Anneroth G, Hansen LS: Variations in keratinizing odontogenic cysts and tumors, *Oral Surg* 54:530-546, 1982.
7. Batsakis JG: *Tumors of the head and neck*, ed 2, Baltimore, 1979, Williams & Wilkins.
8. Bone R: Cystic lesions of the maxilla, *Laryngoscope* 82:308-320, 1972.
9. Brannon RB: The odontogenic keratocyst: a clinicopathological study of 312 cases. II. Histologic features, *Oral Surg* 43:233-255, 1977.
10. Browne RM: The odontokeratocyst: clinical aspects, *Br Dent J* 128:225-231, 1970.
11. Browne RM: *Investigative pathology of the odontogenic cysts*, Boston, 1991, CRC.
12. Buchner A, Hansen LS: The histomorphologic spectrum of the gingival cyst in the adult, *Oral Surg* 48:532-539, 1979.
13. Chuong R, Donoff RB, Guarlnick W: The odontogenic keratocyst, *J Oral Surg* 40:797-802, 1982.
14. Donatsky O, Hjorting-Hansen E, Philopen HP, Fijerskov O: Clinical, radiographic, and histologic features of the basal cell nevus syndrome, *Int J Oral Surg* 5:19-28, 1976

15. Evans DC, Farndon PA, Burnell LD, et al: The incidence of Gorlin syndrome in 173 consecutive cases of medulloblastoma, *Br J Cancer* 64(5):959-961, 1991.

16. Fejerskov O, Krough J: The calcifying ghost cell odontogenic tumor or the calcifying odontogenic cyst, *J Oral Pathol* 1:272-278, 1972.

17. Frame JW, Wake MJC: Computerized axial tomography in the assessment of mandibular keratocysts, *Br Dent J* 153:93-96, 1982.

18. Freedman PD, Lumerman H, Gee JK: Calcifying odontogenic cyst, *Oral Surg* 40:93-106, 1975.

19. Gingell JC, Beckman T, Levy BA, Snider LA: Central mucoepidermoid carcinoma, *Oral Surg,* 57:436-440, 1984.

20. Gorlin RJ: Cysts of the jaws, oral floor and neck. In Gorlin RJ, Goodman HW (eds): *Thoma's Oral pathology,* ed 6, St Louis, 1970, Mosby, vol 1.

21. Gorlin RJ: Nevoid basal-cell carcinoma syndrome, *Medicine* 66(2):98-113, 1987.

22. Gorlin RJ, Goltz RW: Multiple nevoid basal cell epithelioma, jaw cysts, and bifid rib: a syndrome, *N Engl J Med* 262:908-912, 1960.

23. Harris M: A review of recent experimental work on the dental cyst, *Proc R Soc Med* 67:1259-1263, 1974.

24. Hartziotis J: Median palatine cyst: report of a case, *J Oral Surg* 24:343-345, 1966.

25. High AS, Hirschmann PN: Age changes in residual cysts, *J Oral Pathol* 15:524-528, 1986.

26. Kakarantza-Angelopoulou E, Nicolatou O: Odontogenic keratocysts: clinicopathologic study of 87 cases, *J Oral Maxillofac Surg* 48(6):593-600; 1990; [Comment in *J Oral Maxillofac Surg* 48(12):1353-1354, 1990.]

27. Killey HC, Kay LW, Seward GR: *Benign cystic lesions of the jaws, their diagnosis and treatment,* ed 3, Edinburgh, 1977, Churchill Livingstone.

28. Kondell PA, Wiberg J: Odontogenic keratocysts: a follow-up study of 29 cases, *Swed Dent J* 12(1-2):57-62, 1988.

29. Lucas RB: *Pathology of tumors of the oral tissues,* ed 4, Edinburgh, 1984, Churchill Livingstone.

30. Lustmann J, Bodner L: Dentigerous cysts associated with supernumerary teeth, *Int J Oral Maxillofac Surg* 17(2):100-102, 1988.

31. MacLeod RI, Soames JV: Squamous cell carcinoma arising in an odontogenic keratocyst, *Br J Oral Maxillofac Surg* 26(1):52-57, 1988.

32. Maxymiw WG, Wood RE: Carcinoma arising in a dentigerous cyst: a case report and review of the literature, *J Oral Maxillofac Surg* 49(6):639-643, 1991.

33. Moskow BS, Seigel K, Zegraelli EV, et al: Gingival and lateral periodontal cysts, *J Periodontol* 41:249-260, 1970.

34. Moskow BS, Weinstein MM: Further observations on the gingival cyst: three case reports, *J Periodontol* 46:176-182, 1975.

35. Nortjé CJ, Farman AG: Nasopalatine duct cyst. An aggressive condition in adolescent Negroes from South Africa? *Int J Oral Surg* 7:65-72, 1978.

36. Partridge M, Towers JF: The primordial cyst (odontogenic keratocyst): its tumor-like characteristics and behavior, *Br J Oral Maxillofac Surg* 25:271-279, 1987.

37. Regezi JA, Courtney RM, Batsakis JG: The pathology of head and neck tumors: cysts of the jaw. XII, *Head Neck Surg* 4:48-57, 1981.

38. Roed-Petersen B: Nasolabial cysts, *Br J Oral Surg* 7:85-91, 1970.

39. Saito I, Suzuki T, Yamamura J, et al: Calcifying odontogenic cyst: case reports, variations, and tumorous potential, *J Nihon Univ School Dent* 24:69-78, 1982.

40. Schwimmer AM, Aydin F, Morrison SN: Squamous cell carcinoma arising in residual odontogenic cyst: report of a case and review of literature, *Oral Surg* 72(2):218-221, 1991.

41. Seward GR: Nasolabial cysts and their radiology, *Dent Pract* 12:154-161, 1962.

42. Seward GR: Dermoid cysts of the floor of the mouth, *Br J Oral Surg* 3:36-47, 1965.

43. Shear M: *Cysts of the oral regions,* Bristol U.K., 1976, John Wright & Sons.

44. Shear M, Altini M: Odontogenic and nonodontogenic cysts of the jaw, *J Dent Assoc South Afr* 38:555-563, 1978.

45. Shear M, Pindborg JJ: Microscopic features of the lateral periodontal cyst, *Scand J Dent Res* 83:103-110, 1975.

46. Siar CH, Ng KH, Murugasu P: Odontogenic keratocyst: a study of 53 cases in Malaysia, *Ann Dent* 45:15-17, 1986.

47. Stockdale CR, Chandler NP: The nature of the periapical lesion: a review of 1108 cases, *J Dent* 16(3):123-129, 1988.

48. Summers GW: Jaw cysts: diagnosis and treatment, *Head Neck Surg* 1:243-256, 1979.

49. Suzuki S: On the lateral enamel strand and the enamel niche in human deciduous front tooth germs. [abstract.] *Bull Tokyo Med Dent Univ* 8:230, 1961.

50. Syrjänen S, Tammisalo E, Lilja R, Syrjänen K: Radiological interpretation of the periapical cysts and granulomas, *Dentomaxillofac Radiol* 11:89-92, 1982.

51. Ten Cate AR: *Oral histology: development, structure, and function,* ed 2, St Louis, 1985, Mosby.

52. Toller PA: Origin and growth of cysts of the jaws, *Ann R Coll Surg Engl* 40:306-336, 1967.

53. Vedtopte P, Practorius F: Recurrence of the odontogenic keratocyst in relation to clinical and histologic features, *Int J Oral Surg* 8:412-420, 1979.

54. Walsh-Waring GP: Nasoalveolar cysts: aetiology, presentation, and treatment, *J Laryngol Otol* 81:263-276, 1967.

55. Weathers DR, Waldron CA: Unusual multilocular cysts of the jaws (botryoid odontogenic cysts), *J Periodontol* 41:249-260, 1970.

56. Wood RE, Nortjé CJ, Padayachee A, Grotepass F: Radicular cysts of primary teeth mimicking premolar dentigerous cysts: report of three cases, *ASDC J Dent Child* 55(4):288-290, 1988.

57. Wright BA, Wysocki GP, Lorder TC: Odontogenic keratocysts presenting as periapical disease, *Oral Surg* 56:425-429, 1983.

58. Wright JM: The odontogenic keratocyst; othokeratinized variant, *Oral Surg* 51:609-617, 1981.

59. Wysocki GP, Brannon RB, Gardner DG, Sapp P: Histogenesis of the lateral periodontal cyst and the gingival cyst of the adult, *Oral Surg* 50:327-334, 1980.

21

STEPHEN R. MATTESON

Benign Tumors of the Jaws

A benign tumor is a new growth resembling the tissue of origin. It typically demonstrates an insidious onset, slow growth, a frequently well-defined mass of regular and smooth outline, a fibrous capsule, and displacement of the adjacent normal tissues. It is usually painless and does not metastasize. Most benign lesions do not endanger life unless they develop in an area that interferes with some vital function or organ.

Growth disturbances lacking the capacity for limitless proliferation are not true neoplasms but rather are *hyperplasias* or *hamartomas*. Hamartomas are abnormal new growths of tissue in their usual location that cease growing along with the tissues of the associated part (e.g., an odontoma). Tumors that continue to grow indefinitely (e.g., the ameloblastoma) are *neoplasms*. Because benign tumors are painless, many are discovered during routine radiographic examination. They may also be found on radiographs obtained to investigate a swelling or mass observed by the patient, suggested by the history, or detected by a physical examination. Only a few benign jaw tumors infiltrate or invade the adjacent normal bone for any considerable distance beyond the radiographic tumor margin, for example, ameloblastoma. Although such destructive lesions are benign (because they usually do not mestastasize), they are locally aggressive and tend to recur because their complete removal is surgically complicated.

After the clinical detection of a tumor and the procurement of adequate radiographic views, it is important to analyze the radiographic image critically and systematically. Radiographic signs are significant features of a tumor that show on the film, lend strong evidence for the type of tumor, and sometimes provide a specific diagnosis. For example, the appearance of periapical cemental dysplasia or an odontoma is so characteristic that a specific interpretation can be made from the film alone. Other tumors resemble one another and can be categorized only as benign with either an aggressive or a nonaggressive nature. It is possible to make the final diagnosis of such lesions only after biopsy. Even then, a diagnosis may require all appropriate clinical, radiologic, histopathologic, and laboratory data.

The radiographic image provides information about the tumor for analysis: location, three-dimensional anatomic relationships, radiodensity, size, shape, architecture of the tumor tissue, configuration of lesional borders, and effect of the lesion on adjacent structures (e.g., bony cortex, teeth, or periosteum). Early in the diagnostic workup of a tumor, it is important to identify the lesion tentatively as benign, aggressive benign, or malignant. Such a designation leads to a set of well-planned diagnostic and therapeutic steps.

Because of the specific anatomic predilection of many tumors, the location of a particular neoplasm is extremely important in its differential diagnosis. For example, odontogenic lesions occur naturally in the alveolar processes where tooth formation occurs. Vascular lesions may develop along the mandibular canal, arising from the inferior mandibular artery. Cartilaginous tumors occur in jaw locations where residual cartilaginous cells lie. The radiodensity of benign tumors is an important feature that lends evidence to the behavior of the lesion. Benign tumors may be radiolucent, mixed radiolucent and radiopaque, or radiopaque. Lesions that contain internal calcification in the form of calcified flecks, septa, or patterned compartments are usually benign because tumor calcification results from organized biochemical processes that occur in benign lesions and not malignant ones. In that both benign and malignant tumors may be radiolucent, it is necessary to differentiate between them by using other radiographic features. The shape of a tumor and the configuration of its borders may indicate the benign nature of the lesion. Regularity of tumor shape, round or oval, and well-defined borders are strong evidence that the lesion is benign. Often, benign lesions are encapsulated and enlarge gradually by formation of additional tissue. Tumor borders are, therefore, relatively smooth and well defined radiographically and sometimes demonstrate hyperostotic edges.

The manner in which a tumor affects adjacent tissues may also signal that it is benign. A benign tumor exerts pressure on neighboring structures, resulting in the displacement of teeth or bony cortices. Benign tumors may bodily displace nearby teeth in a fashion similar to orthodontic movement. For example, as a slowly expanding benign tumor mass approaches the inferior border of the mandible, the cortex becomes expanded or bowed outward from simultaneous resorption of bone along the inner cortex and bone formation along the outside cortical surface by the periosteum. Through this remodeling process, the cortex maintains its continuity between tumor and the surrounding soft tissues.

Roots of teeth may be resorbed by both benign and malignant tumors. This feature can assist in the differentiation of lesions that do or do not absorb roots. For example, most fibroosseous lesions do not cause root resorption. Tumors especially likely to do so are the ameloblastoma, ossifying fibroma, central giant cell granuloma, and squamous cell carcinoma. Benign tumors and cysts tend to resorb the adjacent root surfaces in a smooth fashion and only along the adjacent edge of the tumor. Malignant jaw tumors, however, tend to surround the entire root and, if resorption occurs, the entire root surface contracts into an altered conical form that has been described as spiked. The latter effect may occur with molar roots because of infiltrative carcinoma of the maxillary sinus.

The ensuing discussion considers bony hyperplasias separately from tumors because they are more functional in origin and behavior (with perhaps a genetic component[48]) than neoplasias. The benign neoplasias are separated into odontogenic tumors, lesions of tooth-germ origin, and nonodontogenic tumors.

HYPERPLASIAS

Bony hyperplasias are growths of new bone with normal architecture that occur on the skull and facial skeleton (e.g., the relatively common tori and exostoses). Although they are slow growing and of limited growth potential, they may continue to increase in size for variable periods until undergoing spontaneous arrest. They never seem to regress in size, however. Exostoses that frequently occur in specific locations on the jaws are tori. The *torus palatinus*, for example, occurs in the central portion of the hard palate, which is the most common site for an exostosis on the facial skeleton. The *torus mandibularis* develops on the lingual surface of the mandible, the next most common location for an exostosis, above the mylohyoid line, between the body and the alveolar process in the incisor-canine-premolar (seldom molar) area. Both mandibular and palatine tori usually appear before the age of 30 years, and growth often begins at the onset of puberty.[67] These exostoses are functionally determined.[48]

Torus palatinus

Clinical features. The torus palatinus, the most common of the exostoses, occurs in about 20% of the population, although various studies[18,88] have shown marked differences in racial groups. It develops about twice as often in women as in men and more often in Native Americans and Eskimos.[53] Although it may be discovered at any age, it is rare in children. Its development usually begins in young adults before age 30. The base of the bony nodule extends along the central portion of the hard palate, and the bulk reaches downward into the oral cavity. The torus palatinus varies in size and shape and has been described as flat, spindled, nodular, or mushroomlike (Fig. 21-1). A normal mucosa covers the bony mass and may appear pale and occasionally ulcerated when traumatized. Patients are frequently unaware of its presence, and those who do discover it may insist that it occurred suddenly and has been growing rapidly. Removal may be necessary if an upper denture is to be made.

Radiographic features. On a maxillary periapical or panoramic radiograph, the relatively dense radiopaque shadow of a palatal torus lies below and is attached to the hard palate. It may be superimposed on the apical areas of the maxillary teeth, especially if the torus has developed in the middle or anterior regions of the palate (Fig. 21-1). The border of the opaque shadow is usually well defined because the surface of the torus is compact bone (Fig. 21-2). The image of a palatal torus projecting over the roots of the maxillary molars may resemble that of the zygoma.

An occlusal radiograph provides a good demonstration of a palatal torus (Fig. 21-3). Its image is oval, and both the radiopaque border of compact

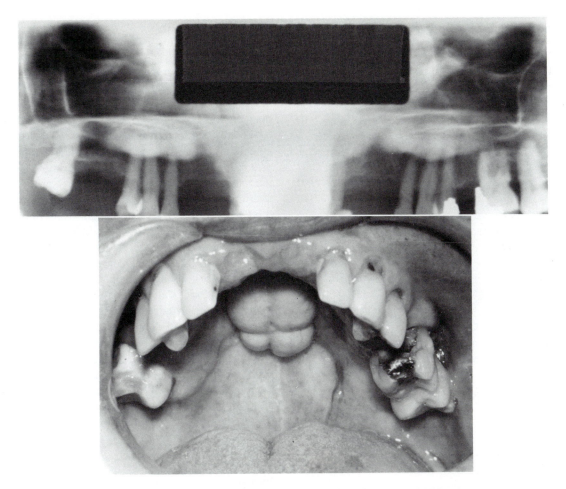

FIG. 21-1. Torus palatinus. (Courtesy Dr. Ronald Baker, Chapel Hill NC.)

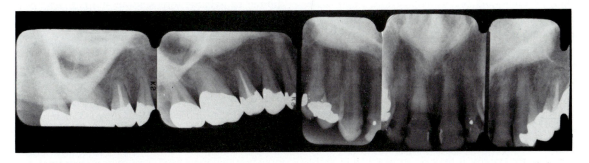

FIG. 21-2. Torus palatinus, seen as a dense opacity in the superior portion of each periapical radiograph in this region of the maxilla.

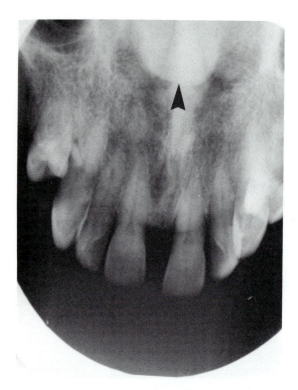

FIG. 21-3. Image of a palatal torus *(arrowhead)* on an occlusal projection.

bone and the less dense interior area of medullary bone are usually apparent.

Torus mandibularis

Clinical features. Tori on the lingual surface of the mandible have a lower incidence than those on the palate, occurring in about 8% of the population. They develop singly or multiply, unilaterally or bilaterally (usually bilaterally), and most often in the premolar region. The size is also variable, ranging from an outgrowth that is just palpable to one that contacts a torus on the opposite side. In contrast to the torus palatinus, the torus mandibularis develops later, being first discovered in middle-aged adults. There is no difference in its sexual predilection from that of palatine tori. Whether the presence of this entity correlates with that of the palatine torus is not clear. As its counterpart in the palate, it may occur more frequently in those of Mongoloid ancestry. Genetic and environmental factors seem to be involved in the development of this entity, but masticatory stress is reported as an essential factor underlying its formation. The high prevalence among Eskimos and other subarctic peoples who make extraordinary chewing demands on their teeth seems to support

this suggestion. Also, patients with a torus mandibularis have, on average, more teeth present than those without a torus.[24] Recognition of mandibular tori relies on their appearance and location. Their presence bilaterally reinforces this impression. Removal may be necessary if a lower denture is planned.

Radiographic features. On mandibular periapical radiographs, the torus mandibularis appears as a radiopaque shadow, usually superimposed on the roots of premolars and molars and occasionally over a canine or incisor. Usually it lies over about three teeth (Fig. 21-4). The images of these overgrowths are usually not as well defined from the adjacent normal bone as those of the palatal variety. Also, the distinction between cortical bone and cancellous bone is not as apparent as in the case of palatine tori. Mandibular tori are sharply demarcated anteriorly on periapical films and are less dense and less well defined as they extend posteriorly.

On occlusal projections, a mandibular torus appears as a radiopaque, homogeneous, knobby protuberance from the lingual surface of the mandible (Fig. 21-5). The border between it and the bone is not sharp but somewhat continuous, suggesting that the exostosis is not a growth on the bone but part of the bone.

Exostoses

Clinical features. Small exostoses may also develop on the facial surface of the maxillary alveolar process at the border between the attached gingiva and the vestibular mucosa, usually in the canine or molar area. They are less common than mandibular or palatine tori, seldom attain a large size, and may be solitary or multiple. Their shape is nodular, pedunculated, or flat prominence on the surface of the bone; because of their small size, they are seldom of clinical significance while teeth are present. They are covered with a normal mucosa and are bony hard to palpation. There are no published data indicating that they occur more often in either sex or what their actual incidence might be. Like the other exostoses described previously, they appear to be more prevalent in Native Americans.

Radiographic features. Radiographically, an exostosis generally appears as a circumscribed, smoothly contoured, somewhat rounded radiopaque mass (Fig. 21-6). Some, however, may have poorly defined borders that blend radiographically into the surrounding normal bone. Although

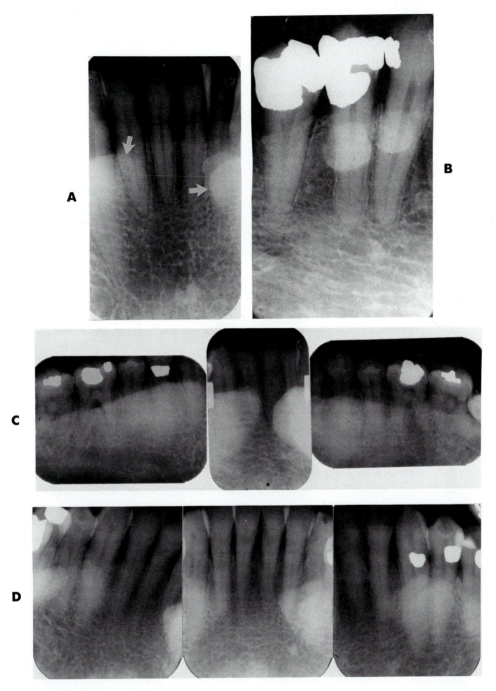

FIG. 21-4. Mandibular tori are usually seen as dense radiopacities in the canine, **A,** and premolar, **B,** regions. **C,** Large mandibular tori from the molar region to the midline. **D,** Note the common appearance of mandibular tori on these anterior periapical radiographs.

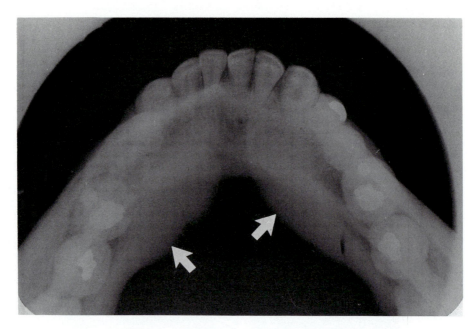

FIG. 21-5. Bilateral mandibular torsi as seen on an occlusal radiograph.

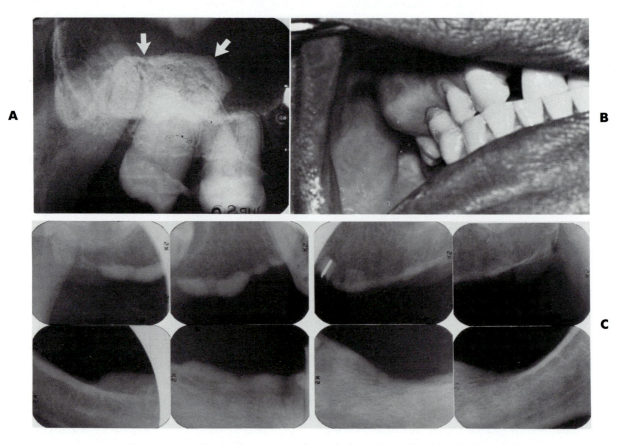

FIG. 21-6. Exostoses. **A,** Opaque bony exostosis on the buccal alveolar ridge in the molar region. **B,** Buccal exostosis in another patient. **C,** Alveolar exostoses in the molar regions (periapical films). (**A** courtesy Dr. A. Shawkat, Radcliff, Ky; **B** courtesy Dr. R. Langlais, San Antonio; **C** courtesy Dr. B. Glass, San Antonio.)

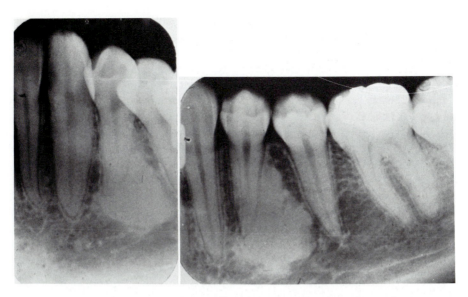

FIG. 21-7. Opaque area of osteosclerosis between the roots of premolars.

large exostoses can show interior medullary bone, most often they consist only of cortical bone.

Enostoses

Enostoses are the internal counterparts of exostoses. They are localized growths of compact bone that extend from the inner surface of cortical bone into the cancellous bone.

Clinical features. Enostoses are more common in the mandible than in the maxilla. They occur most often in the premolar-molar area, although there is no correlation between them and the presence or absence of teeth. They are asymptomatic.

Radiographic features. The radiographic image of an enostosis is a single isolated radiopacity that has borders that are usually diffuse but may be well defined. The trabeculae blend with those of the adjacent normal bone. No trace of a radiolucent margin or capsule lies in the sclerotic area.

Differential diagnosis. It is difficult to distinguish between an enostosis and a periapical idiopathic osteosclerosis (Fig. 21-7); however, doing so is not of clinical importance because neither condition requires treatment. Few other lesions have the dense opaque appearance of either enostosis or periapical idiopathic osteosclerosis. *Periapical cemental dysplasia* has a lucent margin; *hypercementosis* and *cementoblastoma* both develop around the roots of teeth, *osteosarcoma* and *chondrosarcoma* show evidence of a radiolucent component, as do *osteoblastoma* and *metastatic osteoblastic (prostatic) carcinoma*.

Management. Most sclerotic enosteal lesions go unrecognized and are not of clinical importance. If a lesion is suspected as being one of the serious osteoblastic diseases listed in the differential diagnosis, it should be periodically examined for evidence of growth. If increasing size of a lesion arouses suspicion, the tissue in question must be excised for microscopic examination.

ODONTOGENIC TUMORS

Odontogenic tumors arise in the tissues of the odontogenic apparatus. These tissues consist of two main groups, and tumors that derive from each group are similarly classified; the ectodermal (epithelial) odontogenic tumors, the mesodermal (connective tissue) odontogenic tumors, and the mixed or composite (ectodermal-mesodermal) odontogenic tumors. Odontogenic tumors constitute 1 in 50,000 of all tumors[7] and 1.3% to 15% of all oral tumors.[62,72] The ensuing presentation organizes benign jaw tumors according to their tissues of origin. This format should assist the reader in learning to correlate the radiographic appearance of tumors with the underlying pathologic basis of the disease process.

Ameloblastoma

The ameloblastoma represents about 1% of all oral ectodermal tumors and 11% of odontogenic tumors.[58,99] It is an aggressive neoplasm that apparently arises from remnants of the dental lamina and dental organ (odontogenic epithelium), and its histologic appearance is similar to that of the early cap-stage ameloblastic elements of developing teeth.[26] It does not histodifferentiate to the stage of enamel formation. An untreated tumor may grow to great size yet usually remain localized. As it develops, it causes bony expansion and possibly erosion of the cortical plate. Local invasion of the adjacent soft tissues may follow. True metastases are rare (1% to 5%) but are a serious aspect of the tumor.[91] Metastasis to the lung occurs probably via the hematogenous route. This tumor may also spread to more distant sites,[94] including the mediastinum, spleen, kidney, liver, brain, and lymph nodes. A malignant form, ameloblastic carcinoma, has been reported.[65]

Clinical features. There is a slight predilection for this lesion to occur in men, and it develops more often in blacks. Although it may occur in the young (3 years) and in individuals older than 80 years,[58] most patients are between 20 and 50, with the average age at discovery about 40 years.[78] Most ameloblastomas (80%) develop in the molar-ramus region of the mandible but may extend to the symphyseal area; most that occur in the maxilla are in the third molar area, followed by the maxillary sinus and floor of the nose. Although ameloblastoma in the maxilla is the most dangerous primary location for this lesion,[10] delay in recognition of maxillary ameloblastomas is common, and the time from onset of symptoms to treatment is often years.[15] The tumor is frequently discovered during a routine dental examination.

Although ameloblastomas grow slowly and there are few, if any, symptoms in the early stages, the patient subsequently notices gradually increasing facial asymmetry. Swelling of the cheek, gingiva, or hard palate has been reported[77] as the chief complaint in 95% of untreated maxillary ameloblastomas. The mucosa over the mass is normal, but teeth in the involved region may be displaced and become mobile. Pain and paresthesia, fistula or ulcer formation, and tooth mobility are not features generally, although they have been described.[80,96] As the tumor enlarges, palpation may elicit a bony hard sensation or crepitus as the bone thins. If the lesion destroys overlying bone, the swelling may feel firm or fluctuant when cystic degeneration has occurred. Tumors that develop in the maxilla may extend into the paranasal sinuses, orbit, nasopharynx, or a vital structure at the base of the skull.[93] Recurrence rates are higher in older patients and in those with multilocular lesions.[95] As seen with other jaw tumors, local recurrence, whether detected radiographically or histologically, may have a more aggressive character than the original tumor.[97] Nasal obstruction and epistaxis occur primarily in previously treated patients.[77]

Radiographic features. The radiographic image of an ameloblastoma varies according to the stage of its development and whether it has perforated into adjacent soft tissues. In its early stage of development, the lesion is well defined and, indicative of its slow growth, is frequently delineated by a hyperostotic border. Although its radiographic appearance is customarily described as multilocular, the radiolucent area in bone may also be unilocular (Fig. 21-8). There is a greater tendency for advanced cases to develop a configuration suggestive of compartments in the bone separated by distinct septa that reach into the radiolucent area (Fig. 21-9). In some cases the number and arrangement of septa may give the area a honeycomb (numerous small compartments) or soap bubble (larger compartments of variable size) appearance (Fig. 21-10). In advanced cases, when the cortex has been eroded in one or more areas, the perforated cortical plates may contribute to a multilocular appearance. The early ameloblastoma, however, is more likely to be a well-circumscribed, monocystic lesion that develops in the mandible of a younger patient and is not likely to recur.[51] It may be so typically cystlike that if the radiolucent area is associated with the crown of an unerupted or displaced tooth its appearance is that of a dentigerous cyst. Likewise, if the tumor has involved the roots of a functioning tooth, it resembles a radicular cyst (Fig. 21-11). There is also a more pronounced tendency for an ameloblastoma to cause extensive root resorption than is observed with other lesions[86] (Fig. 21-12). Occasionally an ameloblastoma forms from the epithelial lining of a dentigerous cyst. This is a mural ameloblastoma[27] (Fig. 21-13). An occlusal radiograph may demonstrate expansion and thinning of the cortical plate over the affected area, but, notably, a thin "eggshell" of bone usually persists (Fig. 21-14). Perforation of bone is a late feature.

Computed tomography (CT) and magnetic resonance imaging (MRI) are useful modalities for the examination of an ameloblastoma. CT not only may suggest the diagnosis and demonstrate the anatomic location of a lesion but also may help to detect encroachment into such vital regions as the floor of the mouth, infratemporal fossa, and submandibular region.[76] It is useful in determining perforation of the mandibular cortical plates caused

Text continued on p. 438.

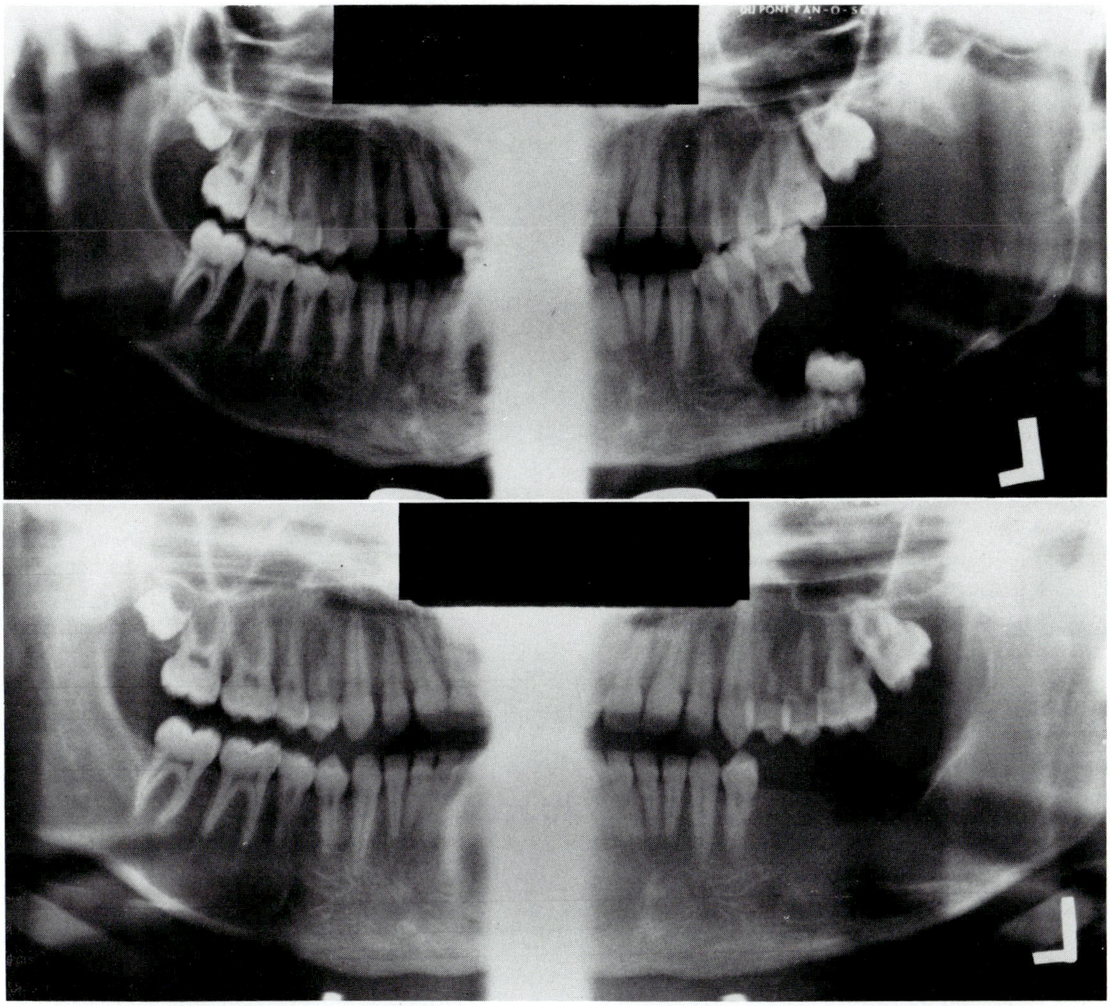

FIG. 21-8. Mural ameloblastoma. **A,** Cystic lesion, showing expansion of the mandible up to the mandibular notch, displacement of the mandibular second molar, and root resorption of the lower left first molar. **B,** Appearance after surgical treatment and subsequent healing. (Courtesy Dr. E.J. Burkes, Chapel Hill, NC.)

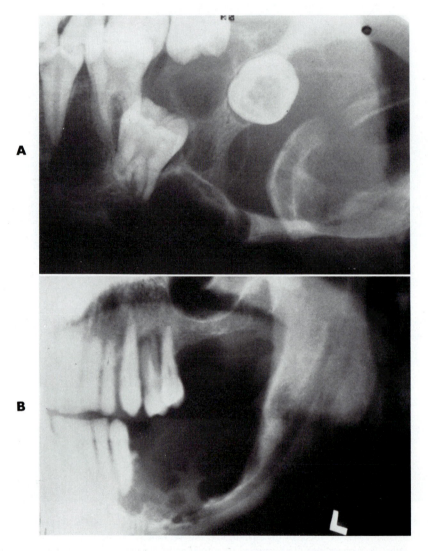

FIG. 21-9. Ameloblastoma. **A,** Multilocular lesion, showing gross displacement of the second and third molars. **B,** Another multilocular lesion. (Courtesy Dr. W. Via, Chapel Hill NC.)

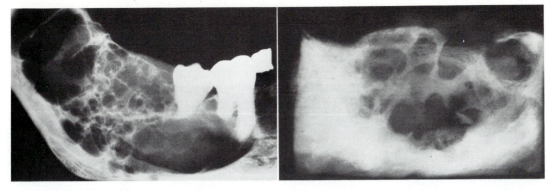

FIG. 21-10. Lateral radiographs of ameloblastoma, radiographs of surgical specimens. **A,** Multiple small cavities with root resorption. **B,** Multiple cavities with poorly defined borders.

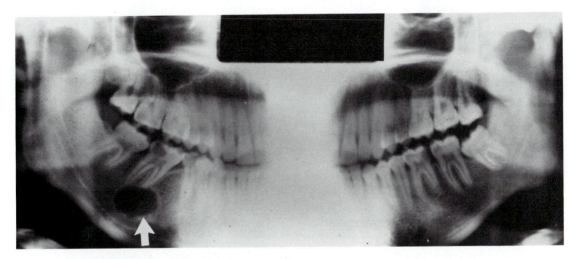

FIG. 21-11. Recurrent ameloblastoma with well-defined margins simulating a radicular cyst. (Courtesy Dr. E.J. Burkes, Chapel Hill NC.)

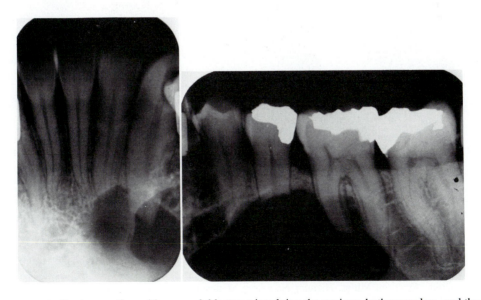

FIG. 21-12. Root resorption with an ameloblastoma involving the canines, both premolars, and the first molar.

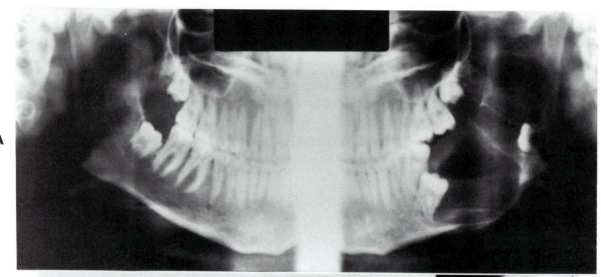

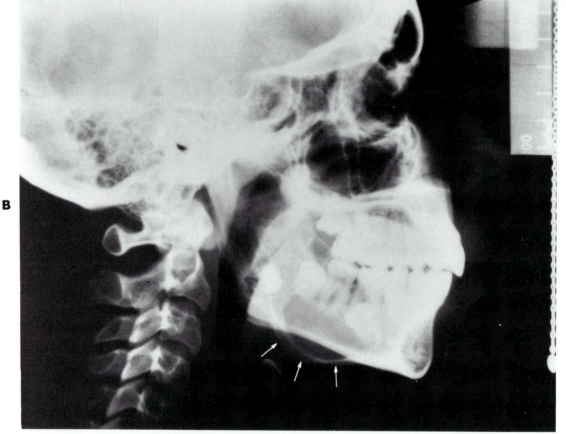

FIG. 21-13. Mural ameloblastoma. **A,** Note the expansion of its bony cortical borders, the displacement of teeth, and the presence of septa within the lesion (panoramic radiograph). **B,** On this lateral cephalometric radiographic, the *arrows* indicate inferior expansion of the lesion. (**A** and **B** courtesy Dr. John Miller, Hickory NC; from Matteson SR, et al: *Dent Radiogr Photogr* 57(1-4):1-84, 1985.)

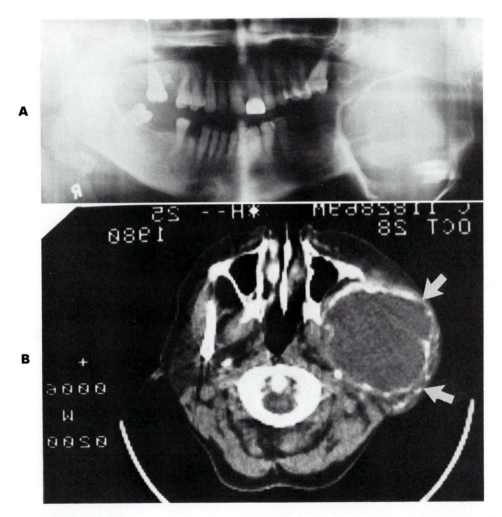

FIG. 21-14. Massive ameloblastoma with preservation of the cortical margin. **A,** Panoramic radiograph. **B,** CT scan at the level of the maxillary sinuses and upper third of the mandibula ramus. *Arrows* show the lateral tumor margin. Note the normal ramus on the opposite side, the maxillary sinuses, and the atlas, and dens. *Continued.*

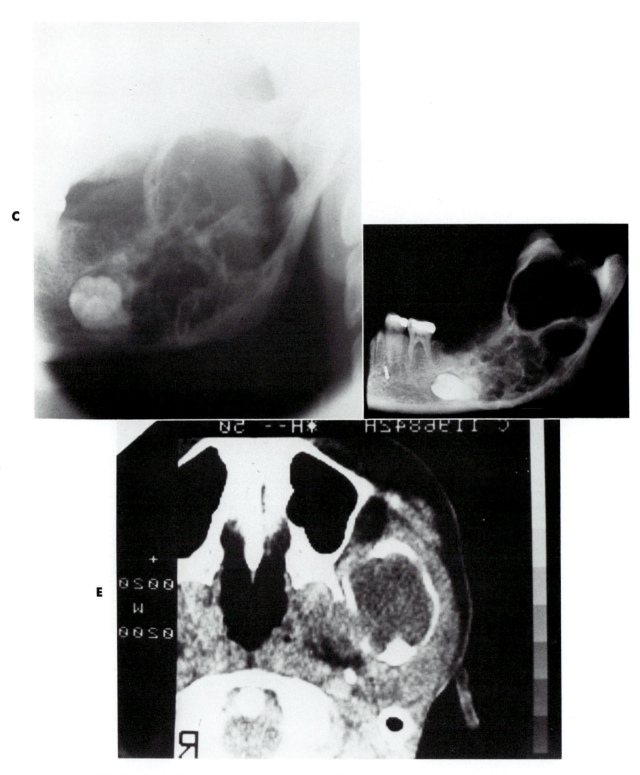

FIG. 21-14, cont'd. Another patient. **C**, Lateral oblique view. **D**, Resected specimen. **E**, CT scan through the midramus.

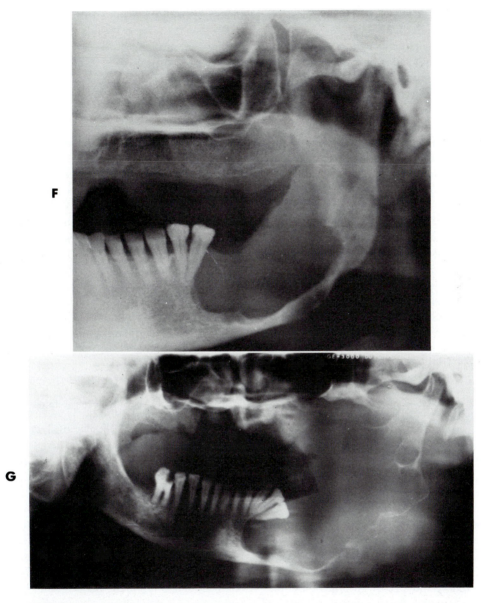

FIG. 21-14, cont'd. F, Large lesion. **G,** Same lesion 2 years later after the patient refused treatment. Note the loss of cortical bone on the anterior surface. (**F** and **G** courtesy Dr. B. Gratt, Los Angeles.)

by rapid enlargement of an ameloblastoma.[43] MRI helps to clarify evaluation of the tumor–normal tissue interface and is superior to CT in the assessment of recurrent disease. It is a useful supplement to CT in the presurgical and follow-up assessment of ameloblastoma.[42]

Differential diagnosis. When an ameloblastoma is small and unilocular, its appearance may share common radiographic characteristics with many lesions—including residual cyst, traumatic bone cyst, keratocyst, lateral periodontal cyst, giant cell granuloma, and odontogenic myxoma. All except the *residual cyst* and *lateral periodontal cyst* tend to occur in persons in their midtwenties or before; the *ameloblastoma* usually develops in older patients. The *giant cell granuloma* generally occurs anterior to the molars, the *lateral periodontal cyst* in the incisor-canine-premolar region of the mandible, and the *ameloblastoma* in the molar region. More advanced ameloblastomas have a dense multilocular appearance similar to that of an *odontogenic myxoma.* The differentiation of these two lesions might subsequently be influenced by a history of a missing tooth. The odontogenic myxoma is extremely rare and frequently associated with an unerupted tooth or one that has failed to develop. Also, the septa dividing the image of a myxoma are usually finer than those in an ameloblastoma.

Management. Whatever surgical procedures are used to treat an ameloblastoma, the surgeon must consider the tendency of the neoplasm to invade adjacent bone beyond its apparent margins. CT and MRI are useful in determining the location of tumor margins. If the ameloblastoma is relatively small, it may possibly be removed completely by an intraoral approach and without a full-thickness resection of the jaw. If it is extensive, however, its excision will probably require en bloc resection of the jaw. Although megavoltage radiotherapy can reduce the size of an ameloblastoma (primarily the part that has expanded the jaw or broken into the soft tissues), it does not appear to be an appropriate treatment for operable ameloblastomas. Its main use is for inoperable tumors, especially in the posterior maxilla.[6,32]

Adenomatoid odontogenic tumor

The origin of adenomatoid odontogenic tumor (AOT, formerly known as *adenoameloblastoma*) is still in doubt. It is an odontogenic epithelial tumor that most likely is a hamartoma and not a neoplasm.[17] It represents 3% of odontogenic tumors and is a developmental overgrowth of odontogenic tissue[19] that is not related to the ameloblastoma. This distinction is important because the surgical treatment for AOT requires only localized removal rather than the more extensive eradication required for an ameloblastoma.

Clinical features. The AOT is a relatively rare lesion[36] that appears in individuals ranging in age from 5 to 50 years; however, some 70% occur in the second decade (teens), average age 16 years.[99] The tumor has a 2:1 female predominance, with at least 75% occurring in the maxilla. Topographically there are central (97.2%) and peripheral (2.8%) AOTs, with two types of central lesions[66]: follicular (those associated with an embedded tooth) and extrafollicular (those with no embedded tooth). Approximately 73% of the central lesions are follicular, which are diagnosed somewhat earlier than the extrafollicular type, probably because the failure of the associated tooth to erupt is noted. The incisor-canine-premolar region is the usual area involved in both jaws, more than 90% in the incisor region. A frequent and notable feature is that the tumor surrounds the entire tooth, most commonly a canine.[99] The tumor is slow growing and, as it enlarges, there is a gradually increasing painless swelling or asymmetry frequently associated with a missing tooth.

Radiographic features. The usual radiographic image of the follicular AOT is a well-defined unilocular radiolucency associated with an unerupted tooth. The appearance may be similar to that of a dentigerous (follicular) cyst although, as with other odontogenic tumors, the outline of the lesion may extend beyond the crown of the impacted tooth. The border of the radiolucency is frequently sclerotic. Radiographically, radiopacities develop in about two thirds of cases.[66] One tumor may be completely radiolucent (Fig. 21-15), another contain faint radiopaque foci (Fig. 21-16), and some will show dense clusters of radiopacities (Fig. 21-17). Microscopic studies verify that the size, number, and density of small radiopacities in the central radiolucency of the lesion vary from tumor to tumor, and seem to increase with age. A radiograph will demonstrate that as the tumor enlarges it displaces the roots of adjacent teeth although root resorption is rare (Fig. 21-18).

Differential diagnosis. The differential diagnosis for the AOT should include the pericoronal radiolucencies: *dentigerous cyst, ameloblastoma,*

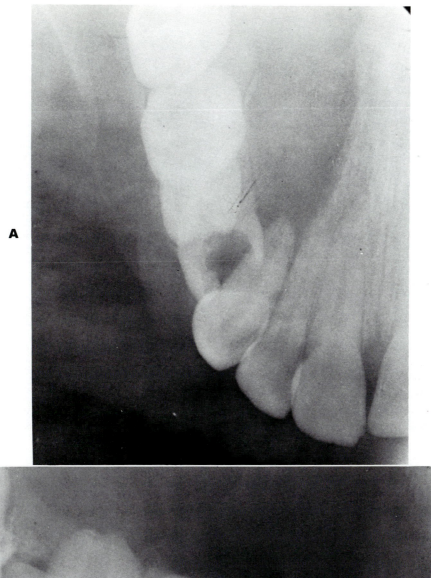

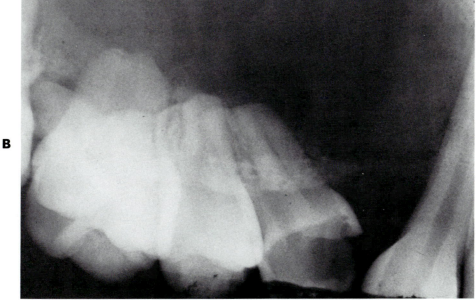

FIG. 21-15. Adenomatoid odontogenic tumor in the maxilla without evidence of calcification. An occlusal view, **A,** periapical view, **B,** and Waters view, **C,** show opacification of the right sinus. Note the expansion of the lateral wall of the sinus *(arrow).* (Courtesy Dr. R. White, Chapel Hill, NC.)

Continued.

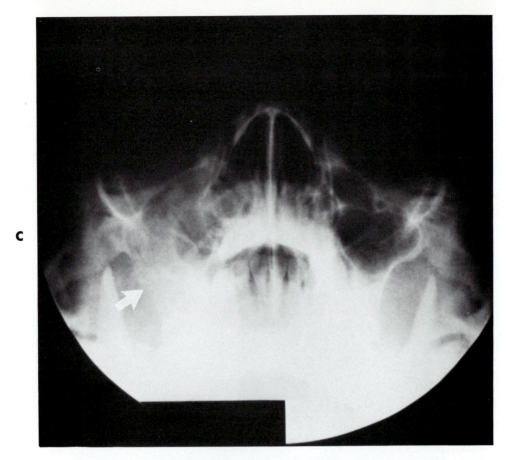

FIG. 21-15, cont'd. For legend see page 439.

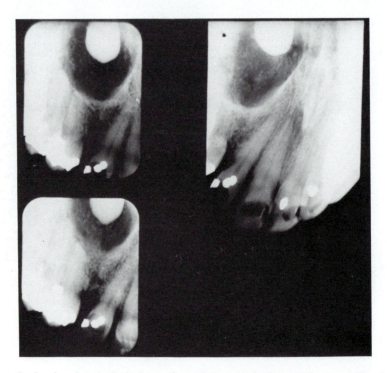

FIG. 21-16. Occlusal and periapical views of an adenomatoid odontogenic tumor showing opaque foci in the radiolucent space around the maxillary canine. (Courtesy Dr. L. Hollender, Göteborg, Sweden.)

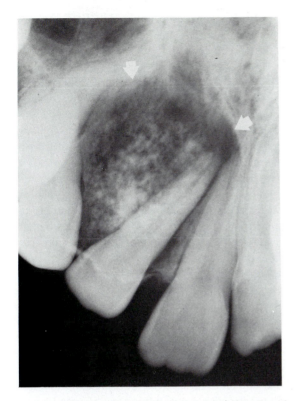

and *ameloblastic fibroma*. However, the combination of a relatively early age of occurrence, a predilection for the anterior region of the jaws, and a tendency to surround more than just the crown of the unerupted tooth with which it generally associates should prompt assignment of the highest probability to the adenomatoid odontogenic tumor.

Management. Conservative surgical excision is adequate because the tumor is not locally invasive, is well encapsulated, and is separated easily from the bone.[2]

FIG. 21-17. Adenomatoid odontogenic tumor in the region of the maxillary canine, showing multiple opaque foci and displacement of the canine and lateral incisor. (Courtesy Dr. R. Howell, Lincoln, Neb.)

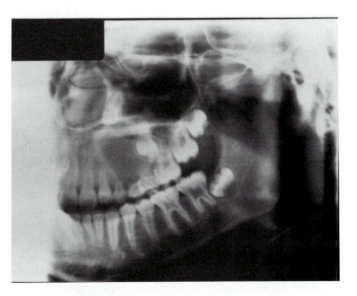

FIG. 21-18. Adenomatoid odontogenic tumor. Portion of panoramic radiograph of lesion in anterior left maxilla. Maxillary left canine and premolar have been displaced superiorly by tumor. Premolar is absent. (Courtesy Dr. E.J. Burkes, Chapel Hill NC. From Matteson, SR, Tyndall, DA, Burkes, EJ, and Jacoway, JR: Seminars in advanced oral radiology, *Dent Radiol Photogr* 57(1-4):1-84, 1985.)

Calcifying epithelial odontogenic tumor

The calcifying epithelial odontogenic tumor (CEOT, also known as *Pindborg tumor*) is a rare lesion of distinctive microscopic appearance that appears to arise from either reduced enamel epithelium or dental epithelium.[30]

Clinical features. The CEOT, which represents about 1% of odontogenic tumors, behaves much like an ameloblastoma; it is locally invasive with a high recurrence rate and is found in about the same age group.[33] This similarity even extends to the occurrence of rare extraosseous lesions.[98] The neoplasm is somewhat more common in men, and patients range in age from 8 to 92 years with an average about 42 years (considerably younger in men and somewhat older in women).[68] Like the ameloblastoma, this tumor has a definite predilection for the mandible, with a ratio of at least 2:1, and most develop in the premolar-molar area, with a 52% association with an unerupted or impacted tooth.[69] Cortical expansion is a regular feature, and about the only symptom, although one case in which the patient described an associated mild paresthesia has been reported.[54] Palpation of the swelling reveals a hard tumor that may be quite well defined or diffuse. Maxillary cases more often occur with swelling.[60]

Radiographic features. Early in the development of the CEOT, radiographs in about half of the cases reveal a radiolucent area around the crown of a mature unerupted tooth. The appearance mimics that of a dentigerous cyst[33] or even an ameloblastoma. The radiolucent, cystlike area may or may not be well delineated (Fig. 21-19). In some tumors the nature of the boundary may change from well defined to diffuse. Later, probably as the result of a maturation process, the radiograph reveals a unilocular or multilocular cystic lesion with numerous scattered radiopaque foci of varying size and density. The most characteristic and diagnostic finding is the appearance of radiopacities close to the crown of the embedded tooth.[69] In addition, small, thin, opaque trabeculae may cross the radiolucency in many directions. Radiographically, the lesion may resemble driven snow.

Differential diagnosis. Although one should consider all radiolucent lesions with radiopaque foci in the differential diagnosis of a CEOT,[99] its radiographic features most resemble central odontogenic fibroma, keratinizing and calcifying odontogenic cyst, odontoma (intermediate stage), and adenomatoid odontogenic tumor. They can be differentiated from the CEOT by their clinical features.

Management. Because the CEOT behaves clinically like an ameloblastoma, it should be treated like one.

Mixed tumors (ectodermal-mesodermal)

Odontoma. Odontomas are hamartomatous malformations of odontogenic tissue that demonstrate various states of histodifferentiation and morphodifferentiation. They apparently result from an extraneous bud of odontogenic epithelial cells from the dental lamina. Depending on the level of differentiation, they may contain various formations of dental tissues (enamel, dentin, cementum, and sometimes pulp or follicular tissue). The structural relationship of the component tissues may vary from nondescript masses of dental tissue (*complex odontoma*) to multiple well-formed teeth (*compound odontoma*). In a rare type of odontoma, the ameloblastic odontoma, some of its odontogenic epithelial component fails to histodifferentiate. This tissue continues to proliferate into undifferentiated ameloblastoma-like epithelium that mixes with the usual tissues in the tumor. A fourth, even less common variety, the ameloblastic fibroodontoma (discussed later in this chapter), can be identified histologically.[44] In one series of more than 700 odontogenic tumors, 67% of lesions were compound or complex odontomas and 4% were either ameloblastic odontomas or ameloblastic fibroodontomas.[72]

Clinical features. The odontoma is the most common (67%) odontogenic tumor,[72] and it often interferes with the eruption of a permanent tooth (Fig. 21-20).[73] There is no sex predilection, and most lesions begin to form while the normal dentition is developing (Fig. 21-21). Odontomas develop and mature while the corresponding teeth are forming and cease development when the associated teeth complete development. Most odontomas occur in the second decade of life. Odontomas rarely form with primary teeth.[83] If untreated, they persist; they are discovered throughout life. The compound odontoma is about twice as common as the complex, and more (62%) of the compound variety occur in the incisor-canine areas of the maxilla. In contrast, the complex odontomas are usually (70%) in the mandibular first and second molar area.[13] Although the compound variety forms equally among men and women, 60% of the complex odontomas occur in women.[99] Compound odontomas seldom cause bony expansion or exceed a normal tooth crown in size; most are between 1 and 3 cm in diameter. Most odontomas are discovered before the age of 20 years because of de-

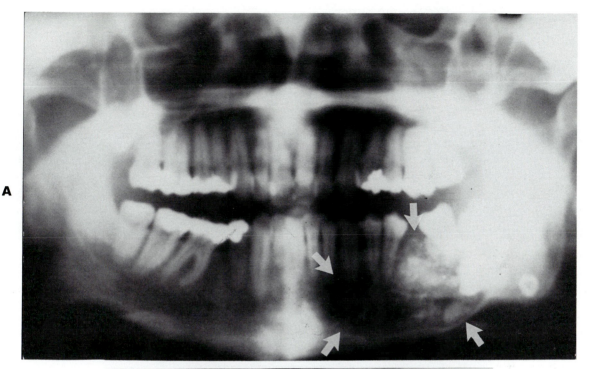

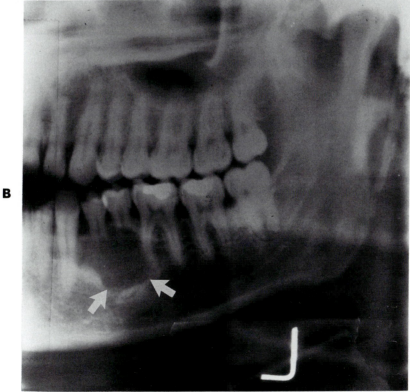

FIG. 21-19. Pindborg tumor *(arrows)*. In **A** it appears as a mixed radiolucent-radiopaque lesion associated with an unerupted tooth. In **B** it has caused resorption of the mandibular premolar roots. (**A** courtesy Dr. M. Gornitsky, Montreal; from Langlais RP, Bentley KC: *Exercises in dental radiology*. Vol 2. *Advanced oral radiographic interpretation,* Philadelphia, 1979, WB Saunders; **B** courtesy Dr. J.R. Jacoway, Chapel Hill, NC.)

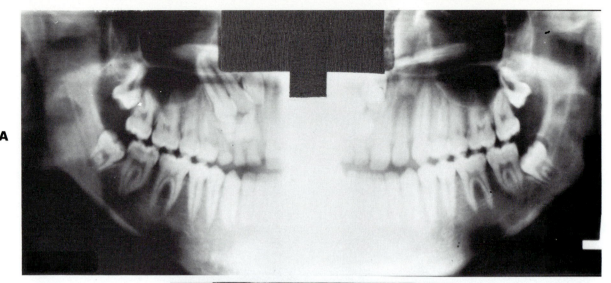

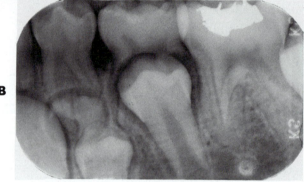

FIG. 21-20. Odontomas. **A,** Compound odontoma preventing eruption of the maxillary right canine, lateral incisor, and central incisor. **B,** Another compound odontoma in the mandibular premolar region preventing eruption of a premolar. (**A** from Matteson SR, et al: *Dent Radiogr Photogr* 57 [1-4]:1-84, 1985.)

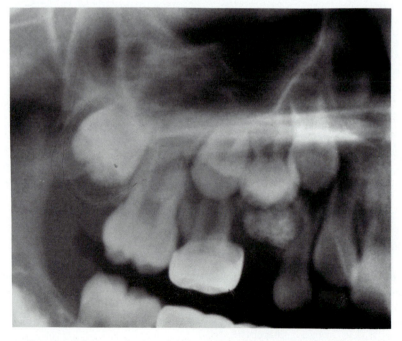

FIG. 21-21. Complex odontoma in the mixed dentition stage. This lesion, formed during development of the dentition, is blocking the eruption of a premolar.

layed eruption of adjacent teeth, retained primary teeth, or swelling.[3] Pathologic changes such as impaction, malpositioning, diastema, aplasia, malformation, and devitalization of adjacent teeth are associated with 70% of odontomas.[13]

Ameloblastic odontoma (AO, also known as odontoameloblastoma) is a clinically aggressive, rare, benign, odontogenic neoplasm characterized by the simultaneous occurrence of an ameloblastoma and complex odontoma, both of which may show recurrence following inadequate removal. They seem to appear in children early in the second decade of life, probably more often in boys,[44] with a slightly greater incidence in the mandible. They are frequently discovered during routine dental examination or routine investigation of the cause of a missing tooth. They cause bony expansion and destruction of the cortex, displacement of the teeth, and often mild pain.[82] They have clinical similarities to both the odontoma (age at time of diagnosis) and ameloblastoma (location, expansion, and recurrence rate).[52]

A related but extremely rare lesion, the *ameloblastic fibroodontoma,* consists of elements of an ameloblastic odontoma and a compound odontoma. Some suggest it represents a stage in the maturation of the ameloblastic fibroma and that this lesion may be more locally aggressive than the more common odontomas. However, there is little likelihood that this tumor could be recognized radiographically (Fig. 21-22).

Radiographic features. The compound odontoma demonstrates a number of toothlike structures (Fig. 21-23). The radiographic appearance of the complex odontoma is that of a well-defined radiolucent area containing an irregular mass or masses of calcified tissue (Fig. 21-24). The contents of these lesions are largely radiopaque. The extent to which the radiopaque structures occupy the radiolucent area and their variation in density, imparted by the distribution of enamel and dentin, vary from tumor to tumor. The complex odontoma usually forms in association with an unerupted canine, generally in the vicinity of the crown. This suggests that its origin is an extra bud of the dental lamina. The borders of both lesions are well defined but vary from smooth to irregular and may have a hyperostotic border.

The radiographic density of the ameloblastic odontoma may be radiopaque and similar to a complex odontoma or may be mixed radiolucent and radiopaque. This difference depends on the proportion of soft and hard tissue contained within the lesion. Radiographic evidence of bone expansion, destruction, tooth displacement, and resorption is possible. There is also a tendency for the radiopaque portion of the lesion to occupy a relatively smaller proportion of the lesion than in the odontoma (Fig. 21-25).

Differential diagnosis. The toothlike appearance of the radiopaque structures within the well-defined radiolucent lesion leads to the easy recognition of the compound odontoma. However, the calcified structures within the complex odontoma may be so nondescript that the radiographic appearance may be difficult to distinguish from a cementifying or ossifying fibroma, adenomatoid odontogenic tumor, calcifying odontogenic cyst, periapical cemental dysplasia, or calcifying epithelial odontogenic tumor. The complex odontoma differs from cementifying or ossifying fibromas because of the tendency of the complex odontoma to associate with unerupted molar teeth and by its tendency to be more radiopaque than the fibromas. The odontomas may also develop at a much younger age than the fibromas. The adenomatoid odontogenic tumor is rarely as opaque as a complex odontoma, and usually forms with maxillary canines. Periapical cemental dysplasia is usually smaller than a complex odontoma and occurs usually in the mandibular anterior region of the middle-aged adults. The calcifying epithelial odontogenic tumor is rare, usually less opaque, and usually develops in midlife.

Management. Complex and compound odontomas should be removed by simple excision because they do not recur and are not locally invasive. It is important not to injure the adjacent periodontium during their surgical removal.[89] Inasmuch as the accompanying epithelium may form cysts and neoplasms, the surgeon should be careful that it is entirely removed. The ameloblastic odontoma and ameloblastic fibroodontoma should be treated as if they were ameloblastomas because of their aggressive behaviors.[52]

Ameloblastic fibroma. The ameloblastic fibroma is a mixed odontogenic tumor arising from both epithelial and mesenchymal elements of the tooth germ. Although it is less common than the ameloblastoma, it does not rate the description of a rarity.

Clinical features. An ameloblastic fibroma is completely benign. There is no complete agreement relative to sex predilection, but most occur between the ages of 5 and 20 years, during the period of tooth formation, with the average being

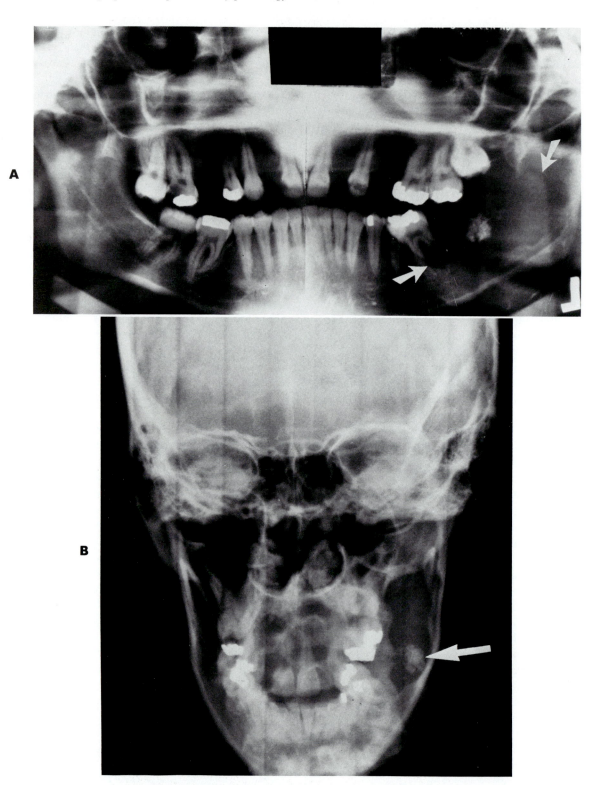

FIG. 21-22. Ameloblastic fibroodontoma shown as a large radiolucency with a small area of calcification in the left mandibular molar region. **A,** In this panoramic view *arrows* point to the anterior and posterior margins of the lesion. **B,** This posteroanterior view shows the lesion with a central opacity *(arrow)*. (**A** and **B** courtesy Dr. E.J. Burkes, Chapel Hill, NC.)

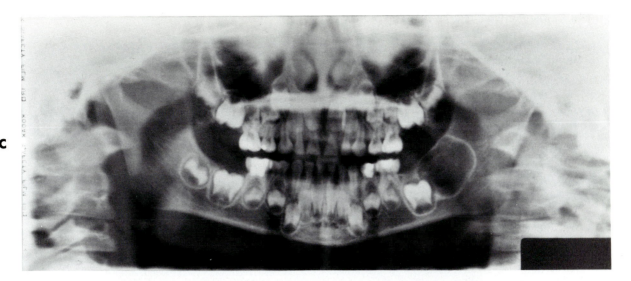

FIG. 21-22, cont'd. C, Another ameloblastic fibroodontoma in the left posterior mandible. (**C** courtesy Dr. Karl Kliner, Columbia SC; from Matteson SR, et al: *Dent Radiogr Photogr* 57 [1-4]:1-84, 1985.)

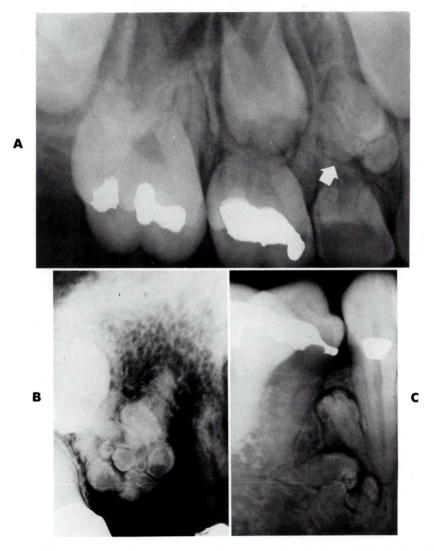

FIG. 21-23. Odontomas. **A** to **D,** Compound odontomas with multiple toothlike bodies. **E,** A developing odontoma (periapical films). The film on the *right,* made 9 months after that on the *left,* shows progressive calcification of the lesion. **F,** Compound odontoma in the maxillary premolar region (occlusal radiograph). (**A** courtesy Dr. W. Via, Chapel Hill, NC.) *Continued.*

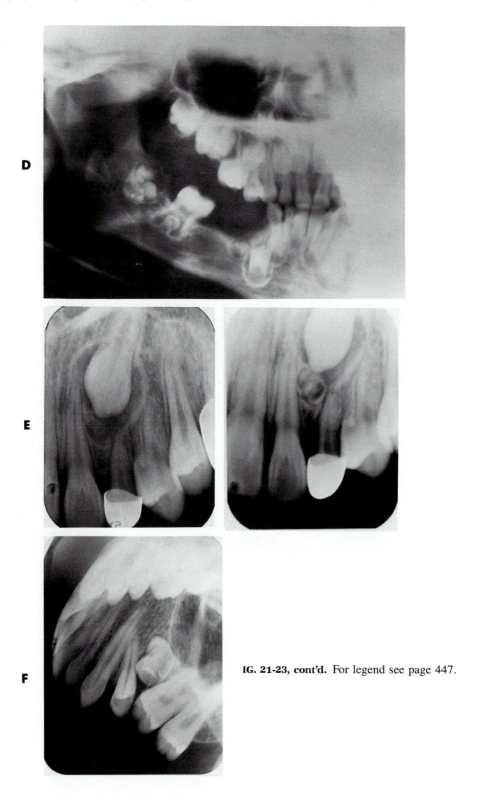

IG. 21-23, cont'd. For legend see page 447.

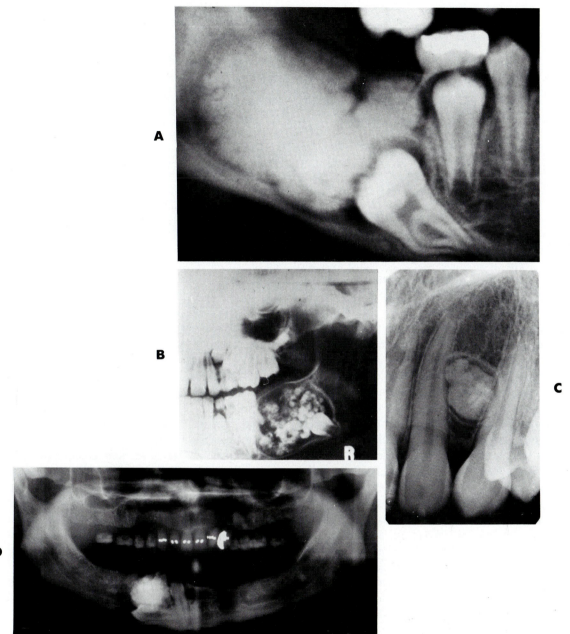

FIG. 21-24. Complex odontomas. **A,** Note the radiolucent space around the calcified mass. **B** and **C,** Peripheral cortical margin around a calcified mass. **D,** Complex odontoma in the anterior mandible (panoramic radiograph). Three impacted teeth are associated with this mass in an otherwise edentulous patient. (**C** courtesy Drs. A.G. Farman, Louisville KY; C.J. Nortjé, Tygerberg, Cape Province, South Africa; and R.E. Wood, Toronto.)

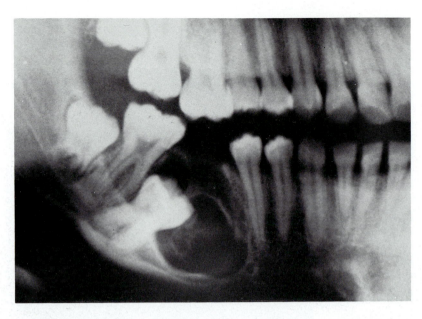

FIG. 21-25. Ameloblastic odontoma associated with the crown of an impacted mandibular first molar. (Courtesy Dr. E.J. Burkes, Chapel Hill, NC.)

about 15 years. However, some patients in their forties and fifties have been reported.[92] They usually develop in the premolar-molar area of the mandible and produce a painless, slow-growing expansion of the cortical plate and migration of the involved teeth (Fig. 21-26). In some cases the tumor may involve the ramus and extend forward to the premolar-molar area. Although the most frequent symptom is swelling or occlusal pain, the tumor may be discovered on a routine dental radiograph. It may be associated with a missing tooth.

Radiographic features. Radiographically, the ameloblastic fibroma closely resembles a simple ameloblastoma. The image of an ameloblastic fibroma may be either unilocular or multilocular (Fig. 21-27), and it may be associated with either an unerupted tooth or be in an area where the tooth failed to develop.[44] Its borders are well defined, and those associated with teeth may be difficult to distinguish from dentigerous cysts. However, in some cases there is a tendency for this tumor to appear as an outgrowth from the dental follicle rather than a symmetrical enlargement encompassing the crown, characteristic of the dentigerous cyst (Fig. 21-28). An expanded, intact cortical plate is frequently apparent on the radiograph.

Differential diagnosis. The ameloblastic fibroma may appear as a unilocular or multilocular lesion, usually in teenagers. The differential diagnosis includes central giant cell granuloma, aneurysmal bone cyst, odontogenic myxoma, central hemangioma, keratocyst (from a supernumerary tooth), and ameloblastoma. Distinguishing features that help to differentiate the ameloblastic fibroma are as follows: The giant cell granuloma, odontogenic myxoma, and central hemangioma have a finer trabeculation with a honeycomb or tennis racket pattern. The giant cell granuloma occurs more anteriorly, and none of the three necessarily associates with a tooth. In addition, the central hemangioma may show local gingival bleeding and rebound mobility of a tooth or teeth. By definition, the keratocyst usually produces a thick, yellowish, granular fluid. Finally, the ameloblastoma develops in a much older age group.

Management. Ameloblastic fibroma is benign, and the rate of recurrence is low.[38] Simple excision is the treatment of choice in most cases.

Mesodermal tumors

Odontogenic myxoma. The odontogenic myxoma (odontogenic fibromyxoma, myxofibroma) is uncommon, representing about 3% to 6% of the odontogenic tumors. It is a locally aggressive but nonmetastasizing neoplasm that probably arises from a developing tooth's primitive mesenchymal structures, including dental papilla, dental follicle, periodontal ligament, or odontogenic epithelial rests.[22] This entity develops only in the bones of

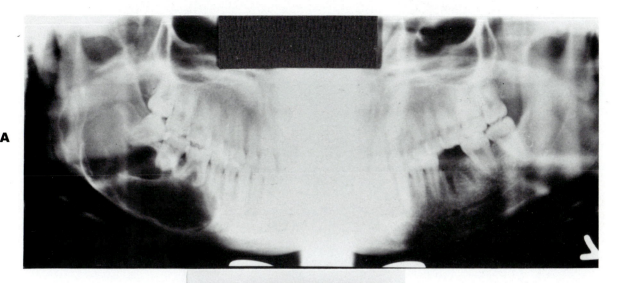

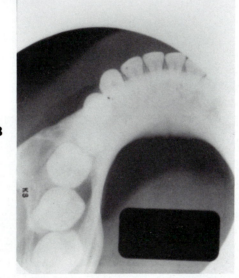

FIG. 21-26. Large ameloblastic fibroma in the right mandibular body and ramus, seen as a radiolucency on a panoramic radiograph. **A,** and occlusal projection, **B.** (**A** and **B** courtesy Dr. J. Winslow, Rocky Mount NC; from Matteson SR et al: *Dent Radiogr Photogr* 57[1-4]:1-84, 1985.)

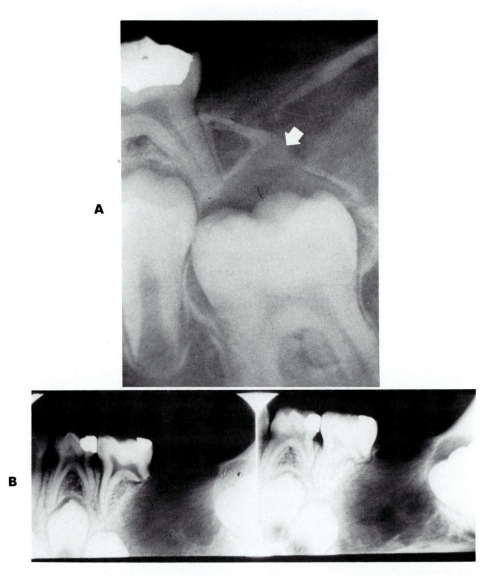

FIG. 21-27. Ameloblastic fibroma, appearing as a unilocular outgrowth of the first molar follicle, **A,** or as a multilocular growth stimulating resorption of the distal root of the primary molar, **B.** (**A** courtesy Dr. R. White, Chapel Hill NC; **B** courtesy Dr. L. Hollender, Seattle.)

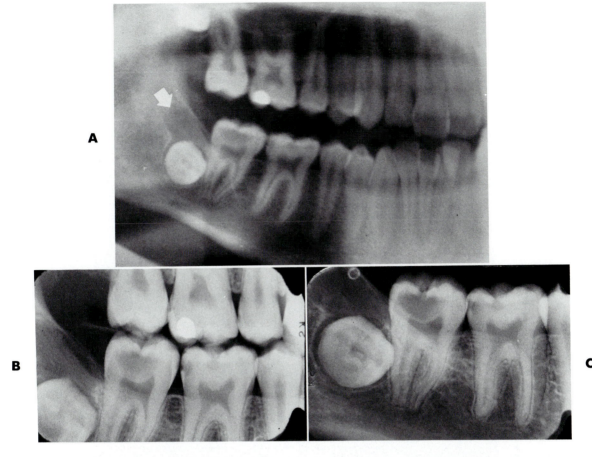

FIG. 21-28. An ameloblastic fibroma, seen as a faint radiolucency above the follicle of this unerupted third molar (*arrow* in **A**), grows superiorly and distally on a panoramic radiograph, **A,** bitewing, **B,** and periapical, **C,** view. (**A** to **C** courtesy Dr. G. Sanders, La Crosse, Wisc.)

the facial skeleton.[99] The concept that this lesion develops from odontogenic rather that nonodontogenic mesenchyme is supported by the facts that it only appears in the jaws, it affects young persons, it is related with a tooth that failed to erupt or is missing, and in some cases, odontogenic epithelium can be detected microscopically.[101]

Clinical features. If the odontogenic myxoma has a sex predilection, it slightly favors females; although it occurs at any age, more than half have occurred in individuals between the ages of 10 and 30 years, and it rarely occurs before age 10 or after age 50.[35] It more commonly affects the mandible by a margin of 3 to 1. In the mandible these tumors occur in the premolar and molar areas and only rarely in the ramus and condyle (non-tooth-bearing areas). Myxomas in the maxilla rarely affect the anterior area and usually involve the alveolar process in the premolar and molar regions and the

zygomatic process of the maxilla; they may also invade the maxillary sinus and cause exophthalmos.[22] The tumor is frequently associated with a congenitally missing or unerupted tooth.[90] The growth rate of this neoplasm is slow, and associated pain is variable.[78] Eventually the tumor causes expansion and becomes huge if unattended. When the tumor expands in a tooth-bearing area, it displaces and loosens teeth, but root resorption is rare. Recurrence rates of up to 25% have been reported. This high rate may result from the lack of encapsulation of the tumor, its poorly defined boundaries, and the extension of nests or pockets of myxoid (jellylike) tumor into trabecular spaces, where they are difficult to detect and remove surgically.[20]

Radiographic features. Radiographically, the destructive, expansive nature of the odontogenic myxoma may be apparent. It may be either uni-

FIG. 21-29. Odontogenic myxoma. **A,** Large lesion in body of mandible. **B,** Occlusal view shows buccal expansion of lesion. **C,** Periapical view shows angular trabecular pattern. **D,** Surgical specimen from same patient.

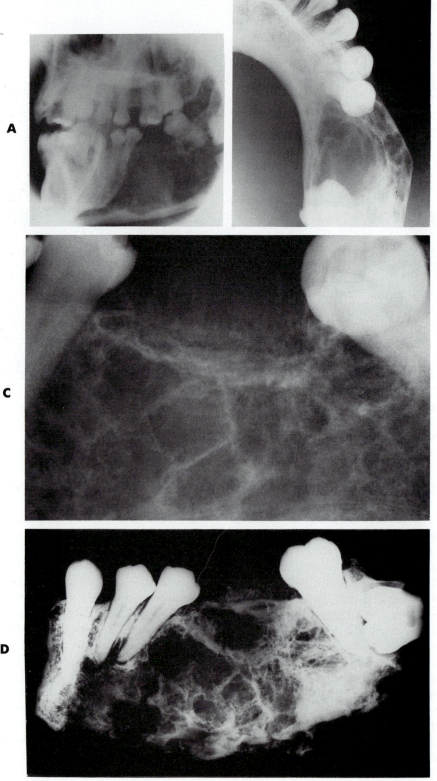

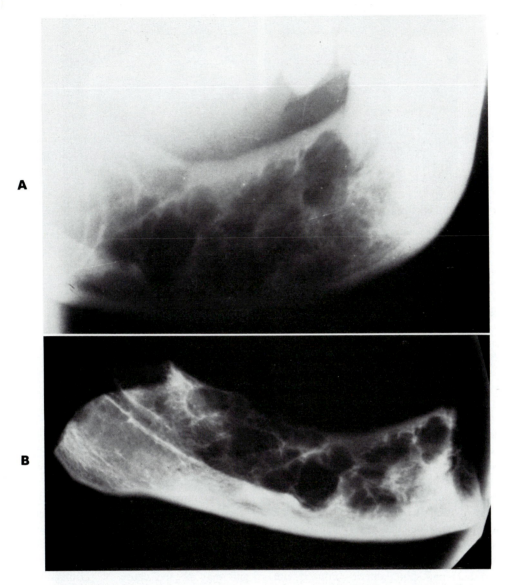

FIG. 21-30. Odontogenic myxoma with ill-defined borders. **A,** Lateral oblique radiograph. **B,** Lateral radiograph of a surgical specimen.

locular or multilocular, although some describe it as typically multilocular,[16] especially after it has enlarged.[8] Although the locules are usually small and uniform with the typical honeycomb effect, the arrangement of the trabeculae may also suggest the strings of a tennis racket (Fig. 21-29). When it occurs pericoronally with an impacted tooth, it is most likely to have a cystlike unilocular outline, although it may have a mixed radiolucent-radiopaque image. Often exceptionally fine septa cross the radiolucent areas, producing a wispy soap bubble appearance. The radiolucent area is usually well defined, and it is common for it to have a corticated margin. However, the outline of some lesions is

poorly defined (Fig. 21-30). In addition, the lesion frequently scallops between the roots of adjacent teeth, and the roots may rarely show resorption.[58] CT and MR imaging enhance the visualization of the anatomic extent of the lesion and better define the tumor–normal tissue interface. Accordingly, these advanced imaging procedures may enhance surgical treatment planning[21] (Fig. 21-31).

Differential diagnosis. Because the radiographic image of most odontogenic myxomas is a multilocular radiolucency, the differential diagnosis should include all lesions that may produce such a pattern: ameloblastoma, central giant cell granuloma, central giant cell lesion of hyperparathy-

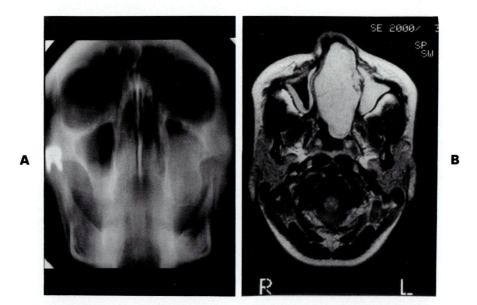

FIG. 21-31. Myxoma. **A,** A coronal tomogram shows clouding of the left maxillary sinus with expansion of the sinus borders laterally and inferiorly. **B,** A MR image (axial plane) through the maxillary sinuses shows a high-density area in the right sinus, representing the myxoma. (**A** and **B** courtesy Drs. A.G. Farman, Louisville KY; C.J. Nortjé, Tygerberg, Cape Province, South Africa; and R.E. Wood, Toronto.)

roidism, cherubism, aneurysmal bone cyst, metastatic tumor to the jaw, and central hemangioma.

Initially the central giant cell granuloma has a low probability because of its usual anterior location in the mandible. An ameloblastoma is also unlikely because this lesion usually occurs with an older age distribution than the myxoma. An image of fine honeycomb trabeculation (typical of some myxomas) also is unlikely in an ameloblastoma. Cherubism occurs in a younger age group and is bilateral, so this tumor should not be confused with myxoma. The giant cell lesion of hyperparathyroidism can be eliminated from consideration if the patient has no history of kidney disease and normal serum chemistry. Metastatic carcinoma can be given a low rank on the basis of the usual older age for such development and if there is an absence of a primary tumor in any other area. The aneurysmal bone cyst is rarer than the myxoma and usually tender or painful. The intrabony (central) hemangioma may arise in the same age group and location and have a similar radiographic appearance as the myxoma. However, it is not associated with a missing tooth, nor is the myxoma associated with the pumping tooth syndrome. Aspiration of blood from the lesion should differentiate between these two; aspiration of a myxoma is nonproductive. The most important and difficult differential diagnosis includes the myxoid liposarcoma secondarily invading the jaws, fibrosarcoma with myxoid changes, and the rare primary liposarcoma in bone. Histologic evaluation is essential in the final diagnosis.[35]

Management. The tumor is treated by resection with a generous amount of surrounding bone to assure removal of myxomatous tumor that infiltrates the adjacent marrow spaces. Radiation therapy is probably of no value in its management[22] and may be the cause of postirradiation sarcomas.[101] With appropriate treatment, prognosis of the odontogenic myxoma is good.

Benign cementoblastoma. The benign cementoblastoma is most likely a neoplasm of cementum derived from the periodontal ligament. It is produced by functioning cementoblasts. They produce a relatively large bulbous mass of cementum on the roots of a tooth. Most commonly this tumor develops with permanent teeth but rarely with primary teeth.[12]

Clinical features. Although statistical data suggest that this tumor is uncommon,[28] many believe it occurs more frequently than published accounts indicate.[58] The lesion is more frequent in males than in females. The ages of the reported patients range from 12 to 65 years, although most patients are younger than 25. There is no racial predilection.

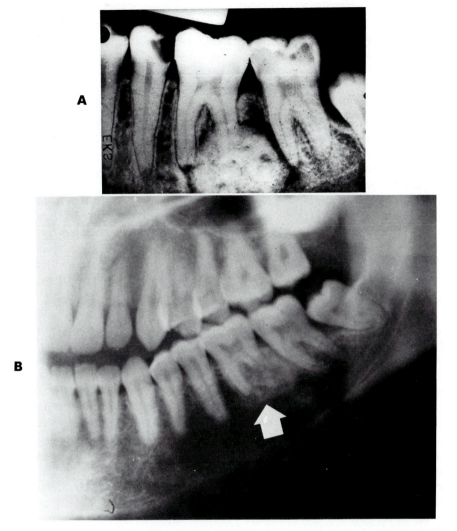

FIG. 21-32. Cementoblastoma, appearing as a dense opacification with a radiolucent border on this periapical radiograph, **A,** and on a panoramic projection (from another patient), **B,** *(arrow).* (**A** courtesy Dr. L. Hollender, Seattle; **B** courtesy Dr. C.Q. Cherry, Wilmington NC.)

It is usually a solitary lesion, occurs more often in the mandible, and forms on a second premolar or first molar. The lesion is slow growing but may eventually displace teeth. The involved tooth is vital. The tumor grows slowly, forming a mass at the roots. In some cases it may cause expansion of the jaw. Associated pain seems to vary from patient to patient.[1]

Radiographic features. The radiographic image of a benign cementoblastoma is a well-defined radiopacity usually attached to the root of a premolar or molar (Fig. 21-32). There is usually a radiolucent halo (zone) at the border of the calcified mass. The density of the cementum mass usually obscures the outline of the enveloped root. If the

root outline is apparent, it always shows some resorption. An occlusal radiograph will demonstrate its expansile nature.

Differential diagnosis. The differential diagnosis for benign cementoblastoma should include periapical cemental dysplasia, chronic focal sclerosing osteomyelitis, periapical osteosclerosis, and hypercementosis. However, the clinical and radiographic features usually allow differentiation of the benign cementoblastoma from these other periapical radiopacities. It is intimately associated with the root of a tooth, larger than hypercementosis, and separated from the surrounding bone by a radiolucent rim.

Management. The tumor is apparently self-limiting and does not recur after enucleation. Simple exicision and extraction of the associated tooth are sufficient treatment.[16] In some cases the tumor may be amputated from the tooth, which is then treated endodontically.[74]

NONODONTOGENIC TUMORS

The ectodermal and mixed ectodermal-mesodermal benign nonodontogenic tumors are tumors of neural tissue. Benign intraosseous nerve tumors arise from the nerve sheaths and from the nerve fibers in combination with their supporting tissues. These are the neuromas, neurofibromas, and neurilemomas. Although they are rare, most occur in the jaws, especially in the body and ramus of the mandible.[25,71] That most nerve sheath tumors occur in the mandible may be because the mandibular canal conveys a larger neurovascular bundle for a longer distance than does any other bony canal.

Ectodermal

Neurilemoma (schwannoma). The central neurilemoma is of neuroectodermal origin, arising from the Schwann cells that make up the inner layer covering the peripheral nerves. Although rare, it is the most common of the nerve tumors.

Clinical features. The neurilemoma is slow growing, occurs at any age from young to old, and occurs with equal frequency in both sexes. The lesion most often involves the mandible, with fewer than 1 in 10 cases occurring in the maxilla. There are few symptoms except those that relate to location and size of the tumor. The usual complaint is a "lump in the jaw." They usually occur singly, and the jaw expansion may lead to perforation and a mass that is firm to palpation. Being solid tumor tissue, they are nonproductive on aspiration. Although pain is uncommon, unless the tumor encroaches on adjacent nerves, paresthesia may arise with these bony lesions. Pain, when present, usually develops at the site of the tumor, and the paresthesia occurs distal to the tumor.

Radiographic features. The radiographic features of the neurilemoma are usually a round or oval radiolucent area of bone destruction posterior to the mental foramen. If the tumor protrudes from the mental foramen, there may be an erosive lesion on the surface of the jawbone from pressure caused by the overlying tumor. The expanding tumor may cause root resorption of adjacent teeth. In keeping with its slow rate of growth, the margins are well defined, cystlike, and occasionally hyperostotic. There may be loculations or areas of cortical ero-

sion that suggest a multilocular nature. It may resemble an ameloblastoma.[4,87] The radiographic features are not distinctive.

Differential diagnosis. Because the neurilemoma, like the other nerve sheath tumors, has few if any distinctive features and may also have a multilocular radiographic image, a differential diagnosis would be unwieldy and not generally rewarding. Only when the lesion is small and confined to a clear expansion of the inferior alveolar dental canal is the neural nature of the lesion suggested.

Management. Excision is usually the treatment of choice because malignant change in the neurilemoma probably does not occur. These lesions generally do not recur if completely removed. A capsule is usually present, facilitating surgical removal. However, periodic examination is indicated to monitor for recurrence.

Neuroma. Despite its name, the neuroma (also known as amputation neuroma or traumatic neuroma) is not a neoplasm. Rather, this lesion is an overgrowth of a severed nerve attempting to regenerate when scar tissue or malalignment of a fractured nutrient canal blocks its distal end. As a result, the proliferating nerve forms an unorganized collection of nerve fibers composed of varying proportions of axons, perineural connective tissue, and Schwann cells. The nerve damage may be the result of mechanical or chemical irritation of the nerve due to fracture, orthognathic surgery, removal of a tumor or cyst, extrusion of endodontic cement, dental implants, or tooth extraction.[5,40,41,45,64]

Clinical features. The central neuroma is a slow-growing reactive hyperplasia that seldom becomes large, rarely more than 1 cm in diameter. Larger lesions destroying a considerable amount of bone have been described.[37] They may cause varying symptoms, including severe pain as a result of pressure applied as the tangled mass enlarges in its bony cavity or as the result of external trauma. The patient may have reflex neuralgia, with pain referred to the eyes, face, and head.

Radiographic features. Radiographic features of a neuroma relate to the extent and shape of the proliferating mass of neural tissue. When the mass grows larger than the size of trabecular spaces, it appears as a radiolucent area in bone with well-defined borders. It may occur in various shapes, depending on how the resistance offered by the surrounding bone affects its expansion. In the mandible it usually forms in the mandibular canal, which should help distinguish it from a cyst.

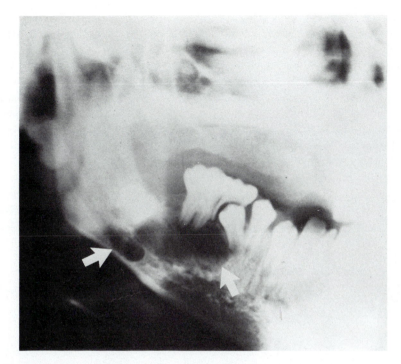

FIG. 21-33. Neurofibroma *(arrow)* in an 11-year-old boy with von Recklinghausen's disease. (Courtesy Dr. P. Boyne, Loma Linda Calif; from Langland OE, et al: *Principles and practice of panoramic radiology,* Philadelphia, 1982, WB Saunders.)

Differential diagnosis. The presence of a painful or extremely sensitive cystlike radiolucency in the bone and a history of fracture or surgery in the same region suggests a neuroma.

Management. Treatment is recommended because the neuroma tends to continue to enlarge. It may also cause pain. Regardless of the nature of the injury that precipitated the development of the neuroma, its simple excision is not commonly followed by recurrence.

Mixed tumors (ectodermal-mesodermal)

Neurofibroma. The neurofibroma is composed of both the connective tissue of the sheath of Schwann and also other components of the peripheral nerves including the axons. As the neurofibroma grows, it incorporates axons. By contrast, the neurilemoma is composed entirely of Schwann cells and grows by displacing axons.

Clinical features. The central lesion of neurofibroma is the same as the multiple lesions that develop in von Recklinghausen's disease. The central lesions may also occur in that syndrome. It occurs at any age, but is usually found in young patients. Its distribution in both jaws tends to be more proximal than the neurilemoma, and it has a

high potential for malignant change. The central neurofibroma may occur in the mandibular canal, in the spongiosa, and below the periosteum. The central lesions may also be multiple, occurring in both jaws simultaneously and expanding and filling the maxillary sinus. Patients with solitary central lesions may infrequently develop brown spots in the skin and, even less frequently, scoliosis.[46] The neurofibroma associated with the mandibular nerve is most likely to produce pain or paresthesia,[63] but fortunately it is rare. It may expand and perforate the cortex, producing swelling that is either hard or firm to palpation.

Radiographic features. There is nothing distinctive about the radiographic appearance of a neurofibroma. A neurofibroma of the inferior dental nerve shows a fusiform enlargement of the canal (Fig. 21-33). The density and size of this tumor are variable, depending on its location, and proportional to the extent of bone destruction. Like the neurilemoma, the margins of the radiolucency are usually sharply defined and may be hyperostotic. However, despite its benign nature and slow growth, some neurofibromas have indistinct margins. The tumors usually appear unilocular, but a multilocular image may occur. Radiographic

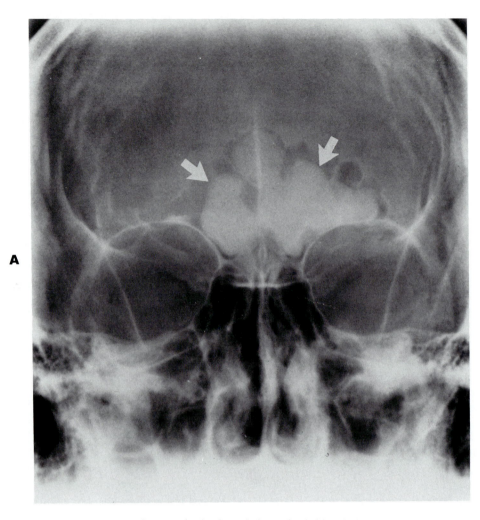

A

FIG. 21-34. Osteoma in the frontal sinus. **A,** Caldwell view *(arrows).*

changes in the jaws associated with neurofibromatosis include enlargement of the mandibular canal, mental and mandibular foramina, and increased incidence of branched mandibular canal.[23]

Differential diagnosis. Lesions localized to the mandibular canal suggest early nerve tumors. When the neurofibroma and the other nerve sheath tumors increase in size beyond the canal, there is so little that is distinctive that differential diagnosis is of little or no potential value. Vascular lesions should also be considered when radiolucent lesions are present along the mandibular neurovascular canal.

Management. Solitary central lesions that have been excised seldom recur. It is wise to reexamine the area periodically because these tumors are not encapsulated. Some undergo malignant change.

Mesodermal tumors

Osteoma. The cause of the slow-growing osteoma is obscure, but it may arise from cartilage or embryonal periosteum. It is not clear whether it is a benign tumor or hamartoma. It occurs almost exclusively in the skull and skeleton of the face on membranous bone. It may occur on more than one bone or with more than one osteoma on a single bone. The tumor of the facial bones may be periosteal or endosteal. The periosteal variety may occur either externally or in sinuses, more common in the frontal and ethmoid than the maxillary sinuses. (See Chapter 26.) Structurally there are three types of osteoma: compact bone, cancellous bone, or a combination of compact and cancellous bone.

Clinical features. The usual location for an os-

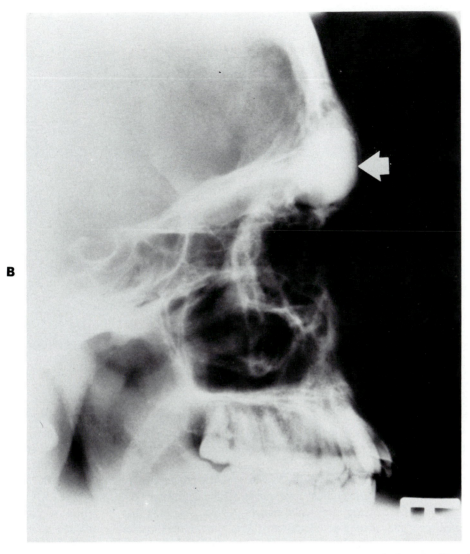

FIG. 21-34, cont'd. B, Lateral view *(arrow)*. (**A** and **B** courtesy Dr. G. Himadi, Chapel Hill, NC.)

teoma of the jaws is on the mandible. It is most frequently on the lingual side of the ramus or on the inferior border below the molars. It occurs at any age, but most frequently in individuals older than 40 years. The only symptom of a developing osteoma is the asymmetry caused by a bony hard swelling on the jaw. Because all three variants of the tumor have a surface of cortical bone, the osteoma is bony hard to palpation. This swelling is painless until its size or position interferes with function. The osteoma attaches to the cortex of the jaw by a pedicle or along a wide base. The mucosa covering the tumor is normal in color and freely movable. The compact or ivory variety develops more often in men, and the highest incidence of

the cancellous lesions is in women. Although most of the osteomas are small, some may become large enough to cause severe damage, especially those that develop in the frontoethmoid region (Fig. 21-34). Rarely, an extraosseous lingual osteoma may occur as a pedunculated solitary mass that arises from the posterior tongue near the foramen cecum, possibly derived from ossified undescended thyroid tissue.[11]

Radiographic features. The radiographic appearance of an osteoma consists of a radiopaque mass with well-defined borders located within a paranasal sinus or associated with the mandible. The mandibular lesion may be exophytic, extending outward into adjacent soft tissue spaces that

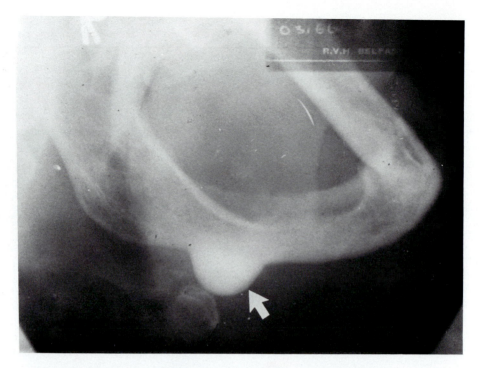

FIG. 21-35. Osteoma of compact bone *(arrow)* on the inferior surface of the mandible.

can be observed on panoramic, periapical, or extraoral radiographs. Those composed solely of compact bone are uniformly radiopaque (Fig. 21-35); those containing cancellous bone show evidence of internal trabecular structure (Fig. 21-36).

Differential diagnosis. The clinical appearance and location of a characteristic bony enlargement of anticipated size and shape, coupled with the radiographic image of a dense radiopaque mass, indicate an osteoma. However, a mature ossifying fibroma, early (small) osteogenic sarcoma, or small chondrosarcoma may occasionally resemble an exostosis or a torus.

Management. Simple excision is appropriate in that tori, exostoses, and peripheral osteomas do not recur after complete removal. However, treatment of these entities may be postponed unless they are causing some undesirable phonetic effect or interfere with the construction or function of a prosthetic device. External osteomas of the mandible may require removal for cosmetic reasons.

Gardner's syndrome. Gardner's syndrome is a hereditary condition characterized by multiple osteomas, cutaneous sebaceous cysts, subcutaneous fibromas, and multiple polyps of the small and large intestine. The associated osteomas appear during the second decade. They are most common in the frontal bone, mandible, maxilla, and sphe-

noid bones.[47] A significant feature of Gardner's syndrome is the predilection of the intestinal polyps to undergo malignant conversion, making early detection of the syndrome important. The presence of the osteomas often precedes the development of the intestinal polyps, so that early recognition of the syndrome may be a lifesaving event. Multiple unerupted supernumerary and permanent teeth in both jaws also occur with Gardner's syndrome (Fig. 21-37), as do central enostoses. Multiple osteomas may also occur on the mandible and in the frontal and maxillary sinuses as isolated findings in the absence of the diseases associated with Gardner's syndrome.[58]

Management. The removal of osteomas is not generally necessary unless the tumors are symptomatic. However, if one of these bony growths is causing masticatory trauma or an intraosseous osteoma is close to the surface in an intended denture-bearing area, surgical removal should be undertaken. The important concern is to refer any patient suspected of having Gardner's syndrome for proctosigmoidoscopy and barium enema to examine for the presence of intestinal polyposis. There is a low but dangerous potential for intracranial complications by osteomas of the sinus walls.

Central hemangioma. The central hemangioma is a benign tumor that occurs most often in

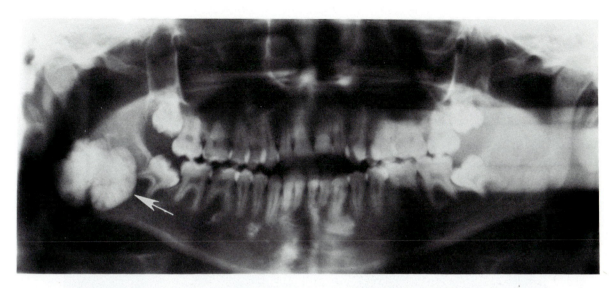

FIG. 21-36. Osteoma *(arrow)*, fixed to the region of the right mandibular angle, showing evidence of some internal trabeculation. (From Matteson SR, et al: *Dent Radiogr Photogr* 57(1-4):1-84, 1985.)

the vertebrae and skull. It rarely develops in the jaws. Fewer than 50 mandibular hemangiomas and a lower number of maxillary lesions have been reported.[31] It may be developmental, as an anomaly of the blood vessels in the marrow spaces, or traumatic in origin.

Clinical features. Hemangiomas are more prevalent in females than males, the ratio being 2:1. They also affect the mandible about twice as often as the maxilla. Although they occur in individuals of all ages, at least 50% form before and during the teen years.[59] Those that occur in the mandible form predominantly in the body and ramus. Enlargement is slow, producing a nontender expansion of the jaw over several months or years. The swelling may or may not be painful, is not tender, and usually is bony hard. Pain, if present, is probably throbbing. Some tumors may be compressible or pulsate, and a bruit may be detected on auscultation. There may be anesthesia of the skin supplied by the mental nerve. The lesion may cause loosening and migration of teeth in the affected area. There may be bleeding from the gingiva around the neck of the affected teeth, and these teeth may demonstrate rebound mobility. When depressed into their sockets, the teeth return to their original position within several minutes. Aspiration produces arterial blood that may be under pressure and detected through the syringe plunger.

Radiographic features. A hemangioma of bone appears radiographically as an osteolytic defect that may take many forms, especially in the mandible. The mandibular lesion is usually not as well defined as those in other bones. The locules formed in the maxilla by the central hemangioma resemble enlarged trabecular spaces, and the trabeculae are coarse, dense, and well defined (Fig. 21-38). The most often observed radiolucencies are multicystic and frequently have a soap bubble or honeycomb appearance that results from a fine trabeculation within the locules. Other lesions may present linear trabeculations or be radiolucent (Fig. 21-39). Coarsely multilocular regions of rarefaction that accompany cortex expansion to the thickness of paper may mimic a giant cell tumor of the jaws. However, some investigators believe that the loculations produced by the hemangioma are smaller and interspersed with a fine fibrillar network.[59] In addition, a projection that demonstrates the expanding lesion in profile may show the sunray or sunburst image.[57] The roots of teeth in the invaded area are frequently resorbed, and phleboliths—small areas of calcification or concretions found in a vein— occasionally occur in the lesion (Fig. 21-40). Phleboliths develop from thrombi, caused by slowing of peripheral blood flow, that become organized and mineralized. They consist of calcium phosphate and calcium carbonate.[75] However, because the lesion is so variable in appearance and has such a lethal potential, the dif-

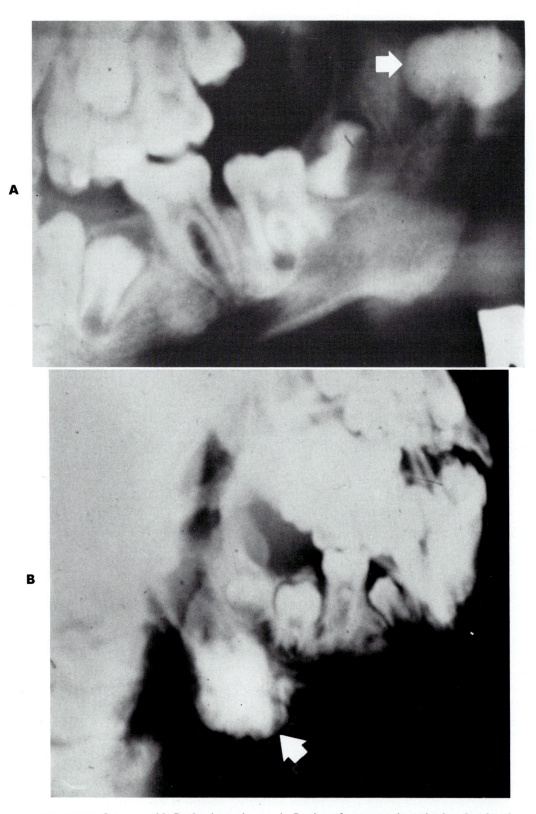

FIG. 21-37. Osteoma with Gardner's syndrome. **A,** Portion of a panoramic projection showing the lesion *(arrow)* associated with the mandible. **B,** Lateral oblique projection of the mandible with the osteoma *(arrow)* on the mandibular ramus. (Courtesy Dr. R. Bays, Augusta, Ga.)

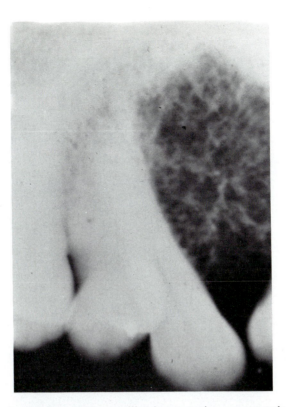

FIG. 21-38. Hemangioma in the anterior maxilla, demonstrating a coarse trabecular pattern. (Courtesy Dr. E.J. Burkes, Chapel Hill, NC.)

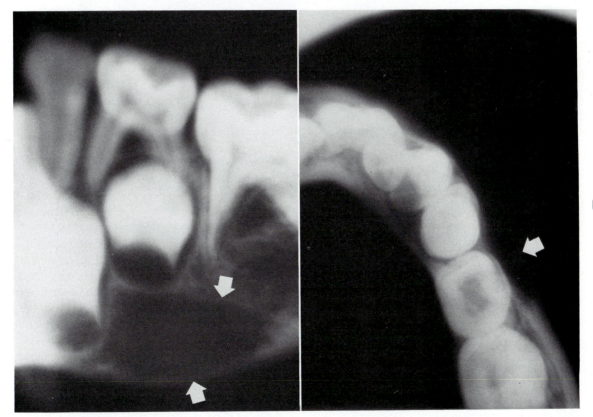

A

B

FIG. 21-39. Vascular lesion. **A,** Note the radiolucency in the mandible below the developing first premolar *(arrows)*. **B,** An occlusal projection shows the expansion, with loss of the buccal cortex *(arrow)*. (**A** and **B** courtesy Dr. R. White, Chapel Hill, NC.)

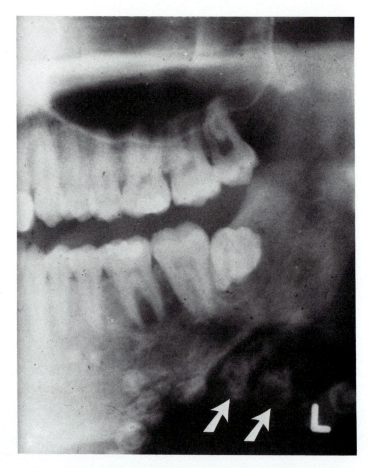

FIG. 21-40. Soft tissue hemangioma with phleboliths *(arrows)*.

ferential diagnosis for all rarefactions in the jaws should include central hemangioma in spite of its low recurrence rate.

Differential diagnosis. Regard any multilocular radiolucent lesion in the jaws as a potentially dangerous lesion and endeavor to eliminate the possibility of a central hemangioma. Initially, the clinical features of the central hemangioma should be noted or determined not to exist. Aspiration of the area will establish whether the radiolucency in question is a vascular tumor. If not, the differential diagnosis for a multilocular radiolucency of the jaws should consider central giant cell granuloma, giant cell lesion of hyperparathyroidism, aneurysmal bone cyst, ameloblastic fibroma, odontogenic myxoma, ameloblastoma, metastatic tumors, and cherubism. The traumatic bone cyst and keratocyst are both generally more radiolucent and have borders that are better defined.

Management. Treatment of a central hemangioma should be accomplished without delay be-

cause trauma that disrupts the integrity of the affected jaw may result in lethal exsanguination of the patient. Specifically, embolization (introduction of inert materials into the lesion by vascular route), surgery (en bloc resection with ligation of external carotid artery), and sclerosing techniques have been used singly or in combination.

Arteriovenous fistula. The arteriovenous fistula (also known as arteriovenous shunt or malformation), an uncommon lesion, is a direct communication between an artery and a vein that bypasses the intervening capillary bed. It usually results from trauma, but in rare instances may be a developmental anomaly. An arteriovenous shunt may occur anywhere in the body, in soft tissue, or in the alveolar ridge, as well as central in the jaw. Apparently the head and neck are the most common locations. Recognition of the hemorrhagic nature of these lesions is of utmost importance because extraction of an associated tooth may be immediately followed by life-threatening bleeding.[100]

Clinical features. The clinical appearance of a central arteriovenous shunt can be quite variable, depending on the extent of bone or soft tissue involvement. The lesion may expand bone, and there may also be a mass in the extraosseous soft tissue. The soft tissue swelling may have a purplish discoloration. Palpation or auscultation of the swelling may reveal a pulse. Then again, neither the bone nor the soft tissue may be expanded, and no pulse may be clinically apparent. Aspiration will produce blood.

Radiographic features. Although the radiographic appearance of the arteriovenous fistula is not distinctive, central lesions or those in the soft tissue that erode bony surfaces cause well-defined (cystlike) resorptive lesions in the bone. The central lesions may be multilocular. It is most common for the lesion to develop in the ramus and retromolar area of the mandible and to involve the mandibular canal. The wall of the shunt may contain radiographically apparent calcified material that may suggest the nature of the lesion.

Angiography, a radiographic procedure carried out by injecting radiopaque dye into vessels and making radiographs when the dye is located in the vasculature, is useful for demonstrating the size and extent of a vascular tumor of the jaw. It displays an abnormal collection of vessels located in the suspected area, with many vessels feeding and draining the lesion (Fig. 21-41). Angiography demonstrates the nature of the vascular derangement, its relationship to the bone defect, and associated abnormal arterial and venous vasculature (Fig. 21-42).

Differential diagnosis. The differential diagnosis should include the multilocular lesions that occur, with hemangioma and ameloblastoma assigned a relatively high priority. In addition, consider the radicular and dentigerous cyst. Usually the soft tissue hemangioma does not involve bone, which may help to distinguish it.

Management. The arteriovenous fistula is treated surgically. Surgical intervention should be initiated only in the hospital after ligation of the external carotid artery and with blood transfusion available.

Chondroma. The chondroma is a benign cartilaginous tumor. It is relatively common in certain other areas of the skeleton, but seldom found in the jaws.[70] Those that develop in the oral tissues grow slowly and are locally invasive. Even though both the mandible and maxilla are membrane bones, they do contain vestigial cartilage, and the tumor may arise from these cartilage cells and from the cartilage-forming connective tissue in these bones.

Clinical features. The incidence of chondroma in the jaws is highest during the fifth and sixth decades, but it may occur at any age, as evidenced by its discovery in infants and children. If there is a sexual predilection, males seen to be slightly favored.[9] It may develop in either jaw, but seems to slightly favor the anterior region of the maxilla. Those in the mandible most often develop in the premolar-molar region and at the symphysis. They also occur in the condyle and coronoid process.[58] The reason for the preferential development of the tumor in these areas is a matter of debate.[34,79] The tumors usually become apparent as a painless mass, the growth rate of which varies among patients. As the tumor grows, the involved teeth become loose and may be lost; this may be an early symptom. Tumors that involve the condyle and coronoid process may interfere with mandibular function.

Radiographic features. The destructive nature of the chondroma becomes apparent in the irregular radiolucent nature of its image. The border may be well defined or ragged and poorly defined. It may also develop opacities in the osteolytic area, which produces a mottled appearance (Fig. 21-43). Radiographs may also reveal resorption of involved tooth roots. However, the radiographic image of chondroma is not pathognomonic but suggestive of a number of lesions.

Differential diagnosis. Lesions whose radiographic appearance is similar to chondroma include chondrosarcoma, osteogenic sarcoma, osteoblastic metastatic carcinoma, ossifying subperiosteal hemangioma, fibrous dysplasia, and peripheral fibroma with calcifications. The age of the patient, history of trauma, presence or absence of a primary tumor, pain, and the general order of the lesion's appearance help to differentiate the chondroma from these other lesions.

Management. Inasmuch as such a high percentage of chondrosarcomas result from malignant change in chondromas, the tumor assumed to be a chondroma should be excised with a wide margin of normal tissue. This may cause the surgeon some conflict between the requirements for complete removal and avoidance of undue mutilation.

Osteoblastoma. There appears to be increasing agreement that if the osteoblastoma and osteoid osteoma (see the following section) are different lesions, they differ only in size and minor morphologic features.[16] Both are rare in the jaws, ac-

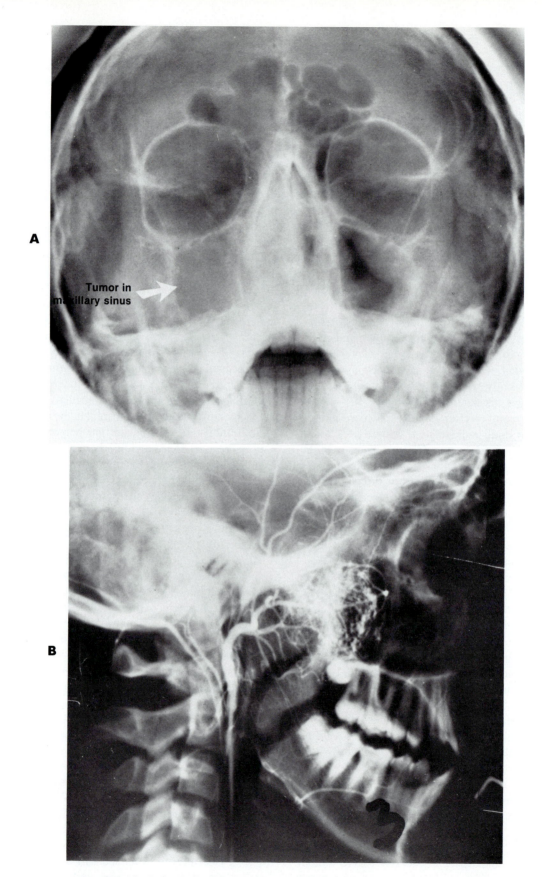

FIG. 21-41. Vascular lesion in the right maxillary sinus. **A,** A Waters projection shows the opacified maxillary antrum *(arrow)*. **B,** Note the tumor vasculature on this angiogram. (**A** and **B** courtesy Dr. G. Himadi, Chapel Hill NC.)

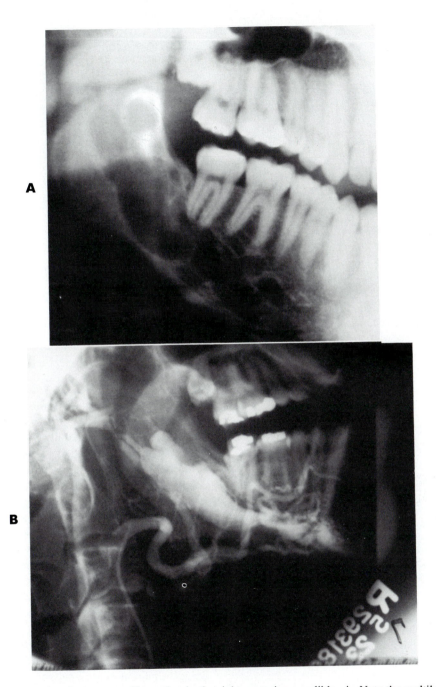

FIG. 21-42. Arteriovenous malformation in the right posterior mandible. **A,** Note the multilocular radiolucency along the course of the mandibular neurovascular canal in this segment from a panoramic radiograph. **B,** Radiopaque dye is distributed throughout the lesion (external carotid angiogram). (From Kelly DE, et al: *J Oral Surg* 35:387-393, 1977.)

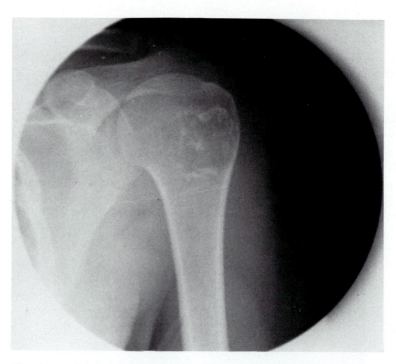

FIG. 21-43. Chondroma of the head of the humerus, showing areas of flocculent opacification within a large defect with circumscribed borders. (Courtesy Department of Radiology, Baylor Hospital, Dallas.)

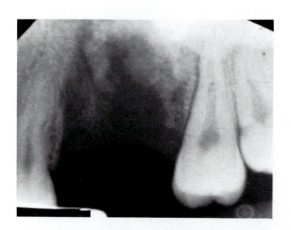

FIG. 21-44. Osteoblastoma in a 21-year-old man with a history of pain for 3 months. Note the evidence of bone formation and the diffuse margins. (Courtesy Dr. B. Gratt, Los Angeles.)

counting for about 10% of these lesions.[47] The male to female ratio is 2:1, and the average age is 17 years, with most lesions occurring in the second and third decades of life.[81] Lesions in the jaws are more frequent in the tooth-bearing regions of the mandible. Clinically, patients often report pain and swelling of the affected region. There are also some descriptions that indicate the minor histologic differences. For example, the osteoid trabeculae in the osteoblastoma are generally larger (broader and longer, with wider trabecular spaces than the osteoid osteoma). The osteoblastoma is also usually more vascular and less painful, and it has more osteoclasts. In addition, the benign osteoblastoma is considered a more aggressive lesion.[14] On the level of their ultrastructures, both lesions are essentially similar or at least closely related.

Radiographic features. The radiographic appearance of the osteoblastoma is quite variable. The tumor may be entirely radiolucent (Fig. 21-44) or show varying degrees of calcification. The borders may be diffuse or show some sign of a cortex. Mandibular lesions have been reported that show a central calcified mass surrounded by a radiolucent halo or sunray pattern.[81]

Differential diagnosis. If the radiographic appearance of an osteoblastoma is lucent with ill-defined borders, it may suggest infection or malignancy. When the lesion is sclerotic, it is easier to recognize. The osteoid osteoma can be differentiated from the benign osteoblastoma by its more eccentric radiolucency with sclerotic borders. This feature, the sclerotic border, is given more weight

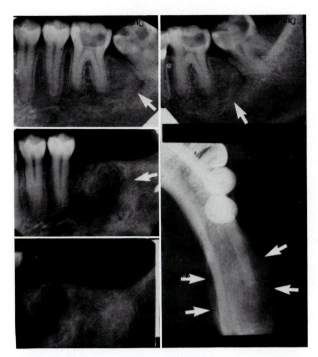

FIG. 21-45. Osteoid osteoma *(arrow)*, appearing as a mixed radiolucent-radiopaque lesion in the molar region and causing expansion of the buccal and lingual cortex of the mandible *(arrows)*. (Courtesy Dr. A. Shawkat, Radcliff Ky.)

than the size of the lesion because a sclerotic lesion indicates osteoid osteoma even if it is larger than 1 cm.[14] Symptoms are not a specific aid for diagnosis.

Management. Treatment is by curettage or local excision, which relieves the pain. Recurrences have been described, and a few are suspected of becoming sarcomas or at least of being initially unrecognized low-grade osteosarcomas.[61]

Osteoid osteoma. Osteoid osteoma is a benign tumor that is rare in the jaws. Its true nature is not known, but some investigators think it is a variant of osteoblastoma.[84,85] The tumor has an oval or roundish tumorlike core, usually only about 1 cm in diameter; some may reach 5 or 6 cm.[55] This core consists of osteoid and newly formed trabeculae within highly vascularized osteogenic connective tissue. It may develop within the cancellous bone or near or within the cortex; it is usually intracortical.[49] In the spongiosa, a thin rim of sclerotic bone develops around the core, but when intracortical the cortex becomes dense, thickened, and hard for a considerable distance beyond the core.

Clinical features. Osteoid osteomas occur most frequently in young persons, usually males between the ages of 10 and 25 years, seldom after 40 years or before 4 years. This condition affects at least twice as many males as females. Most of the lesions occur in the femur and tibia, whereas the jaws are rarely involved. In those that do occur in the jaws, somewhat more develop in the body of the mandible.[39,50] Severe pain in the bone is characteristic. In addition, the soft tissue over the involved bony area may be swollen and tender.[29]

Radiographic features. The radiographic appearance of osteoid osteoma is a small ovoid or round radiolucent area (core) surrounded by a rim of sclerotic bone (Fig. 21-45). The central radiolucency may have some radiopaque foci. The lesion is most common in the cortex of the limb bones. In an occlusal projection, the overlying cortex is thickened by new bone being formed subperiosteally. The presence of tooth images superimposed over the lesion and the possibility of associated idiopathic osteosclerosis complicate the interpretation of radiographs of cases that develop in the jaws, compared with the images seen in other bones.[14]

Differential diagnosis. The osteoid osteoma is rare in the jaws. A clinician suspecting that a sclerotic lesion is an osteoid osteoma should also consider sclerosing osteitis, ossifying fibroma, monostatic fibrous dysplasia, and periapical cemental dysplasia. The presence of a central radiolucency usually eliminates enostosis or osteosclerosis. If a diagnosis cannot be made with confidence at this point, further effort should be made to rule out other rare entities that may share features with osteoid osteoma: osteogenic sarcoma, chondroblastoma, ameloblastoma, cementifying fibroma, and benign osteoblastoma.[29,56]

Management. Complete excision is the currently recommended treatment, as it often relieves the pain and cures the disease. Although spontaneous remission may occur in some cases, there are insufficient data for identifying such cases in advance.

SPECIFIC REFERENCES

1. Abrams AM, Kirby JW, Melrose RJ: Cementoblastoma: a clinico-pathologic study of seven new cases, *Oral Surg Oral Med Oral Pathol* 38:394-403, 1974.
2. Abrams AM, Melrose RJ, Howell FW: Adenoameloblastoma: a clinical pathologic study of ten new cases, *Cancer* 22:175-185, 1968.
3. Acton CH, Savage NW: Odontomes and their behavior: a review, *Aust Dent J* 32:430-435, 1987.
4. Agha FP, Lilienfeld RM: Roentgen features of osseous neurilemmoma, *Radiology* 102:325-326, 1972.

5. Appiah-Anane S: Amputation neuroma: a late complication following sagittal split osteotomy of the mandible, *J Oral Maxillofac Surg* 49:963-967, 1990.

6. Atkinson CH, Harwood AR, Cummings BJ: Ameloblastoma of the jaw: a reappraisal of the role of megavoltage irradiation, *Cancer* 53:869-873, 1984.

7. Baden E: Odontogenic tumors, *Pathol Annu* 6:475-568, 1971.

8. Batsakis JG: *Tumors of the head and neck,* ed 2, Baltimore, 1979, Williams & Wilkins.

9. Batsakis JG, Dito WR: Chondrosarcoma of the maxilla, *Arch Otolaryngol* 75:55-61, 1962.

10. Batsakis JG, McClatchey DK: Ameloblastoma of the maxilla and peripheral ameloblastoma, *Ann Otorhinolaryngol* 92:532-533, 1983.

11. Bernard PJ, Shugar JM, Mitnick R, et al: Lingual osteoma, *Arch Otolaryngol Head Neck Surg* 115:989-990, 1989.

12. Berwick JE, Maymi GF, Berkland ME: Benign cementoblastoma, *J Oral Maxillofac Surg* 48:208-211, 1990.

13. Bodin I, Julin P, Thomsson M: Odontomas and their pathological sequels, *Dentomaxillofac Radiol* 12:109-114, 1984.

14. Brady CL, Bronne RM: Benign osteoblastoma of the mandible, *Cancer* 30:329-333, 1977.

15. Bredenkamp JK, Zimmerman MC, Mickel RA: Maxillary ameloblastoma: a potentially lethal neoplasm, *Arch Otolaryngol Head Neck Surg* 115:99-104, 1989.

16. Byers PD: Solitary benign osteoblastic lesions of bone osteoid osteoma and benign osteoblastoma, *Cancer* 22:43-57, 1968.

17. Cahn LR: Discussion of Thoma, K., *Oral Surg Oral Med Oral Pathol* 8:441-444, 1955.

18. Chew CL, Ton PH: Torus palatinus: a clinical study, *Aust Dent J* 29:245-248, 1984.

19. Cina MT, Dahlin DC, Gares RJ: Ameloblastic adenomatoid tumors: a report of four new cases, *Am J Clin Pathol* 39:59-65, 1936.

20. Cohen MA, Hertzanu Y: Myxofibroma of the maxilla: a case report with computed tomogram findings, *Oral Surg Oral Med Oral Pathol* 61:142-145, 1986.

21. Cohen MA, Mendelsohn DB: CT and MR imaging of myxofibroma of the jaws. *J Comput Assist Tomogr* 14:281-285, 1990.

22. Cuestas-Carnero R, Bachur RO, Gendelman H: Odontogenic myxoma: report of a case, *J Oral Maxillofac Surg* 46:705-709, 1988.

23. D'Ambrosia JA, Langlais RP, Young RS: Jaw and skull changes in neurofibromatosis, *Oral Surg Oral Med Oral Pathol* 66:391-396, 1988.

24. Eggen S, Natvig B: Relationship between torus mandibularis and number of present teeth, *Scand J Dent Res* 94:233-240, 1986.

25. Eversole LR: Central benign and malignant neural neoplasms of the jaws: a review, *J Oral Surg* 27:716-721, 1969.

26. Eversole LR: *Clinical outline of oral pathology: diagnosis and treatment,* ed 2, Philadelphia, 1984, Lea & Febiger.

27. Eversole LR, Leider AS, Strub D: Radiographic characteristics of cystogenic ameloblastoma, *Oral Surg Oral Med Oral Pathol* 57:572-577, 1984.

28. Eversole LR, Sabes WR, Dauches VG: Benign cementoblastoma, *Oral Surg Oral Med Oral Pathol* 36:824-830, 1973.

29. Farman AG, Nortjé CJ, Gratepass F: Periosteal benign osteoblastoma of the mandible: report of a case and review of the literature pertaining to benign osteoblastic neoplasms of the jaws, *Br J Oral Surg* 14:12-22, 1976.

30. Franklin CD, Pindborg JJ: The calcifying epithelial odontogenic tumor: a review and analysis of 113 cases, *Oral Surg Oral Med Oral Pathol* 42:753-765, 1976.

31. Gamez-Aravjo JJ, Toth BB, Luna MA: Central hemangioma of the mandible and maxilla: review of a vascular lesion, *Oral Surg Oral Med Oral Pathol* 37:230-238, 1974.

32. Gardner DG: Radiotherapy in the treatment of ameloblastoma, *Int J Oral Maxillofac Surg* 17:201-205, 1988.

33. Garguilo EA, Ziter WD, Mastrocula R: Calcifying epithelial odontogenic tumor: report of case and review of literature, *J Oral Surg* 29:862-866, 1971.

34. Geschickter CF: Tumors of the jaws, *Am J Cancer* 24:90-126, 1935.

35. Ghosh BC, and others: Myxoma of the jaw bones, *Cancer* 31:237-240, 1973.

36. Giansanti JS, Someren A, Waldron CA: Odontogenic adenomatoid tumor (adeno-ameloblastoma), *Oral Surg Oral Med Oral Pathol* 30:69-88, 1969.

37. Gibilesco JA, Turlington EG: *Stafne's oral roentgenographic diagnosis,* ed 5, Philadelphia, 1985, WB Saunders.

38. Gorlin RJ, Chaudhry AP, Pindborg JJ: Odontogenic tumors: classification, history, pathology, and clinical behavior in man and domesticated animals, *Cancer* 14:73-101, 1961.

39. Green GW Jr, Natiella JR, Spring PN Jr: Osteoid osteoma of the jaws: report of a case, *Oral Surg Oral Med Oral Pathol* 26:342-351, 1968.

40. Gregg JM: Studies of traumatic neuralgias in the maxillofacial region: surgical pathology and neural mechanisms. *J Oral Maxillofac Surg* 48:228-239, 1990.

41. Hecht SS: Amputation neuroma, *Oral Surg Oral Med Oral Pathol* 10:475-479, 1957.

42. Heffez L, Mafee MF, Vaiana J: The role of magnetic resonance imaging in the diagnosis and management of ameloblastoma, *Oral Surg Oral Med Oral Pathol* 65:2-12, 1988.

43. Hertzanu Y, Mendelsohn DB, Cohen M: Computed tomography of mandibular ameloblastoma, *J Comput Assist Tomogr* 8:220-223, 1984.

44. Hooker SP: Ameloblastic odontoma: an analysis of twenty-six cases, *Oral Surg Oral Med Oral Pathol* 24:375-376, 1967.

45. Huber CG, Lewis D: Amputation neuromas, *Arch Surg* 1:85-113, 1920.

46. Hunt JC, Pugh DG: Skeletal lesions in neurofibromatosis, *Radiology* 76:1-20, 1961.

47. Huvos A: *Bone tumors: diagnosis, treatment and prognosis,* Philadelphia, 1979, WB Saunders.

48. Hylander WL: The adaptive significance of Eskimo craniofacial morphology. In Dahlberg AA, Graber TM, editors: *Craniofacial growth and development,* The Hague, 1977, Monton.

49. Jacobson SA: *The comparative pathology of the tumors of bone,* Springfield, Ill, 1971, Charles C Thomas.

50. Jurgens PE: Osteoid osteoma of the mandible: report of case, *J Oral Surg* 26:129-132, 1968.

51. Kahn MA: Ameloblastoma in young persons: a clinicopathologic analysis and etiologic investigation, *Oral Surg Oral Med Oral Pathol* 67:706-715, 1989.

52. Kaugars GE, Miller ME, Abbey LM: Odontomas. *Oral Surg Oral Med Oral Pathol* 67:172-176, 1989.

53. Kolas J and others: The occurrence of torus palatinus and torus mandibularis in 2,478 dental patients, *Oral Surg* 6:1134-1141, 1953.

54. Langlais RP, Bentley KC: *Advanced oral radiographic interpretation,* vol 2, Philadelphia, 1979, WB Saunders.

55. Lichtenstein L: *Bone tumors,* ed 4, St Louis, 1972, Mosby.

56. Lichtenstein L, Sawyer WR: Benign osteoblastoma, *J Bone Joint Surg [Am]* 46:755-765, 1964.

57. Loring MF: Hemangioma of the mandible: diagnosis and therapy, *Arch Otolaryngol* 85:648-652, 1967.

58. Lucas RB: *Pathology of tumors of the oral tissues,* ed 4, New York, 1984, Churchill Livingstone.

59. Lund BA, Dahlin DC: Hemangiomas of the mandible and maxilla, *J Oral Surg* 22:234-242, 1964.

60. Marannda G, Gourgi M: Calcifying epithelial odontogenic tumor (Pindborg tumor): review of the literature and case report, *J Can Dent Assoc* 52:1009-1012, 1986.

61. Merryweather R, Middlemiss JH, Somerkin NG: Malignant transformation of osteoblastoma, *J Bone Joint Surg* 62:381-384, 1980.

62. Mosadomi A: Odontogenic tumors in an African population, *Oral Surg Oral Med Oral Pathol* 40:502-521, 1975.

63. Oringer MJ: Neuroma of the mandible, *Oral Surg Oral Med Oral Pathol* 1:1135-1136, 1948.

64. Peszkowski MJ, Larsson A: Extraosseous and intraosseous oral traumatic neuromas and their association with tooth extraction, *J Oral Maxillofac Surg* 48:963-967, 1990.

65. Phillips SD, Corio RL, Brem J, Mattox, D: Ameloblastoma of the mandible with intracranial metastasis, *Arch Otolaryngol Head Neck Surg* 118:861-863, 1992.

66. Philipsen HP, Reichart PA, Zhang KH et al: Adenomatoid odontogenic tumor: biologic profile based on 499 cases, *J Oral Path Med* 20:149-158, 1991.

67. Pindborg JJ: Tumors of the jaws (benign and malignant). In Tiecke RW, editor: *Oral Pathology,* New York, 1965, McGraw-Hill.

68. Pindborg JJ: The calcifying epithelial odontogenic tumor: review of literature and report of extraosseous case, *Acta Odontol Scand* 24:419-430, 1966.

69. Pindborg JJ, Vedtofte P, Reibel J, Praetorius F: The calcifying epithelial odontogenic tumor: a review of recent literature and report of a case, *APMIS Suppl* 23:152-157, 1991.

70. Potdar GG, Srikhande SS: Chondrogenic tumors of the jaws, *Oral Surg Oral Med Oral Pathol* 30:649-658, 1970.

71. Prescott GH, White RE: Solitary central neurofibroma of the mandible: report of case and review of the literature, *J Oral Surg* 28:305-309, 1970.

72. Regezi JA, Kerr DA, Courtney RM: Odontogenic tumors: an analysis of 706 cases, *J Oral Surg* 36:771-778, 1978.

73. Ruprecht A, Batniji S, Neweihi E: The incidence of odontomas in dental patients at King Saud University, *Dentomaxillofac Radiol* 13:77-79, 1984.

74. Ruprecht A, Ross AS: Benign cementoblastoma (true cementoblastoma), *Dentomaxillofac Radiol* 12:31-33, 1983.

75. Sano K, Ogawa A, Inokuchi T, et al: Buccal hemangioma with pheboliths: report of two cases, *Oral Surg Oral Med Oral Pathol* 65:151-156, 1988.

76. Schultz SM, Twickler DM, Wheeler DE, Hogan TD: Ameloblastoma associated with basal cell nevus (Gorlin) syndrome: CT findings, *J Comput Assist Tomogr* 11:901-904, 1987.

77. Sehdev MK, Huvos AG, Strong EW, et al: Ameloblastoma of the maxilla and mandible, *Cancer* 33:324-333, 1974.

78. Shafer WG, Hine MK, Levy BM: *Oral pathology,* ed 4, Philadelphia, 1983, WB Saunders.

79. Shira RB, Bhaskar SN: Oral surgery and oral pathology conference: no. 6, Walter Reed Army Medical Center, *Oral Surg Oral Med Oral Pathol* 16:1255-1260, 1963.

80. Sirichitra V, Dhiravarangkura P: Intrabony ameloblastoma of the jaws, *Int J Oral Surg* 13:184-193, 1984.

81. Smith RA, Hensen LS, Resnick D, Chan W: Comparison of the osteoblastoma in gnathic and extragnathic sites, *Oral Surg Oral Med Oral Pathol* 54:285-298, 1982.

82. Spouge JD: *Oral pathology,* St Louis, 1973, Mosby.

83. Stajcic ZZ: Odontoma associated with a primary tooth, *J Pedod* 12:415-420, 1988.

84. Steiner GC: Ultrastructure of osteoid osteoma, *Hum Pathol* 7:309-325, 1976.

85. Steiner GC: Ultrastructure of osteoblastoma, *Cancer* 39:2127-2136, 1977.

86. Struthers P, Shear M: Root resorption by ameloblastomas and cysts of the jaw, *Int J Oral Surg* 5:128-132, 1976.

87. Sumter TG, Vellios F, Shafer WG: Neurilemmoma of bone, *Radiology* 75:215-222, 1960.

88. Suzuki M, Sakai T: A familial study of torus palatinus and torus mandibularis, *Am J Phys Anthropol* 18:263-272, 1960.

89. Swan RH: Odontomas: a review, case presentation and periodontal considerations in treatment, *J Periodontol* 58:856-860, 1987.

90. Thoma KH, Goldman HM: Central myxoma of the jaw, *Am J Orthod Oral Surg* 33:532-540, 1947.

91. Tomohiko A, Nakajima T, Takeuchi S, et al: Malignant ameloblastoma with metastasis to the skull: report of a case, *J Oral Surg* 39:690-696, 1981.

92. Trodahl JN: Ameloblastic fibroma: a survey of cases from the Armed Forces Institute of Pathology, *Oral Surg Oral Med Oral Pathol* 33:547-558, 1972.

93. Tsaknis PJ, Nelson JF: The maxillary ameloblastoma: an analysis of 24 cases, *J Oral Surg* 38:336-342, 1980.

94. Ueda M and others: Mandibular ameloblastoma with metastasis to the lungs and lymph nodes: a case report and review of the literature, *J Oral Maxillofac Surg* 47:623-628, 1989.

95. Ueno S, Mushimoto K, Shirasu R: Prognostic evaluation of ameloblastoma based on histologic and radiographic typing, *J Oral Maxillofac Surg* 47:11-15, 1989.

96. Ueno S, Nakamura S, Mushimoto K, Shirasu R: A clinicopathologic study of ameloblastoma, *J Oral Maxillofac Surg* 44:361-365, 1986.

97. van Zanten TEG, Golding RP: A case of gigantiform ameloblastoma, *Diagn Imag Clin Med* 55:391-393, 1986.

98. Vap OR, Dahlin DC, Turlington EG: Pindborg tumor: the so-called calcifying epithelial odontogenic tumor, *Cancer* 25:629-636, 1970.

99. Wood NK, Goaz PW: *Differential diagnosis of oral lesions,* ed 4, St Louis, 1991, Mosby.

100. Worth HM, Stoneman DW: Radiology of vascular abnormalities in and about the jaws, *Dent Radiol Photogr* 52:1-23, 1979.

101. Zachariades N, Papanicolaou S: Treatment of odontogenic myxoma, *Ann Dent* 6:34-37, 1987.

22

Malignant Disease of the Jaws

Although cancer has probably afflicted us for as long as we have existed, we have been aware of it for only about 200 years. Cancer was of little concern to humans when they were dying early as a result of war, famine, and epidemic diseases. However, with time and the conquest of most causes of early death, cancer has become one of the most common causes of death in the elderly, accounting for about 20% of all deaths.

Cancer is a major health problem in the United States—approximately 700,000 new cancers are diagnosed annually—and is second only to heart disease as a cause of death. Oral cancers account for approximately 2% to 3% of all cancers diagnosed in the United States.[43] They are two to three times as common in men as in women.[49] These oral lesions are about 90% squamous cell carcinomas, 5% adenocarcinomas, and 4% sarcomas.[86] More than half of the squamous cell cancers of the oral cavity are well advanced when they are discovered.[9] This is the malignant lesion most likely to produce radiolucent lesions of the jaws. Patients infected with human immunodeficiency virus (HIV) are more at risk of developing oral cancers.[41] In the last 40 years, the 5-year survival rate for oral cancer has increased little.[8] In fact, the 5-year survival rate for advanced oral cancer is even worse than for many diseases such as melanoma and colon and breast cancer.[19] An oral squamous cell carcinoma no more than 2 cm in diameter has probably metastasized (spread to a distant site), and the 5-year survival rate is about 30% regardless of treatment.[59]

MALIGNANT LESIONS
Characteristics

Malignant lesions in bone cause radiographically recognizable disruption of the normal anatomy in an area. Although both benign and malignant bony lesions may be destructive, they are usually distinguishable radiographically by their growth char-acteristics and influence on surrounding tissues.

Lesion borders. Benign lesions characteristically have well-defined borders. There is a sharp demarcation between the destruction produced by the lesion and the normal radiographic appearance of the adjacent structures (Fig. 22-1). Further, because of their nonaggressive growth, they tend to be round or oval. In contrast, malignant lesions exhibit ill-defined borders (Fig. 22-2). When the margins are irregular and ragged, it may be impossible to establish the exact limits of the malignant lesion on the radiograph because the area of normal tissue gradually blends into the disease. This appearance suggests tumor infiltrating bone along alternate areas that offer reduced resistance to its penetration. It is usually possible to determine radiographically whether a lesion is malignant or benign. Evidence of new bone formation distinguishes sarcomas from carcinomas, except in the case of metastatic carcinoma from the prostate gland.

Peripheral tumors are subject to infection. The infection may spread from the tumor and invade the bone, superimposing its effects on the radiographic changes induced by the tumor. Depending on the circumstances, acute infections cause radiolucent bone destruction, whereas a chronic process causes sclerosing osteitis in the bone next to the tumor. Recognition of this reaction will preclude misidentification and the erroneous conclusion that the tumor is osteogenic. Certain benign processes, such as infections, may also produce lesions with destructive borders that resemble malignant tumors.

Adjacent cortical bone. As the benign lesion grows, it tends to displace the normal structures around it. This has the effect of causing distortion of the bone, usually expansion of the cortex. As the tumor elevates the periosteum, it may stimulate the formation of layers of reactive bone, termed "onion skin" because of its radiographic appearance

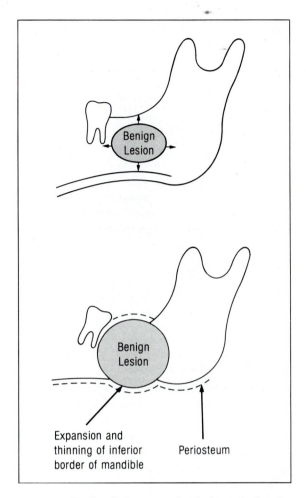

FIG. 22-1. Benign lesions growing in bone tend to be round or oval, and to grow by displacement and expansion of the surrounding structures. (From Matteson SR, et al: *Dent Radiogr Photogr* 57:35-52, 1985.)

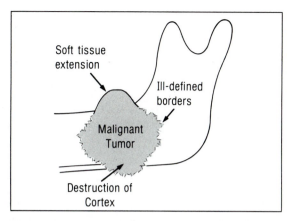

FIG. 22-2. Malignant tumors in bone grow by invasion and destruction of surrounding bone without cortical expansion. (From Matteson SR, et al: *Dent Radiogr Photogr* 57:35-52, 1985.)

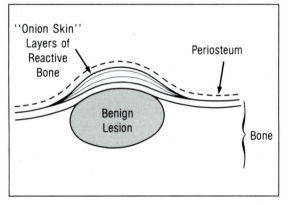

FIG. 22-3. The presence of a benign tumor growing near cortex tends to cause expansion of the cortex and occasionally the formation of layers of reactive bone from elevation of the periosteum. (From Matteson SR, et al: *Dent Radiogr Photogr* 57:35-52, 1985.)

(Fig. 22-3). Malignant lesions, however, grow by invasion and destruction of adjacent structures. There may be a soft tissue mass, but the lesion penetrates and destroys the bony cortex rather than causing expansion. The lesion may grow through the bony cortex so rapidly that it carries portions of the periosteum with it, forming trails of bone and causing a "sunburst" appearance (Fig. 22-4).

Radiodensity. Malignant carcinomas are radiolucent lesions (except in the case of metastatic carcinoma of the prostate gland). The presence of new bone formation usually indicates the presence of sarcoma rather than carcinoma.

Dental involvement. The rapid growth and spread of malignant lesions usually cause them to expand around the roots of teeth, leaving the roots intact and the teeth in position (Fig. 22-5). On occasion, there is evidence of root resorption. Benign lesions, which grow more slowly, are more likely to cause resorption of roots of teeth and displacement of roots (Fig. 22-6).

Radiographic examination

A panoramic radiograph is often used as a preliminary radiograph for suspected malignant lesions of the jaws because of its general availability and broad coverage of the jaws.[60] When malignant lesions of the jaws are identified or suspected, they should be visualized on at least two right-angle views. Make lateral views of lesions involving the

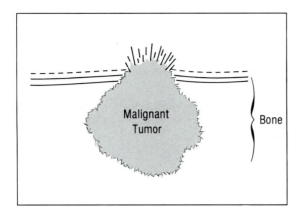

FIG. 22-4. The presence of a malignant tumor growing near cortex tends to cause destruction and occasionally rapid elevation of the bone-forming periosteum, resulting in bony spicules resembling a sunburst. (From Matteson SR, et al: *Dent Radiogr Photogr* 57:35-52, 1985.)

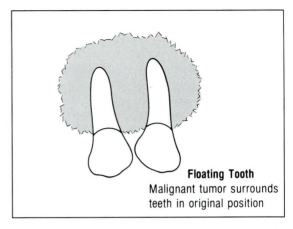

Floating Tooth
Malignant tumor surrounds
teeth in original position

FIG. 22-5. A malignant lesion spreads rapidly, destroying bone but leaving the teeth in position and often without evidence of root resorption. (From Matteson SR, et al: *Dent Radiogr Photogr* 57:35-52, 1985.)

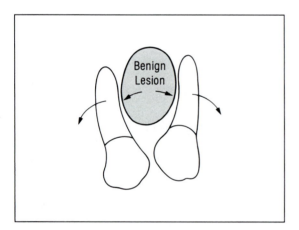

FIG. 22-6. A benign lesion usually grows slowly, causing displacement and resorption of the tooth roots. (From Matteson SR, et al: *Dent Radiogr Photogr* 57:35-52, 1985.)

body or ramus of the mandible using panoramic, lateral oblique, or periapical projections. Examination of these regions mediolaterally may include occlusal, posteroanterior skull, or submentovertex views. Examine the maxilla carefully with posteroanterior cephalometric, Waters, submentovertex, or panoramic projections. Pay particular attention to include all bony margins on each radiograph. Because of the multiple superimposition of structures in this region, it is often desirable to use complex motion tomographic views or computed tomography (CT). CT allows an evaluation of both the extent of the lesion in the soft tissue and the character of the lesion as judged by its interaction with bone.

CARCINOMA
Squamous cell carcinoma

Squamous cell carcinoma is of epithelial origin. It is the most common type of oral cancer. Most arise in the oral mucosa and thus are peripheral lesions that invade the deeper tissues. It spreads by invasion of adjacent soft tissues, nerve trunks, and blood vessels and through bone.[20] Oral lesions often invade the jaws, especially if they originate in areas of the oral mucosa near the underlying bone. Because the chance of successful treatment greatly improves with early detection of carcinomas, clinicians should be alert to identify oral premalignant lesions clinically manifested as either leukoplakia, erythroplakia, or a speckled combination.[8] Lesions that develop in regions at some distance from bone, such as in the cheek, tongue, or floor of the mouth, do not invade bone unless they are neglected and enlarge to the point of bony contact. The verrucose carcinoma is a low-grade, exophytic type of squamous cell carcinoma that seldom invades bone. Only rarely do cases of central squamous cell carcinoma develop within the jaw bones. These apparently originate from malignant transformation of residual islands (nests) of epithelium derived from the dental lamina or from the epithelial lining of dental cysts.[38]

Clinical features. Squamous cell carcinoma in the oral cavity occurs predominantly in men older than age 50. Although the specific cause is unknown, the lesion is more prevalent in heavy smokers, those who abuse alcohol, those who have poor oral hygiene, and possibly those with a history of syphilitic glossitis.[43] The lesion most commonly involves the posterior lateral border of the tongue and lower lip and less frequently the floor of the mouth, alveolar mucosa, palate, and buccal mucosa. Osseous involvement in the jaws is most frequent in the third molar region of the mandible where the developing tumor is relatively close to bone. Small lesions, less than 1 cm, are usually asymptomatic and discovered on routine oral examination. Larger lesions often cause some pain, paresthesia, or swelling that leads to their discovery. Carcinoma in close relation to the teeth may cause loosening or exfoliation and some root resorption of the involved dentition. Carcinoma may also be discovered in edentulous patients when the expanding lesion causes an ill-fitting dental prosthesis. Squamous cell carcinoma spreads by direct extension into surrounding structures and by metastasis. Metastasis is usually through lymphatic channels and to the submental and submandibular lymph nodes. Treatment usually consists of radiation therapy, surgery, or both.

Radiographic features. The radiographic appearance of primary carcinoma* of the jaw is usually that of a destructive lesion. Lesions of the alveolar mucosa may infiltrate and cause erosion of the alveolar bone producing lesions with ill-defined, irregular margins (Fig. 22-7). This appearance of irregular erosion of the bony margin may occur along the entire bony border of the tumor or be restricted to a relatively small area. In some cases, irregular spicules of bone are left behind by the advancing tumor front. When lesions in the mandible become quite large, they may erode into the alveolar canal. Often a radiograph of such a lesion demonstrates the elevated outline of the soft tissue margins of the tumor above the lesion. When the lesion extends to the inferior border of the mandible, a pathologic fracture is likely. Posteroanterior, lateral oblique, and occlusal views are often most useful for demonstrating such fractures.[24] When a lesion lies on the lingual surface of the mandible, erosion of bone may be difficult to detect, especially when the area of erosion is small. CT has been found useful in identifying such areas.[27] CT scanning has also been found useful for detecting and delineating nasopharyngeal carcinomas and for confirming infiltration of tumor to the base of the tongue.[83]

Although the margins of squamous cell carcinoma are characteristically ill defined and radiolucent, occasionally there is a radiopaque zone beyond the lesion margin (Fig. 22-7, *D*) or at its border. In the latter instance, the result is a sharply outlined radiolucency. The radiodensity of the wider, more diffuse, reactive osseous margins may resemble the ground-glass pattern of fibrous dysplasia. However, those that impart a reasonably well-defined hyperostotic border suggest the condensing osteitis that frequently defines chronic granulomatous inflammation.[84] Although the cause of this border is not clear, it may be that the infiltrate of lymphocytic cells characteristically observed in the bone marrow spaces ahead of the invading tumor stimulates a sclerotic change in the bone that is characteristic of chronic inflammation.

The rare central squamous cell carcinoma has the characteristic appearance of a radiolucent lesion with ill-defined borders but is entirely embedded in bone. Occasionally, there are small opacities in the lesion representing small residual islands of bone left behind by the advancing tumor. No evidence of periosteal reaction or new bone formation is evident.

Differential diagnosis. Squamous cell carcinoma must be distinguished from other lesions that can cause diffuse loss of bone. None have unique radiographic characteristics. *Osteomyelitis* or *osteoradionecrosis* may cause lesions radiographically resembling those of squamous cell carcinoma, but these lesions often produce symptoms of infection and show areas of sequestration that help to rule out carcinoma alone. In contrast to squamous cell carcinoma, osteomyelitis may also demonstrate areas of periosteal new bone formation. The radiographic distinction between osteoradionecrosis of the jaw with infection and tumor persistence or recurrence is often difficult. The history and a clinical examination may be instructive, but biopsy may be necessary. Less frequently, malignant salivary gland tumors or radiolucent sarcomas may cause the same radiographic image. Areas of locally destructive bone loss also occur in cases involving *histiocytosis X* (resulting in the "teeth floating in space" appearance), *periodontitis, juvenile periodontitis,* or *Papillon-Lefèvre syndrome.*

Metastatic carcinoma

Metastatic carcinoma is the most common malignant tumor in the skeleton. Metastasis of a primary carcinoma to the jaws from remote sites is relatively rare, representing between 1% and 8%

---

*The term "primary carcinoma" refers to the initial lesion. If the cancer spreads, it results in secondary or metastatic lesions.

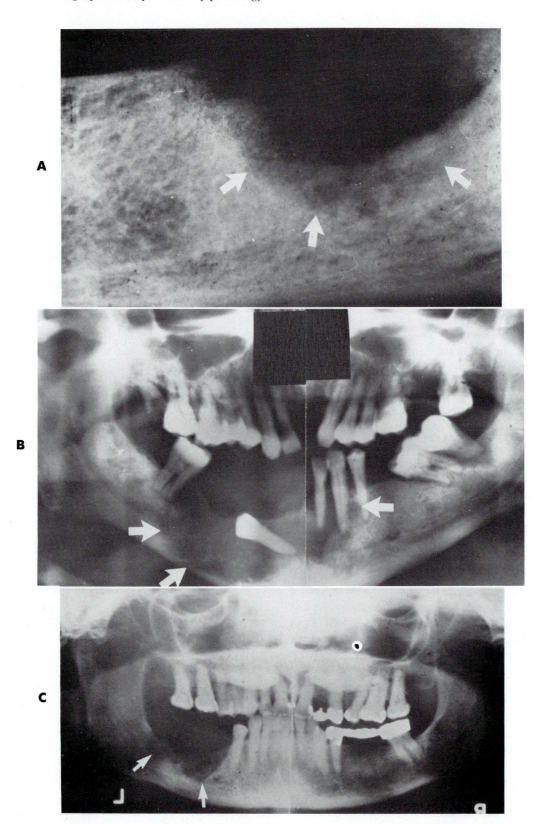

FIG. 22-7. A to **E,** Squamous cell carcinomas *(arrows),* resulting in irregular resorption of bone. Note the soft tissue border of the lesion in **D.** (**B** courtesy Dr. S.R. Matteson, Chapel Hill, NC.)

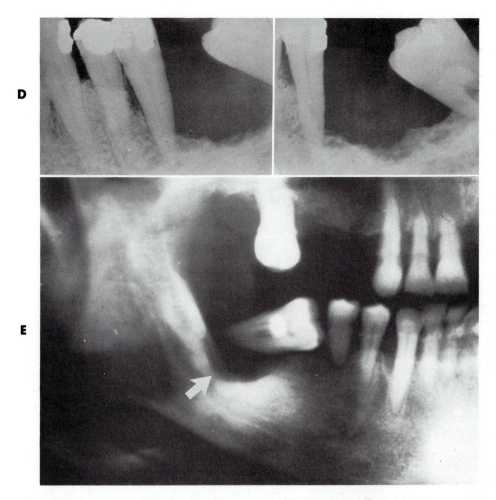

FIG. 22-7, cont'd. For legend see opposite page.

of the malignant tumors in the oral region.[69] Metastatic lesions occur in the jawbones more frequently than in the soft tissues of the mouth.[85] Oral metastasis is usually regarded as a sign that general metastasis is well advanced.[17] Metastatic carcinoma does not include the involvement of the mandible or maxilla by direct extension or infiltration by soft tissue lesions.

Clinical features. Metastatic tumors are second in frequency of occurrence in the jaws only to primary squamous cell carcinoma. They spread to the mandible much more frequently than to the maxilla. The most common site is in the premolar and molar region.[26] Most lesions occur in patients between 40 and 60 years. They most commonly metastasize from primary tumors in the breast, followed in order by the lung, kidney, prostate gland, colon, testis, and stomach.[69] The oral manifestations are frequently the first indication of the disease.[59] Usually such lesions are asymptomatic and

found on routine radiographic examination. Clinical signs, when present, usually include pain followed by paresthesia or anesthesia of the lip or chin. This results from involvement of the mandibular nerve by the lesion. Teeth near the lesion may become loosened or exfoliate and occasionally show evidence of root resorption.[26] In most cases of metastatic carcinoma to the jaw, there are other skeletal metastases and often lung lesions.[26] The prognosis for persons with metastatic lesions to the jaws is poor. Death usually occurs within a short time after the discovery of metastatic lesions in the jaws.[85]

Radiographic features. The usual radiographic appearance of metastatic disease in the jaws is the same as a primary carcinoma. It is a radiolucent lesion with ill-defined, destructive margins.[17] These lesions may be single or multiple, and they vary in size (Fig. 22-8). The appearance of the metastatic lesion is variable, however, sometimes showing areas of bone production (in the case of prostatic and in rare cases from breast and lung carcinoma)[28] and sometimes with fairly well-defined borders.[61] If the lesion is diffuse, it may appear quite similar to osteomyelitis. When the metastatic lesion occurs in the alveolar bone, it may cause loss of the lamina dura leading to mobility or loss of teeth. In such cases, the lesion may resemble advanced periodontal disease. Identification of the lesion is dependent on histologic examination. This may be difficult if the oral lesion is poorly differentiated and especially if the primary lesion has not been detected.

Malignant tumors of salivary glands

Malignant salivary gland tumors make up 10% of all cancers of the oral and perioral tissues (a distant second to squamous cell carcinomas). Most (95%) malignant tumors of the major and minor salivary glands arise in the epithelial elements of these glands.[58] Of all tumors that arise in the major salivary glands, 30% to 40% are malignant; of these, 56% occur in the submandibular gland, 34% in the parotid gland, and 10% in the sublingual gland.[23] Of all the tumors that arise in the submandibular gland, 40% are malignant, as are 30% of those that develop in the parotid gland and 70% in the sublingual gland.[29] Also, from 47% to 85% of tumors that arise in the minor salivary glands

are malignant.[23,29] Approximately 50% of salivary gland tumors arising in children (excluding the quite numerous benign, nonepithelial vascular tumors) are malignant, in contrast to only 25% in adults. Patients with primary benign or malignant salivary gland tumors seem to have a significant increase in second primary tumors. In females, the accompanying tumors are mainly in the breast and bronchus; in the male, the prostate gland and skin are the usual sites.[71] Exposure to radiation is the only factor identified as playing an etiologic role.[73,76] Induced salivary gland tumors are usually benign.

Malignant tumors of the salivary glands include, in order of frequency, mucoepidermoid carcinoma, adenocystic carcinoma, adenocarcinoma, malignant mixed tumor, acinic cell carcinoma, and squamous cell carcinoma.[75] All of the epithelial types of salivary gland tumors may be found within the jaw bones, originating, it is assumed, as the result of metaplasia in epithelial remnants of cysts or in embryologic enclosed salivary gland tissue.[11] These central tumors are generally mucoepidermoid carcinomas.[15] Metastatic involvement of the salivary glands is rare.[10] An interesting comment regarding the nature of salivary gland tumors is credited to Ackerman and del Regato: "The usual neoplasm of the salivary glands is a tumor, the benign variant of which is less benign than the usual

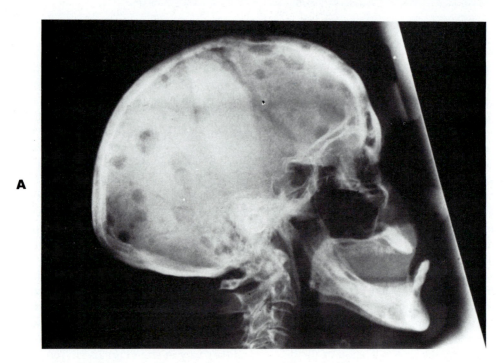

FIG. 22-8. Metastatic carcinomas. **A,** Lesions appearing as multiple radiolucencies in the skull.

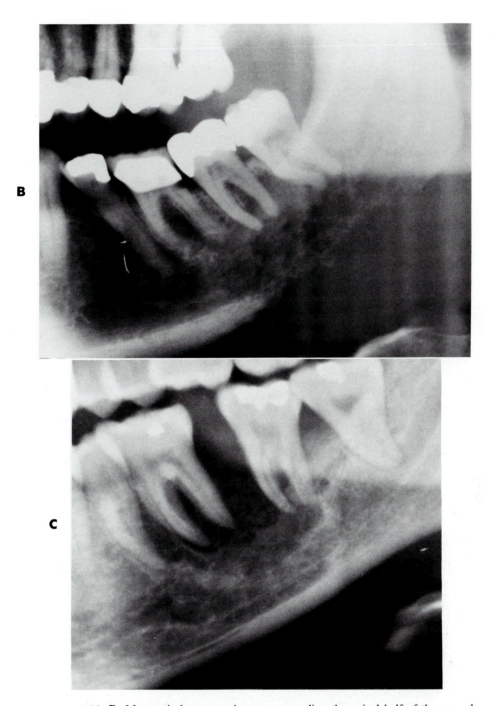

FIG. 22-8, cont'd. B, Metastatic breast carcinoma surrounding the apical half of the second and third molar roots and extending inferiorly. It has destroyed the inferior border of the mandible. **C,** Metastatic renal cell carcinoma that has destroyed the alveolar bone supporting the first and second molars.   *Continued.*

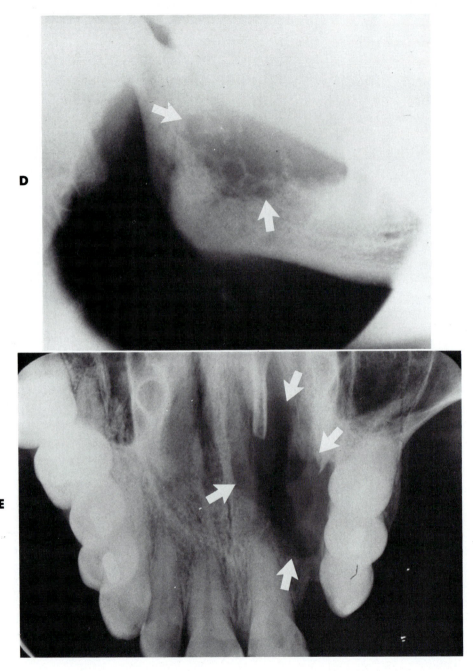

FIG. 22-8, cont'd. D and **E,** Lesions from a gastric carcinoma. (**A, D,** and **E** courtesy Dr L. Hollender, Göteborg, Sweden.)

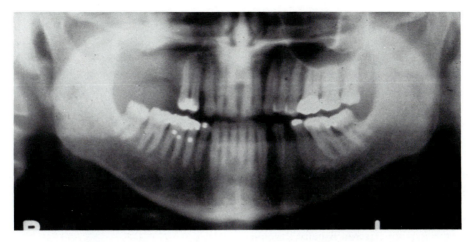

FIG. 22-9. Adenoid cystic carcinoma of the right maxilla. Note the complete opacification of the right antrum and the loss of bony margin of the sinus on the *left* side.

benign tumor, and the malignant variant is less malignant than the usual malignant tumor."[2]

Clinical features. Most malignant salivary gland tumors occur in middle age or later in life. They may arise at any age, however, even in the very young. The range is broad, from 1 to 77 years, with a wide peak throughout the fourth and fifth decades.[11] The highest incidence of central salivary gland tumor, like the peripheral variety, occurs in the female. Most occur in the mandible, in the posterior alveolus, the angle, and ramus, whereas less than half that number arise in the maxillary sinus, palate, and posterior ridges of the maxilla.[11] The tumors are generally slow growing and painless, although those of high-grade malignancy may enlarge rapidly, infiltrate nerves, and cause pain. Metastasis is via the lymphatics. The mucoepidermoid carcinoma is the most frequent variety encountered, and 90% of these occur in the parotid gland.[19] In general, the prognosis for any malignant tumor in the parotid gland is better than for one in the submandibular or minor salivary glands.[39]

Mucoepidermoid carcinoma rarely develops centrally within the jaws.[50] Central mucoepidermoid carcinoma occurs twice as often in females as males and twice as often in the mandible as in the maxilla. It usually develops in the posterior jaws of individuals in their fifth to seventh decades. The tumor usually occurs first as a swelling without pain.

Radiographic features. Because of the proximity of the salivary glands to bone, invasion of the bone by these tumors occasionally occurs. The radiographic image produced when such lesions invade bone cannot be distinguished from periph-eral squamous cell carcinoma. The erosion from the surface into the bone is typically malignant, the border being ragged and poorly defined. Neglected lesions in the hard palate may invade the floor of the maxillary sinus (Fig. 22-9). Mucoepidermoid carcinomas usually appear as multilocular or occasionally unilocular radiolucent lesions with scalloped and reasonably well-defined margins.[58] They may have the appearance of an ameloblastoma. It is most appropriate to image a known or suspected parotid neoplasm with CT, ultrasound, or MR.[21,22,35,53,88]

SARCOMA

Sarcomas are malignant lesions that arise within the connective tissues. The lesions are less common than carcinomas and usually occur in young people. Their spread is usually by direct extension or through the bloodstream. They generally have a poor prognosis. Sarcomas generally occur as rapidly growing masses that cause irregular destruction of bone with indistinct margins. They may be entirely lytic or form radiopaque calcifications. The most common of these is osteosarcoma, followed by chondrosarcoma.

Osteosarcoma

Osteosarcoma is the most common malignant tumor of bone. It arises from relatively undifferentiated bone-forming mesenchymal tissue. Its cause is unknown. Although osteosarcoma is a rare tumor, involving the jaws in only about 7% of cases, it is the most common type of primary sarcoma arising in the jaws. There are different types of osteogenic sarcomas: sclerosing, osteolytic, and mixed. The sclerosing type forms neoplastic osteoid and bone; the osteolytic type does not form bone. There are few differences in the clinical features of these types, although the osteolytic form is more undifferentiated and may have a more rapid rate of growth.

Cinical features. The mean age of occurrence of osteosarcoma in the jaws is around 30, somewhat older by about 10 to 20 years than for other sites in the body.[4,90] These lesions occur approximately equally in men and women and about equally in the maxilla and mandible.[25,90] In the mandible, the lesion most frequently develops in the body. In the maxilla, lesions usually develop in the antrum or alveolar ridge but not the palate. The tumor is most common in long limb bones, usually the femur or tibia. It occasionally develops in the illiac crest, vertebral column, or jaws, but it may develop anywhere. There is an increased incidence of osteogenic sarcoma in bones that have been irradiated, subject to trauma, or affected by Paget's disease.[6,72,78]

The usual early clinical picture is swelling with a fairly short history as the tumor enlarges, occasionally accompanied by pain.[12,25,45,90] The affected teeth may become loose, and paresthesia may develop.[9] The lesion is extremely serious because it tends to grow rapidly (potential doubling time 32 days)[55] and metastasizes early through the bloodstream to the lungs. Jaw lesions are less likely to metastasize than when they occur in other bones.[94] The usual treatment is early radical surgical removal. The 5-year survival rate depends strongly on the completeness of the tumor's removal and the presence of metastasis. It may be as high as 50% for lesions in the maxilla and some 70% for those in the mandible, although other studies report lower rates.[33] An unusual variant, juxtacortical osteosarcoma, is much less aggressive and has a better prognosis.[14,62]

Radiographic features. Osteosarcoma presents a highly varied radiographic appearance in the jaws. One of the earliest signs is a widening of the periodontal ligament space or a radiolucency around one or more teeth (Fig. 22-10).[48] As the lesion enlarges, it may develop into one of three basic forms: an osteolytic radiolucent appearance, a radiopaque osteoblastic form, or a mixed radiolucent image with radiopaque foci. These three varieties occur with about equal frequency in advanced cases.[48] Typically, the lesion is unicentric and the borders are ill defined, suggestive of its

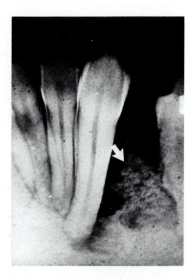

FIG. 22-10. Osteosarcoma with widening of the periodontal ligament space and the production of new bone *(arrow)*.

malignant nature. The lytic variety has ragged borders similar to a carcinoma. The sclerotic portions of the mixed and opaque lesions may show obliteration of the previous trabecular pattern by new bone, imparting a dense granular or sclerotic appearance. The opaque and mixed forms of this lesion frequently show perforation and expansion of the cortical margins. As the tumor grows through the cortex, it elevates the periosteum and may cause the deposition of new bone. This new bone may be apparent in the form of spicules growing at right angles to the bone surface with a "sunray" appearance (Fig. 22-11). This feature is not specific for osteosarcoma or a constant feature of osteosarcoma, being observed in only about a third of osteosclerotic cases. This sunray pattern also occurs in myeloma, metastatic cancer, advanced Ewing's sarcoma, tuberculosis, and other inflammatory diseases. Occasionally this new subperiosteal bone may take the form of "onion peel" lamination.

Chondrosarcoma

Chondrosarcomas are malignant tumors of cartilaginous origin that may arise centrally in bone or peripherally in the periosteum or other connective tissues containing cartilage. These lesions develop from mature cartilage or benign cartilaginous tumors. Most develop from cartilage located in bone, either centrally in the bone (medullary) cavity or peripherally from a cartilage cap of an osteochondroma.[57] Chondrosarcoma is more com-

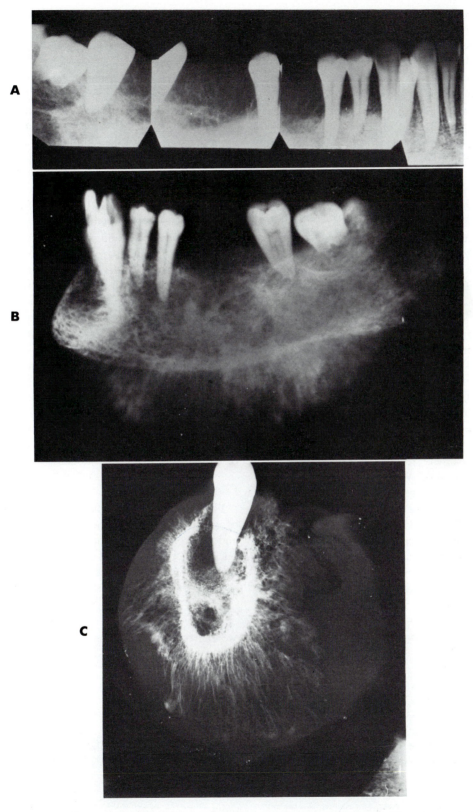

FIG. 22-11. Osteosarcoma in a 25-year-old man, showing sunray spicules of bone on periapical radiographs, **A,** and on resected jaw, **B** and **C.**

mon in the pelvis, ribs, spine, and large limb bones. In the jaws it is relatively rare, accounting for only about 2% of all chondrosarcomas.[58] However, following multiple myeloma and osteosarcoma, it is the third most common primary tumor of the jaws, occurring about half as often as osteosarcoma.[46]

Clinical features. Chondrosarcomas in the jaws occur most often in the maxilla, with fewer lesions developing in the mandible, nasal septum, and paranasal sinuses.[46,91] Mandibular lesions often begin in the premolar-molar regions. The temporomandibular joint is rarely involved.[67] Patients with chondrosarcoma of the jaws are younger than those with the entity elsewhere. It develops in the jaws most often during the second through the sixth decades, with a peak in the third decade (average age about 30 years).[46] A slightly greater number of males are affected, up to a ratio of 2:1.[78] The early tumor is usually painless, with facial asymmetry being the first complaint.[47,85] However, as it slowly enlarges, the swelling on the bone is hard and usually painful.[94] Chondrosarcomas of the jaw may manifest as a slowly increasing gap between adjacent teeth.[51] Teeth adjacent to the lesion may be resorbed, loosened, or exfoliated.[47,85] Chondrosarcomas may arise in previously irradiated normal bone and benign lesions.[44,55] These lesions grow slower than the osteosarcomas and are slower to produce metastases. Treatment is wide surgical excision when possible. When it occurs in the jaws, it has a poorer prognosis than in other bones. In contrast to its behavior in other bones and to osteosarcoma of the jaws, chondrosarcoma of the jaws has a poorer prognosis. Although it rarely metastasizes, death results from its aggressive local infiltration. Recurrences are common.[9]

Radiographic features. The radiographic appearance of chondrosarcoma may be as varied as that of osteosarcoma. Most often the radiographic appearance is that of a malignant tumor, a lytic lesion with poorly defined borders.[46] It may also be sclerotic or mixed (radiolucent-radiopaque), if there is calcification of the neoplastic tissue (Fig. 22-12). Occasionally the area of destruction may appear as an isolated cystlike lesion. Large lobules of cartilage may give the radiolucency a soap bubble appearance, but it may be multiloculated or develop as multiple radiolucencies containing sclerotic foci.[63] The peripheral tumor may show only a portion of its borders in bone, whereas the rest of its mass may be apparent as a hazy image sitting in a ragged defect within the bone. In about 25% of the cases, a sunray pattern may be evident,[48] and in others a ground-glass appearance may be seen. If present, calcifications in chondrosarcoma most often occur in the older part of the tumor and appear as small, dense, irregular islands with a characteristic appearance. As in osteosarcoma, widening of the periodontal ligament may be evident when the lesion involves teeth and is small.[48] As the lesion progresses, resorption of the roots of the included teeth is common.[85] Whereas radiographs will most likely identify the malignant character and location of a chondrosarcoma, it is unlikely that the diagnosis can be made on the basis of the radiographic image alone.

Fibrosarcoma

Fibrosarcoma is a primary malignant neoplasm of either the periosteal, periodontal membrane or endosteal connective tissue that produces collagen but does not form osteoid or bone. It is an uncommon tumor and occurs less frequently than osteosarcoma or chondrosarcoma.

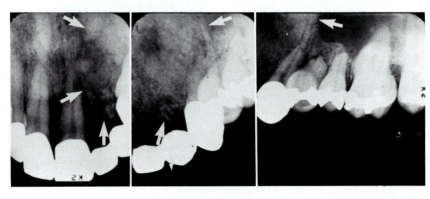

FIG. 22-12. Chondrosarcoma of the anterior maxilla, showing irregular calcification in the tumor *(arrows)*. (Courtesy Dr. L. Hollender, Seattle.)

Clinical features. Oral fibrosarcoma develops centrally in the jaw bones but most often arises in the periosteal tissues.[9] About 13% of those that arise in bone occur in the jaws, most in the mandible (Fig. 22-13).[31] Lesions of the maxilla are quite destructive and invade the antrum.[82] Pain, swelling, and paresthesia are the most common complaints.[87] The mean age of occurrence is 50 years, but it may occur later in life or even in young children. They are most common in the femur or tibia. Most jaw lesions occur in men.[42] As with osteosarcoma, the prevalence of fibrosarcoma is greater in patients with Paget's disease and those who have received therapeutic irradiation of other neoplasms. Early surgical removal is indicated. The 5-year survival is quite variable but is about 40% to 70% for mandibular lesions.[31,87,89]

Radiographic features. The radiographic appearance of fibrosarcoma is that of a destructive lesion and may simulate the osteolytic form of osteosarcoma. Typically, the lesion shows loss of bone with ill-defined borders (Fig. 22-13). The growing tumor may displace teeth and cause root erosion. When the lesion develops from the periosteum, it may cause smooth pressure resorption of the underlying bone.

Ewing's sarcoma

Ewing's sarcoma is a malignancy of bone derived from mesenchymal connective tissue of the marrow.[32] It is an uncommon primary malignancy of the jaws.

Clinical features. Ewing's sarcoma usually occurs between the ages of 5 and 25 years and about twice as frequently in males as females.[92] About 1% to 13% of cases occur in the jaws, usually in the posterior mandible.[92] It is a rapidly growing, highly invasive tumor with early and widespread metastasis. Initially, there is often intermittent pain without palpable disease. Later, the pain becomes continuous and is associated with rapid growth of the tumor and enlargement of bone (with either cortical destruction[79] or expansive growth of the cortex). The painful swellings are usually hard, but occasionally they are soft and fluctuant. The teeth in the area may become mobile, and paresthesia of the lip may develop.[92] The prognosis is poor, most cases leading to death within a few years of diagnosis.[85]

Radiographic features. The radiologic appearance of Ewing's sarcoma is an ill-defined, destructive radiolucent lesion. This lesion may be unilocular or multilocular. Areas of sclerosis may develop around the margins of the lesion. Early in its development, this lesion, with an appearance of mottled rarefaction, may closely resemble an area of osteomyelitis. When the tumor penetrates to the cortex, it may occasionally elevate the periosteum and stimulate it to produce thin layers of bone, resulting in a laminated or onionskin effect along the bone surface. Advanced cases may also occasionally present a sunray pattern.[74] The radiologic appearance of Ewing's sarcoma is complex and not diagnostic.[36]

HEMATOLOGIC NEOPLASMS
Leukemia

Clinical features. Acute leukemias may occur in persons of either sex and at any age. They usually develop in children younger than 5 years and

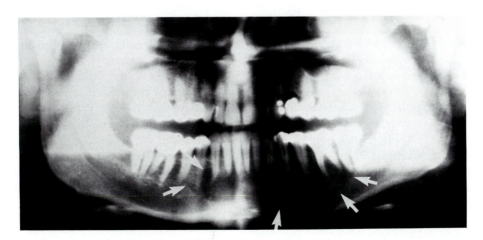

FIG. 22-13. Fibrosarcoma in the mandible, showing large areas of ill-defined bone destruction *(arrows)*.

most often before age 25 months. Chronic leukemias are rare before age 25 years, usually occurring in the fifth through seventh decades. Frequently, leukemic cells infiltrate the gingiva, particularly if gingivitis or periodontal disease is present, and the result is gingival hyperplasia. Because the infiltration of cells occurs in areas of chronic irritation, the oral manifestations usually do not develop in edentulous individuals or very young patients.

Radiographic features. Osteolytic changes occur in more than half of the leukemias involving children. The findings may be those of periodontal disease, destruction of the alveolar bone, loss of the lamina dura, and loosening of the teeth.[80] Also, the body of the mandible may show generalized bone loss as a result of the patient's diminished capacity to resist the periodontal infection. When there are infiltrates of leukemic cells in the jaws, the appearance is that of ill-defined, diffuse radiolucent lesions resembling periapical inflammatory disease.[30] Local dental causes must be ruled out to make this interpretation. In some cases, the leukemic cells destroy the spongiosa and penetrate through the cortex. The result is a focal reaction below the periosteum. New bone deposits in layers parallel with the cortex and is apparent in the radiograph as white lines separated by dark lines (onion peel effect).

IMMUNOLOGIC NEOPLASMS

Neoplasia of the immune system involves cells of the lymphoreticular system, including lymphocytes and histocytes, plasma cells, and intermediate forms.

Malignant lymphoma

Malignant lymphomas are a group of immunologic neoplasms (Hodgkin's disease, lymphosarcoma, or primary lymphoma of bone) that arise in lymphoid tissue. However, some of these tumors may also arise in nonlymphoid tissue such as the gingiva and palate. Lymphosarcoma and primary lymphoma of bone usually occur in the oral cavity as primary tumors. Hodgkin's disease rarely develops in the jaws. These lesions usually do not cause radiographic findings. Malignant lymphomas arising in the oral cavity (primary lymphoma of bone and lymphosarcoma) that do spread to bone cause irregular bone loss in the area of the lesion. Typically, the radiolucent lesions have diffuse, ill-defined margins and are entirely lytic.[34,77] The most common regions are the posterior maxilla and mandible.[37]

Burkitt's lymphoma

Burkitt's lymphoma is a B-lymphocyte malignancy. It was originally detected in children in tropical regions, most often east central Africa, where it is the most common malignant tumor of childhood.[85] However, this disease is now observed in the United States and the rest of the world. Although the African and non-African tumors are histologically identical,[1] there are several important differences between the two varieties. In the African form, the jaw is involved in at least 75% of all cases, and abdominal manifestations* are seen less frequently.[65] In American cases, abdominal lymphoma is usually the primary lesion and only 18% or less of individuals have jaw lesions.[81] As the age of the patient increases, there is a reversal of this distribution of the two varieties, with a greater tendency for the African form to initiate in the abdomen and for the American form to be detected first in the jaws.[7,56] In the African cases, there is usually gross distortion of the face, but this is less frequent in the United States.[56] There is strong serioepidemiologic and experimental evidence implicating Epstein-Barr virus (a member of the herpes group) in the development of this tumor.[70] Both forms respond well to chemotherapy and radiation, but the African tumor characteristically relapses, with poor prognosis.[66] Individuals who do not receive treatment are not likely to survive longer than 3 to 6 months; younger children frequently survive longer than older children. Remission occurs in more than 90% of patients who receive aggressive chemotherapy, but two thirds of patients who have advanced disease when the therapy is initiated relapse.[85]

Clinical features. When these tumors occur in the jaws, any or all quadrants may be involved.[5] The American form usually involves only one quadrant, whereas the African form often involves more than one quadrant.[3,81] Almost all occur in the molar areas. Maxillary lesions may spread rapidly to the floor of the orbit. The tumor has no predilection for any racial group.[18] The age of peak incidence in patients with the African form is 5 to 7 years; with the American form, the peak is 10 to 12 years.[70] This condition is two to four times more prevalent in boys than girls. Loosening, displacement, or mobility of the primary teeth without

---

*Diffuse proliferation of malignant lymphoid cells obscures and destroys the structure of enlarging organs such as the kidney, liver, adrenal glands, gonads, and visceral lymph nodes. Peripheral lymph nodes are infrequently involved, even in terminal cases.

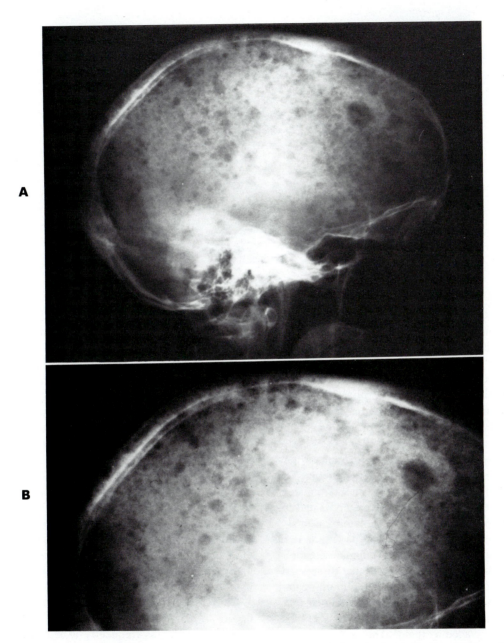

FIG. 22-14. Multiple myeloma, seen as multiple radiolucent lesions in the skull, (**A** and **B**), and in the ribs and humerus, **C.** (**B** and **C** courtesy Dr. L. Hollender, Seattle.)

Continued.

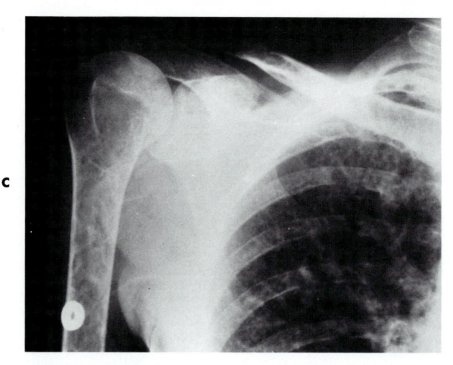

FIG. 22-14, cont'd. For legend see page 489.

any apparent local cause is the usual first sign of a tumor. There may also be premature appearance of the first permanent molars and toothache. The gingiva and mucosa next to the affected teeth become swollen, ulcerated, and necrotic. Swelling of the jaw soon follows, and paresthesia and anesthesia may be observed as the tumor invades the nerve.[3,5]

Radiographic features. Radiographs may show the earliest signs of Burkitt's lymphoma. The earliest radiographic features are small radiolucent foci scattered throughout the affected area and involving the trabecular bone and lamina dura.[3,52] The lesion also may cause loss of the lamina dura around erupted teeth.[70,93] Subsequent radiographs of the expanding lesion will show that these small foci have coalesced and formed large multilocular, irregular radiolucencies with poorly defined margins. The crypts of developing teeth may enlarge as they are invaded by tumor. The tumor may also destroy the cortex around developing teeth and displace unerupted tooth buds distally. As the lesion grows, it may cause marked expansion of the bone, stimulating new periosteal bone formation at its periphery that may produce the sunray appearance.[68] In addition, erosion or perforation of the cortex may occur.[30] Teeth may be resorbed or shed prematurely. Maxillary lesions should be investi-

gated with CT to examine the involvement of the sinus and orbit.[93]

Differential diagnosis. Initially Burkitt's lymphoma must be distinguished from an *acute infection* or *osteomyelitis*. However, the lack of symptoms or a cause for infection, as well as failure of local treatment in the face of continuing osteolysis and tooth displacement, should suggest another diagnosis.

Multiple myeloma

Multiple myeloma is a neoplasm in which there is proliferation of a single clone of abnormal plasma cells in the bone marrow. The proliferating plasma cells eventually replace the normal bone marrow and cause the clinical signs and symptoms. It may affect any part of the skeleton.

Clinical features. Multiple myeloma usually occurs in adults between the ages of 40 and 70 years, and twice as frequently in men. In severe cases, practically every bone may become involved. Pathologic fracture occurs in about 20% of cases.[40] Weakness and pain often accompany the lesions, especially in the back and thorax. Laboratory results that contribute to the identification of the tumor include progressive anemia, elevated sedimentation rate, and increased serum monoclonal immunoglobulins, which reverse the albumin-globulin ratio and elevate the total plasma protein. Plasma cells usually occur in the peripheral blood, and Bence Jones protein occurs in the urine of at least half of patients.

Patients with multiple myeloma have involvement of the jaws in up to 70% of the cases when radiographs are used.[40] Oral manifestations may be the initial sign of systemic disease in about 14% of patients with multiple myeloma.[40] The most frequent lesion sites are the posterior body, angle, and ramus of the mandible.[16] Lesions in the oral cavity may produce pain in the teeth or jaws, paresthesia, swelling, soft tissue mass, mobility or migration of teeth, hemorrhage, or pathologic fracture. The oral cavity may also show secondary signs of bone marrow involvement such as pallor of the oral tissues, intraoral hemorrhage, and susceptibility to infections.[40]

Radiographic features. The usual appearance of multiple myeloma is multiple small, well-defined radiolucencies without a sclerotic border, producing the impression of a punched-out defect. Occasionally the borders of these lesions may display a thin sclerotic rim, and even areas of opacification have been reported.[13] These lesions are usually bilateral and may become confluent, forming larger areas of bone destruction. Although not always present, cranial lesions are common. Skull radiographs should be obtained in suspected cases (Fig. 22-14). Such lesions may resemble metastatic carcinoma. Less frequently, multiple myeloma may demonstrate large lytic lesions with ill-defined ragged borders,[54] or generalized rarefaction of the skeleton in advanced cases.[64]

REFERENCES

1. Abaza NA, Iczkovitz ML, Henefer EP: American Burkitt's lymphoma manifested in a solitary submandibular lymph node, *Oral Surg* 51:121-127, 1981.
2. Abrams AM, Melrose RJ: Why we are failing with oral cancer, *J Am Soc Prevent Dent* 4:24-29, 1974.
3. Adatia AK: Dental tissues and Burkitt's tumor, *Oral Surg* 25:221-234, 1967.
4. Ajagbe HA, Junaid TA, Daramola JO: Osteogenic sarcoma of the jaw in an African community: report of twenty-one cases, *J Oral Maxillofac Surg* 44:104-106, 1986.
5. Anavi Y, Kaplinsky C, Calderon S, Zaizov R: Head, neck, and maxillofacial childhood Burkitt's lymphoma: a retrospective analysis of 31 patients, *J Oral Maxillofac Surg* 48:708-713, 1990.
6. Ballantyne A: Late sequelae of radiation therapy in cancer of the head and neck with particular reference to the nasopharynx, *Am J Surg* 130:433-436, 1975.
7. Banks PM, Arseneau JC, Graknick HR, et al: American Burkitt's lymphoma: a clinicopathologic study of 30 cases: II, pathologic correlations, *Am J Med* 58:322-329, 1975.

8. Barker BF, Dunlap CL: Oral cancer: life or death, *Mo Dent Assoc J* 62:29-31, 1982.
9. Batsakis JG: *Tumors of the head and neck,* ed 2, Baltimore, 1979, Williams & Wilkins.
10. Batsakis JG: The pathology of head and neck tumors: the occult primary and metastases to the head and neck, part 10, *Head Neck Surg* 3:409-423, 1981.
11. Batsakis JG, Regezi JA: The pathology of head and neck tumors: salivary glands, part 2, *Head Neck Surg* 1:167-180, 1978.
12. Bertoni F and others: The Istituto Rizzoli-Beretta experience with osteosarcoma of the jaw, *Cancer* 68:1555-1563, 1991.
13. Blaguiere RM, Guyer PB, Buchanan RB, Gallager PJ: Sclerotic bone deposits in multiple myeloma, *Br J Radiol* 55:591-593, 1982.
14. Bras J, Donner R, van der Kwast W, et al: Juxtacortical osteogenic sarcoma of the jaws, *Oral Surg* 50:535-544, 1980.
15. Browand B, Waldron C: Central mucoepidermoid tumors of the jaws: report of nine cases and review of the literature, *Oral Surg* 40:631-643, 1975.
16. Bruce KW, Royer RQ: Multiple myeloma occurring in the jaws: a study of 17 cases, *Oral Surg* 6:729-744, 1953.
17. Bucin E, Andreasson L, Bjorlin G: Metastases in the oral cavity: case reports, *Int J Oral Surg* 4:321-325, 1982.
18. Burkitt D, Wright D: Geographical and tribal distribution of the African lymphoma in Uganda, *Br Med J* 1:569-573, 1966.
19. Cancer statistics 1982, *CA* 32:15, 1982.
20. Carter RL: Patterns and mechanisms of spread of squamous carcinomas of the oral cavity, *Clin Otolaryngol* 15:185-191, 1990.
21. Casselman JW, Mancuso AA: Major salivary gland masses: comparison of MR imaging and CT, *Radiology* 165:183-189, 1987.
22. Cesteleyn L, Smith RG, Akuamoa-Boateng E, et al: Current diagnosis and therapy of parotid tumours, *Acta Stomatol Belg* 88:157-170, 1991.
23. Chang CH: Radiation therapy. In Rankpow RM, Polayes IM, editors: *Diseases of the salivary glands,* Philadelphia, 1976, WB Saunders.
24. Ciola B: Pathologic fractures of the mandible following invasive oral carcinomas, *Oral Surg* 46:725-731, 1978.
25. Clark J, Unni K, Dahlin D, Devine D: Osteosarcoma of the jaws, *Cancer* 51:2311-2316, 1983.
26. Clausen F, Poulsen H: Metastatic carcinoma to the jaws, *Acta Pathol Microbiol Scand* 57:361-374, 1963.
27. Close LG, Merkel M, Burns DK, Schaefer SD: Computed tomography in the assessment of mandibular invasion by intraoral carcinoma, *Ann Otol Rhinol Laryngol* 95:383-388, 1986.
28. Cohen B: Secondary tumors of the mandible, *Ann R Coll Surg Engl* 23:118-130, 1958.
29. Cornog JL, Gray SR: Surgical and clinical pathology of salivary gland tumors. In Rankow RM, Polayes IM, editors: *Diseases of the salivary glands,* Philadelphia, 1976, WB Saunders.
30. Curtis AB: Childhood leukemias: initial and oral manifestation, *J Am Dent Assoc* 83:159-164, 1971.
31. Dahlin D, Luins J: Fibrosarcoma of bone: a study of 114 cases, *Cancer* 23:35-41, 1969.
32. Dahlin DC, Coventry MB, Scanlon PW: Ewing's sarcoma: a critical analysis of 165 cases, *J Bone Joint Surg* 43a:185-192, 1961.

33. Dahlin DC, Unni KK: Osteosarcoma of bone and its important recognizable varieties, *Am J Surg Pathol* 1:6-72, 1977.

34. Daramola J, Ajagbe H: Presentation and behavior of primary malignant lymphoma of the oral cavity in adult Africans, *J Oral Med* 38:177-179, 1983.

35. Da-Xi S, Hai-Xiong S, Qiang Y: The diagnostic value of ultrasonography and sialography in salivary gland masses, *Dentomaxillofac Radiol* 16:37-45, 1987.

36. deSantos LA, Jing B-S: Radiographic findings of Ewing's sarcoma of the jaw, *Br J Radiol* 51:628-687, 1978.

37. Eisenbud L and others: Oral presentations in non-Hodgkin's lymphoma: a review of 31 cases, *Oral Surg* 57:272-280, 1984.

38. Elzay RP: Primary intraosseous carcinoma of the jaws, *Oral Surg* 54:299-303, 1982.

39. Eneroth C-M: Salivary gland tumors in the parotid gland, submandibular gland, and the palate region, *Cancer* 27:1415-1418, 1972.

40. Epstein J, Voss N, Stevenson-Moore P: Maxillofacial manifestations of multiple myeloma: an unusual case and review of the literature, *Oral Surg* 57:267-271, 1984.

41. Epstein JB, Silverman S Jr: Head and neck malignancies associated with HIV infection, *Oral Surg Oral Med Oral Pathol* 73:193-200, 1992.

42. Eversole L, Schwartz W, Sabes W: Central and peripheral fibrogenic and neurogenic sarcoma of the oral regions, *Oral Surg* 36:49-62, 1973.

43. Fedele DJ, Jones JA, Niessen LC: Oral cancer screening in the elderly, *J Am Geriatr Soc* 39:920-925, 1991.

44. Feintuch TA: Chondrosarcoma arising in a cartilaginous area of previously irradiated fibrous dysplasia, *Cancer* 31:877-881, 1973.

45. Forteza G, Colmenero B, Lopez-Barea F: Osteogenic sarcoma of the maxilla and mandible, *Oral Surg Oral Med Oral Pathol* 62:179-184, 1986.

46. Garrington GE, Collett WK: Chondrosarcoma: I, a selected literature review, *J Oral Pathol* 17:1-11, 1988.

47. Garrington GE, Collett WK: Chondrosarcoma: II, chondrosarcoma of the jaws: analysis of 37 cases, *J Oral Pathol* 17:12-20, 1988.

48. Garrington GE, Scofield HH, Cornyn J, Hooker S: Osteosarcoma of the jaws, *Cancer* 20:377-391, 1967.

49. Gerson SJ: Oral cancer, *Crit Rev Oral Biol Med* 1:153-166, 1990.

50. Gingell J, Beckerman T, Levy B, Snider L: Central mucoepidermoid carcinoma, *Oral Surg* 57:436-440, 1984.

51. Hackney FL, Aragon SB, Aufdemorte TB, et al: Chondrosarcoma of the jaws: clinical findings, histopathology, and treatment, *Oral Surg* 71:139-143, 1991.

52. Hupp J, Collins F, Ross A, Muall R: A review of Burkitt's lymphoma, *J Maxillofac Surg* 10:240-245, 1982.

53. Isaza M, Ikezoe J, Morimoto S, et al: Computed tomography and ultrasonography in parotid tumors, *Acta Radiol* 30:11-15, 1989.

54. Kaffe I, Ramon Y, Hertz M: Radiographic manifestations of multiple myeloma in the mandible, *Dentomaxillofac Radiol* 15:31-35, 1986.

55. Krolls SO, Shaffer RC, O'Rear JW: Chondrosarcoma and osteosarcoma of the jaws in the same patient, *Oral Surg* 50:146-149, 1980.

56. Levine PH and others: American Burkitt's lymphoma registry: a progress report, *Ann Intern Med* 83:31-36, 1975.

57. Lichtenstein L: *Bone tumors*, ed 4, St Louis, 1972, Mosby.

58. Lucas RB: *Pathology of tumors of the oral tissues*, ed 4, New York, 1984, Churchill Livingston.

59. Mashberg A: Erythroplasia vs. leukoplakia in the diagnosis of early asymptomatic oral squamous cell carcinoma, *N Engl J Med* 297:109-110, 1977.

60. Matteson SR, Tyndall DA, Burkes EJ, Jacoway JR: The radiology of benign and malignant lesions, *Dent Radiol Photogr* 57:35-52, 1985.

61. Meyer I, Shklar G: Malignant tumors metastatic to mouth and jaws, *Oral Surg* 230:350-362, 1965.

62. Millar BG, Browne RM, Flood TR: Juxtacortical osteosarcoma of the jaws, *Br J Oral Maxillofac Surg* 28:73-79, 1990.

63. Mirra JH: *Bone tumors: diagnosis and treatment*, Philadelphia, 1980, JB Lippincott.

64. Moseley JE: *Bone changes in hematologic disorders*, New York, 1963, Grune & Stratton.

65. Nkrumah FK, Perkin IV: Burkitt's lymphoma: a clinical study of 110 patients, *Cancer* 37:671-676, 1976.

66. Nonoyama M and others: Epstein-Barr virus DNA in Hodgkin's disease: American Burkitt's lymphoma and other human tumors, *Cancer Res* 34:1228-1231, 1974.

67. Nortjé CJ, Farman A, Grotepass F, Van Zyl J: Chondrosarcoma of the mandibular condyle: report of a case with special reference to radiographic features. *Br J Oral Surg* 14:101-111, 1976.

68. O'Connor GT: Malignant lymphoma in African children, *Cancer* 14:270-283, 1961.

69. Oikarinen VJ, Calonius PEB, Sainio P: Metastatic tumors to the oral region: I, an analysis of cases in the literature, *Proc Finn Dent Soc* 71:58-65, 1975.

70. Patton LL, McMillan CW, Webster WP: American Burkitt's lymphoma: a 10-year review and case study, *Oral Surg Oral Med Oral Pathol* 69:307-316, 1990.

71. Pogrel MA, Hansen LS: Second primary tumor associated with salivary gland carcinoma, *Oral Surg* 58:71-75, 1984.

72. Pons A, Arlet J, Alibelli M, et al: Malignant degeneration of fibrous bone dysplasia: general review, apropos of two cases, *Ann Radiol (Paris)* 17:713-720, 1974.

73. Preston-Martin S, White SC: Brain and salivary gland tumors related to prior dental radiography: implications for current practice, *J Am Dent Assoc* 120:151-158, 1990.

74. Rapoport A, Sobrinho J, de Carvalho M, et al: Ewing's sarcoma of the mandible, *Oral Surg* 44:89-94, 1977.

75. Regezi JA, Sciubba JJ: *Oral pathology: clinical-pathologic correlations*, Philadelphia, 1989, WB Saunders.

76. Rice DH, Batsakis JG, McClatchey KD: Postirradiation malignant salivary gland tumor, *Arch Otolaryngol* 102:699-670, 1976.

77. Robbins KT, Fuller L, Manning J, et al: Primary lymphoma of the mandible, *Head Neck Surg* 8:192-199, 1986.

78. Roca A, Smith J, Jing B: Osteosarcoma and periosteal osteogenic sarcoma of the maxilla and mandible, *Am J Clin Pathol* 54:625-636, 1970.

79. Roca A, Smith IL, MacComb WS, et al: Ewing's sarcoma of the maxilla and mandible: study of six cases, *Oral Surg* 25:194-203, 1968.

80. Ruprecht A, Arora B: Involvement of the mandible in leukemia, *Dentomaxillofac Radiol* 7:27-30, 1978.

81. Sariban E, Donahue A, Magrath I: Jaw involvement in American Burkitt's lymphoma, *Cancer* 53:1777-1782, 1984.

82. Saw D: Fibrosarcoma of maxilla, *Oral Surg* 47:164-168, 1979.

83. Schaefer S, Merkel M, Diehl J, et al: Computed tomographic assessment of squamous cell carcinoma or oral pharyngeal cavities, *Otolaryngology* 108:688-692, 1982.

84. Schwartz S, Shklar G: Reaction of alveolar bone to invasion of oral carcinoma, *Oral Surg* 24:33-37, 1967.

85. Shear M, Alstini M: Clinical and histological aspects of oral malignancies, excluding squamous cell carcinomas and salivary gland tumors. In van der Wall I, Snow GB, editors: *Oral oncology,* Boston, 1984, Martinus Nijhoff.

86. Silverman S, Galante M: *Oral cancer,* San Francisco, 1976, University of California Press.

87. Slootweg P, Muller H: Fibrosarcoma of the jaws, *J Maxillofac Surg* 12:157-162, 1984.

88. Som PM, Shugar JM, Sacher M, et al: Benign and malignant parotid pleomorphic adenomas: CT and MR studies, *J Comput Assist Tomogr* 12:65-69, 1988.

89. Taconis WK, van Rijssel TG: Fibrosarcoma of the jaws, *Skeletal Radiol* 15:10-13, 1986.

90. Tanzawa H, Uchiyama S, Sato K: Statistical observation of osteosarcoma of the maxillofacial region in Japan: analysis of 114 Japanese cases reported between 1930 and 1989, *Oral Surg Oral Med Oral Pathol* 72:444-448, 1991.

91. Weiss WW Jr, Bennett JA: Chondrosarcoma: a rare tumor of the jaws, *J Oral Maxillofac Surg* 44:73-79, 1986.

92. Wood RE, Nortjé CJ, Hesseling P, Grotepass F: Ewing's tumor of the jaw, *Oral Surg Oral Med Oral Pathol* 69:120-127, 1990.

93. Wood RE, Nortjé CJ, Hesseling P, and Mouton S: Involvement of the maxillofacial region in African Burkitt's lymphoma in the Cape Province and Namibia, *Dentomaxillofac Radiol* 17:57-60, 1988.

94. Worth HM: *Principles and practice of oral radiologic interpretation,* Chicago, 1972, Mosby.

23

in collaboration with DONALD D. BLASCHKE

Diseases of Bone Manifested
in the Jaws

This chapter considers diseases of bone (other than tumors) that appear in the jaws. These lesions develop from some disorder of one of the components of the osseous tissue. Chapter 24 considers systemic conditions that originate outside bone but that may be seen in bone. In most cases the cause of lesions of bone is unknown. Some of these diseases are localized and usually singular (e.g., simple bone cyst or giant cell granuloma); others may appear in multiple bones (e.g., fibrous dysplasia or Paget's disease); still others are systemic, affecting all bones (for example, osteopetrosis). The lesions described in this chapter involve the jaws and may be seen by the general dentist. Most of these conditions have a fairly benign course, but some may cause considerable disability; osteopetrosis in its severest form leads to early death. The dentist must recognize these lesions so that appropriate therapy may be provided.

FIBRO-OSSEOUS LESIONS

Fibro-osseous lesions are a group of conditions that replace normal bone with benign fibrous tissue containing variable amounts of mineralization. Some of these lesions may be of periodontal ligament origin (periapical cemental dysplasia, ossifying or cementifying fibroma), whereas others are not (fibrous dysplasia).[66,67] Florid osseous dysplasia and cherubism are also members of this family of fibro-osseous diseases. The terminology for these lesions is quite variable among institutions and geographic areas, and the criteria for their classification are not well defined.

Fibrous dysplasia

Fibrous dysplasia of bone appears to be a localized benign developmental anomaly of the skeletal system. Its cause is unknown. It arises from bone-forming mesenchyme in the spongiosa and develops by the proliferation of fibrous tissue. Within the fibrous tissue irregular trabeculae form and increase in number and size as the lesion matures. Generally, the affected site shows evidence of fibrosis, bone resorption, cortical expansion, and osseous formation.

Clinical features. Fibrous dysplasia encompasses three clinical forms. *Monostotic fibrous dysplasia,* the form found in the majority of affected jaws,[71] by definition involves only one bone and presents no extraskeletal effects other than occasional pigmented skin lesions. The most frequent sites (in order) are ribs, femur, tibia, maxilla, and mandible.[43] The maxilla is involved almost twice as often as the mandible.[16] *Polyostotic fibrous dysplasia* involves multiple bones and is divided into two forms: the less severe *Jaffe's type* and the more severe *Albright's syndrome.*[54] The most frequently involved bones are the femur, skull, and tibia.[43] Jaffe's type of polyostotic fibrous dysplasia appears with multiple bone involvement and often areas of increased skin pigmentation called "café-au-lait" spots. Albright's syndrome, in addition to these features, commonly includes various endocrine disturbances such as precocious puberty, goiter, hyperthyroidism, hyperparathyroidism, Cushing's syndrome, and acromegaly.[37] The monostotic form of fibrous dysplasia accounts for about 70% of cases and the polyostotic form about 30%.[43]

Fibrous dysplasia is usually found in young persons, generally in children younger than 10 years. Monostotic disease is typically discovered in a slightly older age group than the polyostotic form. Studies of the sex distribution of fibrous dysplasia show no sexual predilection except for Albright's

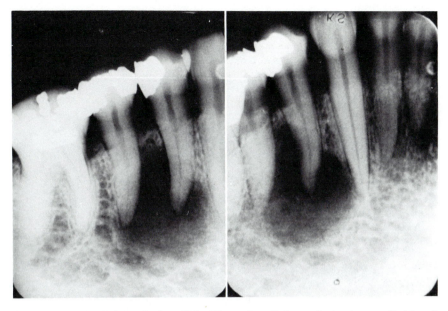

FIG. 23-1. Fibrous dysplasia in the mandible. The early radiolucent lesion has resulted in a loss of alveolar bone and lamina dura around the teeth. (Courtesy Dr. L. Hollender, Seattle.)

syndrome, which is detected almost exclusively in females.[43] Symptoms of the disease may be mild or not present at all, and the discovery of monostotic fibrous dysplasia is occasionally the result of an incidental radiographic finding. The polyostotic variety is more likely to affect entire limbs and to result in crippling deformities or fractures.[43] The bone and skin lesions of both polyostotic forms tend to be predominantly unilateral. Usually the skeletal lesions become static with the cessation of growth, but proliferation may continue, particularly in the polyostotic form.[27,29,43] Sarcomatous changes are unusual but have been reported.[11,45]

Jaw involvement occurs in a minority of all cases of fibrous dysplasia, although the incidence of jaw involvement is higher in the polyostotic forms. The lesions develop more commonly in the maxilla than in the mandible, with most of the changes occurring in the posterior regions. The anterior maxilla is least frequently involved.[66] Patients with jaw involvement may first complain of unilateral facial swelling or an enlarging deformity of the alveolar process. Pain and pathologic fractures are not often encountered. Craniofacial lesions may lead to anosmia (loss of the sense of smell), deafness, or blindness.

Radiographic features. The overall radiographic appearance of fibrous dysplasia varies with the degree of the lesion's maturation. Early lesions, usually found in young patients, tend to be radiolucent, with relatively well-defined borders (Fig. 23-1). The bony defect is often unilocular, but occasionally bony septa may be apparent, creating the impression of a multilocular cavity.

Dysplastic bone trabeculae increase in number and size as a lesion matures. The predominantly radiolucent appearance changes to a smoky, mottled radiopacity (Fig. 23-2). Within the lesion, replacement of fibrous tissue by trabeculae of approximately equal size continues to the point that the radiographic appearance may simulate ground glass or have an orange peel or pebbled appearance (Fig. 23-3). This type of homogeneous radiopaque appearance is most frequently seen in the maxilla[44] and is considered to be a radiographic sign strongly suggestive of the disease. It is the most common radiographic appearance of fibrous dysplasia. The actual degree of opacity of a particular lesion depends on the number and size of the newly formed internal trabeculae. As with the radiolucent form, the borders of the lesion often blend gradually into normal bone.

Alternatively, fibrous dysplasia may demonstrate areas of whorled, amorphous, partially calcified material that are fairly well circumscribed.[9] Other varieties of the lesion may be sclerotic (Fig. 23-4), cystlike (unilocular or multilocular), or pagetoid, showing areas of increased density and lucency such as in Paget's disease (Fig. 23-5). The radiolucent, unilocular, cystlike variety is more

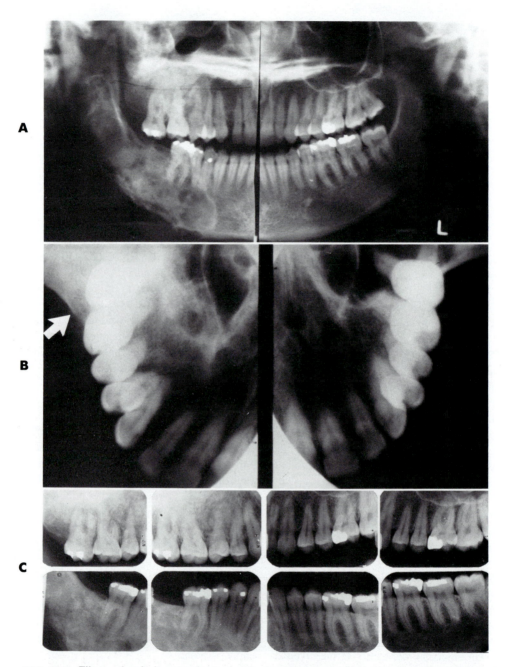

FIG. 23-2. Fibrous dysplasia occurring as a mixed appearance in the jaws. **A,** Note the lesions in the right maxilla and mandible (panoramic radiograph). **B,** There is expansion of the maxilla *(arrow)*, with increased density of trabecular bone on the affected side (occlusal projection). **C,** The periapical views show increased density of bone on the affected side.

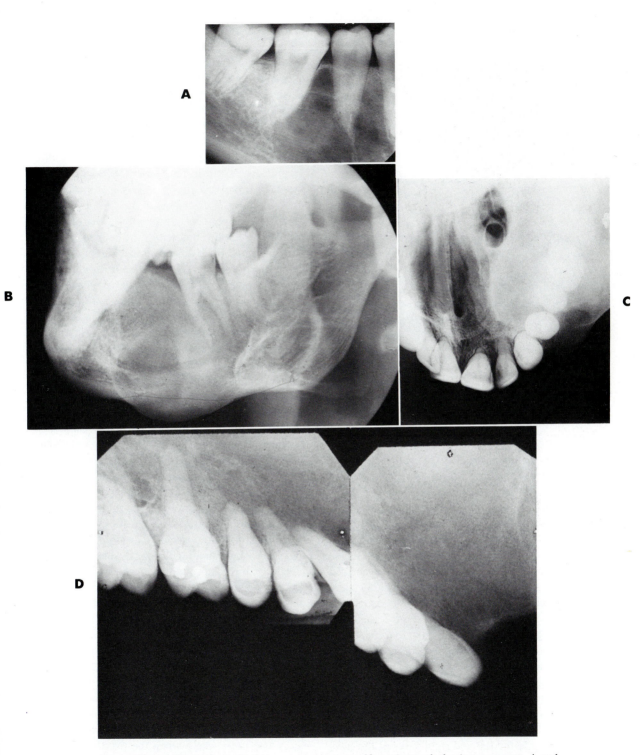

FIG. 23-3. Fibrous dysplasia in the jaws may present a uniform (ground-glass) appearance. **A** and **B,** Lesions in the mandible. **C** to **F,** Unilateral expansion in the maxilla. (**A** to **C** courtesy Dr. H. Worth, Vancouver BC; **D** courtesy Dr. H. Abrams, Los Angeles.)

Continued.

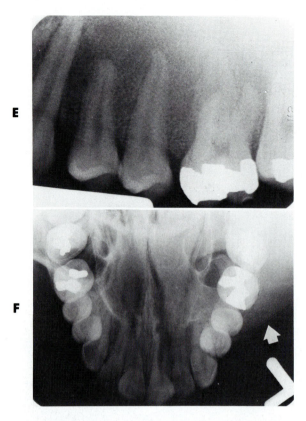

E

F

FIG. 23-3, cont'd. For legend see page 497.

common in the mandible. Also, a chalky type composed of dense, amorphous material has been described.[9]

The radiographic margins of fibrous dysplasia are variable and probably relate to the size and maturity of the lesion. Smaller, osteolytic lesions, generally seen in younger patients, tend to have fairly definite and possibly even circumscribed margins.[23] As lesions become more opaque, there is a tendency for the margins of the altered bone within the lesion to blend imperceptibly with the surrounding normal bone. Thus, the margins of the larger, more radiopaque lesions characteristically fade gradually.

In the jaws, bony expansion of fibrous dysplasia usually extends to the buccal and distal areas. If the inferior border of the mandible becomes displaced, it is usually also thinned. In less severe cases, compare the left and right sides of the jaws to detect subtle differences in size, density, and expansion. If a lesion of fibrous dysplasia occurs within the maxilla and is of moderate to large size, it usually encroaches on or obliterates the maxillary sinus. Fibrous dysplasia of the jaws may produce

tilting and bodily displacement of teeth. It may also cause resorption of roots and destruction of developing teeth. Frequently there is loss of the lamina dura.[44]

Although conventional radiographs are usually adequate to establish a diagnosis of fibrous dysplasia, computed tomography (CT) is often useful to establish the extent of facial lesions and is particularly helpful in evaluation of orbital involvement.[42]

Differential diagnosis. Most of the radiographic diagnostic difficulty associated with fibrous dysplasia involves younger persons, those most likely to have an early and active form of the disease. In such patients, fibrous dysplasia often appears as a radiolucency with well-defined, discrete bony margins. Such an appearance might also suggest *central giant cell granuloma, simple bone cyst,* or *aneurysmal bone cyst,* all lesions compatible with young age. Among these entities, however, fibrous dysplasia would be the most likely diagnosis if the defects were multifocal (involving two or more sites in a single affected bone) or polyostotic. The presence of prominent cortical bulging or displacement of teeth essentially eliminates simple bone cysts from further consideration. Aneurysmal bone cyst is a rare lesion, often identified by a hemorrhagic aspirate. Giant cell granuloma typically has faint, wispy trabeculae coursing through it, whereas the internal calcifications that may occur in fibrous dysplasia tend to be stippled or granular in appearance.

The presence of a radiolucent (fibrous) capsule and radiopaque cortex distinguishes *ossifying fibroma* from mature, essentially radiopaque fibrous dysplasia. Longstanding fibrous dysplasia typically blends with the surrounding normal bone. Radiographic differentiation between mature fibrous dysplasia and *Paget's disease* (described later in this chapter) might be difficult except that the typical age range is so different for the two diseases. Active fibrous dysplasia is uncommon in middle and older age groups, whereas Paget's disease is distinctly rare in adolescents and young adults. Although both bone diseases favor maxillary involvement, Paget's disease is much more likely to involve either jawbone *bilaterally.* Fibrous dysplasia is also more likely when the maxillary sinuses show significant bony obliteration.

Management. Observe patients carefully and consider surgery in the presence of severe clinical manifestations such as reduction in the size of the optic or auditory canals. Conservative osseous con-

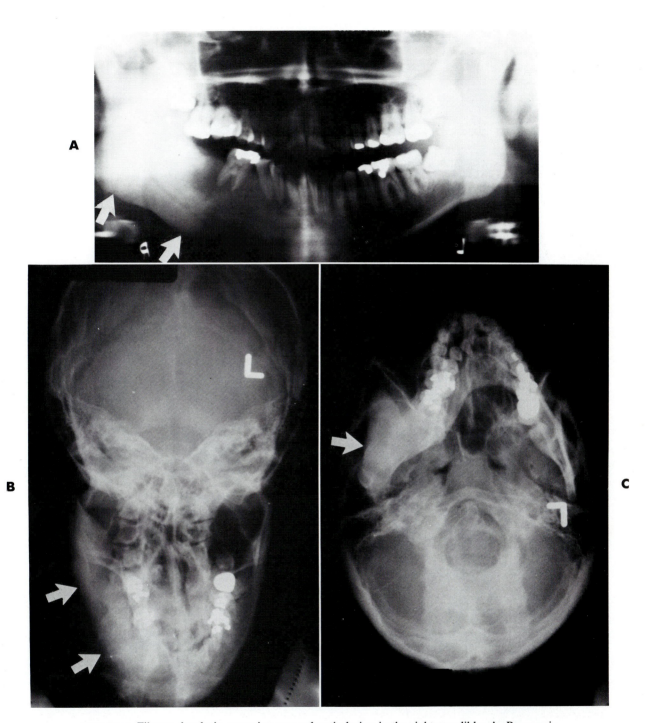

FIG. 23-4. Fibrous dysplasia occurring as a sclerotic lesion in the right mandible. **A,** Panoramic, **B,** Towne, and **C,** submentovertex projections demonstrate a dense thickening of the trabeculae and enlargement of the mandible *(arrows).*   *Continued.*

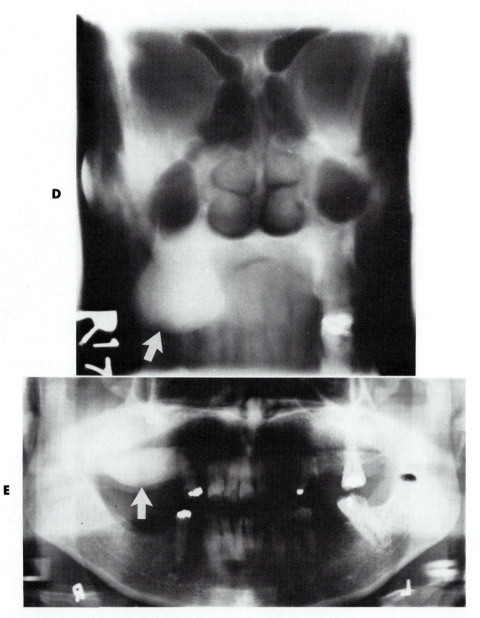

FIG. 23-4, cont'd. In another patient, **D** and **E,** a facial tomogram and a panoramic radiograph demonstrate the sclerotic lesion of fibrous dysplasia in the right maxilla *(arrow).*

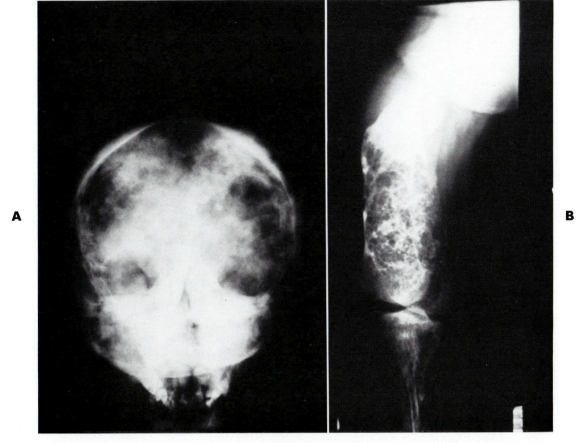

FIG. 23-5. Fibrous dysplasia. **A,** Pagetoid lesions in the skull. **B,** Gross enlargement of and multilocular growth in the tibia. (Courtesy Dr. L. Hollender, Seattle.)

touring has been used for cosmetic correction, usually delayed until after the cessation of· skeletal growth. Radiation therapy is contraindicated because of the possibility of inducing malignant transformation.[57]

Periapical cemental dysplasia

Periapical cemental dysplasia (PCD) (also known as cementoma, fibrocementoma, sclerosing cementoma, periapical osteofibrosis, or periapical fibro-osteoma) is believed to be a reactive fibro-osseous lesion derived from odontogenic cells in the periodontal ligament. It may be quite closely related to ossifying and calcifying fibromas.[67,68]

Clinical features. Periapical cemental dysplasia is one of the more commonly encountered non-inflammatory pathologic entities of the jaws. The lesions typically occur during middle age (the mean age is 39 years).[28] They are nine times more frequent in females than in males and are almost three times more common in blacks than in whites.[28] The condition has a predilection for the periapical bone of the mandibular anterior teeth, and there is a tendency for the lesions to be multiple.

The involved teeth are vital, and there is no history of pain or sensitivity in the associated teeth. Lesions are usually discovered as an incidental finding during a periapical or panoramic radiographic examination made for other purposes. PCD rarely enlarges within the jawbone to the extent of being clinically palpable.

Histologic features. Histologic changes correlate with the maturity of the lesion. Early in a lesion's course, an enlarging mass of fibrous tissue replaces periapical bone. The fibrous tissue usually retains continuity with the periodontal ligament tissue. Later, small round or ovoid calcifications form within the fibrous mass near the involved root surface. These depositions are composed of bone, cementum, or a nondescript "cementum-like bone."

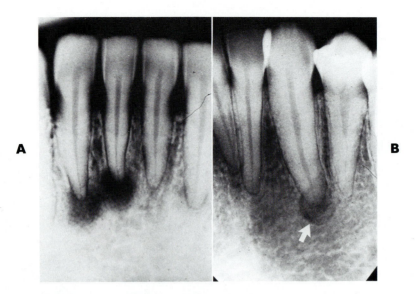

FIG. 23-6. Periapical cemental dysplasia: radiolucent stage. **A,** Loss of the lamina dura around the central incisor. **B,** Presence of part of the lamina dura *(arrow).*

The calcific foci tend to coalesce as they enlarge, although some foci remain separated permanently.

Radiographic features. The radiographic appearance of periapical cemental dysplasia demonstrates one of the following generally sequential stages:

Stage 1: Radiolucent (fibrous). The appearance of the periapical bone is identical to that seen in routine periapical rarefying osteitis (Fig. 23-6). (Vitality tests of involved teeth are mandatory during this stage.)

Stage 2: Mixed stage: Minute radiopacities develop within the radiolucent periapical lesions. As this stage progresses, the small radiopacities may coalesce (Fig. 23-7). The overall radiolucency usually does not enlarge further.

Stage 3: Radiopaque (calcified stage): Lesions that reach this stage have undergone substantial or complete opacification (Fig. 23-8). A radiolucent capsule (which may be very thin) always surrounds the opacity and separates it from the adjacent normal bone.

The radiographic margins of PCD vary from well defined to poorly defined, exactly as do the margins of periapical inflammatory disease secondary to pulpal necrosis. With PCD, however, the radiographic margins *tend* to be fairly distinctive. The lamina dura of adjacent teeth are, with few exceptions, discontinuous in the area of the lesion. An occasional lesion, however, may be separated a millimeter or so from the nearest periodontal ligament space by an intact, intervening lamina dura.

Differential diagnosis. Periapical cemental dysplasia is usually a fairly straightforward diagnosis made by its radiographic presentation and the presence of a vital tooth. The lesion's usual occurrence in middle-aged black women, its usual site of involvement in the mandibular incisor periapical bone, its tendency toward multiplicity, its course of development, and radiographic appearance are all characteristic. The most likely error in radiographic diagnosis, that of confusing early PCD with *periapical rarefying osteitis* secondary to a necrotic pulp, should not occur if the clinician tests the vitality of the tooth in question. Table 23-1 compares characteristics of four fibro-osseous lesions of periodontal ligament origin of the jaws.[15,40,41,69]

Less common problems in differential diagnosis can include confusion between mature (essentially radiopaque) PCD and *complex odontoma*. Around both lesions there is generally a fibrous radiolucent capsule and sclerotic bony rim. Both lesions radiographically present a calcified interior of rather nondescript form. The complex odontoma, however, usually occurs in third molar regions, develops in childhood and adolescence, and is typically more highly radiopaque (because it contains elements of enamel). Long-term serial radiographs would likely demonstrate maturation of the PCD lesion but a static appearance for the odontoma.

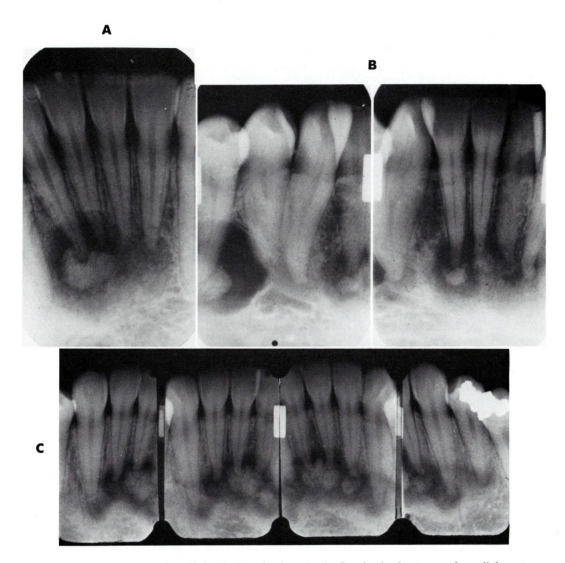

FIG. 23-7. Periapical cemental dysplasia: mixed stage. **A,** Opacity in the center of a radiolucent cavity. **B,** Multiple radiolucent regions containing radiopaque foci. **C,** Multiple radiopaque foci and a surrounding radiolucent zone.

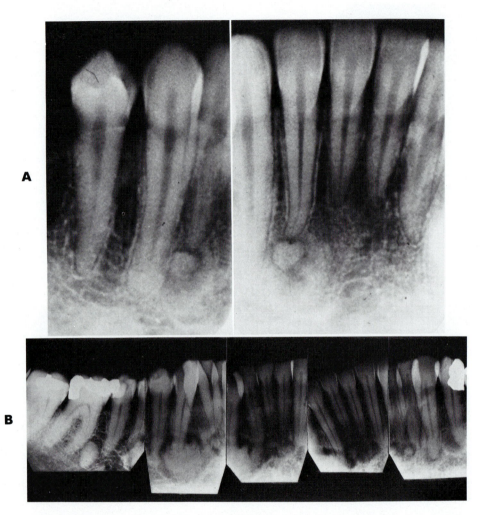

FIG. 23-8. Periapical cemental dysplasia: radiopaque stage. **A,** Opaque lesion with a thin radiolucent border. **B,** Multiple opacities with radiolucent capsules.

TABLE 23-1. Characteristics of four fibro-osseous lesions of periodontal ligament origin

Characteristic	Periapical cemental dysplasia	Cementifying and ossifying fibroma	Florid osseous dysplasia	Cementoblastoma
Growth pattern	Reactive	Benign neoplasm	Reactive	Benign neoplasm
Number of stages	Three	Three	Three	Three
Shape	Somewhat rounded	Somewhat rounded, maybe multilocular	Diffuse multiquadrant	Somewhat rounded (bulbous)
Number of lesions	Solitary or multiple	Solitary	Diffusely distributed throughout jaws	Solitary
Growth	Usually <1 cm diameter	Grow; if untreated may expand jaw	Hard buccal or labial expansion; usually no facial asymmetry	1-8 cm diameter; hard lingual-buccal expansion usual; occasional facial assymmetry; unlimited growth (0.5 cm/yr)
Root involvement	No root resorption or displacement	Root resorption or displacement uncommon	No root resorption or displacement	Related roots resorbed (50%); may be root displacement
Radiographic appearance	Well defined; third radiopaque stage has distinctive radiolucent halo	Well defined; third radiopaque stage has distinctive radiolucent halo	Less well defined; coalescing radiopaque masses obscure segments of radiolucent halo	Well defined; third radiopaque stage has distinctive radiolucent halo
Race	Mostly in blacks	Whites, 50%; Hispanics 25%	Mostly in blacks	No racial predilection
Sex	Mostly in females	If sexual predilection, slightly female	Mostly in females	If sexual predilection, slightly male
Onset	Seldom before fourth decade	Third or fourth decade	Fifth or sixth decade	Especially young; 10-72 years; most before 25 years
Jaw location	90% in mandible	70%-90% in mandible	Any quadrant, usually all four	Most in mandible (80%-85%)
Tooth vitality	Vital teeth	Vital teeth	Vital teeth	Vital teeth; usually fused with (and surrounding) root
Tooth location	Usually periapical incisors; usually distinct from roots	Periapical molar-premolar; may be superimposed with roots	Throughout jaws, only alveolar process affected	Molar–second premolar area (80%)
Symptoms	Asymptomatic	Asymptomatic when small	Approximately half have vague, intermittent dull pain, like toothache	May be associated with dull or vague pain
Composition	Probable cemental tissue	Probable cemental tissue	Probably cemental tissue	Bone or cementum
Complications	None	None	Low-grade osteomyelitis with sequestra; usually in patients with dentures	None

Finally, PCD differs from a *benign cemento-blastoma* as the latter physically connects to (indeed, is a *part* of) a tooth root surface. The cemento-blastoma appears radiographically much like a round, enlarging root mass. The benign cemento-blastoma often enlarges to the extent that it produces palpable swelling of the cortical surfaces. PCD, by contrast, is virtually always distinct from an associated root surface and does not cause bulging of the bone surfaces. The benign cemento-blastoma most frequently develops around the roots of mandibular premolars and molars.

Management. Biopsies are not needed except in highly unusual cases. Treatment is not required because the condition is harmless and self-limiting.

Ossifying fibroma, cementifying fibroma, and cemento-ossifying fibroma

Ossifying fibroma, cementifying fibroma, and cemento-ossifying fibroma are characteristically *encapsulated* lesions consisting of highly cellular fibrous tissue in which bone formation occurs. These lesions may show locally aggressive behavior. There is no clear-cut distinction between ossifying fibroma, cementifying fibroma, and cemento-ossifying fibroma. Rather, view these fibro-osseous lesions as part of a spectrum of related conditions arising from periodontal ligament tissue.[67] The clinical behavior of the group is variable. Even with identical histopathologic appearances, such lesions can be either very benign or locally aggressive. Management of this condition depends on clinical findings and radiologic evidence of bone-destroying activity.

Clinical features. The ossifying fibroma is an unusual lesion. It can occur at any age but is usually found in young adults. Females are more frequently affected than males. The disease is usually asymptomatic at the time of discovery except for occasional facial asymmetry. Displacement of the teeth may be an early clinical feature. Because the lesion is usually slow growing, the bony cortices and covering mucosa remain intact. In rare cases rapid growth may occur, especially in young children. Most such conditions are discovered during routine dental examination. Deformity of the involved jaw may be the only symptom. Persons other than the patient may be the first to notice the facial deformity because of its usual slow, innocuous growth. These lesions continue to enlarge after cessation of normal skeletal growth, unlike monostotic fibrous dysplasia.[29]

The ossifying fibroma appears mostly in the facial bones, usually the mandible.[53] In the maxilla, it occurs most often in the canine fossa and zygomatic arch area. When ossifying fibroma involves the maxillary sinus, it may completely fill the sinus cavity and expand the sinus walls. In the mandible, ossifying fibroma frequently develops inferior to the premolars and molars.

Histologic features. The histologic appearance of ossifying fibroma is similar to that of fibrous dysplasia. A large number of fibroblasts with flat, elongated nuclei are present within a network of interlacing collagen fibers. A common feature is the presence of "Chinese character" n-shaped islands of bone or calcification distributed throughout the connective tissue, somewhat similar to the trabeculae in fibrous dysplasia. Although the histologic appearance may be indistinguishable from fibrous dysplasia, the lesion itself is encapsulated and behaves as a neoplasm.

Microscopically, the ossifying fibroma and cementifying fibroma are very similar. However, the cementifying fibroma has a greater tendency to form more cementum-like material that is more ovoid and more heavily calcified than that produced by the ossifying fibroma. In the ossifying fibroma, the calcified material is more spiculated and reminiscent of woven bone, with that at the periphery being more lamellar in appearance.

Radiographic features. The radiographic density of the ossifying fibroma is dependent on its stage of development. Bone destruction that occurs early in lesion formation causes a unilocular radiolucent defect within the bone (Fig. 23-9). Subsequent calcification that takes place within the lesion results in the appearance of radiopaque foci (Fig. 23-10). The radiopaque calcified areas tend to coalesce, and the lesion may become very radiopaque after several years (Fig. 23-11). The radiographic appearance may be radiolucent, radiopaque, or a mixture. Growth tends to be concentric within the medullary part of the bone, with outward expansion approximately equal in all directions. This expansion may result in osseous deformity. In such cases, the margins become thinned but remain intact.[53]

The borders of the ossifying fibroma are usually well defined. A thin radiolucent line representing a fibrous capsule separates the mixed-density lesion from surrounding bone. Sometimes the bone next to the lesion may develop a hyperostotic border. A thin shell of bone usually forms along the lesion's

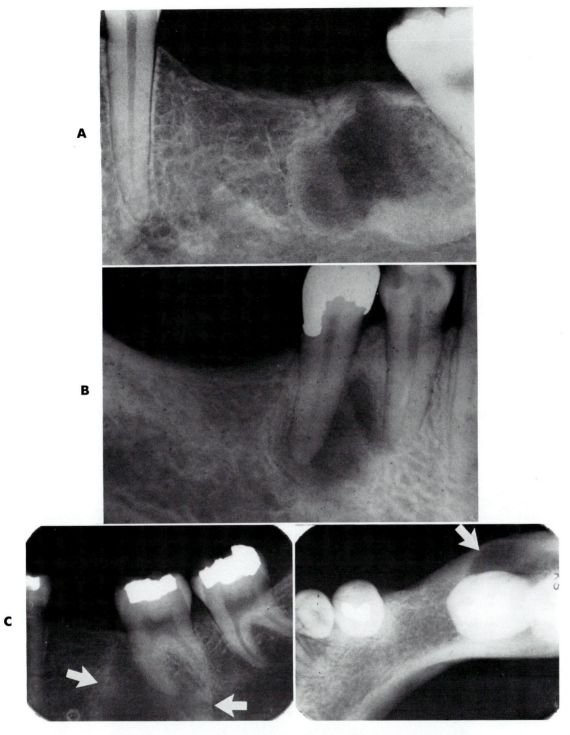

FIG. 23-9. Ossifying fibromas: radiolucent stage. **A,** Edentulous region with radiopaque margins of a radiolucent lesion. **B,** Premolar region with a radiolucent defect. **C,** Molar region showing an area of lysis *(arrows)*. Note the buccal expansion in the occlusal view *(arrow)*. (**A** and **C** courtesy Dr. R. Howell, Chapel Hill, NC; **B** courtesy Dr. L. Szerlip, Morristown, NJ.)

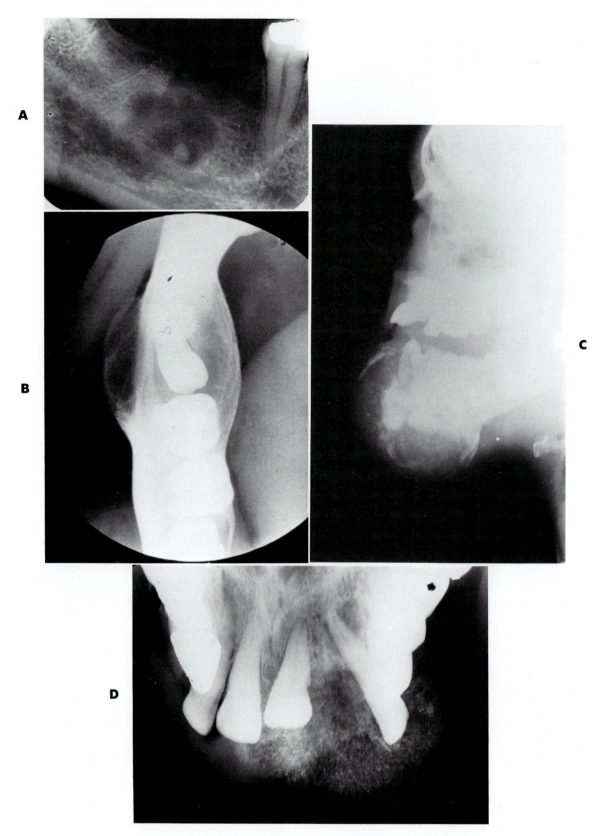

FIG. 23-10. Ossifying fibromas. **A,** Small area of radiopaque foci in a radiolucent lesion. **B,** Expansile lesion with internal trabeculation. **C,** Expansile lesion with multiple foci of calcification. **D,** Expansile lesion of the maxilla with an extensive trabecular pattern. (**B** courtesy Dr. L. Hollender, Seattle; **D** courtesy Dr. L. Szerlip, Morristown, NJ.)

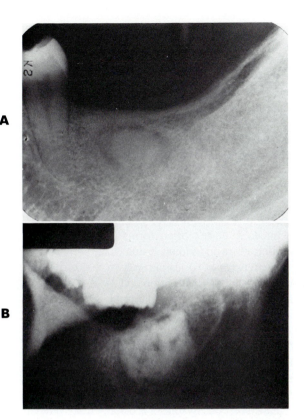

A

B

FIG. 23-11. Ossifying fibromas. **A,** Dense lesion with a peripheral radiolucent rim. **B,** Cementifying fibroma, demonstrating a dense central portion with a radiolucent capsule.

border just inside the radiolucent capsule. As the ossifying fibroma grows, it displaces or destroys nearby structures. Teeth are displaced away from the lesion, and root resorption may range from mild to severe. The teeth remain vital.

Differential diagnosis. The differential diagnosis of ossifying fibroma necessarily includes both radiolucent lesions and those with a mixed radiolucent-radiopaque appearance. The differential diagnosis of radiolucent lesions is discussed in the section on ameloblastoma in Chapter 21. The differential diagnosis of the more *common lesions* of mixed radiolucency and radiopacity includes ossifying fibroma, cementoma, myxoma, and calcifying cysts. The more *rarely occurring lesions* with mixed radiodensity are the adenomatoid odontogenic tumor, the calcifying epithelial odontogenic tumor (Pindborg), osteoblastoma, osteoid osteoma, and osteogenic sarcoma. Paget's disease and condensing osteitis can usually be eliminated from the differential diagnosis because they lack a surrounding radiolucent capsule.

Entities with mixed radiolucent and radiopaque appearance consist of a noncalcified soft tissue component associated with and sometimes interspersed with a calcified portion. Mature PCD lesions that have not completely calcified are mixed radiolucent and radiopaque and may be confused with ossifying fibroma. Lesion peripheries are often well defined and may be surrounded by a radiolucent line. PCD, however, is diagnosed by its anterior location and its association with vital teeth. Similar lesions within the bone not associated with teeth are identified only by microscopic examination.

The *adenomatoid odontogenic tumor* is a rare lesion that usually develops in association with an impacted maxillary canine in a young patient. The tumor borders are regular. A mixed density lesion in these circumstances suggests the presence of this lesion. The rare *calcifying epithelial odontogenic tumor* is most commonly a tumor with mixed radiodensity occurring in the posterior body and ramus of the mandible. The *osteoblastoma* and the *osteoid osteoma* contain bone material and present a mixed radiographic appearance. Both form in the inferior aspect of the mandible, the osteoblastoma being the larger and more aggressive tumor.

Osteogenic sarcoma may present an appearance of radiopacity and radiolucency resulting from both the destruction and formation of bone that is characteristic of this tumor. Ill-defined lesion borders and periosteal bone formation with bony spicules aligned at right angles to the host bone are tumor characteristics. *Paget's disease* in the jaw is characterized by enlargement of the affected bone, radiolucent involvement during early stages, and mixed radiopaque and radiolucent areas formed as the disease advances, commonly referred to as the "cotton-wool" appearance.

The differentiation of ossifying fibroma from *fibrous dysplasia* is important. Complete removal of ossifying fibroma is indicated, whereas the management of fibrous dysplasia usually consists of surgery only in extreme cases. Clinically, both lesions are hard and firm. The radiographic appearance of fibrous dysplasia reveals a homogeneous radiopaque area with an internal architecture that is evenly granular and obliterates normal marrow spaces. The internal structure of ossifying fibroma is either radiolucent or mixed radiolucent and radiopaque. The appearance of the borders of the lesions is also a differentiating radiographic feature. In fibrous dysplasia, the borders are ill defined and gradually blend into the surrounding normal bone over a distance of about a centimeter. In the ossifying fibroma, however, the peripheries are usually well defined and regular. Root resorption is a characteristic of ossifying fibroma that is not typical of fibrous dysplasia. The early ossifying fibroma can resemble a cyst, small ameloblastoma, or myxoma.

Management. The prognosis of ossifying fibroma is favorable, with surgical enucleation of the encapsulated mass the treatment of choice. Even if it has reached appreciable size, the ossifying fibroma can usually be separated from the surrounding tissue and completely removed. Recurrence following removal is unlikely.

Florid osseous dysplasia

Florid osseous dysplasia (FOD) is the most common cause of generalized radiopacities in the jaws.[14] It is also known as gigantiform cementoma and florid cemento-osseous dysplasia. FOD appears to be a widespread form of PCD.[41] There are several key similarities between FOD and PCD, including age, sex, racial profiles of patients, and comparable radiographic and histologic appearances. Most likely FOD, like PCD, is a reactive type of fibro-osseous bone disease derived from cells in or near the periodontal ligament spaces.

Clinical features. Most patients with FOD are female and middle-aged (the mean being 42 years), although the age range is broad.[41,63] There is a marked predilection for blacks. Usually FOD develops in both jaws simultaneously. If only one jaw is affected, it is more often the mandible. The typical patient's sex, age, race, and site of involvement clearly suggest that this disease and PCD are related, possibly even varying manifestations of the same essential bone disease.

FOD is often discovered incidentally during a radiographic examination of the teeth. Occasionally, patients complain of intermittent, poorly localized pain in the affected bone area with or without associated bony swelling. Clinical features of osteomyelitis, including mucosal ulceration of fistulous tracts with suppuration, may be present. Teeth in the involved bone area are vital unless they are coincidentally affected by other dental disease.

Histologic features. Histologically, FOD displays homogeneous, dense, calcified masses scattered throughout a fibrous matrix. Within an individual calcified mass, bone may be the sole or principal component, with cementum seen in many lesions. Such calcified masses are poorly vascularized, making them susceptible to infections that may be particularly difficult to control. Some of the masses fuse to cementum of adjacent teeth.[22]

Radiographic features. FOD is apparent as a radiolucent area partially filled with one or more dense, radiopaque masses (Fig. 23-12). These radiopaque masses typically have a lobular or lumpy shape and a fluffy, soft, radiopaque character sometimes similar to the "cotton-wool" radiopacity seen in Paget's disease. The masses are qualitatively similar to the radiopacities seen in mature PCD. The margins of the encompassing radiolucent spaces in FOD tend to be fairly regular and well defined. A cortex often forms around at least a portion of an individual lesion. The more mature and extensive FOD lesions consist less of the surrounding radiolucent region and more of the internal radiopaque mass. Similar to PCD, this increasingly radiopaque appearance signifies the final stage in which bone or cementum deposition within the fibrous mass is either considerable or complete. However, in most cases the overall radiographic appearance is that of an amorphous, mixed, radiolucent-radiopaque lesion.

Florid osseous dysplasia is usually discovered as a multiplicity of lesions in one or both jaws, frequently in all four jaw quadrants. Individual lesions typically do not exceed 3 cm in diameter by the time active growth diminishes and the size becomes static. These lesions often coalesce as they enlarge. They principally develop in the alveolar processes of the jaws. In the mandible, the lesions lie superior to the mandibular canal in most cases,[39] although some lesions may extend deep into the mandibular ramus or the maxillary sinuses.

A significant number of FOD lesions also develop concurrent simple bone cysts.[38] Such combined lesions have prominent areas of radiolucency within the overall limits of the lesion (Fig. 23-13). The presence of a simple bone cyst within FOD is suggested if repeat radiographs reveal that a radiolucent cavity is enlarging over a period of months. There may be hypercementosis of tooth roots in affected areas of bone, as well as fusion of some radiopaque masses to tooth roots.

Differential diagnosis. FOD often has a distinctive radiographic appearance, especially if a panoramic view supplements periapical projections. The panoramic projection is particularly helpful in providing an overall estimation of lesion sites in the four jaw quadrants and in visualizing some of the larger lesions in their entirety. There are few pathologic entities that would likely pro-

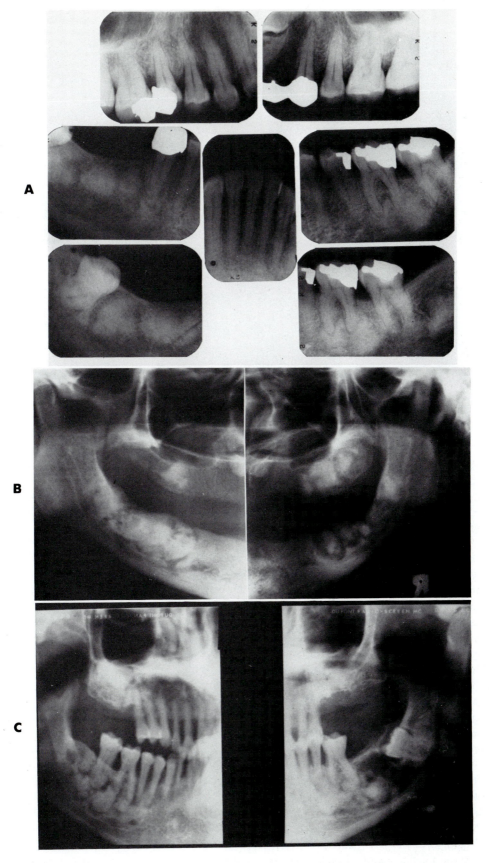

FIG. 23-12. Florid osseous dysplasia. **A,** Multiple radiopaque lesions in periapical regions throughout the jaws. **B,** Radiopaque lesions in all quadrants showing radiolucent borders. **C,** Radiopaque lesions in all quadrants. (Courtesy Dr. H. Abrams, Los Angeles.)

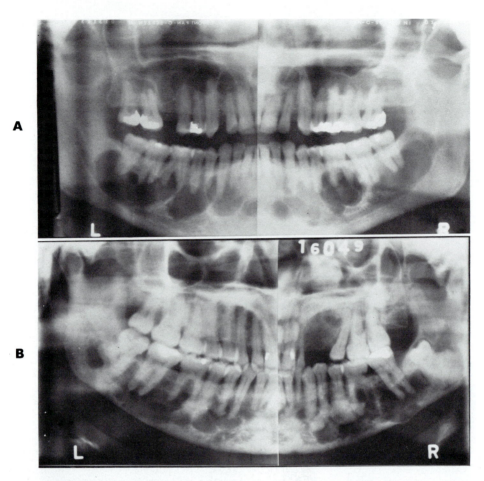

FIG. 23-13. Florid osseous dysplasia associated with traumatic bone cysts. **A,** Mostly cystic lesions with only sparse opacifications. **B,** Large cystic areas associated with multiple radiopaque foci. (Courtesy Dr. H. Abrams, Los Angeles.)

duce the typical radiographic appearances of FOD, that is, multiple radiopaque masses scattered throughout most or all the jaw quadrants, each lesion surrounded by a radiolucent capsule and a cortical rim. Because the condition mostly occurs in middle-aged women, typically black, the overall combination becomes almost pathognomonic. Nevertheless, the clinician should attempt to exclude Paget's disease and osteopetrosis from the differential diagnosis in those unusual cases in which the sclerotic masses are exceptionally florid and dense. *Paget's disease* demonstrates no radiolucent capsule around the radiopaque portions of the lesion. In addition, Paget's disease usually develops as a polyostotic disease. For example, when it occurs in either jaw, it is almost always present in the skull. Also, FOD develops only in the jaws. Skeletal radiographs and a serum test for alkaline phosphatase level should identify Paget's disease

in cases of difficult differentiation. *Osteopetrosis,* by contrast, is a generalized bone disease usually identified on lateral skull radiographs by a profuse thickening of the skull base or calvarium. In addition, osteopetrosis produces *diffuse* bony radiopacities, not ones that simulate masses. Finally, osteopetrosis and Paget's disease both cause enlargement of involved bone areas, a feature not often observed in FOD.

Management. If the FOD lesions are asymptomatic, they do not require treatment. However, if teeth are present, it is important for the patient to initiate and maintain an effective oral hygiene program because removal of teeth from patients with FOD often results in poor healing. These sclerotic jaws are relatively susceptible to osteomyelitis.[63] Jaws expanded by FOD lesions may require bone recontouring before denture construction.

Cherubism

Cherubism is a rare, inherited fibro-osseous bone disease that affects only the jaws. The term "cherubism" reflects the characteristic chubby, cherubic facial appearance of affected children. The bilateral enlargement of the mandible in this condition does produce a full, round lower face similar to that of cherubs portrayed in Renaissance religious paintings.

Clinical features. Cherubism develops in early childhood between the ages of 2 and 6 years. The most common presenting sign is a painless bilateral enlargement of the lower face. The enlarged posterior region of the lower jawbone is firm and hard to palpation. The overlying mucosa is intact and nonpainful. There may be enlargement of the submandibular lymph nodes, but there are no systemic abnormalities. Inasmuch as most young children have somewhat naturally chubby faces, parents may not appreciate the abnormality until there is an obvious progression of the mandibular swellings. In many cases, bilateral enlargement of the maxilla gradually follows. Severe swellings of this kind in the maxilla, when present, contribute to the cherubic analogy by causing a pulling or stretching of the skin of the cheeks. This in turn depresses the lower eyelids, exposing a thin line of sclera and causing an "eyes raised to heaven" look. Occasional unilateral lesions have been reported.[47]

Radiographic features. The radiographic picture of cherubism presents multiple cystlike radiolucencies of the mandible, less often of the maxilla (Fig. 23-14). In both jaws, the size and growth patterns of the lesions are fairly symmetrical bilaterally. Also typical is the initiation of bone destruction near the angles of the mandible, with later expansion of the lesions posteriorly into the rami and anteriorly into the mandibular body. Occasionally, there may be extension of the lesion into the condylar head.[3] If the maxilla does become involved, it typically lags behind the mandible in its degree of involvement.

Radiographically, the lesions of cherubism are multilocular cavities that tend to coalesce as they enlarge. The lesions are typically well defined with cortices around all or most of the radiolucencies. Expansion of the buccal and lingual cortical plates, obvious on clinical examination, is convincingly demonstrated radiographically on both occlusal and frontal (PA) mandibular projections. Cortical perforation is uncommon. Maxillary lesions enlarge into the maxillary sinuses.

The destructive central jaw lesions profoundly affect the developing permanent dentition. It is common to see marked displacement of numerous tooth buds and dental follicles. Cystlike lesions may even destroy outright one or more developing tooth buds before enamel calcification. The most commonly affected teeth are the mandibular second and third molars. Erupted deciduous teeth in the areas of the bone involvement often exfoliate prematurely.

Differential diagnosis. The typical patient with cherubism is a child or a young adolescent with bilateral posterior mandibular bulges, often with displaced or missing permanent teeth, and with few or no symptoms associated with the jaw swellings. The patient's parents usually confirm that the time of disease discovery was within the characteristic age span of 2 to 6 years and occasionally that another family member has the condition. Thus, even before the first radiographs are seen, cherubism may be a prohibitive favorite in the differential diagnosis.

Fibrous dysplasia can be substantially excluded from the differential diagnosis by the bilaterality of the cystic bone defects. Other solitary lesions such as *giant cell granuloma* and *aneurysmal bone cyst* can often be dismissed for the same reason. The only multifocal bone disease that could reasonably be expected to present well-defined jaw radiolucencies and thus cause differential difficulty is *nevoid basal cell carcinoma syndrome*. This syndrome often occurs with multiple keratocysts within the posterior portions of the jaws. It does not, however, produce the facial swelling characteristic of cherubism. Individual keratocysts are likely to be unilocular and asymmetrical in size. Further, patients with this syndrome often have the characteristic cutaneous abnormality (nevoid basal cell carcinomas) or bifid rib anomalies seen on a chest radiograph. Apart from this syndrome, it is doubtful that multiple *dentigerous cysts,* which may have a familial basis for transmission, would be confused with a disease as unusual as cherubism.

Management. Suspected cherubic lesions should be biopsied. The managing clinician should be aware, however, that the distinctive *radiographic* features are often more diagnostic than the histopathologic findings. The consensus regarding treatment of cherubic lesions is to delay surgical procedures because the cystlike defects usually become static and may regress during adolescence and adulthood.[35] Conservative surgical methods,

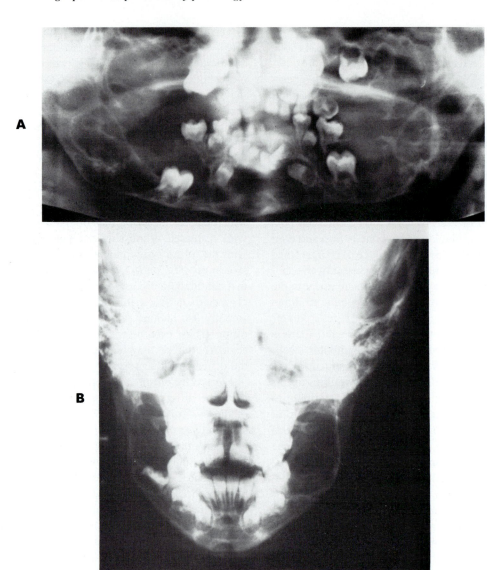

FIG. 23-14. Cherubism. **A,** Multilocular lesion in all quadrants causing displacement of the teeth. **B,** A PA radiograph shows lytic expansile lesions in the mandible. (**A** courtesy Dr. B. Gratt, Los Angeles.)

however, may be employed to improve serious cosmetic problems in the early phase of the disease. Although early surgical recontouring carries the risk of recurrence,[17] this possibility is less likely after age 20.

REACTIVE LESIONS
Central giant cell granuloma

The central giant cell granuloma is fairly common in the jaws. It is a nonneoplastic bone disease, probably reactive to some unknown stimulus. It consists primarily of fibroblasts, numerous vascular channels, multinucleated giant cells, and macrophages. Whether it has a definite relationship with the *benign giant cell tumor* of the general skeleton remains unproved and the topic of fairly long-standing controversy.

Clinical features. The central giant cell granuloma of the jaws is a lesion of adolescents and young adults. At least 60% of cases occur in persons younger than age 20 years, and 74% occur in persons 30 years of age or younger.[68] Lesions develop in the mandible twice as frequently as in the maxilla, with the anterior half of the mandible showing the greatest incidence of involvement. Most mandibular lesions occur anterior to the first molars (i.e., the regions formerly occupied by the deciduous teeth), with a fairly high percentage (21%) crossing the symphysis.[68]

The most common presenting sign of central giant cell granuloma is painless swelling.[30] Typically this swelling is first detected by the patient or the patient's parents, who notice an asymmetry in facial appearance. Palpation of the suspect bone area may elicit tenderness. Alternatively, the abnormality may be disclosed as a purely incidental finding during an oral radiographic examination made for an unrelated purpose. The growth of this lesion is usually slow, although it may sometimes be rapid and create the suspicion of a malignancy. Developing lesions are usually painless and without paresthesia. In only about 25% of the cases is the lesion accompanied by pain. Teeth in the area of the lesion may become mobile but maintain their vitality.

Radiographic features. The radiographic picture of central giant cell granuloma is quite variable. Incipient lesions may be no larger than a centimeter in diameter and simulate a small odontogenic cyst (Fig. 23-15). Such unilocular lesions usually show no evidence of internal structure or trabeculation. As giant cell granuloma grows, however, it often assumes a multilocular appearance (Fig. 23-16). Most multilocular giant cell granulomas show bony trabeculae within the lesion. These internal septa, which may give the lesion a multilocular appearance, tend to be mildly wavy on close inspection. The septa have a wispy, delicate quality.[71] Such multilocular lesions often result in an uneven, variable bulging or undulation of the cortical contour (Fig. 23-17). Large giant cell granulomas may occupy the whole of one mandibular body and extend past the midline to the opposite side. When giant cell granulomas involve the maxillary sinus, they may erode or expand bone, and have the appearance of a tumor or mucocele.[48] CT evaluation of lesions in the maxilla assists in demonstrating extension of the lesion into adjacent structures. For large lesions, CT examination also helps to evaluate soft tissue extension.[7]

Because this lesion grows relatively slowly, it usually produces a fairly clear radiographic margin. However, although most lesions have margins that are well defined but not corticated, the margins of some are corticated, and the margins of others are poorly defined.[7,30]

Central giant cell granulomas generate sufficient pressure as they enlarge within the medullary bone to resorb the lamina dura of adjacent teeth. They

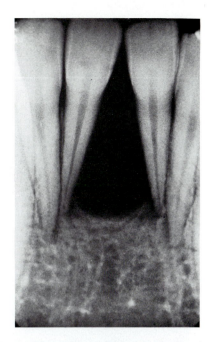

FIG. 23-15. Giant cell granuloma in the anterior mandible without evidence of internal trabeculation. (Courtesy Dr. E.J. Burkes, Chapel Hill, NC.)

may also displace tooth follicles and tooth roots, commonly resulting in divergence of roots next to the lesion.[7] These lesions may also resorb neighboring tooth roots. They have nearly the same propensity to resorb tooth roots as do ameloblastomas.

Differential diagnosis. Because giant cell granulomas occur as solitary, noncalcifying, soft tissue masses within the spongy portion of the jaws, like several other entities, there is occasional difficulty with the differential diagnosis. The physical mechanism by which giant cell granuloma produces a central mandibular bone defect (i.e., by pressure resorption of surrounding trabeculae) is apparently identical to the growth mechanism of *ameloblastoma, odontogenic myxoma, aneurysmal bone cyst,* and *ossifying fibroma.* All produce relatively well-defined unilocular or multilocular radiolucencies within the jaws.

In practice, however, the most difficult differentiation is between giant cell granuloma and *ameloblastoma.* There are several useful guidelines for the diagnostician. First, ameloblastoma is uncommon in the younger age range most susceptible to giant cell granuloma. Second, ameloblastoma more often develops in the posterior mandible, whereas giant cell granuloma tends to occur near or anterior to the first molar area. Third, ameloblastoma radiographically demonstrates an internal structure of

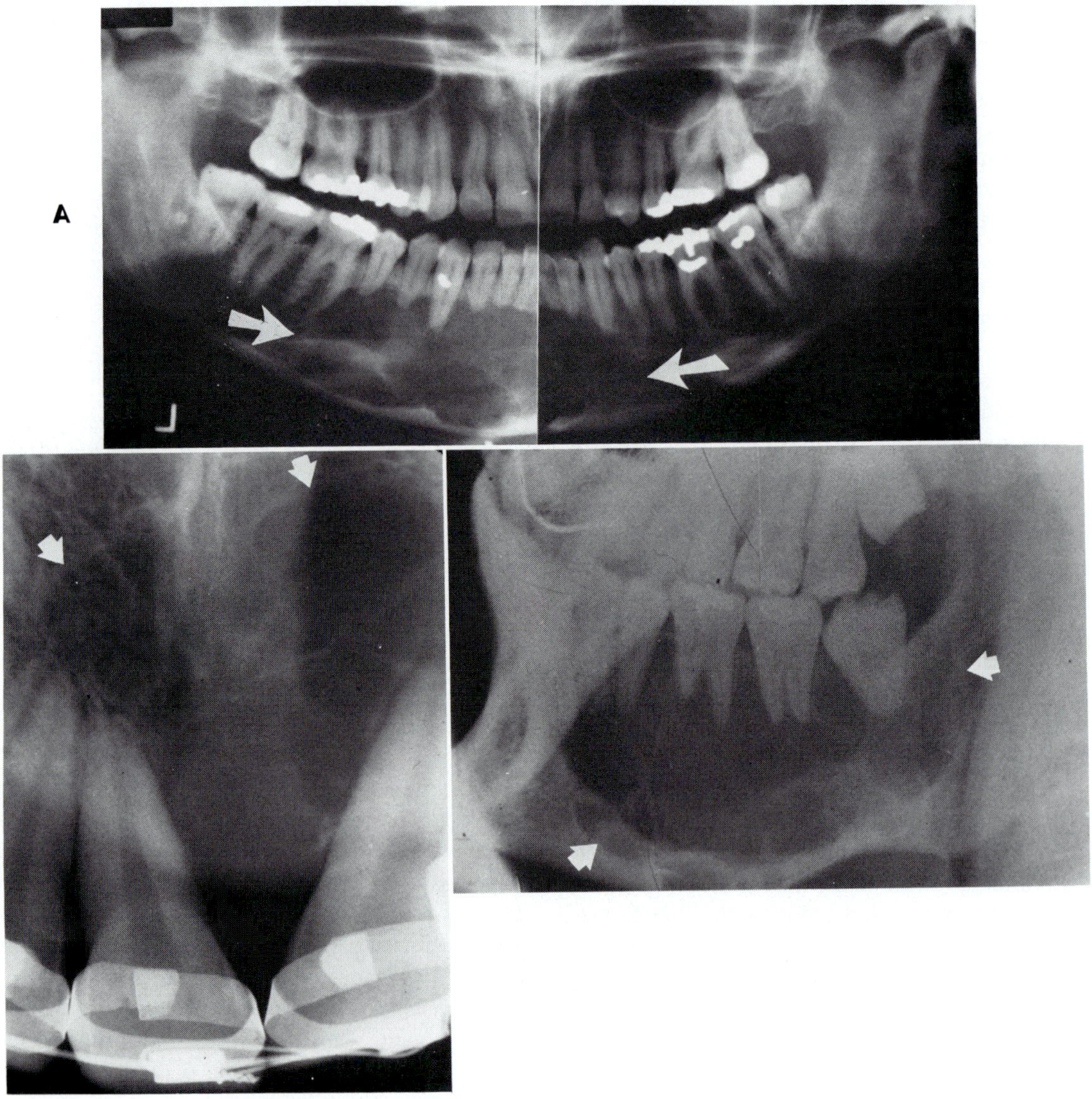

FIG. 23-16. Giant cell granulomas. **A,** Large multilocular lesion in anterior mandible. **B,** Multilocular lesion in the maxilla. **C,** Multilocular pattern in the body of the mandible. (**A** courtesy Dr. W. Via, Chapel Hill, NC; **C** courtesy Dr. R. White, Chapel Hill, NC.)

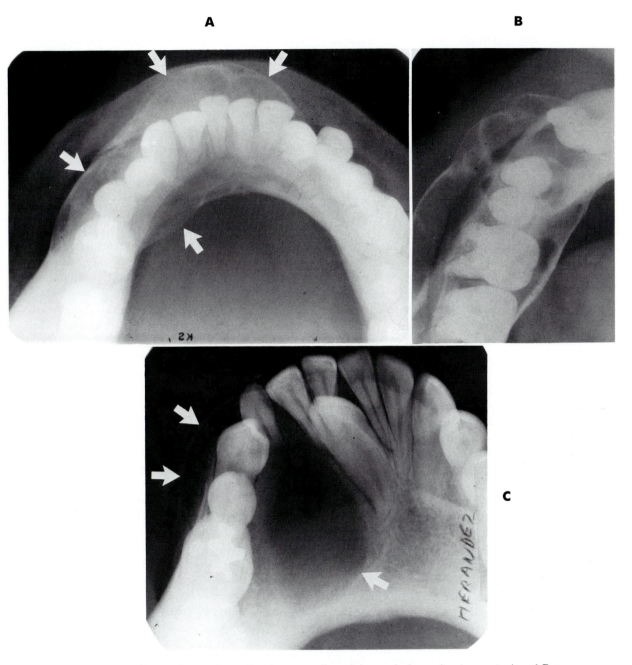

FIG. 23-17. Giant cell granuloma showing expansion of the cortical margins *(arrows)*. **A** and **B**, Note the uneven expansion of the cortical plates and the presence of septa in the lesions. **C,** The canine has been displaced across the midline.

relatively thick, curved, archlike septa, whereas giant cell granuloma has lighter, wispy septa. Finally, ameloblastoma is more often multiloculated than the giant cell granuloma, which is prone to simple unilocularity. Note, however, that these radiographic distinctions are virtually impossible to make if the radiolucent lesion in question is small or incipient.

Aneurysmal bone cyst may appear radiographically identical to giant cell granuloma but does not have a particular tendency to occur in the anterior mandible. Aspiration of lesion contents can often separate these two possibilities. Also, the aneurysmal bone cyst is a rare lesion in comparison with the incidence of giant cell granuloma. A unilocular odontogenic myxoma may simulate a giant cell granuloma. Myxoma, however, is more commonly multiloculated and typically has a honeycomb pattern of intersecting septa. In addition, the clinician usually notes either a missing or an impacted tooth associated with the myxoma, a finding not likely seen with the giant cell granuloma. *Simple bone cyst* can usually be excluded if radiographs demonstrate a splaying apart or bodily movement of adjacent tooth roots or significant expansion of overlying bone cortices. Further, radiographic evidence of a significant number of septa within the lesion largely excludes simple bone cysts.

Last, it is usually radiographically possible to distinguish a fluid-filled *odontogenic cyst* from a soft-tissue, tumor-like lesion such as giant cell granuloma or ameloblastoma. There are two pertinent rules both described by Worth[71]: First, if there is even a *hint* of internal septa within a lesion, one can, with a single exception, rule out cyst. The slightest spicule of bone protruding from a lesion's radiographic margin into its lumen is strong evidence against the presence of a cyst. (The only exception is very large cystic jaw lesions, those occupying a major part of a mandibular body or ramus. In this rare situation, even dentigerous cysts may display partially loculating internal septa.) Second, the type of expansion of bony cortical plates resulting from fluid-filled cysts differs from that caused by growing soft tissue masses. An occlusal radiograph of an odontogenic cyst—which enlarges at a slow, deliberate rate by hydraulic expansion—demonstrates a regular, smooth bony expansion of the cortical plates. The enlarging giant cell granuloma or ameloblastoma, by contrast, produces a scalloped, undulating bulging of the cortices as a result of variable tissue growth rates.

The radiographic image of *brown tumors of hy-*

perparathyroidism is identical to that of central giant cell granuloma. An accurate diagnosis is complicated by the fact that both lesions have similar histopathologic presentations. It is therefore necessary to assay the serum for elevated calcium levels in patients with suspected central giant cell granuloma in order to rule out hyperparathyroidism.

Management. Treatment of the central giant cell granuloma is by enucleation or curettage. Some surgeons treat lesions larger than 2 cm in diameter by partial resection of the jaw. Recurrence is uncommon, particularly for the smaller lesions.

Aneurysmal bone cyst

Aneurysmal bone cyst (ABC) is most likely a reactive lesion of bone, an osseous dysplasia.[12] The name of this entity is misleading in that it does not contain vascular aneurysms and it is not a true bony cyst. Its etiology is unclear. One opinion is that it represents an exaggerated, localized, proliferative response of vascular tissue in bone. It may be related to central and peripheral giant cell granuloma, which it resembles in some ways, including the histologic presence of giant cells. This lesion occasionally develops in association with other primary lesions. Others argue that it is a secondary lesion developing from primary lesions in bone, most frequently central giant cell granuloma or fibrous dysplasia.[13,62] The lesion is not neoplastic in that it does not have an independent, uncoordinated growth capable of unlimited proliferation.

Clinical features. Although aneurysmal bone cyst may develop in adults, it is mainly an abnormality of older children and adolescents. More than 90% of reported jaw lesions have been in individuals younger than age 30 years.[61,64] There appears to be a predilection for females in the cases reported for all bones and for those involving the jaws.[24] The mandible is somewhat more commonly involved than the maxilla (3:2), and the molar region far more commonly involved than the anterior region.[25] Aneurysmal bone cyst is primarily an abnormality of the long tubular bones (where about 50% of all reported cases occur) and the vertebral bodies (about 20%).[8,64] It is rare in the jaws.[13]

The jaw aneurysmal bone cyst usually presents as a fairly rapid bony swelling (usually buccal or labial). Pain is an occasional complaint, and the involved area may be tender to palpation. The patient does not experience inferior alveolar nerve or mental nerve paresthesia. In lesions that clinically and radiographically resemble aneurysmal bone cysts, needle aspiration should be performed before biopsy. Bruits are not typically ausculated, in contrast to the bony hemangioma.

Radiographic features. The aneurysmal bone cyst is an expansile, osteolytic process within an affected bone and is radiolucent (Fig. 23-18). There are three stages of development: an initial stage characterized by an ill-defined lytic area, a growth phase showing an enlarged area of bone destruction with early signs of peripheral cortication, and finally a mature stage showing bony expansion, cortication, and faint septa coursing through the lesion in a random pattern (Fig. 23-19).[4] These are not true septa but rather ridges of bone protruding from the inner cortex of the lesion wall. There are also free bands of bone within the lesion. This lesion occurs more often as a unilocular radiolucency. The term "soap bubbles" may aptly describe an occasional multi-loculated radiographic appearances. Many of these lesions at the time of detection have a faint bony cortex, although usually not around the entire defect. Aneurysmal bone cyst, like central giant cell granuloma, demonstrates margins somewhat less regular and distinct than those of an odontogenic cyst but more discrete than those of a central malignancy. As the aneurysmal bone cyst enlarges to more than a few centimeters in anteroposterior dimension, it also produces expansion of the buccal and lingual cortical plates. Its appearance is not diagnostic.

When these lesions occur in dentulous portions of the jaws, they generally cause simple tilting or bodily displacement of an erupted tooth or an unerupted developing tooth. Aneurysmal bone cyst may also produce some degree of external root resorption, although it does not devitalize an affected tooth.

Differential diagnosis. Preoperative diagnosis of aneurysmal bone cyst is difficult because of their rarity and similar appearance to other lesions.[65] Because aneurysmal bone cysts predominantly occur in patients younger than 20 years of age, *ameloblastomas* as a group may be largely excluded. *Giant cell granulomas,* however, often develop in a similar young age group. Needle aspiration of all moderately large, non-tooth-associated radiolucencies in the jaws is, therefore, recommended. A hemorrhagic aspirate favors the diagnosis of aneurysmal bone cyst. If an audible bruit over the involved bone area is heard, or if there is bleeding from around necks of neighboring teeth, a *central hemangioma* is more likely present, especially if the hemorrhagic aspirate is profuse.

Management. Surgical curettage and partial resection are the primary forms of treatment for aneurysmal bone cysts. The recurrence rate is fairly high, ranging from 19% to about 50% after curettage,[25,61] and 11% following resection.[24] This indicates the need for careful follow-up. Massive hemorrhage is sometimes a complication of surgery.

OTHER LESIONS OF BONE
Simple bone cyst

Simple bone cyst (also called *traumatic bone cyst, hemorrhagic bone cyst, extravasation cyst, progressive bone cavity, solitary bone cyst,* or *unicameral cyst*) is not a true cyst. It lacks an epithelial lining, and surgical exploration often reveals it to be empty (i.e., devoid of fluid). The "cyst" part of the name derives from its radiographic appearance,

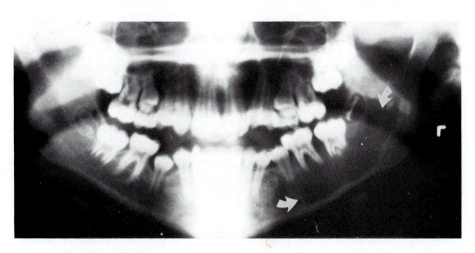

FIG. 23-18. Aneurysmal bone cyst in the body of the mandible of a child.

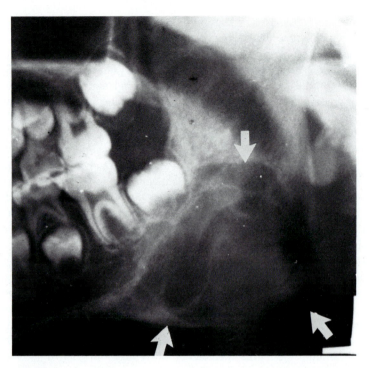

FIG. 23-19. Aneurysmal bone cyst in the angle of the mandible, demonstrating internal septa. (Courtesy Dr. H. Abrams, Los Angeles.)

which is similar to the appearance of a true cyst. The cause of the lesion is unknown. Although some have speculated that it develops in response to trauma, the rate of trauma in patients with this lesion is equivalent to that in the general population.[36]

Clinical features. There is growing evidence that simple bone cysts develop in two patient populations:[31,51] One group consists of children or young adults with a mean age of 17. In this younger group, lesions are more likely in males (about 2:1), and most form in the mandible. The older group of patients has a mean age of 42 and are usually women (4:1). This group of patients usually develops lesions in the mandible, but about 25% of the lesions are in the maxilla. About half the teeth related to these lesions had loss of lamina dura with exposure of the roots inside the lesion. In this older group about half the lesions are multiple, and most develop in association with radiopaque lesions such as hypercementosis, periapical cemental dysplasia, or florid osseous dysplasia.

The simple bone cyst is asymptomatic in most cases, but occasionally there may be evidence of pain or tenderness. Cortical swelling or tooth movement is unusual. The teeth in the affected region are usually vital, but nonvital teeth have

been reported.[36] Most of these lesions are discovered by chance during radiographic examination. Needle aspiration is usually unproductive. When aspiration is productive, it usually produces only a few milliliters of straw-colored or serosanguineous fluid. On occasion surgeons find the bony cavity filled with fluid.

Radiographic features. Simple bone cysts appear on radiographs of the younger group of patients as radiolucent lesions with well-defined to moderately defined borders. There may be evidence of a hyperostotic border around the entire lesion, but often in some areas such a border is lacking. There is no radiographic evidence of internal bone such as residual trabeculae or septa. Although simple bone cysts usually develop around the tooth apices, they may occur in any dentulous region. They may superimpose with tooth roots or "scallop" superiorly between the roots. Their size may vary considerably, sometimes extending around many teeth (Fig. 23-20). The radiographic feature most characteristic of this cyst is the *scalloped superior or occlusal margin,* where it extends between the roots of teeth (Fig. 23-21). Only occasionally are the lamina dura of involved teeth lost, and even less frequently are adjacent roots resorbed. These lesions occasionally cause cortical

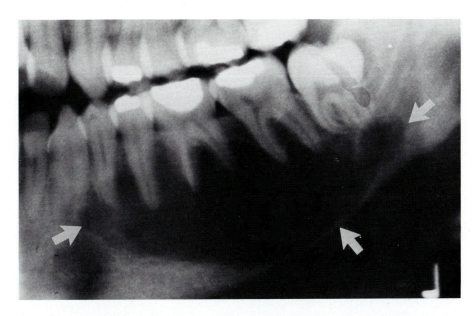

FIG. 23-20. Traumatic bone cyst seen as a lytic lesion in the body of the mandible, thinning the inferior cortex.

expansion. When expansion does occur, it is usually buccally and is generally slight. The surface is smooth, the cortical plates intact, and pathologic fracture does not result (Fig. 23-22). Most cases are unilocular with fairly regular borders. In the maxilla, the lesion may resemble the floor of the maxillary sinus and be overlooked.[32]

The radiographic characteristics of simple bone cysts in the older group of patients differ from the lesions in the younger group in several respects. In the older group, there are more likely to be multiple lesions, and there are often multiple areas of opacification in the jaws characteristic of florid osseous dysplasia. Teeth are also likely to show evidence of periapical cemental dysplasia. Tooth roots in the lesion also frequently show hypercementosis.[31]

Differential diagnosis. The radiographic image of a simple bone cyst may be similar to other lesions. A *radicular (periapical) cyst* may, in unusual circumstances, simulate a simple bone cyst. The presence of vital teeth, however, quickly rules out this possibility. Further, all true cysts tend to have a more rounded, regular, and more "hydraulic" shape than do simple bone cysts. A *central giant cell granuloma* usually shows evidence of internal bony septa, which the simple bone cyst generally lacks.

Ameloblastomas and *odontogenic myxomas* are usually multilocular. Lesions of *eosinophilic granuloma* and radiolucent *fibrous dysplasia* are not as well corticated as are simple bone cysts. Note that if a simple bone cyst is discovered accidentally while it is still small, it may be impossible to distinguish it radiographically from early forms of some of these lesions. However, thoughtful consideration of the clinical circumstances of the case in question, the results of needle aspiration, and the radiographic picture will lead to the correct diagnosis.

Management. It is important to explore this lesion surgically to rule out the possibility of a more serious condition. When exploration establishes the correct diagnosis, enucleation and curettement of the cavity are usually carried out. Most surgeons make sure to close a blood-filled cavity. The defect should heal readily, eventually demonstrating a normal bony appearance on follow-up radiographs. Periodic follow-up radiographic examinations are important to assure that healing is occurring.[19,33] Instances of self-healing have been described when patients refused treatment.[52]

Paget's disease

Paget's disease (also known as *osteitis deformans*) is a condition in which there is abnormal resorption and apposition of osseous tissue in one or more bones. There is a growing body of evidence that a slow virus infection is the cause of this disease.[46,55] Paget's disease may involve many bones

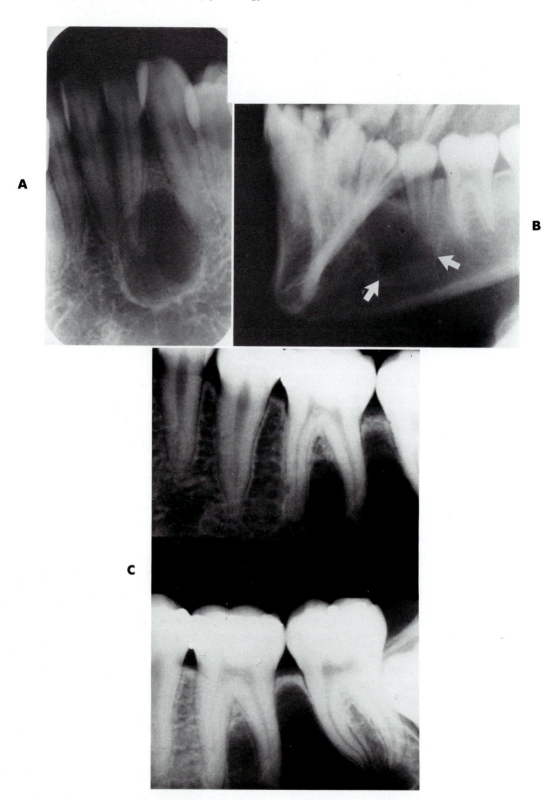

FIG. 23-21. Traumatic bone cysts extending ("scalloping") between tooth roots. **A,** Anterior mandible. **B,** Premolar region. *Arrows* point to the periphery of the lesion. **C,** Posterior mandible. (Courtesy Dr. L. Hollender, Seattle.)

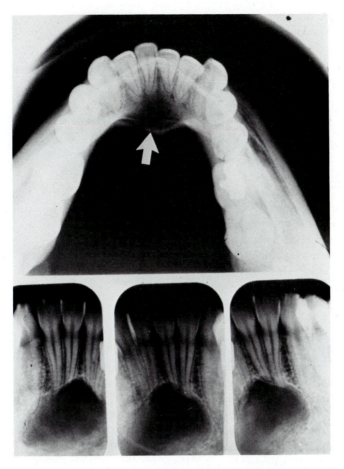

FIG. 23-22. Traumatic bone cyst *(arrow)* causing expansion of the lingual cortical plate of the mandible.

simultaneously, but it is not a generalized skeletal disease. The disease is initiated by an intense wave of osteoclastic activity, with resorption of normal bone resulting in irregularly shaped resorption cavities, followed after a variable period of time by vigorous osteoblastic activity forming woven bone.[18] Paget's disease is seen most frequently in Britain and somewhat less frequently in North America and western Europe; it is rare in Scandinavia and Africa.[1] Several large autopsy and radiologic studies have shown the incidence to be about 3.5% of all persons over age 40 years.[58] The older the age group, the higher the incidence of the disease.

Clinical features. Paget's disease is prone to occur in the axial skeleton, especially the skull, femur, sacrum, and pelvis. The incidence of jaw involvement is fairly low.[26] Paget's disease affects the maxilla about twice as often as the mandible. Nearly every case involving the jaws also affects the skull. Whenever a section of jawbone shows evidence of the disease, the bone is usually affected throughout.[71] Although Paget's disease is fairly symmetrical bilaterally in an involved jaw, occasionally there is significantly greater involvement on one side or the other.

Paget's disease is primarily a disease of later middle and old age. The incidence of involvement in males is approximately twice that of females at age 65 years.[2] Patients with symptoms most commonly complain of a deformity, pain, or both and may have bowing of the legs, curvature of the spine, enlargement of the skull, or a grotesque facial appearance caused by bony deformity. Bone pain is an inconsistent symptom, most often directed toward the weight-bearing bones, and is rare before age 40 years. Paget's disease usually produces enlargement of affected jawbones. In dentulous patients, there may be movement and migration of teeth and consequently malocclusion. In edentulous patients, the dentures may fit poorly. Facial or jaw pain is infrequent. Extraction sites heal slowly. The incidence of jaw osteomyelitis is higher than for nonaffected individuals.[59] Approximately 90% of affected persons have no symptoms.[18]

Patients with Paget's disease often demonstrate markedly elevated levels of serum alkaline phosphatase during osteoblastic phases of the disease. Higher levels of this serum component occur in patients having Paget's disease than in any other known disease state. The elevation appears to be directly proportional to the degree of bone changes as seen on radiographs.[21] Only in the early stages of the disease or in an isolated monostotic case is the alkaline phosphatase level within normal limits. Patients with Paget's disease also often show high levels of hydroxyproline in their urine. This is thought to result from degradation of bone collagen.[50] A bone scan may be indicated to determine the extent of disease.[20]

Patients with Paget's disease usually have a normal life span, but they may have a variety of complications. Foremost is the occurrence of osteogenic sarcoma in a pagetoid lesion. The best estimate is that osteogenic sarcoma develops in less than 1% of all patients with monostotic Paget's disease.[56,58] Patients with polyostotic disease have possibly a 10% chance of incurring the malignant tumor.[56] If this complication does develop, the prognosis is grave. In addition, the clinician must be alert for the development of osteomyelitis in the relatively avascular pagetoid bone. Once such a condition develops, it often spreads rapidly throughout the involved bone and can be highly refractory to antibiotic therapy. Patients with Paget's disease may also have ill-defined neurologic pain as the result of restricted foramina and canals and pathologic fracture of affected bones.

Radiographic features. There are three somewhat separate radiographic stages of Paget's disease, although these often do overlap in the clinical setting:

1. An early radiolucent resorptive stage
2. A granular or ground-glass-appearing second stage
3. A denser, more radiopaque appositional late stage

The early, radiolucent stage of the disease is infrequently discovered in the jaws because the disease usually produces no early symptoms. If the disease is detected in the mandible during this stage, the inferior cortex may appear osteoporotic

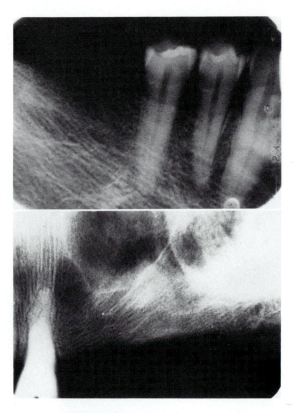

FIG. 23-23. Paget's disease, showing an altered trabecular pattern—linear striations in the mandibular molar region, **A,** and in the maxilla, **B.** (**A** and **B** Courtesy Dr. H.G. Poyton, Toronto, Ontario.)

and possess a laminated structure. Such cortical lamination may also develop in the alveolar bone (Fig. 23-23). Early Paget's lesions have an altered internal bone pattern. The trabeculae reduce in number, run linearly in the direction of the length of the bone, and have few intersections between them.[71] In the skull, early lytic lesions may develop as discrete radiolucent areas termed *osteoporosis circumscripta.*

In the more commonly observed later stages, rounded, radiopaque patches of abnormal bone often occur within individual jaw lesions, giving the impression of cotton wool (Fig. 23-24). As the fluffy, opacified areas become more numerous and enlarge, they tend to coalesce. This cotton wool sign is probably the most characteristic radiographic manifestation of Paget's disease in the skull or jaws. Advanced lesions may become increasingly opaque (Fig. 23-25).

Paget's disease always enlarges an affected bone to some extent, even in the early stages. Often

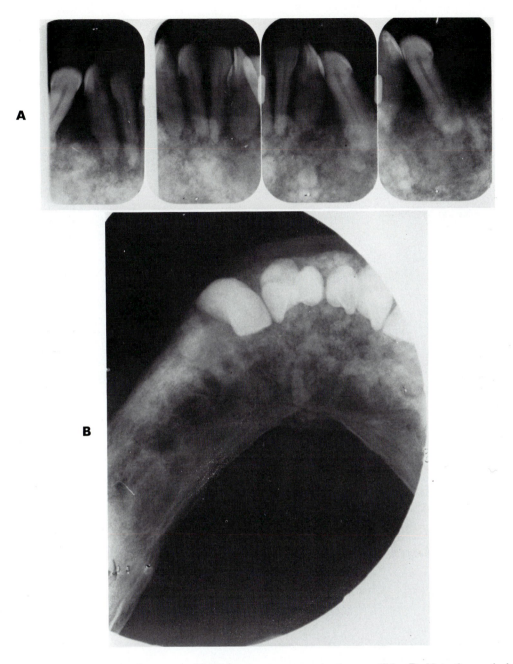

FIG. 23-24. Paget's disease. **A,** Multiple opaque masses in the mandible. **B,** Note the cortical expansion of the mandible.

the bone enlargement is impressive. Prominent pagetoid skull bones may swell to three to four times their normal thickness on a lateral radiograph (Fig. 23-26). The same lateral skull projection may also demonstrate a large, prognathic mandible. Maxillary Paget's disease generally encroaches into the maxillary sinus. Although the sinus floor is invariably involved by this disease, the air space is usually not diminished to a great extent.[71]

In affected jaws, hypercementosis develops on one or more tooth roots (Fig. 23-27). This occurs only following the bony jaw changes. In long-standing, advanced cases of Paget's disease, most of the remaining teeth show this change to some

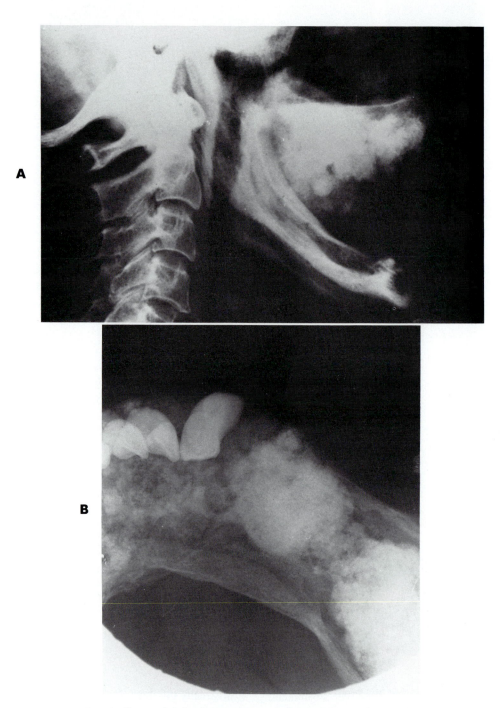

FIG. 23-25. Paget's disease showing opaque lesions in the maxilla, **A,** and mandible, **B.** (**A** courtesy Dr. H.G. Poyton, Toronto, Ontario.)

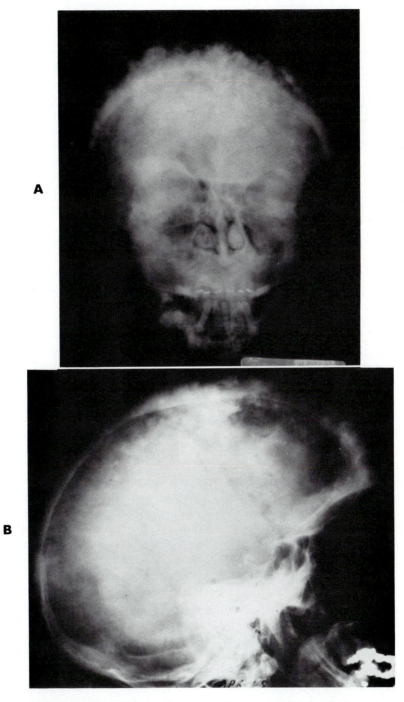

FIG. 23-26. Paget's disease of the skull, demonstrating gross thickening of the calvarium. **A,** PA view. **B,** Lateral view.

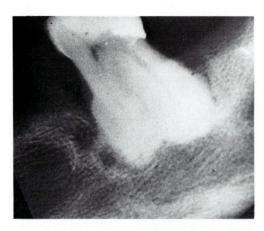

FIG. 23-27. Paget's disease showing hypercementosis of a molar.

extent. Hypercementosis is not known to be induced by any other systemic bone or metabolic disease and is therefore a considerable aid in diagnostic differentiation.[46] Paget's disease may obliterate areas of lamina dura and the periodontal ligament space around both normal and hypercementosed roots, resulting in ankylosis of teeth, but this is an inconsistent finding. During osteolytic phases, progressive resorption of tooth roots rather than hypercementosis has been described.[58] Whatever change takes place in the roots or periapical bone, the teeth remain viable.

The most alarming radiographic indication of osteogenic sarcoma development within a pagetoid lesion is frank dissolution or destruction of bone. This should be distinguished from early, uncomplicated Paget's disease in which the bone may appear noticeably osteoporotic but still have intact outlines. Malignant involvement of pagetoid bone produces actual bone dissolution and other radiographic features common to osteogenic sarcoma, such as invasive margins and intrinsic tumor calcification.

Differential diagnosis. Paget's disease presents a fairly specific radiographic pattern except in early, newly discovered cases. When Paget's disease becomes predominantly osteoblastic and produces obvious radiopacities, it resembles only a few other diseases. There are two radiographic features that, taken together, are virtually pathognomonic of Paget's disease: (1) a dense cotton wool or cotton ball pattern of fluffy, round radiopacities, and (2) enlargement of the one or more bones showing the radiopacities. When one considers, apart from the radiography, that Paget's disease is usually an abnormality of persons in their sixth or later decade of life and that the serum alkaline phosphatase level is usually highly elevated, the radiographic impression is persuasively strengthened.

Because of age differences, *fibrous dysplasia* is not usually confused with Paget's disease. Paget's disease generally occurs more diffusely throughout an involved bone. Further, Paget's disease is much more likely to occur in the jaws bilaterally, is less likely to obliterate the maxillary sinus, and more characteristically produces a cotton ball appearance than does fibrous dysplasia. *Florid osseous dysplasia* may be distinguished from Paget's disease because the former typically presents radiolucent capsules around central sclerotic masses, besides being limited to the jaws. It would be highly unlikely for Paget's disease to be confined to the jawbones. Areas of jaw *osteosclerosis, tori,* or *osteomas* are typically too confined in a relatively small area of bone to simulate the usual appearance of mature Paget's disease.

Management. Current management of Paget's disease is usually medical, using either calcitonin or sodium etidronate.[34] Calcitonin relieves pain and reduces serum alkaline phosphatase levels and osteoclastic activity. Sodium etidronate covers bone surfaces and retards bone resorption and formation. Surgery may be required for the correction of deformities of the long bones and the treatment of fractures.

Osteopetrosis

Osteopetrosis (also called Albers-Schönberg or "marble bone" disease) is a rare bone disease in which abnormal persistence of calcified cartilage is due to an apparent failure of osteoclasts in bone resorption and remodeling. Following development of the skeletal system, the spongy portion of an affected bone continues to form bone until it ultimately becomes a solid block of calcified cartilage. With obliteration of the marrow, there is inadequate space for hematopoiesis. Such bones are also fragile and susceptible to fracture.

Clinical features. There are two forms of osteopetrosis: (1) a more severe, recessive form known as *osteopetrosis congenita,* seen in infants or young children, and (2) a more benign, dominant form known as *osteopetrosis tarda.* The severe congenital form is invariably fatal early in life because of massive hemorrhage, anemia, leukopenia, or rampant bone infection. Such manifestations result from a progressive loss of the bone marrow

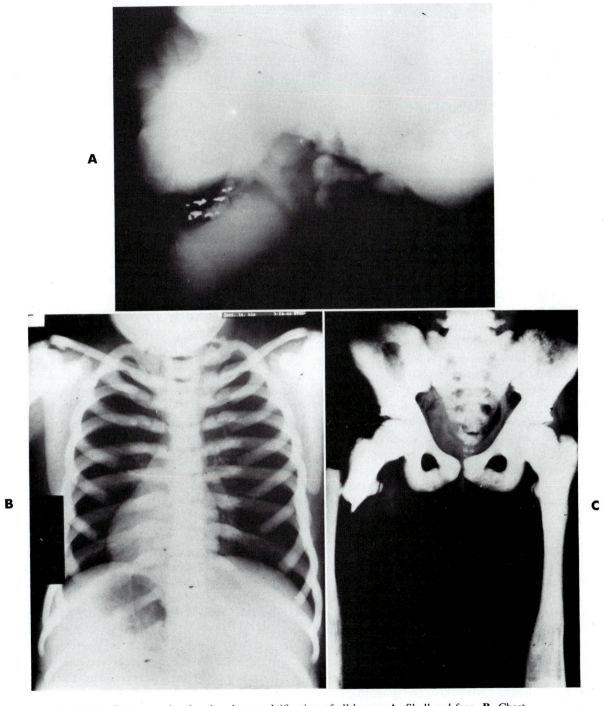

FIG. 23-28. Osteopetrosis, showing dense calcification of all bones. **A,** Skull and face. **B,** Chest. **C,** Pelvis and femora (note the fracture of the proximal right femur).

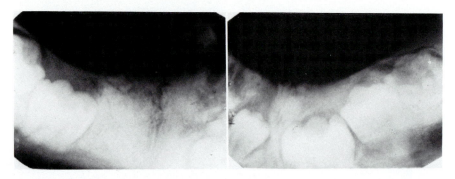

FIG. 23-29. Osteopetrosis, showing dense alveolar bone and embedded, poorly formed, teeth. (Courtesy Dr. H.G. Poyton, Toronto Ontario.)

and its cellular products. This severe form of the disease presents greatly increased bone density as well as entrapment syndromes including hydrocephalus, blindness (resulting from progressive narrowing of the optic canals), deafness, vestibular nerve dysfunction, and facial nerve paralysis.

The benign, tarda form of osteopetrosis is transmitted as an autosomal dominant disorder, is milder, and may be entirely asymptomatic. It may be discovered anytime from childhood into adulthood. The disease may be found as an incidental finding on a dental radiographic examination obtained for unrelated purposes, or it may cause a pathologic fracture of a bone. In some of the more chronic cases, bone pain may be a clinical problem, as may cranial nerve palsies caused by neural compression. Osteomyelitis may complicate this disease because of the relative avascularity of the bone. This problem is more frequent in the mandible, where such bone infections are usually secondary to dental or periodontal disease.[60]

Radiographic features. In the classic radiographic presentation of osteopetrosis, all bones show greatly increased density, which is bilaterally symmetrical. The trabecular patterns of the medullary cavities may be virtually unrecognizable (Fig. 23-28). This stark, radiopaque presentation routinely occurs in the severe, congenita form but is considerably moderated in the tarda form arising later in childhood or in adolescence. The long, tubular bones in osteopetrosis characteristically increase in diameter and tend to be funnel shaped as a result of impairment of normal bone modeling. The vertebrae and the skull base show excessive radiopacity. The increased density throughout the skeleton is homogeneous and diffuse. In severe cases, the observer cannot discern a trabecular pattern nor differentiate the cortex of bone from the

spongy portion. The entire bone may be mildly enlarged.

Dental defects that present radiographic manifestations include delayed eruption and early loss of teeth, missing teeth, malformed roots and crowns, and teeth that are poorly calcified and prone to caries (Fig. 23-29).[10] The normal eruption pattern of the primary and secondary dentitions may be delayed as a result of the exceptional density of the alveolar bone or ankylosis of cementum to bone.[72] The lamina dura surrounding the teeth apparently thickens, as do other minor cortical structures, such as the walls of the mandibular canal. In most cases, however, the increased bone density suggests osteopetrosis. Indeed, moderate to severe osteopetrosis usually produces such extensive radiopacity in the jaws that thin cortical structures such as the lamina dura and the mandibular canal, and in some cases even the dental roots, are not visible at all.

Differential diagnosis. *Sclerosteosis* has a similar radiographic appearance to osteopetrosis but shows a massive increase in the size of the mandible as well as increased girth of the metacarpals and phalanges, giving them a cigar-shaped appearance.[70] Individuals with sclerosteosis do not suffer from bone infection or compromised bone marrow activity but are susceptible to sudden death from damage to the medulla oblongata caused by elevated intracranial pressure.

Infantile cortical hyperostosis can usually be differentiated from osteopetrosis in that infantile cortical hyperostosis often presents (1) a positive history of highly specific soft tissue and bony abnormalities, (2) sites of involvement limited to a few bones in most cases, and (3) the peculiar pattern of mandibular enlargement in which new bone is mainly subperiosteal and confined to the

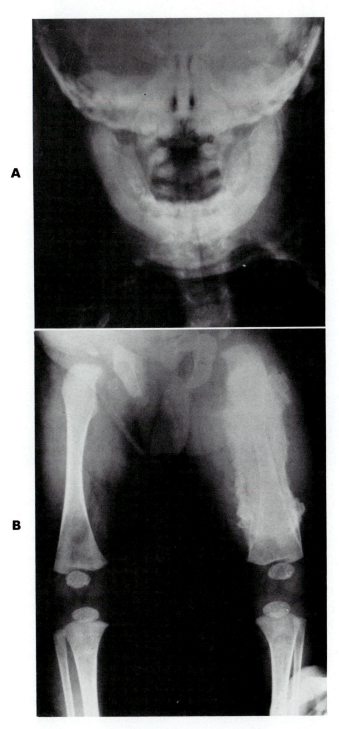

FIG. 23-30. Infantile cortical hyperostosis, showing thickening of the cortex. **A,** Mandible. **B,** Femur. (Courtesy Dr. H. Worth, Vancouver, BC.)

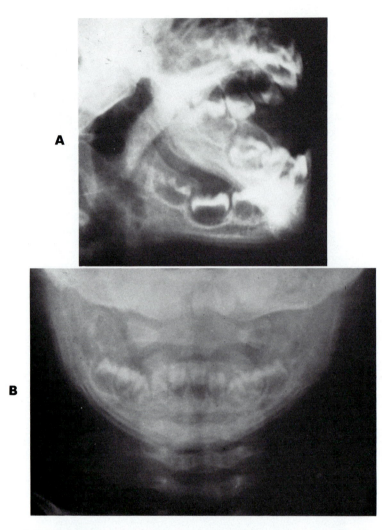

FIG. 23-31. Infantile cortical hyperostosis, showing development of the laminated appearance of the inferior border of the mandible. **A,** Lateral oblique view. **B,** PA view. (Courtesy Dr. H. Worth, Vancouver, BC.)

inferior border. In addition, clinical findings can be quite helpful in making this differentiation; blindness or other cranial neuropathies tend to point to osteopetrosis, whereas fever and hyperirritability are more consistent with infantile cortical hyperostosis.

Other less common conditions that may produce a generalized increase in bone density include pyknodysostosis, craniometaphyseal dysplasia, disphyseal dysplasia, melorheostosis, osteosclerosis of fluoride poisoning, and osteopathia striata.[49]

Infantile cortical hyperostosis

Infantile cortical hyperostosis (ICH, or Caffey's disease) is a perplexing bone-forming disease without a known cause or a definite pathogenesis. A prominent feature of the disease is the unusual cortical thickening observed in certain bones. Inflammatory changes also occur in contiguous soft tissues. The entity may be an infectious disease because many patients have severe and protracted fevers and most have increased erythrocyte sedimentation rates.[6] There is no evidence that the febrile episodes affect the calcification or eruption of the teeth.

Clinical features. ICH occurs equally in males and females. The average onset is at 9 weeks of age and rarely occurs after the fifth month of life. Several cases have even occurred in utero. In most instances, however, the neonate appears well for several weeks before the disease onset. The affected infant usually develops a fever and becomes hyperirritable. Soft tissue swellings develop over areas where bones will later thicken. These soft tissue swellings often have a sudden onset, especially in the facial area, and early in the disease may be very warm and tender. It is of considerable diagnostic significance that the onset of the soft tissue swelling predates the onset of the cortical thickening.[6] Only after the soft tissue changes have subsided and are no longer tender are there positive radiographic findings in the bones. The bones most commonly affected by ICH are (in order of frequency) the mandible, the clavicle, and the ulna. ICH affects the lower jaw bilaterally in almost all cases, although the two sides may demonstrate different degrees of involvement. The maxilla appears to be unaffected altogether.

Radiographic features. The cardinal radiographic feature of mandibular ICH is a thickening of the inferior cortex caused by new bone formation deep to the periosteum (Fig. 23-30). Mandibular lesions may vary widely in extent of involvement and activity. The dentist may observe an overall enlargement of the body of the mandible with a homogeneously increased density throughout. In less prolific cases, the bone thickening involves only the inferior cortex. Occasionally, the new bone forms in layers, giving the inferior cortex a laminated appearance (Fig. 23-31). The normal bony contour of the mandible often shows through the shadow of the dense new bone. After about a year, the disease tends to regress slowly with accompanying moderation of the radiographic changes. Variable degrees of deformity persist for several years after the disease subsides.[5] When asymmetry of the mandible persists, it results in malocclusion of variable severity.

Differential diagnosis. Because no other disease produces the peculiar bony hyperostosis in infants that ICH does, in most cases there is really no danger of misdiagnosis if the observer is familiar with the disease characteristics. Usually a firm diagnosis may be obtained without a biopsy.

Because the cortical hyperostosis is, for the most part, bilaterally symmetrical in the mandible, the disease may be distinguished from exuberant callus formation that occasionally appears as a sequela of *bone fracture* in infants and young children. The latter abnormality is typically unilateral or at least asymmetrical. *Osteomas* rarely develop in such a young age group; even so, multiple mandibular osteomas might rarely simulate the new bone formation of ICH. Although cherubism also produces bilateral deformities, the jaw lesions are multiloc-

ular, expansile radiolucencies, and there is no cortical thickening. Occasionally, the most troublesome diagnostic differentiation comes from osteopetrosis, as noted in the previous section. In ICH the abnormal bone production is subperiosteal, whereas in osteopetrosis it is mostly cancellous. Clinical features of these two diseases and the extent of skeletal involvement should also sufficiently favor one condition over the other.

Management. The condition resolves spontaneously without treatment.

REFERENCES

1. Barker D: The epidemiology of Paget's disease, *Metab Bone Dis Rel Res* 3:231-234, 1981.
2. Barker D, Clough P, Guyer P, Gardner M: Paget's disease of bone in 14 British towns, *Br Med J* 1:1181-1183, 1977.
3. Bianchi SD, Boccardi A, Mela F, Romagnoli R: The computed tomographic appearances of cherubism, *Skeletal Radiol* 16:6-10, 1987.
4. Buraczewski J, Dabska P: Pathogenesis of aneurysmal bone cyst: relationship between the aneurysmal bone cyst and fibrous dysplasia of bone, *Cancer* 28:597-603, 1971.
5. Burbank P, Lovestedt S, Kennedy R: The dental aspects of infantile cortical hyperostosis, *Oral Surg* 11:1127-1137, 1958.
6. Caffey J: *Pediatric x-ray diagnosis,* ed 7, Chicago, 1978, Mosby.
7. Cohen MA, Hertzanu Y: Radiologic features, including those seen with computed tomography, of central giant cell granuloma of the jaws, *Oral Surg Oral Med Oral Pathol* 65:255-261, 1988.
8. Dahlin D, McLeod R: Aneurysmal bone cyst and other nonneoplastic conditions, *Skeletal Radiol* 8:243-250, 1982.
9. Daramola J, Ajagbe H, Obisesan A, et al: Fibrous dysplasia of the jaws in Nigerians, *Oral Surg* 42:290-300, 1976.
10. Dick H, Simpson W: Dental changes in osteopetrosis, *Oral Surg* 34:408-420, 1972.
11. Ebata K, Usami T, Tohnai I, Kaneda T: Chondrosarcoma and osteosarcoma arising in polyostotic fibrous dysplasia, *J Oral Maxillofac Surg* 50:761-764, 1992.
12. Eisenbud L, Attie J, Garlick J, Platt N: Aneurysmal bone cyst of the mandible, *Oral Surg Oral Med Oral Pathol* 64:202-206, 1987.
13. El Deeb M, Sedano H, Waite D: Aneurysmal bone cyst of the jaws, *Int J Oral Surg* 9:301-311, 1980.
14. Emmering TE: Generalized radiopacities. In Wood NK, Goaz PW: *Differential diagnosis of oral lesions,* ed 4, St Louis, 1991, Mosby.
15. Eversole L, Merrell P, Straub D: Radiographic characteristics of central ossifying fibroma, *Oral Surg* 59:522-527, 1985.
16. Eversole L, Sabes W, Rovin S: Fibrous dysplasia: a nosologic problem in the diagnosis of fibro-osseous lesions of the jaws, *J Oral Pathol* 1:189-220, 1972.
17. Faircloth WJ Jr, Edwards RC, Farhood VW: Cherubism involving a mother and daughter: case reports and review of the literature, *J Oral Maxillofac Surg* 49:535-542, 1991.
18. Fame B, Marcel G: Paget's disease: a review of current knowledge, *Radiology* 141:21-24, 1981.

19. Feinberg S, Finkelstein M, Page H, Dembo J: Recurrent "traumatic" bone cysts of the mandible, *Oral Surg* 57:418-422, 1984.

20. Fogelman I, Carr D, Boyle I: The role of bone scanning in Paget's disease, *Metab Bone Dis Rel Res* 3:243-254, 1981.

21. Franck WA, Bress NM, Singer RR, Krane SM: Rheumatic manifestations of Paget's disease of bone, *Am J Med* 56:592-603, 1974.

22. Fun-chee L, Jinn-fei Y: Florid osseous dysplasia in Orientals, *Oral Surg Oral Med Oral Pathol* 68:748-753, 1989.

23. Gibilisco JA, Turlington EG, editors: *Stafne's oral roentgenographic diagnosis*, ed 5, Philadelphia, 1985, WB Saunders.

24. Giddings NA, Kennedy TL, Knipe KL, et al: Aneurysmal bone cyst of the mandible, *Arch Otolaryngol Head Neck Surg* 115:865-870, 1989.

25. Gingell J, Levy B, Becherman T, Tilghman D: Aneurysmal bone cyst, *J Oral Maxillofac Surg* 42:527-534, 1984.

26. Guyer P, Clough P: Paget's disease of bone: some observations on the relation of the skeletal distribution to pathogenesis, *Clin Radiol* 29:412-426, 1978.

27. Hall MB, Sclar AG, Gardner DF: Albright's syndrome with reactivation of fibrous dysplasia secondary to pituitary adenoma and further complicated by osteosarcoma, *Oral Surg* 57:616-619, 1984.

28. Hamner J, Scofield H, Coryn J: Benign fibro-osseous jaw lesions of periodontal membrane origin: an analysis of 249 cases, *Cancer* 22:861-876, 1968.

29. Harrison D: Osseous and fibro-osseous conditions affecting the craniofacial bones, *Ann Otol Rhinol Laryngol* 93:199-203, 1984.

30. Horner K: Central giant cell granuloma of the jaws: a clinico-radiological study, *Clin Radiol* 40:622-626, 1989.

31. Horner K, Forman GH: Atypical simple bone cyst of the jaws: II, a possible association with benign fibro-osseous (cemental) lesions of the jaws, *Clin Radiol* 39:59-63, 1988.

32. Kaffe I, Littner M, Begleiter A, et al: Traumatic bone cyst of the maxilla: a rarity? *Clin Prevent Dent* 5:11-12, 1983.

33. Kaffe I, Littner M, Buchner A: Traumatic bone cyst, *Quint Int* 13:469-472, 1982.

34. Kanis J, Evanson J, Russell R: Paget's disease of bone: diagnosis and management, *Metab Bone Dis Rel Res* 3:219-230, 1981.

35. Katz JO, Dunlap CL, Ennis RL: Cherubism: report of a case showing regression without treatment, *J Oral Maxillofac Surg* 50:301-303, 1992.

36. Kaugars GE, Cale AE: Traumatic bone cyst, *Oral Surg Oral Med Oral Pathol* 63:318-324, 1987.

37. Lipson A, Hsu T: Albright syndrome associated with acromegaly: report of a case and review of the literature, *Johns Hopkins Med J* 149:10-14, 1981.

38. Lucas RB: *Pathology of tumors of the oral tissues,* ed 3, Edinburgh, 1976, Churchill Livingstone.

39. MacDonald-Jankowski DS: Gigantiform cementoma occurring in two populations, London and Hong Kong, *Clin Radiol* 45:316-318, 1992.

40. Makek M, Lello G: Benign cementoblastoma: case report and literature review, *J Maxillofac Surg* 10:182-186, 1982.

41. Melrose RJ, Abrams AM, Mills BG: Florid osseous dysplasia: a clinical-pathologic study of 34 cases, *Oral Surg* 41:62-82, 1976.

42. Mendelshon D, Hertzanu Y, Cohen M, Lello G: Computed tomography of craniofacial fibrous dysplasia, *J Comput Assist Tomog* 8:1062-1065, 1984.

43. Nager G, Kennedy D, Kopstein E: Fibrous dysplasia: a review of the disease and its manifestations in the temporal bone, *Ann Otol Rhinol Laryngol* 91Suppl 92:5-52, 1982:

44. Obisean A, Lagundoye S, Darmola J, et al: The radiologic features of fibrous dysplasia of the craniofacial bones, *Oral Surg* 44:949-959, 1977.

45. Present D, Bertoni F, Enneking WF: Osteosarcoma of the mandible arising in fibrous dysplasia: a case report, *Clin Orthop* 204:238-244, 1986.

46. Rao V, Karasick D: Hypercementosis: an important clue to Paget's disease of the maxilla, *Skeletal Radiol* 9:126-128, 1982.

47. Reade P, McKelar G, Radden B: Unilateral mandibular cherubism: brief review and case report, *Br J Oral Maxillofac Surg* 22:189-194, 1984.

48. Rhea J, Weber A: Giant-cell granuloma of the sinuses, *Radiology* 147:135-137, 1983.

49. Ruprecht A, Wagner H, Engel H: Osteopetrosis: report of a case and discussion of the differential diagnosis, *Oral Surg Oral Med Oral Pathol* 66:674-679, 1988.

50. Russell R, Beard D, Cameron E, et al: Biochemical markers of bone turnover in Paget's disease, *Metab Bone Dis Rel Res* 3:255-262, 1981.

51. Saito Y, Hoshnia Y, Nagamine T, et al: Simple bone cyst: a clinical and histopathologic study of fifteen cases, *Oral Surg Oral Med Oral Pathol* 74:487-491, 1992.

52. Sapp PJ, Stark ML: Self-healing traumatic bone cysts, *Oral Surg Oral Med Oral Pathol* 69:597-602, 1990.

53. Sciubba JJ, Younai F: Ossifying fibroma of the mandible and maxilla: review of 18 cases, *J Oral Pathol Med* 18:315-321, 1989.

54. Shafer WG, Hine MK, Levy BM: *A textbook of oral pathology,* ed 4, Philadelphia, 1983, WB Saunders.

55. Singer F, Millo B: Evidence for a viral etiology of Paget's disease of bone, *Clin Orthop* 178:245-251, 1983.

56. Singer FR: *Paget's disease of bone,* New York, 1977, Plenum.

57. Slow I, Stern D, Friedman E: Osteogenic sarcoma arising in preexisting fibrous dysplasia: report of a case, *J Oral Surg* 29:126-129, 1971.

58. Smith B, Eveson J: Paget's disease of bone with particular reference to dentistry, *J Oral Pathol* 10:233-247, 1981.

59. Sofaer J: Dental extractions in Paget's disease of bone, *Int J Oral Surg* 13:79-84, 1984.

60. Steiner M, Gould A, Means W: Osteomyelitis of the mandible associated with osteopetrosis, *J Oral Maxillofac Surg* 41:395-405, 1983.

61. Struthers P, Shear M: Aneurysmal bone cyst of the jaws: I, clinicopathological features, *Int J Oral Surg* 13:85-91, 1984.

62. Struthers P, Shear M: Aneurysmal bone cyst of the jaws: II, pathogenesis, *Int J Oral Surg* 13:92-100, 1984.

63. Thompson SH, Altini M: Gingantiform cementoma of the jaws, *Head Neck* 11:538-544, 1989.

64. Tillman BP: Aneurysmal bone cyst: an analysis of 95 cases, *Mayo Clin Proc* 43:478-495, 1968.

65. Ueno S, Mushimoto K, Kurozumi T, et al: Aneurysmal bone cyst of the mandible, *J Oral Maxillofac Surg* 40:680-683, 1982.

66. Waldron C, Giansanti J: Benign fibro-osseous lesions of the jaws: a clinical-radiologic-histologic review of sixty-five cases: I, fibrous dysplasia of the jaws, *Oral Surg* 35:190-210, 1973.

67. Waldron C, Giansanti J: Benign fibro-osseous lesions of the jaws: a clinical-radiologic-histologic review of sixty-five cases: II, benign fibro-osseous lesions of periodontal ligament origin, *Oral Surg* 35:340-350, 1973.

68. Waldron CA, Shafer WG: The central giant cell granuloma of the jaws: an analysis of 38 cases, *Am J Clin Pathol* 45:437-447, 1966.

69. Wood N, Goaz P: *Differential diagnosis of oral lesions,* ed 4, St Louis, 1991, Mosby.

70. Wood RE, Kleyn G, Nortjé CJ, Grotepass F: Jaw involvement in sclerosteosis: a case report, *Dentomaxillofac Radiol* 17:145-148, 1988.

71. Worth HM: *Principles and practice of oral radiologic interpretation,* Chicago, 1963, Mosby.

72. Younai F, Eisenbud L, Sciubba JJ: Osteopetrosis: a case report including gross and microscopic findings in the mandible at autopsy, *Oral Surg Oral Med Oral Pathol* 65:214-221, 1988.

24

in collaboration with DONALD D. BLASCHKE

Systemic Diseases Manifested
in the Jaws

Various disorders of components of the endocrine system or other systemic diseases have a generalized adverse effect on the skeletal system. In some instances, the changes seen in the bone are indirect and result from pressure effects of tissue growing in bone, as in sickle cell anemia. In other cases, there is altered metabolism, for example, hyperparathyroidism or hypophosphatasia. An appreciation of these varied conditions aids the dentist in better understanding and managing the dental needs of affected patients.

ENDOCRINE DISORDERS
Hyperparathyroidism

Hyperparathyroidism is an endocrine abnormality in which there is an excess of circulating parathyroid hormone (PTH). An excess of serum PTH stimulates osteoclasts to mobilize calcium from the skeleton, leading to hypercalcemia. In addition, PTH increases renal tubular reabsorption of calcium, further aggravating this condition. Because 99% of the body's calcium is in the skeleton, imbalance of PTH function has a profound impact on the processes of bone formation and resorption.

Primary hyperparathyroidism usually results from a functioning benign tumor of one of the four parathyroid glands, thus producing excess hormone. Less frequently, individuals may have hyperplastic parathyroid glands that secrete excess PTH. The combination of hypercalcemia and elevated serum level of PTH is diagnostic of primary hyperparathyroidism.[2] *Secondary hyperparathyroidism* results from a compensatory increase in the output of PTH in response to hypocalcemia. The underlying hypocalcemia may result from an inadequate dietary intake or poor absorption of vitamin D or from deficient metabolism of vitamin D in the liver or kidney.[2] This condition produces clinical and radiographic effects similar to those of primary hyperparathyroidism.

The incidence of primary hyperparathyroidism is about 0.1%. Blood tests for patients undergoing examination for unrelated medical problems occasionally discover biochemical cases of hyperparathyroidism.[3] An important consequence is that in many persons this disease is being diagnosed earlier, and, as a result, fewer patients have the classic, long-term, devastating bone changes seen in years past.

Clinical features. Women are two to three times more commonly affected by primary hyperparathyroidism than men. The condition occurs mainly in those 30 to 60 years of age. Clinical manifestations of the disease cover a fairly broad range, but most patients have symptoms and signs referable to renal calculi, peptic ulcers, psychiatric problems, or bone and joint pain. These clinical symptoms are mainly related to hypercalcemia.[32] There may be gradual loosening, drifting, and loss of teeth.[40]

Hypercalcemia is the keystone of the diagnosis of this disease.[43] Definite consistent hypercalcemia is virtually pathognomonic of primary hyperparathyroidism. (Rarely, multiple myeloma and metastatic tumors may produce the same serum alterations.) The serum calcium level in patients should be tested at different intervals with suspected hyperparathyroidism because the actual level of circulating calcium in marginal hyperparathyroidism is subject to considerable day-to-day fluctuation. The serum alkaline phosphatase level may also be elevated in hyperparathyroidism. This biochemical change correlates fairly well with the degree of radiologic evidence of bone damage. The alkaline phosphatase assay is a fairly reliable indicator of bone turnover or resorption in various systemic and bone diseases.

Radiographic features. The pathologic effects of an overabundance of PTH on the skeleton are manifested radiographically in four principal categories:

1. *Demineralization of the skeleton.* Bone matrix (osteoid) contains less than the normal amount of calcium, producing unusually radiolucent skeletal images.
2. *Osteitis fibrosa generalisata.** Localized destruction of bone is produced by osteoclastic activity, leaving residual radiolucent areas of fibrosis.
3. *Brown tumors.* Late in the disease, and in about 10% of the cases, so-called brown tumors of bone may develop peripherally or centrally. They appear radiographically as ill-defined radiolucencies. These are giant cell tumors, called brown tumors because the gross specimen is brown or reddish brown.
4. *Pathologic calcifications.* Punctate and nodular calcifications are occasionally observed radiographically in the kidneys and joints.

Only about one in five patients with hyperparathyroidism has radiographically observable bone changes.[43] The earliest and most reliable changes are subtle erosions of bone from the subperiosteal surfaces of the phalanges of the hands, representing a form of osteitis fibrosa generalisata. Most patients with any radiographic evidence of their disease will show some degree of this phalangeal erosion. Skull demineralization, which often develops in this disease, results in bone thinning. In prominent hyperparathyroidism, the entire calvarium has a granular appearance caused by the loss of central (diploic) trabeculae and thinning of the cortical tables. In the jaws, there is often demineralization of the inferior border of the mandible and mandibular canal or thinning of the cortical outlines of the maxillary sinuses.

Occasionally, periapical radiographs reveal loss of the lamina dura in patients (about 10%) with hyperparathyroidism (Fig. 24-1). Depending on the duration and severity of the disease, loss of the lamina dura may occur around one tooth or all the

---

*Because these lesions often appear cystlike on a radiograph, the term "cystica" was applied. When they were later found to be areas of fibrosis, the term "osteitis fibrosa cystica" has been replaced by the more appropriate "osteitis fibrosa generalisata."

remaining teeth. Proved cases of hyperparathyroidism, even those with osseous changes in the hands, do not always show loss of lamina dura.[36,43] Around a particular tooth, the loss may be either complete or partial. If complete, the involved tooth is likely to have an unusually tapered appearance. (The reason for this apparent change in root morphology is that the lamina dura accentuates to a small extent the density of the adjacent tooth root.) Loss of the lamina dura is not a specific sign; it occurs in fibrous dysplasia, Paget's disease, Cushing's syndrome, or osteomalacia.

In cases of suspected hyperparathyroid disease, the dentist should attempt to produce intraoral radiographs that have a normal radiographic density of the teeth. This makes it possible to estimate changes in *bone* radiographic density compared to the teeth. Whereas PTH mobilizes minerals from the skeleton, mature teeth are immune to this systemic demineralizing process. If the teeth present a fairly normal radiographic density but the surrounding bone appears dark or overpenetrated, then hyperparathyroidism is strongly suggested.

Brown tumors of hyperparathyroidism may appear in any bone but are frequently found in the facial bones and jaws, particularly in long-standing cases of the disease. These lesions may be multiple within a single bone or may be polyostotic. Radiographically, brown tumors have variably defined margins and may produce cortical expansion (Fig. 24-2). If solitary, the tumor resembles a central giant cell granuloma (with which they are microscopically identical) or an aneurysmal bone cyst. Concurrent generalized bone demineralization should help in pointing to a diagnosis of hyperparathyroidism. In any case, when in doubt about the presence of a brown tumor within the skeleton, the radiologist or clinician should order assays of serum calcium phosphates and alkaline phosphatase. Classically, serum calcium and alkaline phosphatase are increased and the phosphates decreased.

Management. After successful surgical removal of the causative parathyroid adenoma, almost all radiographic changes revert to normal. The only exception may be the site of a brown tumor, which often heals with bone radiographically more sclerotic than normal.

Hypoparathyroidism and pseudohypoparathyroidism

Hypoparathyroidism is an uncommon condition in which there is insufficient secretion of parathy-

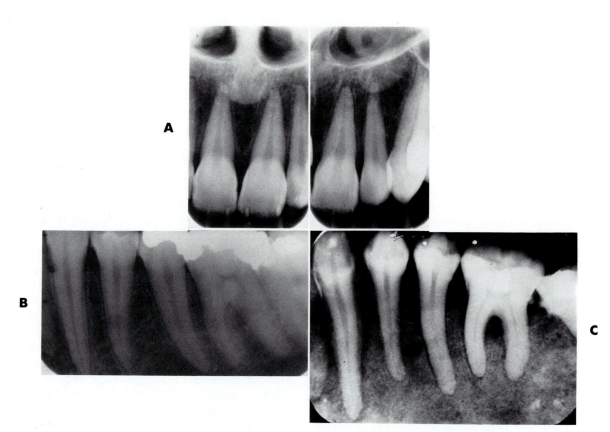

FIG. 24-1. Hyperparathyroidism manifested as demineralization of bone. Note the thinned lamina dura and the loss of trabecular bone. (**C** courtesy Dr. H.G. Poyton, Toronto, Ontario.)

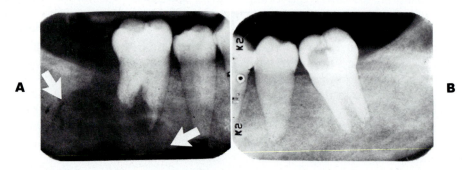

FIG. 24-2. Hyperparathyroidism. **A,** Brown tumor associated with hyperparathyroidism. *Arrows* point to the variable definition of its margins. Note the slight expansion of the cortex adjacent to the first molar. **B,** Ground-glass appearance of the trabecular bone associated with hyperparathyroidism. Note the loss of lamina dura. (Courtesy Dr. E. Millar, Montreal; from Langlais RP, Bentley KC [eds]: *Exercise in dental radiology.* Vol 2. *Advanced oral radiographic interpretation,* Philadelphia, 1979, WB Saunders.)

roid hormone. The usual causes of this condition are many and include surgical damage to parathyroid glands or their vascular supply during thyroid gland procedures, parathyroid damage from radioactive iodine-131 treatment of hyperthyroidism, autoimmune destruction of the parathyroid glands, and developmental and familial hypoparathyroidism (unknown cause). In *Pseudohypoparathyroidism* there is a defect in the response of the tissue target cells to normal levels of parathyroid hormone. The clinical consequences of this condition are similar to those of hypoparathyroidism. These conditions are managed with orally administered supplemental calcium and vitamin D.

Clinical features. Both hypoparathyroidism and pseudohypoparathyroidism produce hypocalcemia, which has a variety of clinical manifestations. Most often this includes sharp flexion (tetany) of the wrist and ankle joints (carpopedal spasm). Some patients have sensory abnormalities consisting of paresthesia of the hands, feet, or around the mouth. Neurologic changes may include anxiety and depression, epilepsy, parkinsonism, and chorea. In chronic forms, there may be a reduction in intellectual capacity. Such a change may result from calcifications within the brain. Some patients show no changes at all. Patients with pseudohypoparathyroidism often have early closure of certain bony epiphyses and thus manifest short stature or extremity disproportions.

When hypoparathyroidism or pseudohypoparathyroidism occurs in children, clinically evident dental effects include hypoplasia of the enamel and delayed eruption.[13,16]

Radiologic features. The principal radiographic change is calcification of the basal ganglia (Fig. 24-3). On skull radiographs, this calcification appears flocculent and paired within the cerebral hemispheres on the posteroanterior view. Radiographic examination of the jaws may reveal dental

enamel hypoplasia, external root resorption, delayed eruption, or root dilaceration (Fig. 24-4).

Hyperpituitarism

Hyperpituitarism results from hyperfunction of the anterior lobe of the pituitary gland, most sig-

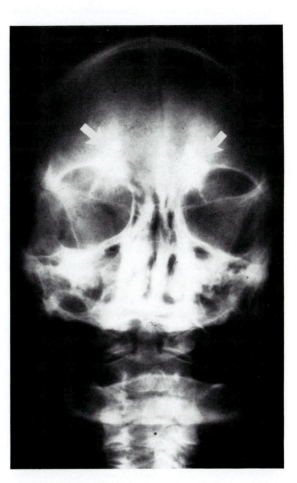

FIG. 24-3. Hypoparathyroidism-induced calcification of the basal ganglia, seen on a PA skull projection. (Courtesy Dr. H.G. Poyton, Toronto, Ontario.)

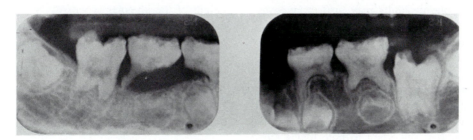

FIG. 24-4. Pseudohypoparathyroidism-induced dental anomalies. (Courtesy Dr. S. Bricker, San Antonio; from Dixter C, et al [eds]: *Exercise in dental radiology.* Vol 3. *Pediatric radiographic interpretation,* Philadelphia, 1980, WB Saunders.)

nificantly with increased production of growth hormone. An excess of growth hormone causes overgrowth of all tissues in the body still capable of growth. The usual cause of this problem is a benign, functioning tumor of the eosinophilic cells in the anterior lobe of the pituitary gland.

Clinical features. When hyperpituitarism occurs in childhood, there is generalized overgrowth of most tissues, a condition termed "giantism." Most soft tissues and bones respond to the excess hormone by enlarging. Active growth occurs in those bones in which the epiphyses have not united with the bone shafts. Throughout adolescence, excessive generalized skeletal growth is the principal manifestation of hyperpituitarism. Childhood and juvenile giants show prominent growth over a prolonged time. These young people may ultimately attain heights of 7 to 8 feet or more, yet exhibit remarkably normal proportions. The eyes and other parts of the central nervous system do not enlarge except in the rare cases in which the condition is manifested in infancy.

Adult hyperpituitarism, called *acromegaly,* has an insidious clinical course, quite different from the clinical profile seen in the childhood disease. In adults, the clinical effects of a pituitary eosinophilic tumor develop quite slowly because many types of tissues have lost the capacity for growth. Most adult bones are incapable of increased growth because of the fusion of the epiphyses with the shafts of the endochondral bones and the fusion of the sutures of the craniofacial bones. In certain bones, however, including the mandible, the excess growth hormone may stimulate articulating surfaces covered with growth-potential cartilage to produce further endochondral bone growth. This type of growth is particularly noticeable in the hand because of the large number of cartilage-covered articulating surfaces in each digit. Mandibular condylar growth may be even more prominent, although similar to the digital enlargement. Excess growth hormone in adults may also produce hypertrophy of some soft tissues. The lips, tongue, and soft tissues of the hands and feet typically overgrow in the acromegalic, sometimes to a striking degree.

Radiographic features. The pituitary tumor responsible for hyperpituitarism often, but not always, produces enlargement ("ballooning") of the sella turcica. It is important to note that a small pituitary tumor can produce prominent clinical manifestations and yet cause no expansion of the sella. Radiography of the sella turcica may there-

fore be negative. Skull radiographs characteristically reveal enlargement of the paranasal sinuses (especially the frontal sinus) and excessive pneumatization of the temporal bone squama and petrous ridges. These air sinuses are more prominent in acromegaly than in pituitary giantism because sinus growth in giantism tends to be more in step with the generalized enlargement of the facial bones. Hyperpituitarism in adults also produces diffuse thickening of the outer table of the skull.

The dental features of *giantism* are interesting in that tooth size is generally normal. The tooth crowns are usually normal in size, although the roots of posterior teeth often enlarge as a result of hypercementosis. Such posterior hypercementosis is probably more reflective of funtional and structural demands on teeth than a primary response to the hormone itself.[22] Because the jaws are enlarged, with consequent lengthening of the dental arches, wide spaces (diastemata) form between the normal-size erupted teeth.

In *acromegaly,* spaces again develop between the teeth as the arch length increases. In contrast to the childhood condition, however, the anterior teeth fan out forward.[46] This may result from an enlarged tongue (macroglossia) pushing outward against the teeth. Others, however, contend that overgrowth of the jaws, and particularly the posterior alveolar bone, results in an anterior open bite that accentuates anterior flaring of the teeth.[46] This sign of incisor flaring is a helpful point of differentiation between acromegalic prognathism and inherited prognathism.

The principal effect of growth hormone on the adult mandible is to cause lengthening of the condylar processes. Excess condylar growth results in lengthening of the ascending ramus and ultimately the body of the mandible (Fig. 24-5). A class III skeletal relationship between the jaws (protruding mandible) is a consistent finding in this disease. There may also be an increase in the thickness and height of the alveolar processes. With downward and forward growth of the mandible, the teeth tend to supererupt secondarily to maintain the occlusal plane at its normal level. Appositional bone growth on the alveolar processes then passively follows the abnormal dental eruption behavior. As mentioned, this supereruption of posterior teeth often develops with hypercementosis.

Hypopituitarism

Hypopituitarism results from reduced secretion of pituitary hormones. It is often the consequence

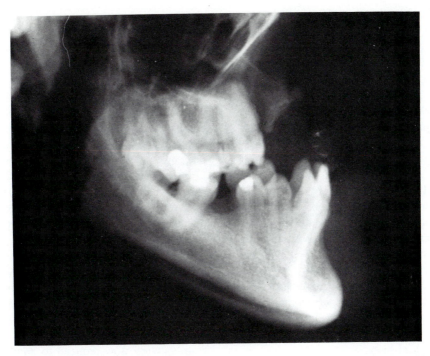

FIG. 24-5. Acromegaly manifested as excessive growth of the mandible, resulting in a Class III skeletal relationship of the jaws.

of growth of pituitary adenomas that compress the pituitary gland or interfere with stalk function. Individuals with this condition show dwarfism but have relatively well-proportioned bodies. Mental development is normal. One study reported a marked failure of development of the maxilla and the mandible.[23] The dimensions of these bones in these adults were approximately those of normal children 5 to 7 years of age. Eruption of the primary dentition occurred at the normal time, but exfoliation was delayed by several years. The crowns of the permanent teeth formed normally, but their eruption was delayed several years. As a rule, there was complete absence of third molar buds. Because in hypopituitarism the tooth crowns are only slightly reduced in size but the jaws, especially the mandible, are small, crowding and subsequent malocclusion often result.

Treatment is usually directed toward removal of the cause or replacement of the pituitary hormones or those of its target gland. The response of the dentition to treatment with growth hormone is variable but seems to parallel skeletal response.[31]

Hyperthyroidism

Hyperthyroidism (also called *thyrotoxicosis*) is a syndrome in which there is excessive production of thyroxin in the thyroid gland. The condition occurs most commonly with diffuse toxic goiter (Graves' disease) and less frequently with toxic nodular goiter or toxic adenoma, a benign tumor of the thyroid gland.[8] Each of these conditions results in increased levels of circulating thyroxin. Excessive thyroxin causes a generalized increase in the metabolic rate of all body tissues.

Patients with hyperthyroidism generally show an advanced rate of dental development and early eruption, with premature loss of the primary teeth. Adults may show a generalized decrease in bone density or loss of some areas of edentulous alveolar bone.

Hypothyroidism

Hypothyroidism usually results from insufficient secretion of thyroxin by the thyroid glands despite the presence of thyroid-stimulating hormone. When this condition occurs in children, it is called *juvenile myxedema;* in the adult it is called *myxedema.*

Clinical features. Juvenile myxedema results in retarded mental and physical development, including delayed fusion of all bony epiphyses. The base of the skull shows delayed ossification, and the paranasal sinuses only partially pneumatize.

Dental development is delayed, and the primary teeth are slow to exfoliate. The maxilla and the mandible are relatively small.

Hypothyroidism in the adult results in myxedematous swelling but not the dental or skeletal changes seen in children. Adult symptoms may range from lethargy, constipation, and cold intolerance to the more florid clinical picture of dull, expressionless face, periorbital edema, large tongue, sparse hair, and skin that feels "doughy" to the touch.

Radiographic features. Radiographic examination of patients with juvenile myxedema reveals delayed closing of the fontanelles and epiphyses. The skull often incorporates numerous wormian bones (accessory bones in the sutures). Examination of the jaws may show thinning of the lamina dura, delayed dental eruption, and short tooth roots. In adult hypothyroidism, periodontal disease and loss of teeth, separation of teeth as a result of enlargement of the tongue, and external root resorption may all be seen.

Diabetes mellitus

Diabetes mellitus is a metabolic disorder that has two primary forms. Type I, insulin-dependent diabetes mellitus (previously known as *juvenile-onset diabetes*), results from an absence or insufficiency of insulin, a hormone normally produced by the beta cells of the islets of Langerhans in the pancreas. Type II, non-insulin-dependent diabetes mellitus, results from insulin resistance. Patients with Type I diabetes have virtually no beta cells (in the islets), whereas patients with Type II diabetes have approximately half the normal number.[30] There has been speculation that an autoimmune response, perhaps in association with a virus, causes diabetes.[30] A shortage of insulin adversely affects carbohydrate metabolism. The principal clinical laboratory signs of the disease are hyperglycemia and glycosuria, both reflecting a complex biochemical imbalance between tissue demand for glucose and the release of this nutrient by the liver.

Clinical features. Untreated diabetes may manifest classic symptoms and signs such as polydipsia (excessive intake of fluids), polyuria (excessive urination), and, in more severe cases, acetone present in the urine and on the breath. This metabolic disorder, if not adequately treated, lowers the body's resistance to infection.

Diabetes may demonstrate a number of adverse effects in the oral cavity. Most prominently, uncontrolled diabetes acts as a continuing factor that predisposes to, aggravates, and accelerates periodontal disease. There is controversy within the dental literature concerning the precise extent of the effects of diabetes mellitus on the periodontium. Diabetes does not directly cause periodontal disease. Many patients with uncontrolled diabetes have normal periodontal tissues. Rather, the general belief is that uncontrolled diabetes predisposes an individual to inflammatory conditions, and, once present, the inflamed periodontium is difficult to treat. Thus, periodontal disease should be considered a complication of diabetes rather than a primary effect. Patients with controlled diabetes do not appear to have more periodontal problems than do normal persons.

Some children with uncontrolled diabetes have increased caries activity, presumably because of a high-carbohydrate diet. After treatment, the level of caries activity reduces, often to lower than normal levels.[30] Another occasional oral complication of diabetes mellitus is xerostomia. This results from salivary flow reduced to about one third of normal. The xerostomia may result from polyuria or decreased blood flow to the salivary glands.[24] Some patients with diabetes have sialism, a symmetric, noninflammatory, nonneoplastic enlargement of the salivary glands.[24] Other findings include increased prevalence of oral candidiasis, tongue mucosal changes, and perhaps oral lichen planus.[24]

Radiographic features. Periodontal disease associated with diabetes is indistinguishable radiographically from periodontal disease in patients without diabetes. Radiographic manifestations range from slight discontinuity or blurring of the cortex of the alveolar crest to wide destruction of the lamina dura and horizontal and vertical interdental bone loss. Mucosal changes are occasionally characteristic of rampant periodontal abscesses. Such periodontal findings may be localized or fairly generalized throughout both dental arches. Alveolar bone resorption is said to increase with the severity of the diabetic condition.[42]

One study of the effects of diabetes on the production of alveolar bone loss in older patients (average age 57 years) found no justification for the contention that diabetes causes increased alveolar bone loss.[28] Its diabetic population showed only a slightly higher percentage of tooth loss from periodontal causes than did a control group. These authors noted that the diabetic state in their patients was, on the whole, milder than that reported in earlier studies and that all the patients in their study were highly motivated persons who practiced good oral hygiene. We may conclude, then, that uncontrolled diabetes mellitus is likely to have some influence on the incidence and severity of periodontal disease. This influence, however, may not be overwhelming, inasmuch as it appears to be outweighed and rendered less damaging by the consistent practice of good oral hygiene.

Cushing's syndrome

Cushing's syndrome arises from an excess of secretion of glucocorticoids by the adrenal glands. This may result from (1) an adrenal adenoma, (2) an adrenal carcinoma, (3) adrenal hyperplasia (usually bilateral), (4) a basophilic adenoma of the anterior lobe of the pituitary gland (Cushing's disease), producing excess ACTH, or (5) by medical therapy with exogenous corticosteroids.

Clinical features. Patients with Cushing's syndrome often show obesity (which spares the extremities), kyphosis of the thoracic spine ("buffalo hump"), weakness, hypertension, striae, or concurrent diabetes. This condition affects females three to five times as frequently as males. Onset may occur at any age but is usually seen in the third or fourth decade.

Radiographic features. The primary radiographic feature of Cushing's syndrome is generalized osteoporosis. Bone deposition is inhibited, whereas osteoclastic action continues unabated. As a consequence, there is osseous demineralization with pathologic fractures often superimposed. The skull can show diffuse thinning accompanied by a mottled appearance. The jaws may show areas of loss of the lamina dura (Fig. 24-6).

ADDITIONAL SYSTEMIC DISEASES MANIFESTED IN THE JAWS
Histiocytosis X

Histiocytosis X is an inflammatory reticuloendothelial condition, possibly a reaction to a viral infection.[25] Although the range of disease severity is quite broad and seems to present a continuous spectrum, histiocytosis X is most likely a single disease with one of three clinical forms: eosinophilic granuloma of bone (monostotic or polyostotic), Hand-Schüller-Christian disease (chronic disseminated histiocytosis X), and Letterer-Siwe disease (acute disseminated histiocytosis X).

In all three disease states there are pathologic accumulations of histiocytes and eosinophilic leukocytes. Eosinophilic granuloma usually appears in the skeleton, although occasional soft tissue le-

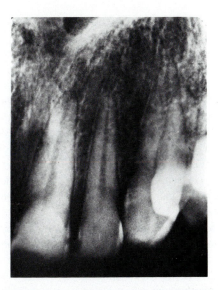

FIG. 24-6. Cushing's syndrome manifested in the jaws as thinning of the lamina dura. (Courtesy Dr. H.G. Poyton, Toronto, Ontario.)

sions may occur. In the chronic disseminated form (Hand-Schüller-Christian disease) and the acute (or subacute) disseminated form (Letterer-Siwe disease), there is involvement of soft tissues and bone. Head and neck lesions are common at initial presentation, and approximately 10% of all patients with histiocytosis X have oral lesions.[2,19] Two thirds of these lesions are intraosseous defects, and one third are soft tissue lesions. Frequently, the oral changes are the first clinical signs of the disease.[9]

Clinical features
Letterer-Siwe disease. Letterer-Siwe disease (acute disseminated histiocytosis X) is a fulminating condition that most often occurs in infants younger than 3 years of age. Soft tissue and bony granulomatous reactions disseminate throughout an affected infant's body. The infant demonstrates intermittent fever, hepatosplenomegaly, anemia, lymphadenopathy, hemorrhages, and failure to thrive. Lesions in bone are rare. Death usually occurs within several weeks of disease onset.

Hand-Schüller-Christian disease. Hand-Schüller-Christian disease (chronic disseminated histiocytosis X) typically beings in childhood, although it may not be fully developed until the third decade of life. It affects males more frequently than females. The early, classic descriptions emphasize a triad of specific abnormalities including bone lesions, diabetes insipidus, and exophthalmos. These three manifestations occur together only in about

10% of reported cases.[12] Usually two of the three abnormalities are found; most commonly observed are osteolytic skull lesions. The course of this disease is chronic, usually with numerous remissions and exacerbations. Usually the earlier the onset and the more rapid the progression, the poorer the prognosis.[9] Although this disease is serious and progressive, adroit medical management may prolong the patient's life for several years. Hand-Schüller-Christian disease often presents oral manifestations. Occasionally, oral changes are the most significant clinical feature of the disease and may even be the chief complaint.[41]

Eosinophilic granuloma of bone. Eosinophilic granuloma usually develops in bony sites (ribs, pelvis, the flat bones of the skull and face, and long bones). Rarely it develops in soft tissues such as the lymph nodes, skin, lungs, and oral cavity (gingiva and palate, especially).[4,26] This condition occurs most often in older children and young adults but may develop later in life.[17] The lesions often form quickly and may cause a dull, steady pain. In the jaws, there may be evidence of bony swelling, a soft tissue mass, gingivitis, bleeding gingivae, pain, or ulceration.[17,19] Loosening or sloughing of the teeth often occurs after the destruction of alveolar bone by one or more eosinophilic granulomas.[39] The sockets of teeth lost to the disease generally fail to heal normally.

Radiographic features. The skull is a more consistent site for eosinophilic granuloma than either of the jaws. One investigator found in a series of 20 general skeletal cases that the mandible was the fourth most common bone to be involved.[48] Eosinophilic granuloma may be solitary or multiple, although within the jaws multiple lesions are more common. The mandible is a more common site than the maxilla; in both jaws, the posterior regions develop lesions more frequently than the anterior regions.

Jaw lesions of eosinophilic granuloma usually occurs as areas of pure osteolysis in or close to the alveolar process. The lesions characteristically destroy the periodontal bone support of one or more teeth, especially in the posterior areas, while producing virtually no resorption of tooth roots (Fig. 24-7). The result is often a distinctive "teeth standing in space" or "floating teeth" radiographic appearance in the region superior to the mandibular canal.

An eosinophilic granuloma is moderately to well defined at its radiographic periphery. Jaw lesions

typically have fairly discrete borders, which are only rarely hyperostotic. They thus have a "punched-out" appearance. The margins may be smooth or somewhat irregular. The margins of these lesions are usually not the hazy, invasive-appearing margins that would prompt a suspicion of malignancy. Bone scans made using ^{99}mTc-labeled diphosphonate readily demonstrate these lesions, thereby disclosing their active osseous metabolism.[10] The radiographic features of these lesions in the vertebral column, ribs, and long bones and the bony lesions of chronic histiocytosis X (Hand-Schüller-Christian disease) and acute histiocytosis X (Letterer-Siwe disease) are all qualitatively similar (Figs. 24-8 and 24-9).

Differential diagnosis. Eosinophilic granuloma may appear radiographically in either jaw as one or more osteolytic defects in or near the alveolar processes. When observing such a radiographic pattern, the first consideration in forming a differential diagnosis should be the patient's age. The number of cases of eosinophilic granulomas of bone discovered in patients older than age 25 years is small. Eosinophilic granuloma is thus not generally a serious radiographic consideration except in children, adolescents, and young adults. Jaw alveolar erosions produced by *oral carcinomas,* which may also have a "teeth standing in space" appearance, tend not to be misdiagnosed as eosinophilic granulomas because these malignant tumors are found in such a decidedly older age group. Besides the consideration of age, the clinician is often able to inspect the oral cavity and visually distinguish the gingival granulomatous lesions of histiocytosis X from epidermoid carcinoma.

The alveolar defect of eosinophilic granuloma typically begins as a scooped out concavity at the alveolar crest, leaving any teeth in the area substantially or completely without periodontal support. This pattern of bone destruction usually appears much like a peripheral lesion eroding into the bone. When this pattern is seen, diseases that are exclusively central can be given less importance in the differential diagnosis. The margins of eosinophilic granuloma are fairly distinct but are virtually never hyperostotic. This lack of cortication would tend to rule out *cysts, giant cell granuloma,* and *traumatic bone cyst* in questionable cases. Condensing osteitis is rare around an eosinophilic granuloma of bone. Such a bony reaction suggests an inflammatory condition such as *severe peri-*

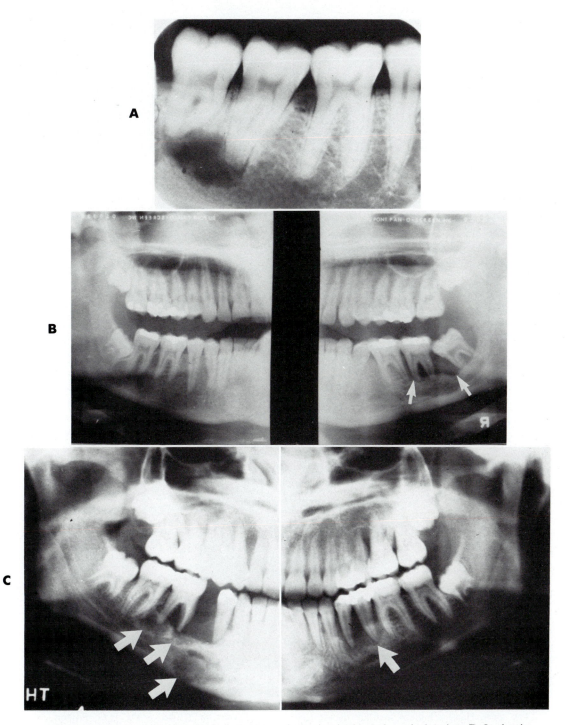

FIG. 24-7. Eosinophilic granuloma in the jaws. **A,** Lesion in the molar apical region. **B,** Lesion in the molar alveolar region *(arrows)*. **C,** Lesions in the alveolar and basal bone *(arrows)*. **D** to **F,** Serial radiographs of a child with anomalous development of the permanent first molar associated with lesion *(arrow)* at 3½, 4½, and 8½ years of age respectively. (**A** courtesy Dr. H. Abrams, Los Angeles; **C** courtesy Dr. B. Gratt, Los Angeles.) *Continued.*

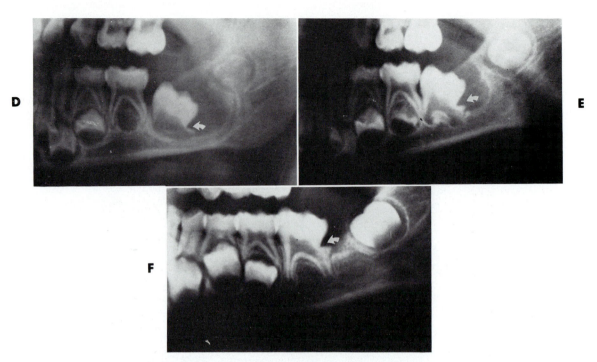

FIG. 24-7, cont'd. For legend see page 545.

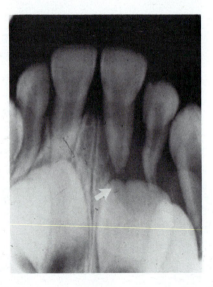

FIG. 24-8. Hand-Schüller-Christian disease *(arrow)* of the maxilla. (Courtesy Dr. H.G. Poyton, Toronto Ontario.)

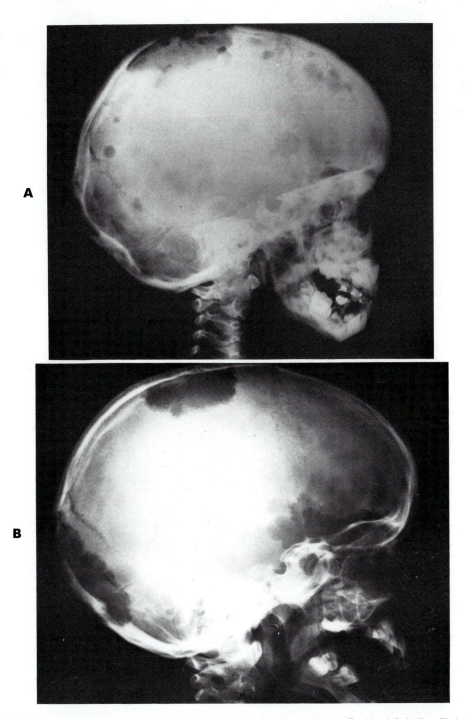

FIG. 24-9. Skull lesions of histiocytosis X. **A,** Letterer-Siwe disease. **B,** Hand-Schüller-Christian disease. (**A** and **B** courtesy Dr. H.G. Poyton, Toronto Ontario.)   *Continued.*

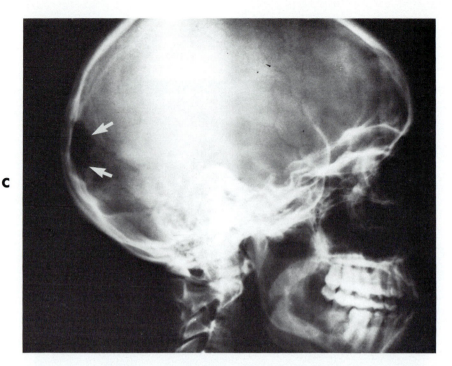

FIG. 24-9, cont'd. C, Eosinophilic granuloma *(arrows).*

odontitis. Finally, because eosinophilic granuloma appears as a pure radiolucency in bone, radiographic evidence of intrinsic septa or calcifications in a given lesion effectively precludes this entity from the differential diagnosis.

The multiplicity of lesions in many cases of eosinophilic granuloma has a tremendous effect in limiting the number of additional diagnostic considerations in a given differential diagnosis. There are, for example, multiple lesions in *cherubism,* but these occur only in the jaws. Accordingly, the presence of multifocal osteolytic lesions within numerous skeletal sites, as so often happens in eosinophilic granuloma, effectively rules out cherubism. Also, swelling of each angle of the mandible usually accompanies cherubism but not eosinophilic granuloma.

Management. A well-conceived radiologic differential diagnosis is critical to both recognition and proper management of this disease. Following the clinical examination and radiographic interpretation, it is important to biopsy the suspected lesion. Treatment of localized lesions usually consists of either surgical curettage or limited radiation therapy, usually in the range of 6 to 10 Gy.[21] Surgical management of jaw lesions is usually preferable because it has the lowest recurrence rate.[19] The earlier eosinophilic granuloma of the mandible

is diagnosed and controlled, the less jeopardy there is to an affected child's or adult's dentition. Delays in recognition may result in one or several teeth being unnecessarily extracted or sloughed as a result of lost bony support.[22] Disseminated disease is treated with chemotherapy.[50]

Osteoporosis

Osteoporosis is "a deficiency of bone tissue, per unit volume of bone."[22] Stated differently, osteoporosis represents a decrease in the physical density of bone, although the bone tissue remains histologically normal. There are two principal types of osteoporosis. The type of bone loss specifically associated with aging, that is, bone loss considered "normal for age," is *primary osteoporosis.* Radiologists have long known that the skeletons of older persons are generally less radiodense than the skeletons of younger persons of equivalent build. With age, bone mass in the skeleton undergoes fluctuation. Bone mass normally increases from infancy to about 35 to 40 years of age, at which time there begins a gradual and progressive decline, decreasing at the rate of about 8% per decade in women and 3% per decade in men.[15] The loss of bone mass with age is so gradual that it is virtually imperceptible until it reaches significant proportions.

Secondary osteoporosis is a reduction of histo-

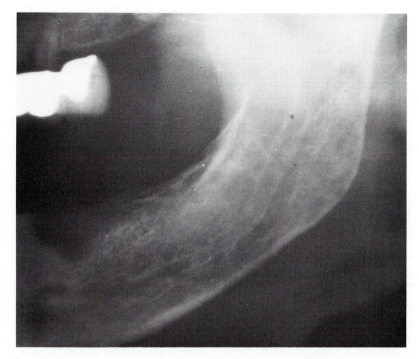

FIG. 24-10. Osteoporosis evident as a loss of the normal thickness and density of the inferior cortex of the mandible.

logically normal bone caused by abnormal or iatrogenic circumstances such as corticosteroid or heparin therapy or conditions such as malnutriton or scurvy.

Clinical features. The most important clinical manifestation of osteoporosis is fracture, usually of the spine or hip in postmenopausal women. The administration of estrogens after menopause prevents cortical and trabecular bone loss and reduces the incidence of fracture in later life.[14]

Radiographic features. The radiographic appearance of primary osteoporosis in older men and women is often referred to as "senile" osteoporosis or, if the affected person is female, "postmenopausal" osteoporosis. Postmenopausal osteoporosis reflects the influence of estrogen insufficiency on rarefaction of the bones. In women, postmenopausal osteoporosis is additive to senile osteoporosis in producing a recognizable radiographic effect.

When osteoporosis is prominent, the most demonstrable radiographic change is a thinning of bone cortices. Thus, the clinician may be able to appreciate osteoporosis in an elderly person by noting a reduction in the density and thickness of the inferior mandibular cortex in comparison with the jawbone in an adolescent or young adult (Fig. 24-

10). As seen on a panoramic film, such a method constitutes a rough appraisal of gross osteoporotic bone loss.

Cancellous (spongy) bone changes are even more difficult to assess than cortical changes. There is a reduction in the overall quantity of trabeculae within the medullary bone. Many of the trabeculae that remain retain their customary density. These trabeculae tend to occur along lines of bone stress. Thus, the greastest numerical reduction of mandibular trabeculae occurs deep within the body or ramus of the bone, as opposed to the alveolar processes where occlusal stresses transfer more readily from the teeth to the bone. Osteoporosis does not significantly alter the characteristic "stepladder" pattern of trabeculae commonly seen in normal alveolar bone.

Rickets and osteomalacia

Rickets and osteomalacia result from inadequate extracellular levels of calcium and inorganic phosphate, minerals required for new bone to calcify properly. Both abnormalities result from a nutritional deficiency of vitamin D. In these diseases, osteoid (the matrix for new bone formation) builds up in excessive amounts because of its failure to mineralize properly. The principal difference between these two diseases is the age of the patient when the disorder is first noted. Rickets occurs in infants and children, whereas osteomalacia develops in adults, persons in whom linear bone growth can no longer occur.

In order for a person to develop rickets or osteomalacia, one of two conditions must be met: lack of vitamin D in the diet or lack of exposure to adequate levels of ultraviolet light. Either a supply of vitamin D or adequate exposure to sunlight will prevent the disease. Ingestion of the vitamin itself is not necessary because the ultraviolet radiation in sunlight activates provitamin D_3, contained in human skin, for conversion to vitamin D_3. In the United States, vitamin D deficiency severe enough to cause noticeable osteomalacia is rare. Rickets, however, is occasionally still seen in certain poor, nutritionally deprived areas.[32]

Rickets and osteomalacia may also result from inadequate absorption or metabolism of vitamin D. Failure to absorb dietary vitamin D may be a result of various gastrointestinal malabsorption problems, such as partial gastrectomy, small bowel disease, or chronic biliary disease. In addition, chronic kidney disease, some types of liver disease, and anticonvulsant therapy may interfere with the metabolism of vitamin D.[32] The vitamin D metabolite 1,25-DHCC is required for calcium absorption from the gastrointestinal tract. These abnormalities have in common a resultant deficiency of the active vitamin D metabolite, and all may produce the characteristic metabolic effects of rickets or osteomalacia. Hypophosphatemic rickets results from renal loss of inorganic phosphate without significant changes in calcium metabolism.

Clinical features

Rickets. In the first 6 months of life, tetany or convulsions are the most common clinical problems resulting from the hypocalcemia of rickets. Later in infancy, the skeletal effects of the disease may be more clinically prominent. Craniotabes, a softening of the posterior of the parietal bones, may be the initial sign of the disease. The wrists and ankles typically swell. Children with rickets usually have short stature and deformity of the extremities. Development of the dentition is delayed, and the eruption rate of the teeth is retarded.[32]

Osteomalacia. Most patients with osteomalacia have some degree of bone pain. Exclusion of rheumatoid arthritis or muscle strain, therefore, may occasionally delay diagnosis of this condition. The majority of patients with osteomalacia have muscle weakness of varying severity. Other clinical features include a peculiar waddling or "penguin" gait, tetany, and greenstick bone fractures. The presence of greenstick fractures (in which one side of a bone is broken and the other side is bent but intact) in adults appears to be unique to osteomalacia. Dental abnormalities are not a feature of this condition.

Radiographic features

Rickets. The earliest and most prominent radiographic manifestation of rickets is a widening and fraying of the epiphyses of the long bones. Because of the relative softness of the altered bones, "bowing" is a characteristic deformity seen in weight-bearing bones such as the femur and tibia. Even after successful medical therapy, such deformities often remain permanently as lasting effects of rickets. Greenstick fractures occur in many patients having rickets.

Several radiographic defects occur in the teeth and jaws of patients with rickets, although all such conditions are uncommon. Some patients show a thinning of jaw cortical structures such as the inferior mandibular border, the walls of the mandibular canal, the lamina dura, or the follicular walls of developing teeth. Such cortical changes in the jaws occur later and are less prominent than the epiphyseal changes in the ribs and long bones. Within the spongy portion of the jaws, the fine trabeculae become reduced in number. In severe cases, the jaws appear overly radiolucent on radiographs made at standard exposure settings.

Rickets in infancy or early childhood may result in hypoplasia of developing dental enamel (Fig. 24-11). If the disease occurs before age 3 years, such enamel hypoplasia is fairly common.[22] Radiographs may reveal this early manifestation of rickets in unerupted and erupted teeth. Radiographs may also document retarded tooth eruption in early rickets.

Osteomalacia. Patients with osteomalacia have thin bones, a result of deficiencies in remodeling. However, this fact contributes little to diagnosis because cortical thickness is so variable among different persons with and without osteomalacia. The radiographic hallmark of osteomalacia in the skeleton is the *pseudofracture,* a poorly calcified, ribbonlike zone extending into bone at approximate right angles to the margin. Such defects appear to be actual fractures of the bone that show an attempt at healing. Osteoid forms in the defect, but, as there is no calcium available to be deposited in the osteoid, the healing process is not complete and the fracture remains apparent radiographically. Pseudofractures occur most commonly in the ribs,

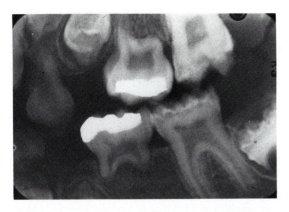

FIG. 24-11. Rickets may cause poor mineralization of the enamel. (Courtesy Dr. H.G. Poyton, Toronto.)

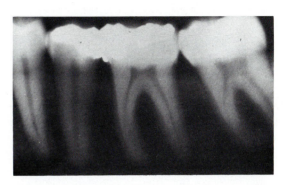

FIG. 24-12. Osteomalacia may cause a loss of density of the alveolar bone and lamina dura.

pelvis, and weight-bearing bones and occasionally in the mandible.

Within the jaws, there may be an overall radiolucent appearance on panoramic projections. Individual bony trabeculae may be sparse and unusually coarse on close examination of intraoral periapical radiographs. In tooth-bearing areas, the lamina dura may be especially thin in individuals with long-standing or severe osteomalacia (Fig. 24-12). When this is evident, hyperparathyroidism should be ruled out as the cause. In most cases of osteomalacia, it is well to remember that *no* radiographic manifestations are apparent in the jawbones. Osteomalacia does not alter the teeth because they are fully developed before the disease onset.

Hypophosphatasia

Hypophosphatasia is a rare inherited disorder in which patients have a low level of serum alkaline phosphatase activity and elevated urinary excretion of phosphoethanolamine.[11] The condition results in the formation of a defective bone matrix. The usual pattern of inheritance is an autosomal dominant mode of disease transmission.

Clinical features. The disease in individuals with homozygous involvement usually begins in utero, and affected patients often die within the first year. These infants demonstrate bowed limb bones and a marked deficiency of skull ossification. Many of these children die of chest infections. Individuals with heterozygote disease show the biochemical defects but a milder disease clinically. These children show poor growth, fractures, and deformities similar to rickets. The skull sutures

close early, resulting in bulging sutures and gyral markings on the internal surface of the skull because of continued underlying brain growth. The skull may assume a brachycephalic shape. There may be a history of fractures, delayed walking, or ricketslike deformities that heal spontaneously. About 85% of these children show premature loss of the primary teeth, particularly the incisors, and delayed eruption of the permanent dentition. This is often the first clinical sign of hypophosphatasia.[20]

Radiographic features. In young children with hypophosphatasia, the long bones show irregular defects and the skull shows poor calcification. In older children with premature closure of the skull sutures, there may be multiple lucent areas on skull films called "gyral" or "convolutional" markings. These markings resemble hammered copper and presumably result from increased intracranial pressure. In adults, there may be a generalized reduction in bone density.

Examination of the jaws reveals a generalized lucency of the maxilla and mandible. The cortical bone and lamina dura are thin, and the alveolar bone may be deficient. Both primary and permanent teeth characteristically show reduced enamel thickness and enlarged pulp chambers and root canals[27] (Fig. 24-13).

Renal osteodystrophy

In renal osteodystrophy, bone changes result from chronic renal failure. Patients with renal osteodystrophy have a defect in the hydroxylation of 25-HCC (a vitamin D metabolite) to 1,25-DHCC, a process that normally occurs in the kidney. The 1,25-DHCC is responsible for the active transport of calcium in the duodenum and upper jejunum. These patients often have hypocalcemia as a result of impaired calcium absorption and hyperphosphatemia resulting from reduction in renal phosphorus excretion. The hypocalcemia, in turn, results in secondary hyperparathyroidism with markedly increased levels of serum parathyroid hormone. Systemic acidosis frequently occurs with this condition.

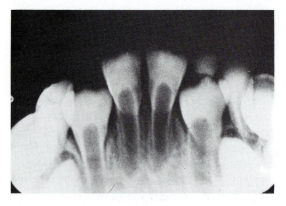

FIG. 24-13. Hypophosphatasia results in teeth with thin enamel, thin root dentin, and large pulp chambers.

Clinical features. The clinical features of renal osteodystrophy are those of chronic renal failure. In children, there may be growth retardation and frequent bone fractures. Adults may experience a gradual softening and bowing of the bones.

Radiographic features. The radiographic features of renal osteodystrophy are quite variable. Some changes are consistent with hyperparathyroidism, including generalized loss of bone density and thinning of bony cortices. The lamina dura may disappear, and the thickness of the cortex at the mandibular angle may be reduced.[5] The rate of bone growth in children is generally slow, and its morphology may be abnormal. Morphometric studies of the mandible viewed on panoramic radiographs also show an increase in the medullary space at the expense of the trabeculae.[45] Other bones may show areas of sclerosis (Fig. 24-14).

Hypophosphatemia

Hypophosphatemia (also called vitamin D–resistant rickets) is a familial (genetic) disease. This condition involves renal tubular disorders such that there is excessive loss of phosphorus. It is inherited in an X-linked dominant fashion. Thus, female patients transmit the disease to half their sons and half their daughters; male patients pass the con-

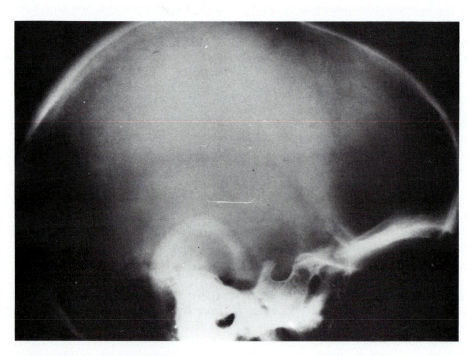

FIG. 24-14. Renal osteodystrophy revealing changes in the trabecular bone of the skull. (Courtesy Dr. H.G. Poyton, Toronto Ontario.)

dition to all their daughters and none of their sons. Hypophosphatemia affects males more severely than females.

Clinical features. Children with hypophosphatemia show reduced growth and ricketslike bony changes. These include bowing of the legs, enlarged epiphyses, and skull changes. Adults have bone pains, muscle weakness, and vertebral fractures.

Radiographic features. In children with hypophosphatemia, radiographic findings are indistinguishable from those of rickets. In adults, the long bones may show persistent deformity, fractures, or pseudofractures. Examination of the jaws of children reveals osteoporotic bone with thinned lamina dura and dental crypts. The teeth may be poorly formed, with thin enamel caps and enlarged pulp chambers and root canals. In addition, there is a high incidence of periapical and periodontal abscesses. When periodontal infections do occur in children with hypophosphatemia, the lesions tend to spread diffusely through the bone.[46] The occurrence of such apparently "uncaused" cases of periapical rarefying osteitis in hypophosphatemia has in the past been a puzzle because the involved teeth are so often free of caries. The most plausible explanation for the periapical lesions is that enlarged pulp horns in these teeth reach nearly to the dentinoenamel junction, and there may be invasion by microorganisms in areas of hypoplastic enamel, leading to pulpal necrosis long before typical caries are recognized.[18] An alternative hypothesis is that the apical lesions are primarily periodontal, owing to the presence of defective cementum.

Progressive systemic sclerosis

Progressive systemic sclerosis (PSS) is a generalized connective tissue disease that causes sclerosis of the skin and other tissues. "Scleroderma" has been used as a descriptive name for this disease that was once thought to be predominantly cutaneous. It is now known, however, that involvement of the gastrointestinal tract, heart, lungs, or kidneys usually results in more serious complications, thus the name "progressive systemic sclerosis." The cause of the disease is unknown.

Clinical features. In most persons with moderate to severe PSS, the involved skin areas have a thickened, hidebound quality. Clinicians note lack of mobility of the skin over the underlying soft tissues, and because of the tautness of facial skin, patients may be able to manage only limited mouth opening. Patients with diffuse disease are also likely to have xerostomia; increased numbers of decayed, missing, or filled teeth; and carious lesions. Further, patients with systemic disease are more likely to have deeper pockets and higher gingivitis scores than patients with disease restricted to the distal extremities.[49] Patients with cardiac and pulmonary problems may have varying degrees of heart failure and respiratory insufficiencies. Renal involvement usually leads to some degree of uremia, with or without hypertension.

PSS is a disease of middle age. The greatest incidence occurs between the ages of 30 and 50 years. It is seen rarely in adolescence or the elderly. Women are affected about three times as often as men.

Radiographic features. The most common oral radiographic manifestation of PSS is an increase in the width of the periodontal ligament (PDL) spaces around the teeth[1,47] (Fig. 24-15). Approximately two thirds of patients with PSS show this change. The PDL spaces affected by PSS usually are at least twice as thick as normal.

Periodontal ligament space change associated with PSS usually affects both anterior and posterior teeth, although the changes are more pronounced around the posterior teeth. There is no significant difference between the incidence of involvement of the maxillary and the mandibular periodontium. The lamina dura around affected teeth remains intact and uninvolved, regardless of any PDL space changes. The specific cause of the PDL space thickening is unknown. Despite the widening of the PDL spaces, the clinician will find that involved teeth are often not mobile and their gingival attachments are usually intact.

A radiographic feature of great potential signif-

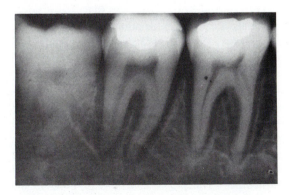

FIG. 24-15. Progressive systemic sclerosis may be manifested as a marked thickening of the periodontal ligament space.

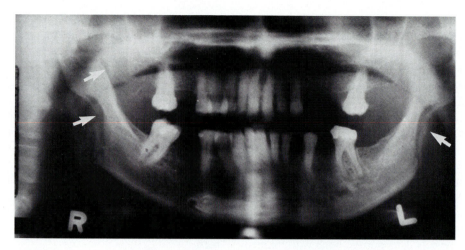

FIG. 24-16. Progressive systemic sclerosis demonstrating a loss of bone in the region of each angle of the mandible *(arrows)*. Note also the amputated right coronoid process *(arrow)*.

icance in some cases of PSS is an unusual pattern of mandibular erosions involving the angles, coronoid process, digastric region, or condyles (Fig. 24-16).[47,49] This type of resorption is typically bilateral and fairly symmetrical. Most of these erosive borders are smooth and sharply defined. In three of six patients with angle resorption in one study, follow-up radiographs were available. In all three cases, progression of the resorption occurred. Further, the coronoid process was either resorbed or amputated in two of six patients who demonstrated concomitant angle resorption and in another patient who did not have angle resorption. Thus, almost half of the patients with the PDL thickening also had some erosive bone changes. This finding suggests that mandibular angle and coronoid erosions, which are apparently asymptomatic, are more widespread in patients having PSS than was previously thought.

Differential diagnosis. The PDL space thickening also occurs in association with *osteosarcoma* of the jaws. However, PDL space thickening with osteosarcoma is not likely to occur evenly around a major portion of a root surface as is PSS involvement. In addition, the likely occurrence of interdental bone destruction associated with a sarcoma would also reduce the likelihood of diagnostic confusion with PSS.

Management. The aforementioned thickening of PDL spaces does not seem to present any clinical difficulties. The progressive loss of bone in the region of the mandibular angle, however, is more serious. It is important to warn patients with PSS

that fracture can occur in this weakened bone. It is wise to obtain initial and periodic panoramic radiography in all patients with PSS to assess mandibular integrity.

Sickle cell anemia

Sickle cell anemia is an autosomal recessive, chronic, hemolytic blood disorder. Patients with this disorder have abnormal hemoglobin (deoxygenated hemoglobins) that under low oxygen tension results in sickling of the red blood cells. The latter have a reduced capacity to carry oxygen to the tissues and, because of damage to their membrane lipids and proteins, adhere to vascular endothelium and clog capillaries.[44] The spleen traps and readily destroys these abnormal red cells. The hematopoietic system responds to the resultant anemia by increasing the production of red blood cells, which requires compensatory hyperplasia of the bone marrow. The expansion of the bone marrow at the expense of spongy bone is the primary radiographic manifestation of sickle cell anemia. Other, rarer hemolytic anemias, such as thalassemia, may also produce similar radiographic evidence in the bones.

The homozygous form of sickle cell anemia occurs in approximately 1 in every 400 black Americans. Although the gene is present in the heterozygous state in about 6% to 8% of blacks, those who manifest this form of the sickle cell trait do not show related clinical findings.

Clinical features. Although symptoms and signs vary considerably, most patients with the disease normally manifest mild, chronic features. There are long, quiet spells of hemolytic latency, occasionally punctuated by exacerbations known as sickle cell crises. During the crisis state, patients often experience severe abdominal, muscle, and joint pain; have a high temperature; and may even undergo circulatory collapse. During milder periods, the patient may complain of fatigability, weakness, shortness of breath, and muscle and joint pain. As in the other chronic anemias, the heart is usually enlarged and there may be a murmur. The disease occurs mostly in children and adolescents. It is compatible with a normal life span, although many patients die of complications of the disease before the age of 40 years.[29]

Radiographic features. The extent of bone changes in sickle cell anemia relates to the degree of hyperplasia of the bone marrow. The resultant thinning of individual cancellous trabeculae and cortices shows best in the vertebral bodies, long bones, skull, and jaws. The skull especially demonstrates the condition as a widening of the diploic space and thinning of the inner and outer tables (Fig. 24-17). There may be a loss of the outer table and a hair-on-end appearance in about 5% of cases.[22] Small areas of infarction may be present within bones after blockage of the microvasculature and are seen radiographically as areas of localized bone sclerosis.[38] Osteomyelitis may complicate sickle cell anemia if infection begins in an area of pronounced hypovascularity. There may also be retardation of generalized bone growth.[34]

The radiographic manifestations of sickle cell anemia in the jaws of adults include general osteoporosis (Fig. 24-18).[29,34] In most cases, the change is mild or moderate, with extreme radiographic manifestations being unusual. As in other bones, the osteoporosis in the jaws is principally a response to the pressure of the expanding marrow within the bone. To a lesser extent, thinning of cortical plates is also responsible for the overall radiolucent appearance of the jaws. Deep within the spongy portions of bone, thin, delicate trabeculae are particularly prone to such pressure resorption, with the heavier internal bony architecture relatively less affected. Portions of bones subjected to greater stresses are more resistant to resorption; in the jaws, the alveolar processes are particularly subject to heavy chewing forces. In the tooth-bearing portions of the jaws, the trabeculae in sickle cell anemia become especially coarse in relation to the rest of the bone and form an accen-

tuated stepladder pattern.[38] These findings of reduced density and coarse trabeculation are not specific to sickle cell anemia.[29]

A recent examination of jaw manifestations of sickle cell anemia in children found the incidence of moderate and severe mandibular changes to be much higher than that reported in earlier studies.[37] Most of these patients showed radiographic evidence of severe bone porosis, and almost half had significant alveolar bone loss. All the children with sickle cell anemia in this study demonstrated noticeable oral radiographic changes, whereas a control population with the same criteria revealed no changes. The authors suggest the feasibility of using dental radiographs as a screening test for the detection of sickle cell anemia. Others have also commented on the greater radiographic sensitivity of jaw changes compared with those of the skull or long bones.[35] Some have found that the marrow hyperplasia associated with sickle cell anemia causes a protrusion of the maxillary alveolar ridge.[6] Dental radiography may thus be useful in the detection of sickle cell anemia in black children and adolescents.

Thalassemia

Thalassemia (also known as *Cooley's anemia, Mediterranean anemia,* and *erythroblastic anemia*) is a hereditary disorder that results in a defect in hemoglobin synthesis. This defect may involve either the alpha- or beta-globulin genes. The resultant red blood cells have a reduced hemoglobin content, are thin, and have a shortened life span. The heterozygous form of the disease (thaslassemia minor) is mild. The homozygous form (thalassemia major) may be severe. A less severe form, thalassemia intermedia, also occurs.

Clinical features. In the severe form of the disease, the onset is in infancy and the survival time may be short. The face develops prominent cheekbones and a protrusive premaxilla. The milder form of the disease occurs in adults.

Radiographic features. The radiographic features of thalassemia generally result from expansion of the ineffective bone marrow to produce more red cells. There is a generalized lucency of the long bones with cortical thinning. Pathologic features may occur. In the skull, there is a marked thickening of the diploic space, especially in the frontal region. The skull shows a generalized granular appearance. Occasionally, radial striations (hair-on-end effect) may develop (Fig. 24-19). The

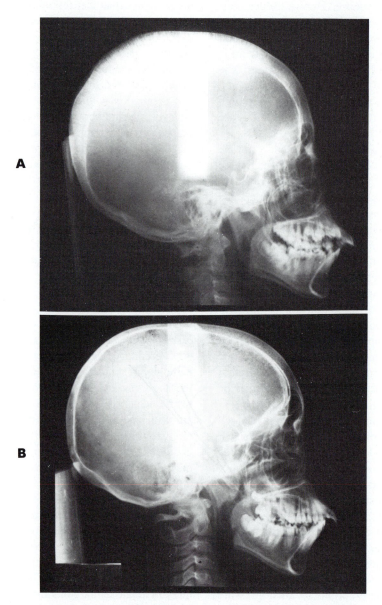

FIG. 24-17. **A,** Sickle cell anemia showing a thickened diploic space and thinning of the skull cortex. **B,** Normal skull for comparison. (**B** courtesy Dr. B. Sarnat, Los Angeles.)

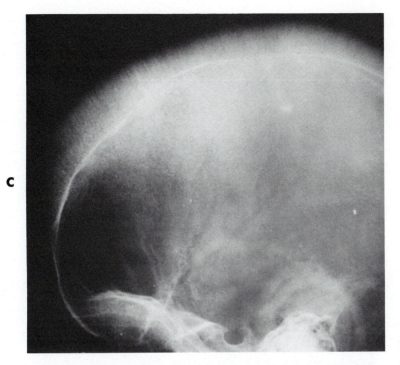

FIG. 24-17, cont'd.   C, Skull showing the "hair-on-end" effect of the cortex. (**C** courtesy Dr. H.G. Poyton, Toronto.)

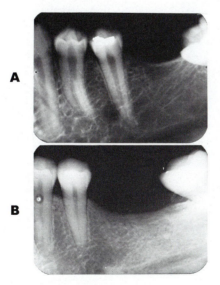

FIG. 24-18.   A, Sickle cell anemia showing enlarged marrow spaces in the mandible. **B,** Normal mandible for comparison. (**A** and **B** courtesy Dr. B. Sarnat, Los Angeles.)

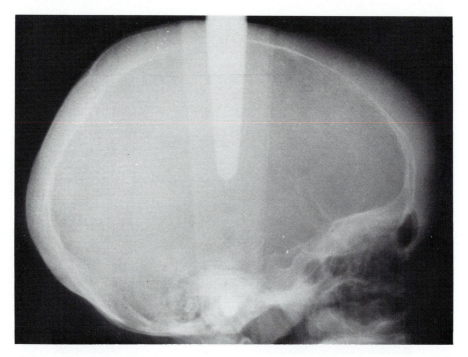

FIG. 24-19. Thalassemia showing a granular appearance of the skull and thickening of the diploic space. (Courtesy Dr. H.G. Poyton, Toronto.)

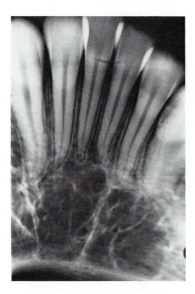

FIG. 24-20. Thalassemia showing thickened trabecular plates and enlarged marrow spaces. (Courtesy Dr. H.G. Poyton, Toronto.)

soft tissue overgrowth within the marrow spaces retards pneumatization of the paranasal sinuses, especially the maxillary sinus.[7]

Examination of the jaws reveals a generalized lucency, with thinning of the cortical borders. The marrow spaces are large, and the trabeculae are large and coarse (Fig. 24-20). The lamina dura is thin, and the roots of the teeth may be short. The premaxilla is often prominent, resulting in malocclusion.[33]

REFERENCES

1. Alexandridis C, White SC: Periodontal ligament changes in patients with progressive systemic sclerosis, *Oral Med Oral Pathol* 58:113-118, 1984.
2. Bilezikian JP: Hyper-and hypoparathyroidism. In Rakel R, editor: *Conn's current therapy,* Philadelphia, 1985, WB Saunders.
3. Boonstra CE, Jackson CE: Serum calcium survey for hyperparathyroidism: results in 50,000 clinic patients, *Am J Clin Pathol* 55:523-526, 1971.
4. Bottomley WK, Gabriel SA, Corio RL, et al: Histiocytosis X: report of an oral soft tissue lesion without bony involvement, *Oral Surg Oral Med Oral Pathol* 63:228-231, 1987.
5. Bras J, van Ooij CP, Abraham-Inpijn L, et al: Radiographic interpretation of the mandibular anglar cortex: a diagnostic tool in metabolic bone loss: II, renal osteodystrophy, *Oral Surg* 53:647-650, 1982.
6. Brown DL, Sebes JI: Sickle cell gnathopathy: radiologic assessment, *Oral Surg Oral Med Oral Pathol* 61:653-656, 1986.
7. Caffey J: Cooley's anemia: a review of the roentgenographic findings in the skeleton, *Am J Roentgenol* 78:381-391, 1957.

8. Cooper D, Wood L: Hyperthyroidism. In Rakel R, editor: *Conn's current therapy,* Philadelphia, 1985, WB Saunders.

9. Cranin AN, Rockman R: Oral symptoms in histiocytosis X, *J Am Dent Assoc* 103:412-416, 1981.

10. Domboski M: Eosinophilic granuloma of bone manifesting mandibular involvement, *Oral Med Oral Pathol* 50:116-123, 1980.

11. Eastman JR, Bixler D: Clinical, laboratory, and genetic investigations of hypophosphatasia: support for autosomal dominant inheritance with homozygous lethality, *J Craniofac Genet Dev Biol* 3:213-234, 1983.

12. Edeiken J, Hodes PJ: *Roentgen diagnosis of diseases of bone,* ed 2, Baltimore, 1973, Williams & Wilkins.

13. Frensilli J, Stoner R, Hinrichs E: Dental changes of idiopathic hypoparathyroidism, *J Oral Surg* 29:727-731, 1971.

14. Gallagher C: Osteoporosis. In Rakel R, editor: *Conn's current therapy,* Philadelphia, 1985, WB Saunders.

15. Garn S, Rohmann C, Wagner B: Bone loss as a general phenomenon in man, *Fed Proc* 26:1729-1736, 1967.

16. Glynne A, Hunter I, Thomson J: Pseudohypoparathyroidism with paradoxical increase in hypocalcemic seizures due to long-term anticonvulsant therapy, *Postgrad Med J* 48:632-636, 1972.

17. Gorsky M, Silverman S, Lozada F, Kushner J: Histiocytosis X: occurrence and oral involvement in six adolescent and adult patients, *Oral Med Oral Pathol* 55:24-28, 1983.

18. Harris R, Sullivan H: Dental sequelae in deciduous dentition in vitamin-D resistant rickets, *Aust Dent J* 5:200-203, 1960.

19. Hartman KS: Histiocytosis X: a review of 114 cases with oral involvement, *Oral Med Oral Pathol* 49:38-54, 1980.

20. Jedrychowski JR, Duperon D: Childhood hypophosphatasia with oral manifestations, *J Oral Med* 34:18-22, 1979.

21. Jones RD, Pillsbury HC: Histiocytosis X of the head and neck, *Laryngoscope* 94:1031-1035, 1984.

22. Keller EE, Stafne EC, Gibilisco JA: Oral radiographic manifestations of systemic disease. In Gibilisco JA, Turlington EG, editors: *Stafne's oral roentgenographic diagnosis,* ed 5, Philadelphia, 1985, WB Saunders.

23. Kosowicz J, Rzymski K: Abnormalities of tooth development in pituitary dwarfism, *Oral Med Oral Pathol* 44:853-863, 1977.

24. Lamey PJ: Darwazeh AM, Frier BM: Oral disorders associated with diabetes mellitus, *Diabetic Med* 9:410-416, 1992.

25. Lichtenstein L: *Bone tumors,* ed 4, St Louis, 1972, Mosby.

26. Loh HS, Quah TC: Histiocytosis X (Langerhans-cell histiocytosis) of the palate: case report, *Aust Dent J* 35:117-120, 1990.

27. Macfarland JD, Swart JGN: Developmental aspects of hypophosphatasia: a case report, family study, and literature review, *Oral Med Oral Pathol* 67:521-526, 1989.

28. Mackenzie RS, Millard HD: Interrelated effects of diabetes, arteriosclerosis and calculus on alveolar bone loss, *J Am Dent Assoc* 54:191-198, 1963.

29. Mourshed F, Tuckson C: A study of radiographic features of the jaws in sickle-cell anemia, *Oral Med Oral Pathol* 37:812-819, 1974.

30. Murrah VA: Diabetes mellitus and associated oral manifestations: a review, *J Oral Pathol* 14:271-281, 1985.

31. Myllarniemi S, Lenko HL, Perheentupa J: Dental maturity in hypopituitarism, and dental response to substitution treatment, *Scand J Dent Res* 86:307-312, 1978.

32. Paterson CR: *Metabolic disorders of bone,* Oxford, 1974, Blackwell Scientific.

33. Poyton HG, Davey KW: Thalassemia: changes visible in radiographs used in dentistry, *Oral Med Oral Pathol* 25:564-576, 1968.

34. Prowler J, Smith E: Dental bone changes occurring in sickle-cell diseases and abnormal hemoglobin traits, *Radiology* 65:762-769, 1955.

35. Robinson IB, Sarnat BG: Roentgen studies of the maxillae and mandible in sickle-cell anemia, *Radiology* 58:517-521, 1952.

36. Rosenberg E, Guralnick W: Hyperparathyroidism: a review of 220 proved cases with special emphasis on findings in the jaws, *Oral Med Oral Pathol* 15(suppl 2):84-92, 1962.

37. Sanger RG, Bystrom EB: Radiographic bone changes in sickle cell anemia, *J Oral Med* 32:32-37, 1977.

38. Sanger RG, Greer R, Averbach R: Differential diagnosis of some simple osseous lesions associated with sickle-cell anemia, *Oral Med Oral Pathol* 43:538-545, 1977.

39. Sigala J, Silverman S, Brody H, Kushner J: Dental involvement in histiocytosis, *Oral Surg* 33:42-48, 1972.

40. Silverman S, Ware W, Gillody C: Dental aspects of hyperparathyroidism, *Oral Med Oral Pathol* 26:184-189, 1968.

41. Sleeper EL: Eosinophilic granuloma: its relationship to Hand-Schuller-Christian and Letterer-Siwe diseases, with emphasis on oral symptoms and findings, *Oral Med Oral Pathol* 4:896-918, 1951.

42. Stahl SS: Roentgenographic and bacteriologic aspects of periodontal changes in diabetics, *J Periodontol* 19:130-132, 1948.

43. Steinbach HL, Gordan GS, Eisenberg E, et al: Primary hyperparathyroidism: a correlation of roentgen, clinical and pathologic features, *Am J Roentgenol* 86:329-343, 1961.

44. Steinberg M: Sickle cell disease. In Rakel R, editor: *Conn's current therapy,* Philadelphia, 1985, WB Saunders.

45. Syrjanen S, Lampainen E: Mandibular changes in panoramic radiographs of patients with end stage renal disease, *Dentomaxillofac Radiol* 12:51-56, 1983.

46. Trapnell DH, Boweman JE: *Dental manifestation of systemic disease,* London, 1973, Butterworth.

47. White SC, Frey NW, Blaschke DD, et al: Oral radiographic changes in patients with progressive systemic sclerosis (scleroderma), *J Am Dent Assoc* 94:1178-1182, 1977.

48. Whitehouse GH: Histiocytosis X: radiological bone changes, *Proc R Soc Med* 64:333-334, 1971.

49. Wood RE, Lee P: Analysis of the oral manifestations of systemic sclerosis (scleroderma), *Oral Med Oral Pathol* 65:172-178, 1988.

50. Zuendell MT, Bowers DF, Kramer RN: Recurrent histiocytosis X with mandibular lesions, *Oral Med Oral Pathol* 58:420-423, 1984.

25

in collaboration with DONALD D. BLASCHKE, and including a section on

Arthrography by ALAN G. LURIE

Temporomandibular Joint

The temporomandibular joint (TMJ or cranio-mandibular joint) is one of the most important joints in the body. Disorders of the TMJ are the cause of most commmon chronic orofacial pain. They are a subclassification of musculoskeletal and rheumatologic disorders. Studies of the incidence of TMJ disorders show that from 28% to 86% of the population display one or more signs or symptoms of TMJ disorder.[88] Symptoms are found equally in men and women, most frequently in the 20- to 40-year-old age group, although females seek treatment about three times more frequently. In many instances, clinical signs are transitory and treatment is not indicated. About 5% of patients have such severe signs and symptoms that TMJ function is compromised and care is indicated.

Optimal radiographic visualization is becoming increasingly important as TMJ disorders are becoming better understood. Imaging of the TMJ is indicated when the clinical examination, history, or both indicate that a recent or progressive pathologic joint condition exists. Examples include trauma, significant dysfunction or alteration in range of motion, sensory or motor alterations, or significant changes in occlusion (anterior or posterior open bite, mandibular shift). Joint imaging is not indicated for joint sounds in the absence of other signs or symptoms.[61]

RADIOGRAPHIC ANATOMY OF TMJ
Condyle

The condyle is a bony ellipsoid structure connected to the ramus of the mandible by a narrow bony isthmus or neck (Fig. 25-1). The condyle is longer lateromedially than anteroposteriorly. The typical condyle has a superior surface that is markedly convex from front to back and gently convex from side to side (pole to pole). The posterior sur-face is also convex, whereas that of the anterior condylar surface is either convex, flat, or concave. Many condyles have a pronounced ridge running from lateral to medial, marking the anteroinferior limits of the articulating area. This ridge is the upper limit of the pterygoid fovea, a small depression on the anterior surface at the junction of the condyle and neck. This is where the superior head of the lateral pterygoid muscle attaches. It should not be mistaken for an osteophyte (spur), which would indicate arthritic joint disease. The average lateromedial condylar length is 20 mm; the anteroposterior diameter of the condyle is about 8 to 10 mm.[122] Although the mandibular and temporal components of the TMJ are calcified by 6 months of age, complete calcification of the cortical borders may not be completed until age 20. Because of this, one may occasionally see radiographs of condyles in children that show little or no evidence of a cortical border. Autopsy studies on young TMJs have revealed condylar articulating surfaces that are smooth and regular in form. A general tendency toward articular surface flattening is associated with stressful loading of the TMJ secondary to lost posterior dental support and increasing age. The condyle is covered in a layer of fibrocartilage that is not seen radiographically.

The long axis of the condyle is not perpendicular to the sagittal plane of the skull. Rather, it is usually angled backward so that the angle formed by the long axis of the condyles and the sagittal plane is between 15 and 33 degrees. Projections of the axes of the two condyles intersect near the anterior border of the foramen magnum (Fig. 25-2).[8,98,122] This information is important to the radiologist, who must adjust the position of the patient's head to align the beam with the long axis of the condyle when performing TMJ tomography.

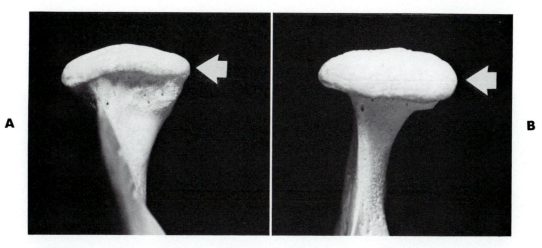

FIG. 25-1. Mandibular condyle. The medial pole *(arrow)* is on the right in each case. **A,** Anterior aspect. **B,** Superior aspect.

Mandibular fossa

The mandibular (glenoid) fossa is composed of the articular fossa and the articular eminence of the temporal bone (Fig. 25-3, *A*). The most lateral aspect of the eminence consists of a protuberance, the articular tubercle. This is principally a ligamentous attachment and accounts for the bulk of the eminence image seen on lateral radiographs, especially on transcranial views. The tubercle is lateral to the articulating surface, and a pronounced tubercular convexity seen radiographically should not be confused with the convexity of the eminence that lies more medially in the joint. The articular tubercle is the anatomic junction where the root of the zygomatic process joins the temporal squama. Like the condyle, the mandibular fossa is covered with a thin layer of fibrocartilage.

The mandibular fossa is on the inferior side of the squamous part of the temporal bone that forms a small portion of the floor of the middle cranial fossa. This thin (translucent) oval layer of cortical bone is all that separates the joint from the intracranial subdural space. The thinness of the roof of the articular fossa, as well as the thinness of the fibrous tissue covering the fossa, suggests that it is not a functional part of the articulation.[66] It is the thicker articular eminence that functions as the stress-bearing part of the joint.

There is considerable variation between individuals in the depth of their articular fossae, varying from rather shallow to deep. The depth of the fossa is a function of the development of the articular eminence. Very young infants do not have a definite eminence and therefore may not demonstrate a fossa at all. However, the articular eminence starts to develop during the first 3 years and reaches mature shape at the time of the mixed dentition. The dimensions of the fossa and eminence vary considerably from person to person.

The posterior limit of the joint is formed by the squamotympanic fissure and its medial extension, the petrotympanic fissure. The superoanterior border of this suture often forms a distinct lip laterally, the postglenoid tubercle (immediately anterior to the external acoustic meatus). Below the fissure, the tympanic portion of the temporal bone forms the major portion of the external auditory canal anterior wall. All aspects of the temporal component of the joint may be pneumatized with small air cells derived from the mastoid air cell complex. Such pneumatization of the articular eminence is seen radiographically in approximately 2% of patients (Fig. 25-3, *B*).[44,104]

Interarticular disk

The interarticular disk (meniscus) is a fibrous connective tissue structure located between the condylar head and articular fossa, dividing the joint into two compartments, one above the other (Fig. 25-4). The disk itself normally occupies only the anterior half of the joint space, with its posterior retrodiskal attachments filling the posterior half. The disk and the posterior attachments are generally referred to as the "soft tissue component" of the TMJ.

When a normal disk is sectioned sagittally

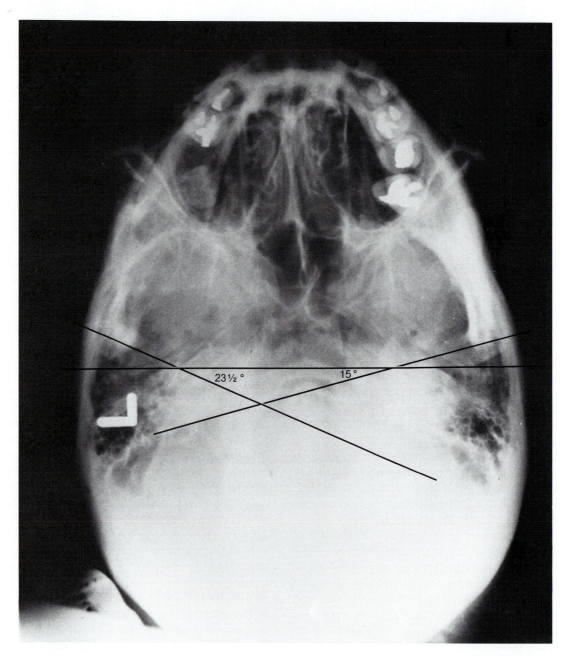

FIG. 25-2. Tracing of angles between the long axis of each condyle and the coronal plane made on a submentovertex projection. For tomographic views the patient should be rotated a corresponding amount to assure an optimum radiographic view of each TMJ.

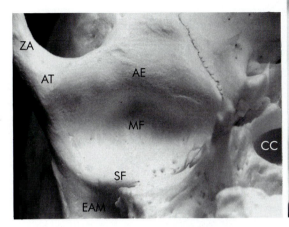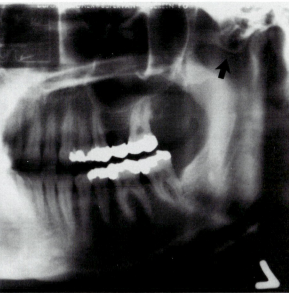

FIG. 25-3. A, Base view of the skull showing the mandibular fossa. *AE,* Articular eminence; *AT,* articular tubercle; *CC,* carotid canal; *EAM,* external auditory meatus; *MF,* mandibular fossa; *SF,* squamotympanic fissure; *ZA,* zygomatic arch. **B,** Pneumatization of the articular eminence with a mastoid air cell (panoramic view). (**B** courtesy Drs. D. Tyndall and S. R. Matteson, Chapel Hill, NC.)

through its center, it appears as a biconcave structure. The central part is the thinnest (1.5 mm), the posterior band is thickest (3 mm), and the anterior band is 2.5 mm. The thin portion in the middle is the area of the disk that normally serves as the articulating cushion between the condyle and the articular eminence. The anterior border of the disk is attached to the superior head of the lateral pterygoid muscle. The posterior band of the disk attaches to the posterior retrodiskal tissues. This junction lies within 10 degrees of vertical above the head of the condyle in normal individuals.[21]

The disk plays a critical role in the function of the temporomandibular joint. As the jaw opens, the condyle moves downward and forward from the mandibular fossa. As the condyle translates forward, the disk also moves forward so that its thin central portion remains between the articulating convexities of the condylar head and the artic-

ular eminence. Laterally and medially the disk is attached to the poles of the condyle, thus helping to assure passive movement of the disk with the condyle. Thus, the condyle and disk both translate forward together under the articular eminence. As the jaw opens, the condyle also rotates against the lower surface of the disk. Upon jaw closing, this process reverses, with the disk moving back with the condyle into the mandibular fossa.

Posterior attachment

The posterior attachment (retrodiskal tissues or zone) consists of a bilaminar region of vascularized and innervated loose fibroelastic tissue. The superior lamina, rich in elastin, inserts into the posterior wall of the mandibular fossa. This stretches and allows the disk to move forward with translation of the condyle. The inferior lamina of the posterior attachment attaches to the posterior sur-

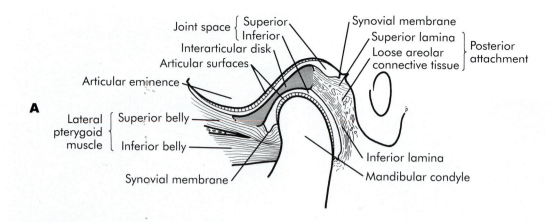

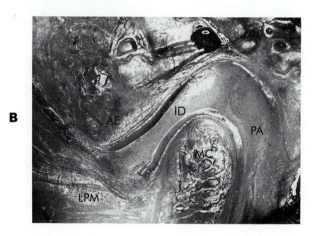

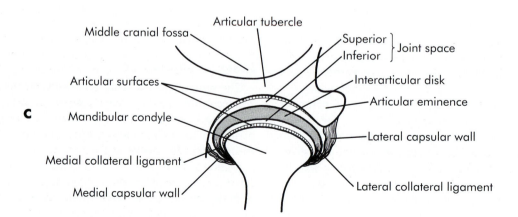

FIG. 25-4. TMJ anatomy. **A** represents a lateral view. **B** is a sectioned cadaver specimen from the same orientation. **C** represents a coronal view. *AE*, Articular eminence; *ID*, interarticular disk; *LPM*, lateral pterygoid muscle; *MC*, mandibular condyle; *PA*, posterior attachment. (Courtesy Dr. W. K. Solberg, UCLA School of Dentistry, Los Angeles.)

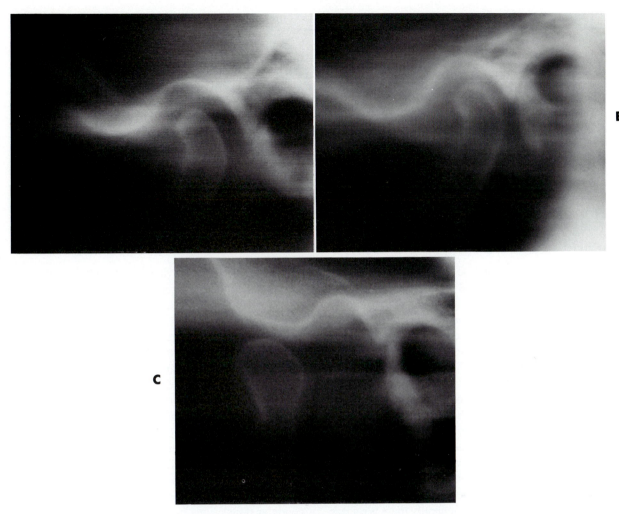

FIG. 25-5. Corrected lateral tomograms. **A,** Closed-mouth view, with the condyles concentrically positioned. **B,** Temporomandibular joint with the condyle retruded. **C,** TMJ with the mouth open and the condyle translated forward just anterior to the articular eminence.

face of the condyle. The posterior attachment is covered with a synovial membrane that secretes the synovial fluid that lubricates the joint. As the condyle moves forward, the tissues of the posterior attachment expand in volume, primarily due to venous distension.[117] As the disk moves forward, tension is produced in the elastic posterior attachment. This tension is thought to be responsible for the smooth recoil of the disk posteriorly as the jaw closes.

Muscles

Of the many muscles involved in mandibular motion, the lateral pterygoid muscle is intimately involved in condylar and disk movement. The inferior belly of the lateral pterygoid inserts into the anterior border of the condylar fovea. It is active primarily during jaw opening, protrusion, and lateral jaw movements. The superior belly of the lateral pterygoid inserts into both the anterior border of the capsule (and thus disk) as well as into the condylar fovea. It is active primarily during jaw closing and is thought to maintain a tension on the disk to balance the retrodiskal elastin.[15]

Joint bony relationships

"Joint space" is the radiographic term for the crescent-shaped radiolucent area between the bony structures of the temporomandibular joint (Fig. 25-5, *A*). This space contains the disk and posterior attachment when the teeth are in occlusion. Only with magnetic resonance imaging (MRI) is it pos-

TABLE 25-1. Comparative capabilities of imaging modalities for the TMJ

| | Disk | | | | Condyle | |
	Position	Perforation	Dynamics	Shape	Cortication	Position
Tomography	No	No	No	No	Yes	Yes
Arthrography	Yes	Yes	Yes	+ / −	Yes	Yes
Transcranial	No	No	No	No	+ / −	No
Transorbital	No	No	No	No	Yes	No
Skull views	No	No	No	No	+ / −	No
Panoramics	No	No	No	No	+ / −	No
MRI	Yes	Yes	Yes	Yes	Yes	Yes
CT	+ / −	No	No	No	Yes	Yes

+ / −, Indicates that the modality offers some information but less than alternative modalities.

sible to discern the precise position of the disk and its posterior attachment in relation to the condyle. A comparison of the radiographic dimensions of several portions of the joint space is often used by clinicians as a guide to determine the position of the condyle within the fossa. Tomograms are a more reliable measure of condylar position than transcranial radiographs.[76]

The position of the condyle within the fossa is variable. The condyle is said to be concentrically positioned when the anterior and posterior aspects of the radiolucent joint space are uniform in width. The condyle is retruded when the posterior joint space width is less than the anterior (Fig. 25-5, *B*), and protruded when the posterior joint space is larger than the anterior. Generally there is a space of about 1.5 to 2 mm between the anterior surface of the condyle and the eminence, 2 to 2.5 mm between the condyle and the roof of the fossa, and 1.5 to 3.2 mm between the condyle and the posterosuperior aspect of the fossa.[15] The diagnostic significance of mild or even moderate condylar retrusion or protrusion is not entirely clear, considering the variability of condyle positions in clinically normal individuals.[8,78] About one half to two thirds of asymptomatic individuals display condylar concentricity, but the rest show substantial variability. This distribution of nonconcentric condyles is more anterior in men and posterior in women. Moderately posterior and anterior condyles may be variants of normal TMJ anatomy and function. It is often helpful to assess the joint space by comparison with the contralateral joint.

Condylar movement

The condyle undergoes a complex movement as the mandible opens. There is both a downward and forward translation (sliding) of the condyle as well as a hingelike rotatory movement. The rotatory movement occurs between the superior surface of the condyle against the inferior surface of the disk. The translatory movement of the condyle results from the sliding movement of the superior surface of the disk against the articular eminence. The actual extent of normal anterior translation of the condyle is highly variable. On full opening, in most individuals the condyle moves downward and forward to the height of the eminence or slightly anterior to it (Fig. 25-5, *C*). Typically the condyle is found within a range of 2 to 5 mm posterior to and 5 to 8 mm anterior to the crest of the eminence.[28] Patients who are not able to open their mouths normally, radiographically show reduced condylar translation. In these patients the condyle may move downward and forward but does not leave the mandibular fossa. Hypermobility of the joint may be suspected if the condyle translates more than 5 mm anterior to the eminence.[11]

IMAGING OF THE TMJ

The TMJ is technically one of the most difficult areas of the body to visualize well because of multiple adjacent osseous structures. For osseous evaluation of the TMJ, frontal and lateral tomography provide the most detailed images. For soft tissue imaging of the TMJ, MRI is used most often. It is replacing arthrography because it is noninvasive and does not result in exposure to ionizing radiation. A summary of the comparative merits of common imaging modalities is shown in Table 25-1.

Tomography

There is nearly universal agreement that tomography (Chapter 13) provides the most definitive radiologic information about the osseous components of the TMJ. This is because a tomographic view provides a radiographic slice through the TMJ. Complex motion tomography (hypocycloidal or spiral motion) is preferable to linear tomography because of the lack of distracting streaking on the image. Tomographic cross-sections of the TMJ are usually made in two orientations with respect to the joint. In one, the head is positioned so that the cross-section is at a right angle to the long axis of the condyle (the lateral view). In the other, the cross-section is parallel to the long axis of the condyle (the frontal view). In that a single tomogram provides information about one specific region of the joint, several serial cross-sections should be made. A complete tomographic examination typically includes three to six closed lateral views. These are made at 2- to 3-mm intervals from the medial pole to the lateral pole. It is also customary to expose a lateral view with the jaw open and a frontal view with the jaw closed or protruded. Tomography is superior to transcranial radiography for demonstrating changes on the articulating surfaces and the position of the condyle within the mandibular fossa.[63,76]

Lateral tomography. The lateral tomographic view offers the best lateral views of the cortical margins of the mandibular condyle, mandibular fossa, and the position of the condyle within the mandibular fossa along with its range of translatory motion (Fig. 25-5, *A* and *C*). The best lateral tomographic views are obtained when the head is positioned to align the central ray along the long axis of the condyle. In some clinics the exact degree of head rotation is established individually for each TMJ to ensure the most precise alignment of the long axis of each condyle. This technique requires that a submentovertex view be obtained as a preliminary film, with plotting of individual condylar angles against the intermeatal (coronal) axis (Fig. 25-2). Condylar angles determined this way will then be used as precise head rotation angles as lateral tomograms are made for the left and right TMJs. A standardized rotation of 25 degrees toward the side of interest is often adequate to produce an approximate profile view of the joint's long axis.

The TMJ radiographs are best made with the patient in an upright posture. The patient should be seated in an adjustable chair or standing at the foot of an upright radiographic table (Fig. 25-6). Upright tomography is requested because of the belief that the delicate bony relationships of the joint should be evaluated in this way instead of lying down, where the joint structures would be displaced by gravity.

During the examination, the patient is asked to bite down firmly on the posterior teeth in a normal bite. When open-mouth projections are desired, the patient should open widely without straining the masticatory muscles and hold this opening posture for the duration of the exposure. Because of the rather long interval of many tomographic exposures (up to 6 seconds), a bite block may be inserted between the patient's anterior teeth to prevent jaw movement.

Frontal tomography. Frontal tomograms are very good for detecting subtle cortical erosions of the superior surface of the mandibular condyle. These views are ideally made with the patient in the upright position. Head rotation is again made before exposure so that the long axis of the condyle and fossa are seen straight on (perpendicular to the course of the central ray). The x-ray beam should be tightly collimated to expose only the joint structures of interest unilaterally, with no attempt to obtain both joints on the same radiographic exposure. It is best to have the patient protrude the lower jaw but keep the teeth in light contact (Fig. 25-7). This has the effect of bringing the condyle forward below the articular eminence so that the condyle may be visualized well. The superior aspect of the condyle will be seen from the lateral pole to the medial pole (Fig. 25-8).

Athrography

Historically, TMJ imaging has been concerned with plain and tomographic demonstrations of the bony components of the joint. However, in patients where there is suspicion of internal derangement— damage to the articular disk and its attaching ligaments and capsular tissues—imaging by other than these traditional films is necessary. The two major techniques that demonstrate various soft-tissue components of the TMJ are MRI and arthrography. Imaging with MRI, described later in this chapter, gives computer-reconstructed images of sections through the TMJ in frontal, axial, and sagittal planes. The anatomic configuration of the disk and its position relative to the condylar head and articular eminence can be shown in open and closed positions. However, it does not show the integrity of the ligaments, the capsule, or the functional movements of the joint soft tissues.

Arthrography has many advantages for imaging TMJ internal derangements.[10,37,85] The advantages of this technique include demonstration of disruptions of the ligament-disk attachments and of capsular integrity, and the ability to image the soft tissues of the joint during function. Although in-

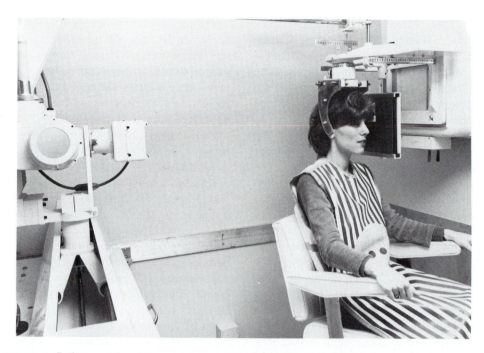

FIG. 25-6. Patient positioned for a lateral tomographic section, showing a 20-degree head rotation to the left to image the left TMJ. In this illustration a linear tomographic unit is being used.

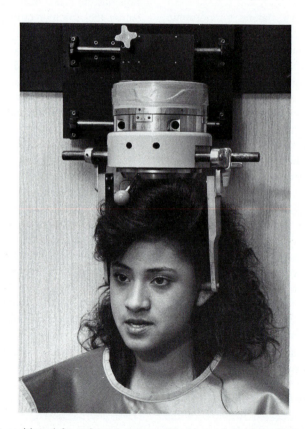

FIG. 25-7. Patient positioned for a frontal tomographic view of the right TMJ, showing the head rotated 20 degrees to the right and the mandible protruded to bring the condyles forward and below the articular eminences.

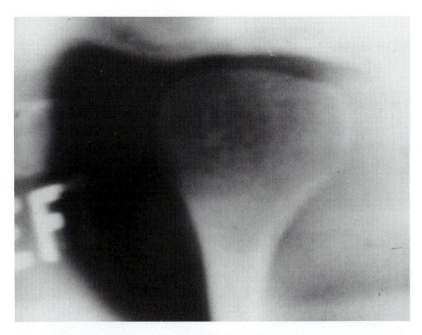

FIG. 25-8. Frontal tomographic section of the mandibular condyle.

vasive, the technique carries minimal risk and discomfort and is considerably less expensive than MRI. It also provides maximal diagnostic information concerning the position and movement of the disk and the integrity of its attachments to the mandible and cranium.

TMJ arthrography involves the injection of a radiopaque contrast agent into one or both joint spaces, thus outlining the space-occupying disk and attachments. Imaging during and following joint space opacification allows clear visualization of the articular disk, the ligamentous attachments, and the capsular integrity in static images or in function on videotape. The use of fluoroscopy, in which the arthrographer can view the examination on a television screen while it is being performed, allows accurate placement of the needle into the joint space and greatly improves the percentage of successful joint space opacifications. TMJ arthrography was infrequently used until recently, when water-based and low-ionic-concentration iodine-containing contrast agents, use of tomography, digital subtraction, videotaping after joint opacification, and improved equipment led to the technique's acceptance as the definitive method for demonstrating TMJ internal derangements.

Indications. The principal indication for TMJ arthrography is suspected internal derangement, most often anterior displacement of the articular disk, with or without reduction. Demonstration of the position of the disk, the integrity of its attachments, and the dynamics of its movement during mandibular function is necessary to diagnose the problem clearly and determine which of the many treatment modalities would be most effective. TMJ arthrography is valuable prior to impending disk surgery.

Temporomandibular joint arthrography should be carried out using sterile procedures: surgical scrub of the preauricular area, draping and isolation of the area, and operator barrier techniques including sterile surgical gloves. This minimizes the risk of introducing an infection into the joint. The following description is for a typical lower joint space arthrogram. Superficial and deep tissues overlying the TMJ are anesthetized with lidocaine (Xylocaine) or mepivacaine, depending on the desired duration of anesthesia. At the final stage of local anesthesia, the needle is inserted into the joint space, usually the lower compartment, and the intracapsular area is anesthetized (Fig. 25-9).

After verification of needle position in the joint space by fluoroscopy,* the joint space is filled with approximately 0.5 cc of iodine-containing radiopaque contrast agent. Once the space is opacified,

---

*Fluoroscopy is an imaging technique in which a continuous or intermittent x-ray beam is used to gather a real-time image. The image is displayed on a monitor, allowing the operator to follow the position of the needle in relation to the osseous structures of the TMJ.

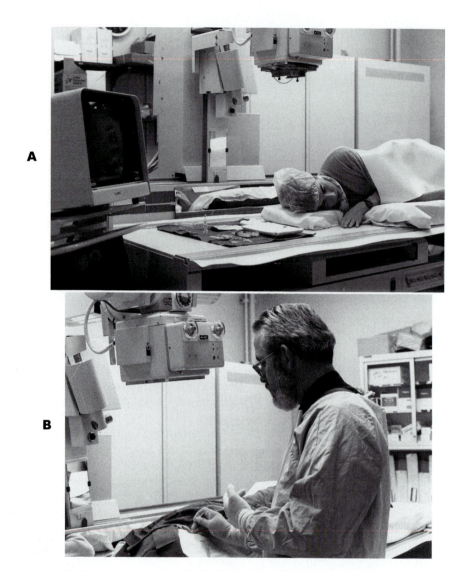

FIG. 25-9. Equipment and setup for TMJ arthrography. **A,** The patient is positioned on the imaging table. The x-ray tube is above the patient and the fluoroscope, connected to a videotape recorder, is below the table. The arthrographer controls the fluoroscope with a foot pedal and views the examination when necessary on the television monitor at the head of the table. The sterile armamentarium—consisting of syringes and needles, connective tubes, local anesthetic, povidone-iodine scrub, contrast agent, and gauze sponges—is located at the patient's head. **B,** Operator and patient following disinfection of the preauricular area and isolation of the field. The needle is about to be inserted for administration of the local anesthetic. The joint space will be filled with contrast agent. **C,** Note the isolated preauricular field and the position of needle insertion superficial to the TMJ. (Courtesy Dr. Alan G. Lurie, University of Connecticut, Farmington.)

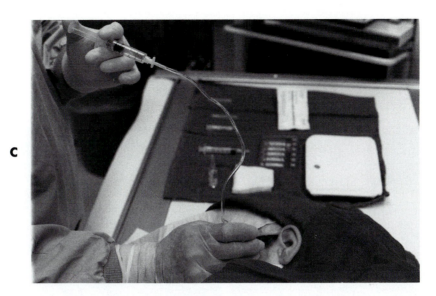

FIG. 25-9, cont'd. For legend see opposite page.

closed, open, and protrusive tomographic images (arthrotomograms) are obtained. With appropriate equipment, one can directly obtain digital subtraction images during the injection† and can make videotapes of the opacified joint during opening, closing, and excursive movements. This procedure generally takes 1 to 2 hours, including time for history and physical examination, preliminary films, patient preparation, anesthesia and contrast injection, image acquisition, cleanup and patient, postprocedure instructions. A variation of this technique, double-contrast arthrography, provides improved visualization of the shape and position of the disk.[111,113] In this technique, dye is injected into the upper and lower joint spaces to coat the surfaces; then it is withdrawn and the spaces are reinjected with air. With this technique the disk is coated with dye and stands out from the dark air-filled joint spaces.

The most common complication of TMJ arthrography is pain in the TMJ area, which may be mild to severe in intensity and 1 to 3 days in duration. This depends on the characteristics of the patient, the amount of internal damage in the patient's joint, and the amount of physical difficulty encountered during the procedure. It may be accompanied by

some masticatory muscle spasm and edema. Most often these problems are controlled with topical ice-pack applications and over-the-counter, non-aspirin nonsteroidal antiinflammatory medications (ibuprofen). Occasionally, stronger pain medication is needed. Intracapsular bleeding, joint infections, and allergic reactions to contrast agents are rare in TMJ arthrography.

In a patient with no internal derangement of the TMJ, the contrast medium easily flows through the upper or lower joint space and clearly outlines the disk and its anterior and posterior attachments. In the closed position, the biconcave disk is the shape of an erythrocyte. Its posterior band is located at or just anterior to the vertex of the condyle (lower compartment, Fig. 25-10, *A* and *C*; upper compartment, Fig. 25-11, *A* and *C*). With the mouth open, the disk is centered over the condyle, with the thin, intermediate zone centered over the condylar vertex (lower compartment, Fig. 25-10, *B* and *D*; upper compartment, Fig. 25-11, *B* and *D*). The contrast agent is confined to the space into which it was injected, which is well demonstrated using digital subtraction radiology (Fig. 25-12). Dynamic videotape images in such patients usually show smooth movements of the disk and smooth redistribution of the contrast agent during opening, closing, and excursive movements.

Transcranial views

Transcranial views provide a reasonably true projection through the long axis of the joint (Fig.

---

†Subtraction radiography, discussed in Chapter 13, allows two images to be compared. Only structures that differ between the two images will be revealed. In this instance, two fluoroscopic images are compared. The image that is changing is that of the dye flowing into the joint space.

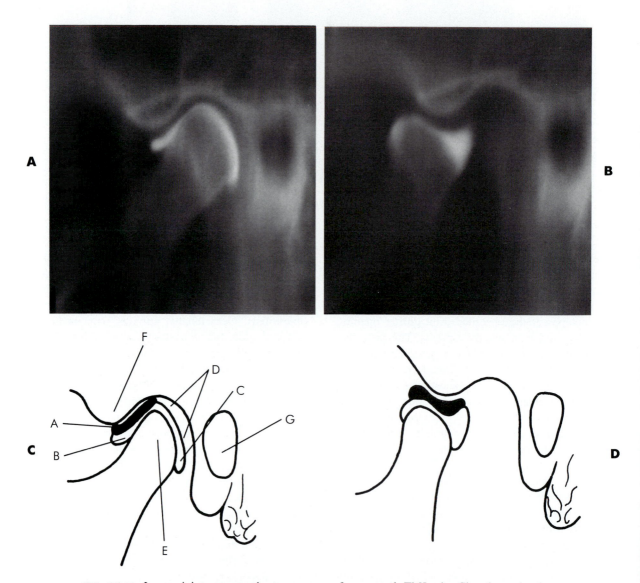

FIG. 25-10. Lower joint space arthrotomograms of a normal TMJ. **A,** Closed-mouth view. **B,** Open-mouth view. The disk can be visualized by observing the superior margin of the contrast agent, which defines the inferior border of the disk and its attachments. **C** and **D** are to help in identifying the structures shown. *A,* Disk; *B,* anterior; and *C,* posterior recesses of the lower compartment, filled with contrast; *D,* bilaminar zone; *E,* head of the condyle; *F,* articular eminence; *G,* auditory canal. (Courtesy Dr. Alan G. Lurie, University of Connecticut, Farmington.)

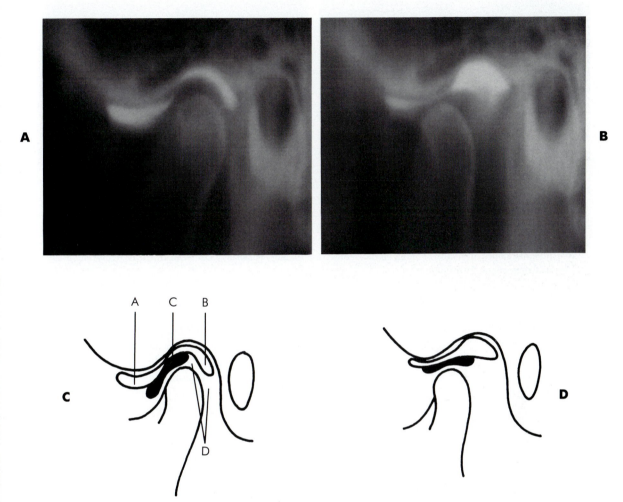

FIG. 25-11. Upper joint space arthrotomograms of the normal TMJ. **A,** Closed-mouth view. **B,** Open-mouth view. The inferior border of the contrast defines the superior border of the disk and its attachments. **C** and **D** are to help in identifying the structures shown. *A,* Anterior and *B,* posterior recesses of the upper compartment, filled with contrast; *C,* disk; *D,* bilaminar zone. The other structures are the same as in Figure 25-10. Note that the position of the disk and its shape are more difficult to assess in this study than in the lower compartment study. (Courtesy Dr. Alan G. Lurie, University of Connecticut, Farmington.)

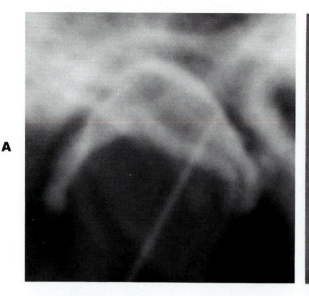 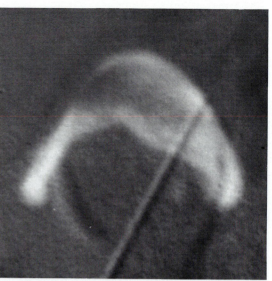

FIG. 25-12. Digital subtraction arthrogram. **A** is a digital transcranial image, and **B,** a digital transcranial subtraction image of the opacified lower joint space in a normal TMJ with the mouth closed. The view is sagittal, and the needle is in the posterior recess of the lower joint space. Subtraction images, obtained at intervals during the filling of the joint space, are useful in demonstrating the integrity of the space. Note the optical removal of bone and the sense of three-dimensionality of the lower space in the subtraction images. (Courtesy Dr. Alan G. Lurie, Univerity of Connecticut, Farmington.)

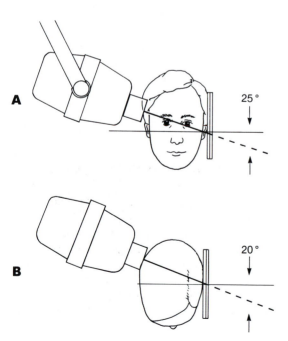

FIG. 25-13. Transcranial projection. The central ray is oriented downward 25 degrees, **A,** and anteriorly 20 degrees, **B,** centered on the TMJ of interest.

25-13). The x-ray film cassette is positioned against the facial skin surface on the side of interest, parallel to the sagittal plane. The x-ray tube is brought into position on the contralateral side of the skull so that the central beam projects downward 25 degrees and anteriorly 20 degrees and is centered on the TMJ. The central beam is projected across the cranium above the petrous ridge of the temporal bone on the film side and exits through the long axis of the condyle. A number of devices are available to assist the operator in aligning the patient, film, and central ray of the x-ray beam. Such a device is necessary to achieve reproducibility of orientation that will permit comparison of images. The routine transcranial radiographic series includes projections of both left and right joints in the closed and wide-open jaw positions (Fig. 25-14).

The observer must remember that the transcranial view displays only the lateral aspects of the condylar head and the articular fossa in profile because of the caudal angulation of the x-ray beam. Thus, transcranial radiography may show minute, subtle bony irregularities on the lateral bony surfaces but is far less instructive of similar changes that occur in the central and medial joint areas.

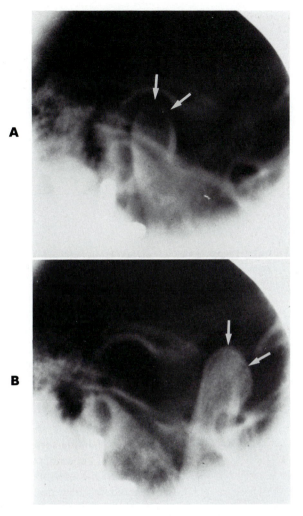

FIG. 25-14. Transcranial projections of the TMJ. In each case the condyle is indicated by arrows. **A,** Mouth closed; **B,** mouth open.

This view is usually compromised by superimposition of the ipsilateral petrous ridge over the condylar neck. Thus, abnormal changes in the condylar neck, such as fracture lines or demineralization, may at times be hidden by the petrous ridge shadow. In addition, there cannot be confidence in the position of the condyle within the fossa demonstrated by this technique because in many TMJs the position of the condyle within the fossa changes from the lateral to medial pole.[23] Further, the apparent position of the condyle in the mandibular fossa changes by varying the horizontal angulation of the x-ray beam.[95] The transcranial view is rapidly being replaced by lateral tomography.

Transorbital views

The conventional frontal TMJ projection that is most routinely successful in delineating the joint with minimal superimpositions is the transorbital (Zimmer) projection.[5] (The transmaxillary projection is similar.) The primary advantages of this projection are the lack of major superimpositions over most of the condylar process, the production of a relatively true frontal projection of the condyle (directing the central ray perpendicular to the long axis of the condyle), and the simplicity with which it is made.

To obtain a transorbital projection of the TMJ, seat the patient upright and tip the head downward about 10 degrees so the canthomeatal line is hor-

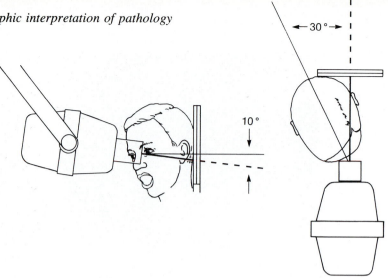

FIG. 25-15. Transorbital projection. The central ray is oriented downward about 10 degrees and laterally about 30 degrees through the ipsilateral orbit, centered on the TMJ of interest.

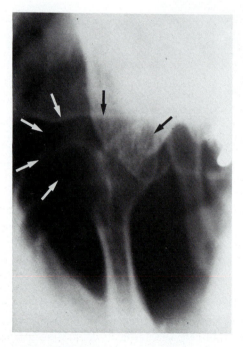

FIG. 25-16. Transorbital view showing the condyle *(arrows)* below the articular eminence. The mastoid process is superimposed on the medial half of the condyle.

izontal (Fig. 25-15). Place the tube head in front of the patient and direct the central ray through the ipsilateral orbit and through the TMJ of interest, exiting from the skull behind the mastoid process. Position the x-ray cassette behind the patient's head so that the central ray is projected to its center and perpendicular to it. Then, ask the patient to open the mouth as wide as possible to move the condyle of interest out of the articular fossa and onto the crest of the articular eminence. This maneuver allows profile visualization of, ideally, the entire lateromedial range of the articulating surfaces of both the condyle and the articular eminence. If the patient cannot open wide, the condylar neck may be well seen on the resultant view, but areas of the joint articulating surfaces will be obscured because of mutual superimposition.

When the transorbital projection is made with the mouth open, the condyle and a major portion of the condylar neck will be visualized and their integrity can be evaluated (Fig. 25-16). The main contribution of the transorbital view is the demonstration of the convex articulating surface of the condyle and the slightly concave or flat, broad ridge of the articular eminence. This is, therefore, the frontal projection of choice when tomography is not available.[72]

Skull views

Three skull projections—the Waters, the submentovertex (SMV), and the reverse-Towne (Chapter 11)—may provide useful information about the joint area in some circumstances. The Towne projection often clearly defines all but the most superior parts of the condylar processes. Thus the Towne view often gives critical diagnostic aid in determining the presence of unilateral or bilateral condylar fractures, especially for fractures running in the sagittal plane. The medial displacement of condylar fragments that occurs in an unfavorable fracture may be optimally demonstrated on this

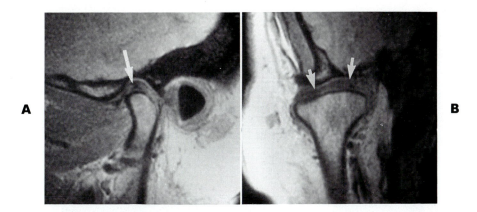

FIG. 25-17. MRI of the normal TMJ. **A,** Closed-mouth view showing the condyle and temporal components. The biconcave disk is located with its posterior band *(arrow)* over the condyle. **B,** Coronal image showing the osseous components and the disk *(arrow)* on top of the condyle. (Courtesy Dr. Per-Lennart Westesson, Department of Radiology, University of Rochester, Rochester, N.Y.)

projection. The Waters view may project the articulating surfaces bilaterally with virtually no compromising superimpositions. With the petrous ridges depressed on the Waters view, the images of the condylar and temporal surfaces of the TMJs are surprisingly clear. However, the bulk of the inferior parts of the condyle are superimposed by the petrous ridges, and the medial joint surfaces are often obliterated by the maxillary posterior teeth. For these reasons, the frontal tomogram is recommended if questionable TMJ findings arise. The SMV view is used primarily to define the angulations of the condyles in the transverse plane of the skull. This information is used to position patients' heads individually for TMJ tomographic procedures as described previously.

Panoramic views

Panoramic radiography (Chapter 12) provides tomographic views of the condyles, rami, and body in one projection. These views are usually of sufficient clarity to evaluate the condyles for gross osseous changes, such as extensive erosions, growths, or displaced fractures. This view is limited because the central ray is not directed through the long axis of the condyle. The relationship of the condyle to the mandibular fossa is also distorted because the mouth is partly open and the mandible is protruded when the radiograph is exposed. Usually the view of the mandibular fossa is inadequate for critical evaluation. As such, this projection is generally not indicated for close examination of the TMJ when the views described previously are

available. A modification of the panoramic method has been described for imaging the TMJ that provides a view with greater resolution and less distortion than conventional panoramic radiography.[13,14] In this method, the patient's head is positioned forward and slightly displaced toward the midline, compared to the usual position.

Magnetic resonance imaging

MRI is an excellent method for imaging the TMJ. It is the only imaging technique that can simultaneously image both the disk and posterior attachment as well as the condyle and mandibular fossa. It is routine to image both joints during a TMJ examination because of the high incidence of bilateral abnormalities in patients with TMJ dysfunction. As with tomography, slices in the corrected lateral orientation as well as corrected frontal views are preferred[30,67,92] (Fig. 25-17). Both open and closed images are used to evaluate the position of the disk. Static images of the joint have been made since the mid-1980s, and more recently motion MRI of the joint during opening and closing has been obtained.[16,74] These are obtained by having patients open their mouths through a series of stepped distances by using rapid image acquisition.

Many pulse sequences have been investigated for examination of the TMJ. Most clinicians use T1-weighted MRI to display the osseous and diskal tissues. T2-weighted images have been found useful to identify joint effusion and inflammatory changes associated with tumors.[30,38,74] Partial flip angle pulse sequences, "fast scan" techniques, are

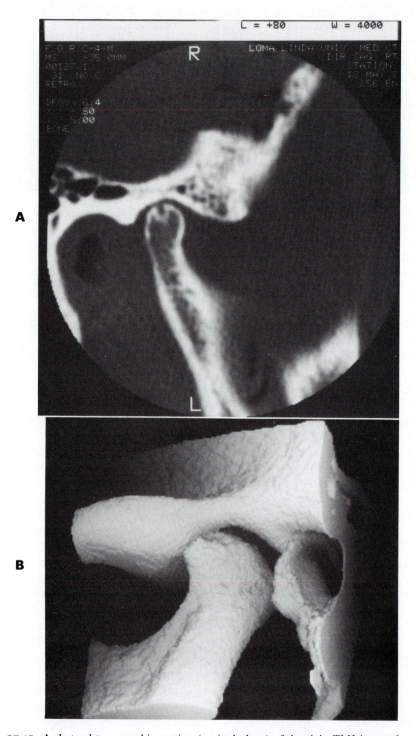

FIG. 25-18. A, Lateral tomographic section (sagittal plane) of the right TMJ in a cadaver demonstrating an area of erosion on the superior surface of the condyle. **B,** Three-dimensional CT reconstruction of the condyle, demonstrating the defect. **C,** Frontal tomogram of the TMJ showing the same erosive lesion on the condylar surface. (**A** courtesy Drs. E. Christiansen and J. Thompson, Loma Linda, Calif.; **B** and **C** courtesy Drs. E. Christiansen, B. Holshouser, A. Reynolds, and S. Goldwasser, Loma Linda, Calif.)

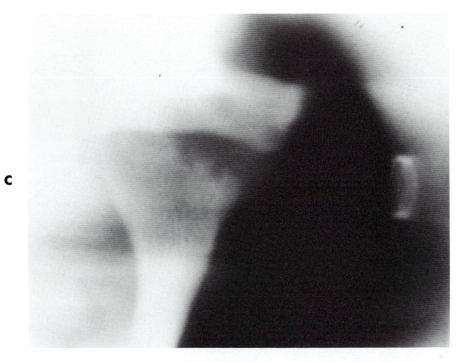

FIG. 25-18, cont'd. For legend, see opposite page.

often used for the motion images, although because of the lower spatial resolution of this method some groups use T1-weighted images for motion studies.[74] Images made with field strengths of 1.5 T provide more diagnostic images for interpretation of disk position, disk configuration, and bony abnormalities than those made on 0.3 T machines.[29] Dual surface coils placed over the patient's TMJs are used to acquire the best images of each joint.

The primary application of MRI for the TMJ is to demonstrate internal derangements of the joint, a major cause of jaw pain and dysfunction.[32] It has been found more accurate than arthrography for determination of disk position.[79] Another frequent use of MRI is to evaluate the joint for joint effusion or damage to the retrodiskal tissues following trauma. It is also useful for postsurgical evaluation of disk position, erosion of the bony components, granulation tissue associated with implants, or excessive fibrosis of the joint capsule. Some observers contend that bony degenerative changes are better seen with MRI than with tomography.[20]

Computed tomography

For a number of years, computed tomography (CT) has been used for evaluation of the TMJ. Its greatest advantage lies in its ability to produce high-quality images of the head of the condyle and the mandibular fossa. High-quality CT images are slightly superior to tomography for revealing subtle TMJ abnormalities.[54] The highest-quality lateral CT views of the TMJ are obtained when the patient is exposed using a direct sagittal technique[33,105] (Fig. 25-18). With this approach, the patient is oriented so that the sagittal plane is oriented parallel to the plane of the section rather than the usual axial scans.

CT is advantageous for evaluating fractures or lesions of the TMJ. Because multiple image slices are typically made, it is possible to produce three-dimensional images reconstructed from the CT data. These images improve the diagnostic value of the CT image, especially to view hidden surfaces (Fig. 25-18).[73,82,83] These images may be useful for surgical treatment planning or evaluation of trauma. Although there has been interest in using CT for evaluation of the soft tissues of the TMJ, this application has largely been replaced by rapid advances in the development of MRI.

PATHOLOGIC CONDITIONS
Internal derangements

The term "internal derangement" implies some abnormality of the soft tissue component of the

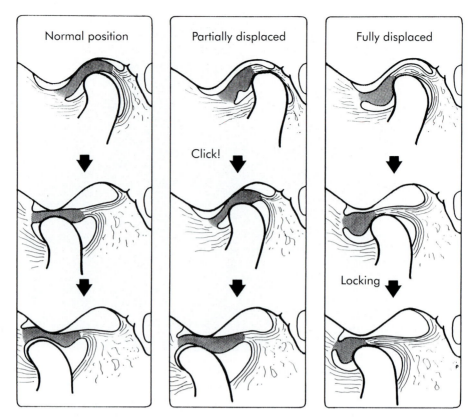

Normal position	Partially displaced	Fully displaced
	Click!	Locking

FIG. 25-19. Position and movement of the disk during jaw opening. Normal position *(left);* partially displaced anteriorly (with reduction, *middle*); fully displaced anteriorly (without reduction, *right*). (Courtesy Dr. W. K. Solberg, UCLA School of Dentistry, Los Angeles.)

joint that interferes with normal function. Clinical signs of internal derangement of the TMJ are found in one fifth of adult patients.[58] The most common type of internal derangement is malposition of the disk. It is usually displaced anteriorly but may be displaced anteromedially, medially, anterolaterally, or laterally. As the condyle translates forward during an opening movement, it initially pushes the disk farther forward but then jumps over the posterior band of the disk (Fig. 25-19). This allows the disk to assume a normal position between the condyle and articular eminence (disk displacement with reduction). In the latter case, the return of the disk to a normal position is signaled with an audible click. On closing, the condyle may again snap under the posterior edge of the disk, again displaced anteriorly and producing a second click. This sequence is termed "reciprocal clicking." Persons who have disk displacement with reduction have reduced movement of the disk against the articular eminence.[75] In more advanced cases, the disk remains anteriorly displaced (disk displacement with-

out reduction) in front of the condyle upon opening, and the range of motion is restricted[40] (Figs. 25-19 and 25-20). The more anterior the disk, the greater the likelihood of irregularities of the articular surfaces.[114] Anterior displacement of the disk has been described in normal volunteers, however, suggesting that it may be a predisposing factor to TMJ dysfunction or a normal variant.[45,116] Patients usually seek care for internal derangement because of pain. When the disk is anteriorly displaced, the condyle often assumes a retruded position in the fossa.[9,84]

The etiology of internal derangement is unknown. It is found much more frequently in young adult women than in men.[118] Internal derangements of the TMJ are a major cause of jaw pain and dysfunction in adults and children,[90] often initiated by an injury to the jaw.[42] About half the patients with internal derangement also have hard tissue changes, and this finding is invariably present when there is perforation of the disk.[112] Some investigators believe that internal derangements may be

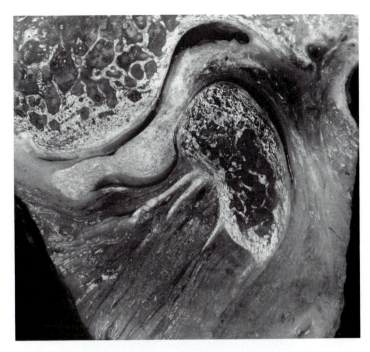

FIG. 25-20. Cadaver TMJ showing anterior displacement of the disk with a loss of normal disk morphology. (Courtesy, Dr. Carol Bibb, UCLA School of Dentistry, Los Angeles.)

an important factor in the cause of osteoarthritis of the TMJ.[38,39]

MRI, like arthrography, is well suited to demonstrate displacement of the disk in the TMJ.[43] It is also used to image postsurgical fibrosis in a symptomatic TMJ.[115] With conventional radiography, individuals with internal derangement of the TMJ often show posterior displacement of the condyles in the mandibular (articular) fossa in the closed position.[9,107] This finding alone is not, however, diagnostic of internal derangement.[28,41,62] Arthrography and MRI may be used to confirm anterior displacement of the disk.

In early internal derangement, the only imaging findings are a displaced disk with reciprocal clicking and possibly a retruded condyle. If this condition persists and advances, then the disk will remain displaced and become deformed.[118] Later, degenerative bony changes become evident (see section on osteoarthritis). Eventually there is perforation through the posterior attachment, and the bony changes continue to become more severe.

Reducing anteriorly displaced disk. In the closed position, the posterior band of the disk is located anterior to the normal position. Its long axis also may be more vertically oriented than in the normal patient. These findings may be visualized directly by MRI (Fig. 25-21) as well as on arthrotomograms (Fig. 25-22, *A*). There may be compression of the posterior recess, giving the contrast media a thinner appearance. The disk usually has a normal shape, although there may be some compression of its long axis. At the start of opening, the disk frequently becomes compressed anterior to the condylar head prior to moving. It then typically resumes a more normal configuration after it reduces to a normal position over the condylar apex upon full opening (Fig. 25-22, *B* and *C*). Closed and open arthrotomograms may appear similar to normal, but a videotape of the patient during mandibular movements with one or both joint spaces opacified often shows a sudden movement of the disk from its anterior position in closed to its normal position in open and back to its anterior position in closed. These sudden movements often coincide with opening, closing, and reciprocal clicks. The dye is usually confined to the compartment(s) in these patients, although capsular tears and ligamentous detachments are occasionally seen.

Nonreducing anteriorly displaced disk. In the closed position, the posterior band of the disk is well forward of the condylar head and may have a variety of peculiar anatomic appearances. These

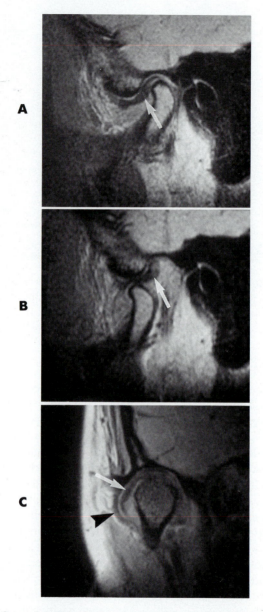

FIG. 25-21. MRI of anterior disk displacement with reduction. **A,** Closed-mouth sagittal view showing the disk with its posterior band *(arrow)* anterior to the condyle. **B,** Open-mouth view showing the normal relationship of disk and condyle and the posterior band of the disk *(arrow)*. **C,** Coronal view showing the disk *(white arrow)* laterally displaced. The joint capsule *(black arrowhead)* is bulging laterally. (Courtesy Dr. Per-Lennart Westesson, Department of Radiology, University of Rochester, Rochester N.Y.)

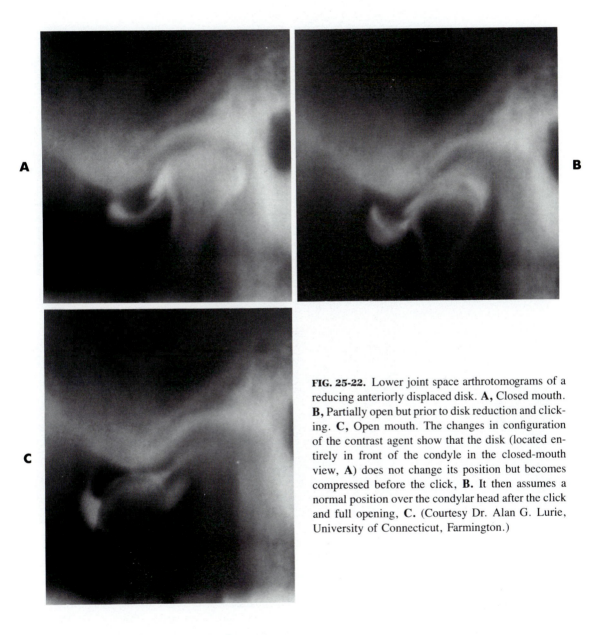

FIG. 25-22. Lower joint space arthrotomograms of a reducing anteriorly displaced disk. **A,** Closed mouth. **B,** Partially open but prior to disk reduction and clicking. **C,** Open mouth. The changes in configuration of the contrast agent show that the disk (located entirely in front of the condyle in the closed-mouth view, **A**) does not change its position but becomes compressed before the click, **B.** It then assumes a normal position over the condylar head after the click and full opening, **C.** (Courtesy Dr. Alan G. Lurie, University of Connecticut, Farmington.)

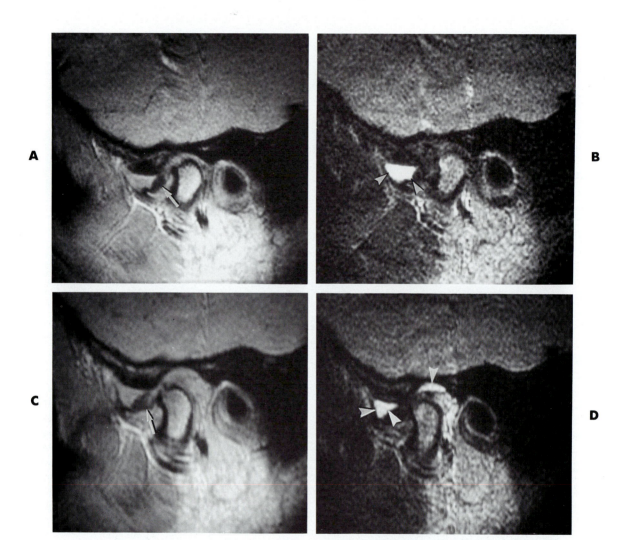

FIG. 25-23. MRI of disk displacement without reduction, in the presence of joint effusion. **A,** The disk *(arrow)* is anteriorly displaced in this closed-mouth view. **B,** A T2-weighted image of the same section shows the collection of joint effusion *(arrowheads)* in the anterior recess of the upper joint space. **C,** Open-mouth view showing the disk anterior to the condyle and the posterior band of the disk *(arrow)*. **D,** This T2-weighted image shows the same layer as **C.** Note the joint effusion *(arrowheads)* in the anterior and posterior recesses of the upper joint space. (Courtesy Dr. Per-Lennart Westesson, Department of Radiology, University of Rochester, Rochester, N.Y.)

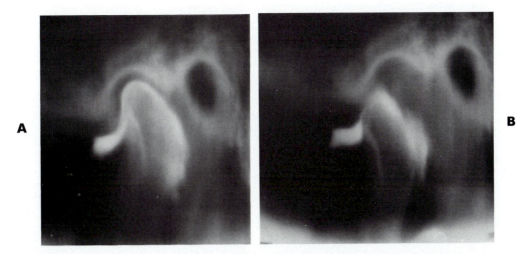

FIG. 25-24. Lower joint space arthrotomograms of a nonreducing anteriorly displaced disk. **A,** Closed position. The disk is located anterior to the condylar head, with its long axis more perpendicular to the Frankfort horizontal plane than in a normal position. **B,** Mouth open. Attempts at opening lead to compression of the disk, represented by a change in the shape of the contrast medium anterior to the condyle. The disk remains anterior to the condyle, and minimal condylar translation occurs. (Courtesy Dr. Alan G. Lurie, University of Connecticut, Farmington).

may be seen directly on MRI (Fig. 25-23) as well as on arthrotomograms (Fig. 25-24, *A*). Contrast agent distribution is variable and largely dependent on the presence or absence of other internal problems such as perforations, capsular tears, and fibrosis. Attempts at opening usually produce some rotation of the condylar head, but the disk remains displaced anteriorly and there is no change in the position of the contrast media (Fig. 25-24, *B*). In cases where the disk is not severely deformed, attempts at opening may compress the disk without its moving. Joint noises are most often absent.

Ligament-disk detachments (perforations). A detachment of the disk from its ligament, usually seen at the posterior band of the disk, results in both joint compartments filling during the initial injection of dye. This is best seen by videofluoroscopy (a video recording of the fluoroscopic images) or by digital subtraction imaging during a single joint space opacification. Contrast medium is seen redistributing between the upper and lower compartments during mandibular movements (Fig. 25-25).

Capsular tears. Capsular tears, as well as perforations, may be accompanied by bleeding into the joint space (hemarthrosis). This may be followed by fibrotic organization of the clot, possibly resulting in restricted condylar movement and unusual distribution of contrast medium as it flows through the involved joint space. If the attachment of the capsule to the condylar neck is compromised, contrast agent flows down the neck of the condyle, an ovious abnormality on any imaging method (Fig. 25-26).

Deviation in form

Deviation in form results from a modification of the normal osseous remodeling of the TMJ. Such abnormal remodeling results from conditions such as excessive stress or joint loading, trauma, or disk displacement. The osseous changes are first seen radiographically as a flattening of the anterosuperior surface of the condyle and possibly of the posterior slope of the articular eminence. These cortical borders are, however, intact and do not show evidence of erosion or cortical irregularity. It is not uncommon to see one joint in a patient showing such changes while the other is normal. Such changes are usually accompanied by changes in the fibrocartilage and may be static for years. The prevalence of such changes is much higher than osteoarthritis (as discussed later in this chapter); thus, this condition does not invariably serve as a precursor of the more advanced condition.[77]

Arthritis

Arthritis is inflammation of a joint. In the case of the TMJ, the cause is not usually known, al-

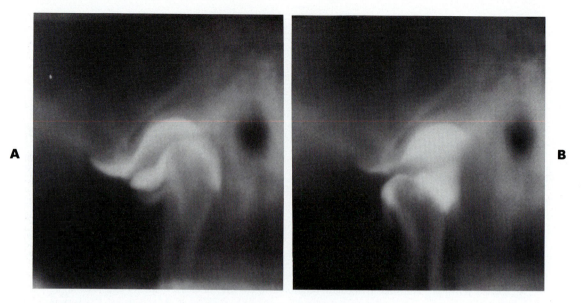

FIG. 25-25. Lower joint space arthrotomograms of a disk in **A,** open position and **B,** closed position, with loss of attachment between the posterior band and the bilaminar zone (perforation). These images were obtained following lower joint space opacification; both lower and upper joint spaces filled simultaneously. Contrast material can be seen redistributing between the compartments in the open and closed images. The disk is anteriorly displaced in the closed position and reduces upon opening. (Courtesy Dr. Alan G. Lurie, University of Connecticut, Farmington.)

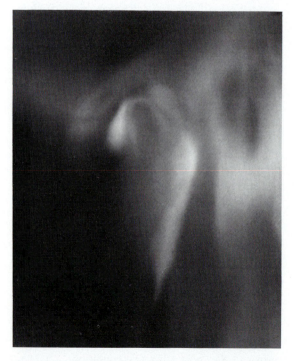

FIG. 25-26. Capsular tear. Lower joint space arthrotomogram of a disk with detachment of the capsule at the posterior neck of the condyle. Contrast material has flowed down the posterior aspect of the condylar neck. (Courtesy, Dr. Alan G. Lurie, University of Connecticut, Farmington.)

though a number of factors may be important, including acute trauma, disk displacement, hypermobility, and loading of the joint such as from bruxism. Although autopsy studies show a correlation between disk displacement and osteoarthritis, some patients have displaced disks without osteoarthritis and others have osteoarthritis with normally positioned disks.[18] Corrected lateral and frontal tomography are the methods of choice for examining the osseous components of the TMJ in these conditions. MRI is recommended when evaluation of the soft tissue component is desired.

Osteoarthritis. Osteoarthritis (degenerative arthritis, osteoarthrosis) is a degenerative process that is the most common form of TMJ disorder originating within the joint. The incidence of osteoarthritis is apparently high, occurring in almost half of those older than 40 years and in as many as 85% of persons older than 70 years.[7,26] However, it is not uncommon for osteoarthritis to occur in the joints of younger individuals as well.[71,90] Most of those demonstrating degenerative articular changes do not have discomfort. The symptoms, if present, are usually unilateral pain over the joint, or the joint may be sensitive only to palpation. There may be limited opening, crepitus, or deviation of the jaw toward the affected side, and the patient may complain of stiffness in the joint as the day wears

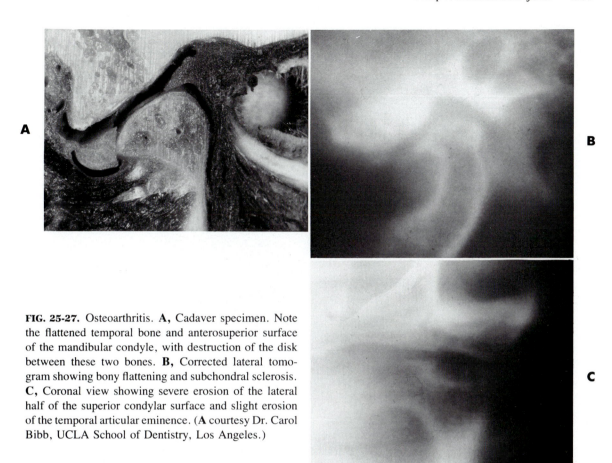

FIG. 25-27. Osteoarthritis. **A,** Cadaver specimen. Note the flattened temporal bone and anterosuperior surface of the mandibular condyle, with destruction of the disk between these two bones. **B,** Corrected lateral tomogram showing bony flattening and subchondral sclerosis. **C,** Coronal view showing severe erosion of the lateral half of the superior condylar surface and slight erosion of the temporal articular eminence. (**A** courtesy Dr. Carol Bibb, UCLA School of Dentistry, Los Angeles.)

on and the joint tires.[12,103] In patients with osteoarthritis of the TMJ, the disk is usually dislocated or perforated.[3,46]

The pathogenesis of osteoarthritis is characterized by the initial destruction of the soft tissue components of the joint and subsequent erosion and hypertrophic changes in the bone. First, the connective tissue covering the condyle, articular eminence, and the disk breaks down. Next, the bony surfaces of the condyle and articular eminence show resorption, and the underlying bone becomes sclerotic. Areas of erosion in the articular surfaces may be seen as irregular cortical margins. The radiographic density of the bony surfaces becomes noticeably increased as a result of subchondral sclerosis (Fig. 25-27). The degenerative changes are most frequently located on the lateral and anterolateral walls of the fossa. The eminence is flattened or almost removed, and the anterior half of the superior convex surface of the condyle is worn to a flat plane. As the articular eminence flattens, the mandibular fossa enlarges and becomes shallower. Osteophytes, small bony outgrowths or spurs, may

also occur on the anterior or superior surface of the condyle, protruding into the joint space, where they are most obvious (Fig. 25-28). As a result of the damaged, thinned disk, narrowing of the joint space is radiographically apparent. As these changes take place, crepitation in the joint becomes apparent and may be accompanied by discomfort.[6,48,49,64,70] Minute areas of degeneration just below the bony surface of the condyle may occasionally be identified by the pathologist. Because of their small size, they are rarely seen by the radiologist. These subchondral cysts (pseudocysts), filled with fibrous tissue, occasionally become large enough to be detected radiographically[31] (Fig. 25-29).

Psoriatic arthritis. The incidence of arthritis in patients with psoriasis is greater than in the general population. In one study, 30% of patients with psoriatic arthritis showed degenerative changes of the TMJ, most frequently erosions, sclerosis, flattening, and osteophytes.[47] These changes are radiographically indistinguishable from osteoarthritis.

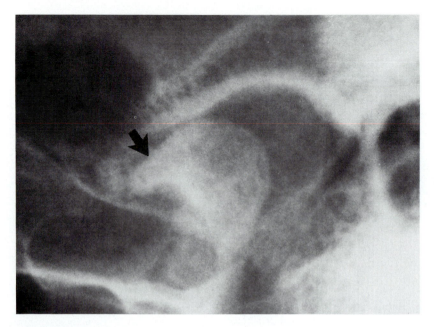

FIG. 25-28. Lateral tomographic view of the TMJ revealing an osteophyte on the anterior surface of the condyle *(arrow)*.

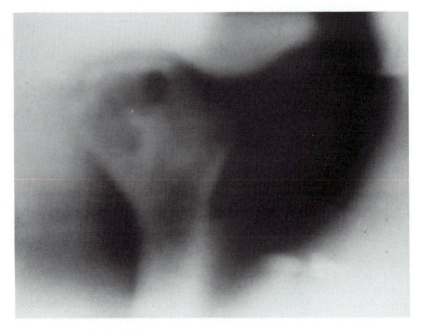

FIG. 25-29. Pseudocyst seen as a radiolucent oval loss of bone in the midsuperior aspect of this coronal view of the mandibular condyle. Note also the erosion of the lateral pole.

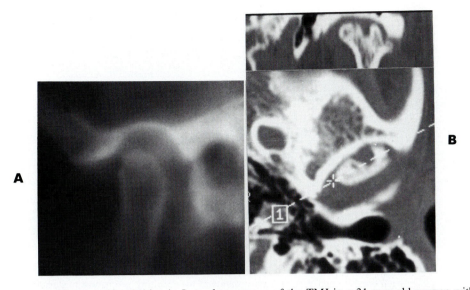

FIG. 25-30. Rheumatoid arthritis. **A,** Lateral tomogram of the TMJ in a 31-year-old woman with rheumatoid arthritis showing a small cortical erosion on the anterior aspect of the condyle. **B,** CT reformatted oblique coronal *(top)* and axial *(bottom)* images in a 26-year-old woman with rheumatoid arthritis showing extensive erosions of the superior and lateral aspects of the mandibular condyle. (Courtesy Dr. Tore A. Larheim, University of Oslo; **A** from El-Mofty S: *Oral Surg* 46:310-317, 1978; **B** from El-Mofty S: *Oral Surg* 33:650-660, 1972.)

Rheumatoid arthritis. In rheumatoid arthritis, the bony components of the TMJ are affected secondary to a granulomatous involvement of its synovial membrane that subsequently spreads to the articular surface of the condyle. This surface is replaced with granulomatous tissue, and small adhesions form between the articular surface and the disk.[7] Rheumatoid arthritis affects individuals over a wide age range, but most often after age 50. Radiographic and clinical signs of the disease are usually diagnosed initially in the small joints of the hands and feet by the time any TMJ involvement is detected. In unselected populations with confirmed rheumatoid arthritis, approximately two thirds or more showed some TMJ changes.[2,56,97] The usual symptoms include bilateral stiffness (in contrast to osteoarthritis, in which unilateral involvement is common), crepitus, tenderness, and swelling over the joint.[2]

The most common radiographic manifestation of rheumatoid arthritis occurring in the TMJ, and that with the greatest statistical significance, is flattening of the head of the condyle (Fig. 25-30). The next most common finding is erosion followed by reduced mobility of the condyle. Reduced mobility is especially related to the duration of the disease in the joint. Erosions of the condyle are present in about two thirds of patients with radiographic abnormalities. They are most common on the anterosuperior condylar surface, although they may also be seen on both the superior and posterior surfaces. Osteophytes are occasionally seen. The mandibular fossa often becomes sclerotic.[2] MRI studies often show disk abnormalities, with the most severe disk changes in patients with the greatest osseous destruction.[55]

Although none of the radiographic changes of rheumatoid arthritis is pathognomonic, in some patients the destructive process may advance far beyond that seen in osteoarthritis. As the rheumatoid destruction progresses, the condylar outline becomes increasingly irregular and ragged. In an advanced stage of disease, the condyle has been described as resembling a sharpened pencil.[93] This radiographic picture is the result of extensive erosions of the condyle on the anterior and posterior surfaces at the attachments of the synovial linings to the surfaces of the bone. Anterior positioning of the condyle within the articular fossa becomes increasingly prominent as the fossa becomes hollowed. In the most severe manifestation of rheumatoid arthritis, the condyle may be completely resorbed, resulting in loss of vertical support and an anterior open bite.

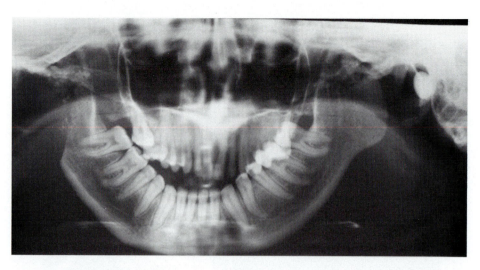

FIG. 25-31. Juvenile rheumatoid arthritis in a 29-year-old man afflicted since age 17. Note the obliteration of each condyle and part of each ramus and the resulting premature posterior contact due to loss of the vertical mandibular height.

Juvenile rheumatoid arthritis. Juvenile rheumatoid arthritis (Still's disease, juvenile chronic polyarthritis) is a chronic synovitis with or without extraarticular manifestations but is accompanied by more systemic features than the adult variety.[26] The systemic features include initial bilateral polyarthritis of both the small and large joints, including the cervical spine, evidenced by neck pain and limited range of movement.[4] The mean age of onset is about 5 years, and in most patients many joints are involved. One or both temporomandibular joints are involved in about 40% of patients.[53] The most common clinical sign in children with TMJ changes is restricted opening of the mouth.[51] Juvenile rheumatoid arthritis may also cause interference with normal condylar growth, leading to a characteristic mandibular retrognathia.[52,99] If the TMJ changes are unilateral, then there will be jaw asymmetry and underdevelopment of the affected side.[96]

Juvenile rheumatoid arthritis produces radiographic manifestations in the TMJ similar to the adult variety. The most common findings are flattening of the articular eminence and erosion of the superior portion of the condyle. On occasion, however, the destructive process may be quite severe, resulting in obliteration of both condyles or even the superior aspect of the mandibular ramus (Fig. 25-31). The severity of the radiographic signs is correlated with the duration and severity of the disease. Persistent deterioration of jaw movement

has been reported to culminate in complete TMJ ankylosis.[59]

Infectious arthritis. Infectious arthritis (septic arthritis) of the TMJ is rare in comparison with degenerative and rheumatoid arthritis. This disease may be caused by direct spread of organisms from an infected mastoid process or (most commonly) through the blood from a distant nidus.[60] Most cases are caused by the hematogenous spread of gonococci or by the direct extension of a middle ear infection. Symptoms include redness and swelling over the joint, severe pain when the joint is moved, inability to place the teeth in occlusion, and large tender cervical lymph nodes. The lymph nodes are not involved in osteoarthritis or rheumatoid arthritis.[27] It may result in ankylosis of the joint or in facial asymmetry if the growth centers are involved.

Again, the early stage of the disease may cause no radiographic manifestations at all. Worth[121] contends that the joint space may be increased by inflammatory distention in the early infective period.[6] Bony changes are seen only later, usually no sooner than 7 to 10 days after onset of the clinical symptoms. Because of the osteolytic effects of infection, the articular cortex of the condyle may become slightly radiolucent. Discontinuities or subtle irregularities of the anterior cortical surface are important radiographic findings. Osteoporosis of the adjacent parts of the condyle or even a major portion of the mandibular ramus may be appreciated

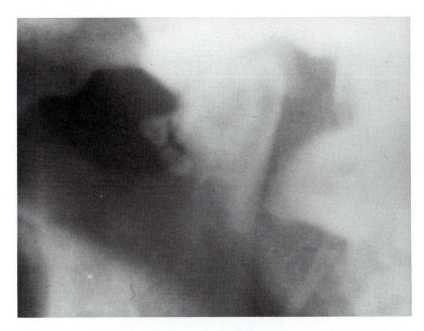

FIG. 25-32. Synovial chondromatosis, seen as opaque bodies lying anterior to the condyle.

in the acute phase of the disease. Later radiographic features may include a peripheral condensing osteitis and approximation of the joint surfaces as the articular cartilage is eroded.

Synovial chondromatosis

Synovial chondromatosis is an unusual condition in which there is dystrophic calcification of the synovial membrane of the TMJ. Histologically, these masses are composed of cartilaginous or osteocartilaginous nodules. They may become loose bodies in the joint spaces (Fig. 25-32). The masses move with the condyle when it translates. These masses are usually detected in patients with TMJ symptoms, but they may be found in asymptomatic individuals.[19]

Trauma

Effusion. Trauma to the TMJ may result in effusion, an influx of fluid into the joint. There may also be swelling of damaged retrodiskal tissues. T2-weighted MR images of a joint with effusion may show a bright signal adjacent to the disk or posterior to the condyle[91] (Fig. 25-23).

Dislocation. Dislocation results when the condyle is forcefully displaced anteriorly out of the articular fossa but remains within the capsule of the joint. This condition is often bilateral. It may be caused by a failure of muscular coordination or

by external trauma. It is well known that the condyle in the open-mouth position may be situated well forward of the eminence in some patients without clinical dislocation. Nevertheless, occasionally the TMJ is clinically dislocated with the condyle situated only minimally anterior to the summit of the eminence. This wide variation in anterior condylar movement during jaw opening maneuvers makes radiographic diagnosis of dislocation by itself inherently hazardous.

Fracture. A recent study demonstrated that fracture of the condylar process accounted for about 18% of 540 mandibular jaw fractures in a survey taken at a large metropolitan general hospital.[50] Unilateral fracture of the condylar process is much more common than bilateral fractures (Fig. 25-33). If a condylar fracture is discovered, appropriate mandibular radiographs must be carefully evaluated to rule out occult fractures of the mandibular body, which occasionally accompany condylar fractures.

Approximately 60% of condylar process fractures show some evidence of fragment angulation and a variable degree of displacement of the fracture ends.[87] Displacement, if present, is characteristically seen radiographically as anterior and medial deviation of the condylar fragment produced by contraction of the lateral pterygoid muscle. Multiple right-angle projections from the lateral, fron-

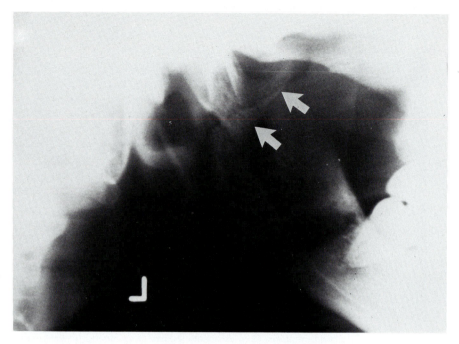

FIG. 25-33. Condylar fracture (infracranial view). *Arrows* point to the fracture margin.

tal, and basilar aspects provide the most confident determination of fragment displacement. CT has also proved excellent for revealing condylar fractures.[34]

The amount of remodeling seen in the TMJ following condylar fracture with medial displacement is quite variable.[57,89] In some cases, the condyle remodels to a form that is essentially normal. In other cases, the condyle and mandibular fossa become flattened, with loss of height on the affected side. The condyle may show degenerative changes including flattening, erosion and osteophytes.[80] Also, bifid condyles may form. Ankylosis may develop in some patients. The changes are more severe if the condyle is displaced.[17] The extent of radiographic and clinical healing is better in young children than in teenagers and better in teenagers than in adults.

Ankylosis

TMJ ankylosis is a relatively rare disability in which there is fusion of the temporomandibular joint. Patients present with a long-standing history of limited jaw opening. TMJ ankylosis is seen primarily in persons younger than 15 years of age.[1,24]

Ankylosis may be caused by a fibrous union of joint parts resulting from previous infection or traumatic injury. Such fibrous adhesions cannot be detected radiographically. In bony ankylosis, the affected joint usually shows degenerative changes. Most unilateral cases are caused by trauma or infection, and only a few were secondary to rheumatoid arthritis. When there is trauma to the condyle of a young child, the condyle may break up into many small, highly osteogenic fragments. This may organize into a fibrosseous mass, eventually converting to a bony ankylosis.[86] The most common cause of bilateral TMJ ankylosis is rheumatoid arthritis, although bilateral fractures may rarely produce this result. Most, if not all, cases of TMJ ankylosis in infancy are secondary to birth injury.[121]

With ankylosis of the TMJ, the radiographic joint space is either partially or completely obliterated. Sometimes a large mass of new bone may be seen obscuring the condyle and the joint space, possibly extending down into the region of the condylar neck (Fig. 25-34). Significantly, no radiographic differences are detected between those cases caused by trauma and those resulting from infection. The formation of new bone may be so extensive as to fuse the condyle to the cranial base.[86,119] Free movement of the affected condyle is impossible in such cases, although the patient may be able to produce several millimeters of interincisal opening.

If TMJ ankylosis occurs before completion of

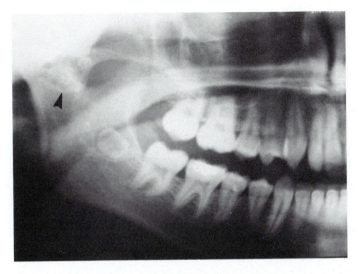

FIG. 25-34. TMJ with bony ankylosis *(arrowhead)* obscuring the joint space and condylar neck (panoramic radiograph). (Courtesy Dr. J.L. Rajchel, Dallas.)

mandibular growth, development of the affected side of the jaw is inhibited. Some degree of mandibular asymmetry is then noted, the severity depending on the patient's age at onset of the condylar damage. Usually the affected side shows a reduction in the length of the body of the mandible and of the ramus.[25] Also there is often elongation of the coronoid process. These data support the concept that mandibular growth is determined in part by response to functional stimulation. An important radiographic finding in these cases is the presence of a prominent antegonial notch on the affected side of the mandible in most patients. This may result from loss of function of the lateral pterygoid muscle.

Ankylosing spondylitis

Ankylosing spondylitis is a chronic inflammatory connective tissue disease that primarily affects the axial skeleton and central joints, including the TMJ. The cause is unknown, but trauma has been ruled out. Although this disease and rheumatoid arthritis share common features, the consensus is that they are distinct entities. The joint stiffness that is a feature of this disease and characteristically results from immobility (during sleep) is typically relieved by heat and exercise. It is more common in men (9:1) and is probably familial. Individuals with ankylosing spondylitis have a higher frequency of radiographic changes of the condyle, including flattening, osteophytes, erosion (Fig. 25-35), and sclerosis, than do control patients.[110] The

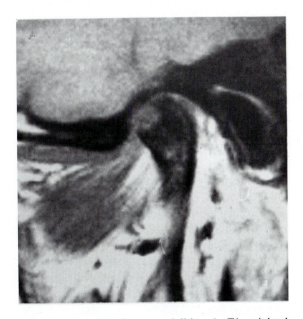

FIG. 25-35. Ankylosing spondylitis. A T1-weighted (600/15) oblique sagittal MRI image of the TMJ in a 25-year-old woman with ankylosing spondylitis shows cortical erosion of the anterior condylar surface and corresponding portion of the temporal bone. No disk is visible, and the interosseous area (of intermediate homogeneous signal intensity) is probably filled with fibrous pannus. Note also the reduced signal intensity of the condylar marrow. (Courtesy Dr. Tore A. Larheim, University of Oslo; from El-Mofty S: *Oral Surg* 46:310-317, 1978.)

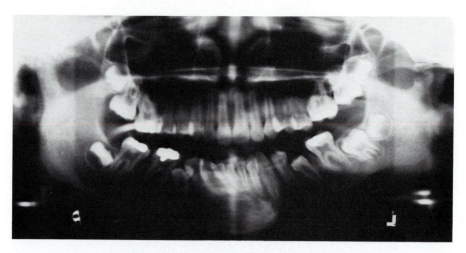

FIG. 25-36. Condylar hypoplasia on the left side, resulting in loss of vertical height of the mandibular ramus.

extent of these findings is correlated with the extent and severity of the disease. The cause of the joint symptoms can be confirmed by demonstrating the rather characteristic radiographic changes in the spine. Intraarticular injections of corticosteroid provide some long-term clinical relief, especially in patients without radiographic signs.[109]

Developmental defects

The developmental defects of the TMJ may be broadly categorized as anomalies of underdevelopment and overdevelopment. In either condition, the most striking radiographic changes in the TMJ are usually seen in the condylar process, although the opposing articular surface of the temporal bone may also exhibit deformity. Condylar articular cartilage provides a site for growth of the mandible. As a result, developmental abnormalities at this location may be manifested by altered growth of the mandibular ramus, body, and even the alveolar process on the affected side. In contrast to the articular and epiphyseal cartilage of long bones, the connective tissue covering permits the condyle to increase in size by both appositional and interstitial growth. As a consequence, this cartilage reacts differently to pathologic stimulae than do other cartilaginous growth centers.[27]

Condylar hypoplasia. Hypoplasia (underdevelopment) of the condyle is generally manifested radiographically by a condylar process and a condyle of reduced size but reasonably normal shape (Fig. 25-36). The condition may be inherited or appear spontaneously or associated with joint disease. Some cases, however, have been attributed

to early injury or destruction of the articular cartilage by birth trauma or infection from adjacent structures, such as the mastoid.[101] Because condylar hypoplasia is usually a component of a mandibular growth deficiency, it is usually associated with an underdeveloped ramus. Often the ipsilateral body of the mandible is also decreased in length. The radiographic appearance of the condyle and mandible is dependent not only on the severity and duration of the process but also on the age of the patient at the time of involvement. The disturbance is much more pronounced if the effect takes place early in life.

In certain prenatal conditions manifesting condylar underdevelopment, for example, hemifacial microsomia and Treacher Collins' syndrome, aural or zygomatic anomalies or both may also be radiographically apparent. If ossicular defects, which may be features of these syndromes, occur, they can be imaged by complex motion tomography of the temporal bone. Antegonial notching of the mandible may be seen in certain developmental abnormalities, such as Treacher Collins' syndrome, hemifacial microsomia, and congenital deformity of the condyle.[6] Because the mandibular ramus may remain relatively short in condylar hypoplasia, while appositional bone growth on the lower border increases the height of the mandibular body, a deep notch in the inferior border of the mandible is produced in front of the attachment of the masseter muscle.[22]

Condylar hyperplasia. Hyperplasia (overdevelopment) of the mandibular condyle is an uncommon event that may occur as a solitary entity

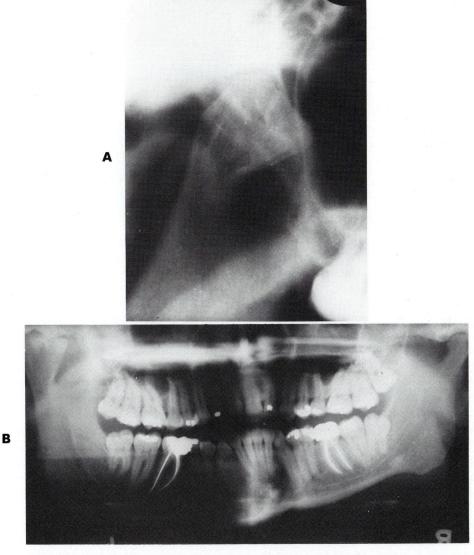

FIG. 25-37. A, Condylar hyperplasia (infracranial projection). **B,** Associated hyperplasia of the ramus and body of the affected side of the mandible (panoramic view).

or be associated with a systemic disorder. When it is an isolated finding, it is probably caused by overactivity of the cartilage or persistent cartilaginous rests, increasing the thickness of the entire cartilaginous and precartilaginous layers. Irritants from an ear infection, abscess of the infratemporal fossa, or osteomyelitis probably act as growth stimulants.[101] In these cases, it is usually limited to one side and is found more frequently in males. Those affected may range in age from childhood to about the fourth decade, and the course is unpredictable. It may progress slowly or rapidly; it may continue to enlarge or become spontaneously arrested. Bi-

lateral condylar hyperplasia is encountered in such developmental abnormalities as hyperpituitarism (giantism in children, acromegaly in adults) and Paget's disease.

Patients with condylar hyperplasia typically have facial asymmetry with deviation of the mandible to the opposite side. In other cases, there may be excessive vertical lengthening of the ramus but without deviation of the chin. Usually the defect is noted during childhood. Surgical correction is usually recommended.[36]

The diagnostic differentiation between hyperplasia and neoplasm involving the condyle, such as osteochondroma, may be impossible to make without critical radiographic evaluation. On one hand, hyperplasia is usually seen radiographically as a generalized enlargement of the condyle with or without some distortion in the shape of the process (Fig. 25-37). On the other hand, the radiographic picture of a localized growth or mass on an otherwise normal-appearing condyle may be the only sound basis for a diagnosis of osteochondroma. Although it is common for the hyperplastic condyle to have an abnormal radiographic contour, a fairly normal cortical thickness and trabecular pattern are usually present. The hyperplastic abnormality may be confined to the condyle, but it is more common for the condylar neck to be enlarged also as a result of a derangement in the bone-remodeling process. Lengthening of the mandibular ramus is typically associated with condylar hyperplasia.

Neoplasia

Benign and malignant neoplastic lesions originating in or involving the TMJ are rare.[72] Such lesions may develop in any component of the joint: the bone of the condyle or articular fossa, the disk, or the capsule. Tumors of the TMJ area grow slowly and attain considerable size before becoming clinically noticeable.[120] They also initially present symptoms that frequently mimic TMJ dysfunction, so radiographs should be examined to exclude the possibility of neoplasia, however slight.[68]

Benign tumors. Benign tumors involving the TMJ include osteoma, osteochondroma, chondroma, chondroblastoma, fibromyxoma, benign giant cell lesion, and synovial chondromatosis. Of these, the first three are the most common. Such tumors in the TMJ are indeed rare. Of 3200 head and neck tumors seen over 20 years in one clinic, only seven were proved cases of tumor of the condyle. Three were osteomas and three were reported as benign giant cell tumors.[69] When such lesions occur, they simulate unilateral condylar hyperplasia clinically by showing (1) facial asymmetry, (2) malocclusion, and (3) prognathic deviation of the mandible to the opposite side.[94] This observation is in keeping with the fact that the condyle is endochondral bone. Benign giant cell lesions also should be considered because they are known to have a predilection for cartilaginous bone.

As mentioned previously, the differentiation between condylar osteoma, osteochondroma, and condylar hyperplasia is occasionally difficult.

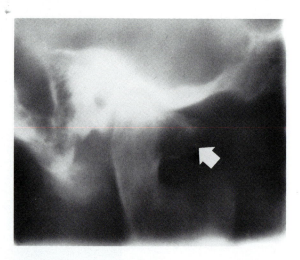

FIG. 25-38. Lateral tomographic view of the TMJ showing a globular osteochondroma on the anterior condylar surface *(arrow)*.

There are two possible areas of differentiation: (1) osteoma and osteochondroma are not as common as hyperplasia, and (2) osteoma and osteochondroma usually occur radiographically as bulbous, globular expansions of the condyle[102] (Fig. 25-38). The characteristic condylar shape and proportions are better preserved in condylar hyperplasia. The radiographic distinction between these tumors and hyperplasia is important because different treatment and follow-up considerations may apply.

Osteochondroma of the coronoid process is rare.[35,121] This deformity may be seen as a bulbous, mushroom-shaped enlargement of the coronoid process. The lesion usually causes progressive limitation of mandibular opening. Such a tumor is typically nonpainful and should be considered in cases of false ankylosis in which the TMJs appear radiographically normal. The Waters projection is the most advantageous conventional view of the coronoid process from the frontal aspect. Tomography or panoramic radiography provides good lateral views, and the SMV projection offers a good basilar view.

Benign tumors and cysts of the mandible may cause considerable destruction of the ramus. It is striking, however, that they usually do not involve the condyle. Ameloblastoma, for example, may involve the entire ramus, yet generally spares the condyle.

Malignant tumors. Primary intrinsic malignant tumors of the TMJ, which are extremely rare, include chondrosarcoma, synovial sarcoma, and fibrosarcoma of the joint capsule.[81] Primary malignant tumors extrinsic to the joint but extending into it are generally direct extensions of parotid salivary gland or other regional carcinomas. Metastatic tumors that invade the condyle through its separate blood supply have also been described.[102] Whereas malignant processes in this region as a rule destroy bony margins, benign lesions typically do not (with the exception of the rather characteristic erosions in rheumatoid arthritis). Chondrosarcoma may be seen as an indistinct, essentially radiolucent enlargement of the condyle with discrete calcifications.[65,106]

Although the coronoid process is membranous bone, a small cap of cartilage develops at its tip at about 4 months of development, only to disappear by the sixth intrauterine month.[100,108] Persistent rests from this transient growth cartilage probably lead to these tumors.

REFERENCES

1. Aggarwal S, Mukhopadhyay S, Berry M, Bhargava S: Bony ankylosis of the temporomandibular joint: a computed tomography study, *Oral Surg Oral Med Oral Pathol* 69:128-132, 1990.
2. Åkerman S, Kopp S, Niler M et al: Relationship between clinical and radiologic findings of the temporomandibular joint in rheumatoid arthritis, *Oral Surg Oral Med Oral Pathol* 66:639-643, 1988.
3. Åkerman S, Kopp S, Rohlin M: Macroscopic and microscopic appearance of radiologic findings in temporomandibular joints from elderly individuals: an autopsy study, *Int J Oral Maxillofac Surg* 17:58-63, 1988.
4. Athreyas BH: Juvenile rheumatoid arthritis. In Rose LF, Kaye D, editors: *Internal medicine for dentistry,* St Louis, 1983, Mosby.
5. Bean L, Petersson A, Svensson A: The transmaxillary projection in temporomandibular joint radiography, *Dentomaxillofac Radiol* 4:13-18, 1975.
6. Becker MH, Coccaro PJ, Converse JM: Antegonial notching of the mandible: an often overlooked mandibular deformity in congenital and acquired disorders, *Radiology* 121:149-151, 1976.
7. Blackwood HJJ: Arthritis of the mandibular joint, *Br Dent J* 115:317-326, 1963.
8. Blaschke DD, Blaschke TJ: A method for quantitatively determining temporomandibular joint bony relationships, *J Dent Res* 60:35-43, 1981.
9. Brand JW: Temporomandibular joint arthrography. In Delbalso AM, editor: *Maxillofacial Imaging,* Philadelphia, 1990, WB Saunders.
10. Brand JW, Whinery JG Jr, Anderson QN, Kennan KM: Condylar position as a predictor of temporomandibular joint internal derangement, *Oral Surg Oral Med Oral Pathol* 67:469-476, 1989.
11. Buckingham RB, Braun T, Harinstein DA et al: Temporomandibular joint dysfunction syndrome: a close association with systemic joint laxity (the hypermobile joint syndrome), *Oral Surg Oral Med Oral Pathol* 72:514-519, 1991.
12. Chalmers IM, Blair GS: Is the temporomandibular joint involved in primary osteoarthrosis? *Oral Surg* 38:74-79, 1974.
13. Chilvarquer I, McDavid WD, Langlais RP et al: A new technique for imaging the temporomandibular joint with a panoramic x-ray machine: part I, description of the technique, *Oral Surg Oral Med Oral Pathol* 65:626-631, 1988.
14. Chilvarquer I, Prihoda T, McDavid WD et al: A new technique for imaging the temporomandibular joint with a panoramic x-ray machine: part II, positioning with the use of patient data, *Oral Surg Oral Med Oral Pathol* 65:632-636, 1988.
15. Christiansen EL, Thompson JR: *Temporomandibular joint imaging,* St Louis, 1990, Mosby.
16. Conway WF, Hayes CW, Campbell RL: Dynamic magnetic resonance imaging of the temporomandibular joint using FLASH sequences, *J Oral Maxillofac Surg* 46:930-938, 1988.
17. Dahlstrom L, Kahnberg KE, Lindahl L: 15 years follow-up on condylar fractures, *Int J Oral Maxillofac Surg* 18:18-23, 1989.
18. deBont LG, Boering G, Liem RSB et al: Osteoarthritis and internal derangement of the temporomandibular joint: a light microscopic study, *J Oral Maxillofac Surg* 44:634-643, 1986.
19. deBont LGM, Liem RSB, Boering G: Synovial chondromatosis of the temporomandibular joint: a light and electron microscopic study, *Oral Surg Oral Med Oral Pathol* 66:593-598, 1988.
20. Donlon WC, Moon KL: Comparison of magnetic resonance imaging, arthrotomography and clinical and surgical findings in temporomandibular joint internal derangements, *Oral Surg Oral Med Oral Pathol* 64:2-5, 1987.
21. Drace JE, Enzmann DR: Defining the normal temporomandibular joint: closed-, partially open-, and open-mouth MR imaging of asymptomatic subjects, *Radiology* 177:67-71, 1990.
22. DuBrul EL: *Sicher's oral anatomy,* ed 7, St Louis, 1980, Mosby.
23. Eckerdahl O, Lundberg M: Temporomandibular joint relations as revealed by conventional radiographic technique: a comparison with the morphology and tomographic images, *Dentomaxillofac Radiol* 8:65-70, 1979.
24. El-Mofty S: Ankylosis of the temporomandibular joint, *Oral Surg* 33:650-660, 1972.
25. El-Mofty S: Mandibular features of patients with temporomandibular ankylosis, *Oral Surg* 46:310-317, 1978.
26. Gibilisco JA: Management of temporomandibular joint disorders associated with systemic disease. In Gelb H, editor: Symposium on temporomandibular joint dysfunction and treatment, *Dent Clin North Am* 7:457-478, 1983.
27. Greenberg MS: Septic arthritis of the temporomandibular joint. In Rose LF, Kaye D, editors: *Internal medicine for dentistry,* St Louis, 1983, Mosby.
28. Hansson LG, Hansson T, Petersson A: A comparison between clinical and radiologic findings in 259 temporomandibular joint patients, *J Prosthet Dent* 50:89-94, 1983.
29. Hansson LG, Westesson PL, Katzberg RW et al: MR imaging of the temporomandibular joint: comparison of images of autopsy specimens made at 0.3 T and 1.5 T with anatomic cryosections, *Am J Roentgenol* 152:1241-1244, 1989.

30. Hasso AN, Christiansen EL, Alder ME: The temporomandibular joint, *Radiol Clin North Am* 27:301-314, 1989.

31. Hecker R, Eversole LR, Packard HR et al: Symptomatic osteoarthritis of the temporomandibular joint: report of a case, *J Oral Surg* 33:780-783, 1975.

32. Helms CA, Kaplan P: Diagnostic imaging of the temporomandibular joint: recommendations for use of the various techniques, *Am J Roentgenol* 154:319-322, 1990.

33. Hoffman DC, Berliner L, Manzione J et al: Use of direct sagittal computed tomography in diagnosis and treatment of internal derangements of the temporomandibular joint, *J Am Dent Assoc* 113:407-411, 1986.

34. Horowitz I, Abrahami E, Mintz S: Demonstration of condylar fractures of the mandible by computed tomography, *Oral Surg* 54:263-268, 1982.

35. James RB, Alexander RW, Traver JG: Osteochondroma of the mandibular coronoid process, *Oral Surg* 37:189-195, 1974.

36. Jonck L: Facial asymmetry and condylar hyperplasia, *Oral Surg* 40:567-573, 1975.

37. Kaplan PA, Helms CA: Arthrography of the inferior joint space of the temporomandibular joint. In Westesson PL, Katzberg RW, editors: *Cranio clinics international: Imaging of the temporomandibular joint,* Baltimore, 1991, Williams & Wilkins.

38. Katzberg RW: Temporomandibular joint imaging, *Radiology* 170:297-307, 1989.

39. Katzberg RW, Keith DA, Guralnick WC et al: Internal derangements and arthritis of the temporomandibular joint, *Radiology* 146:107-112, 1983.

40. Katzberg RW, Keith DA, Guralnick WC et al: Correlation of condylar mobility and arthrotomography in patients with internal derangements of the temporomandibular joint, *Oral Surg* 54:622-627, 1982.

41. Katzberg RW, Keith DA, ten-Eick WR, Guralnick WC: Internal derangements of the temporomandibular joint: an assessment of condylar position in centric occlusion, *J Prosthet Dent* 49:250-254, 1983.

42. Katzberg RW, Tallents RH, Hayakawa K et al: Internal derangements of the temporomandibular joint: findings in the pediatric age group, *Radiology* 154:125-127, 1985.

43. Katzberg RW, Westesson PL, Tallents RH et al: Temporomandibular joint: MR assessment of rotational and sideways disk displacements, *Radiology* 169:741-748, 1988.

44. Kaugars GE, Mercuri LG, Laskin DM: Pneumatization of the articular eminence of the temporal bone: prevalence, development, and surgical treatment, *J Am Dent Assoc* 113:55-57, 1986.

45. Kircos LT, Ortendahl DA, Mark AS, Arakawa M: Magnetic resonance imaging of the TMJ disk in asymptomatic volunteers, *J Oral Maxillofac Surg* 45:852-854, 1987.

46. Kirk WS Jr: A comparative study of axial corrected tomography with magnetic resonance imagery in 35 joints, *Oral Surg Oral Med Oral Pathol* 68:646-652, 1989.

47. Kononen M, Kilpinen E: Comparison of three radiographic methods in screening of temporomandibular joint involvement in patients with psoriatic arthritis, *Acta Odontol Scand* 48:271-277, 1990.

48. Kopp S, Rockler B: Relationship between clinical and radiographic findings in patients with mandibular pain or dysfunction, *Acta Radiol Diagn* 20:465-477, 1979.

49. Kopp S, Rockler B: Relationship between radiographic signs in the temporomandibular joint and hand joints, *Acta Odont Scand* 37:169-175,1979.

50. Kruger GO: *Textbook of oral and maxillofacial surgery,* ed 5, St Louis, 1979, Mosby.

51. Larheim TA, Dale K, Tveito L: Radiographic abnormalities of the temporomandibular joint in children with juvenile rheumatoid arthritis, *Acta Radiol Diagn* 22:277-284, 1981.

52. Larheim TA, Haanaes HR, Ruud AF: Mandibular growth, temporomandibular joint changes and dental occlusion in juvenile rheumatoid arthritis, *Scand J Rheumatol* 10:225-233, 1981.

53. Larheim TA, Hoyeraal HM, Stabrun AE, Haanaes HR: The temporomandibular joint in juvenile rheumatoid arthritis: radiographic changes related to clinical and laboratory parameters in 100 children, *Scand J Rheumatol* 11:5-12, 1982.

54. Larheim TA, Kolbenstvedt A: Osseous temporomandibular joint abnormalities in rheumatic disease: computed tomography versus hypocycloidal tomography, *Acta Radiol* 31:383-387, 1990.

55. Larheim TA, Smith HJ, Aspestrand F: Rheumatic disease of the temporomandibular joint: MR imaging and tomographic manifestations, *Radiology* 175:527-531, 1990.

56. Larheim TA, Storhaug K, Tveito L: Temporomandibular joint involvement and dental occlusion in a group of adults with rheumatoid arthritis, *Acta Odontol Scand* 41:301-309, 1983.

57. Lindahl L, Hollender L: Condylar fractures of the mandible: II, a radiographic study of remodeling processes in the temporomandibular joint, *Int J Oral Surg* 6:153-165, 1977.

58. Lundh H, Westesson PL: Clinical signs of temporomandibular joint internal derangement in adults, *Oral Surg Oral Med Oral Pathol* 72:637-641, 1991.

59. Martis CS, Kerakosis DT: Ankylosis of the temporomandibular joint caused by Still's disease, *Oral Surg* 35:462-466, 1973.

60. Mayne JG, Hatch GS: Arthritis of the temporomandibular joint, *J Am Dent Assoc* 79:125-130, 1969.

61. McNeill C, Mohl ND, Rugh JD, Tanaka TT: Temporomandibular disorders: diagnosis, management, education, and research, *J Am Dent Assoc* 120:253-263, 1990.

62. Mejersjo C, Hollender L: TMJ pain and dysfunction: relation between clinical and radiographic findings in the short and long term, *Scand J Dent Res* 92:241-248, 1984.

63. Mongini F: The importance of radiography in the diagnosis of TMJ dysfunctions: a comparative evaluation of transcranial radiographs and serial tomography, *J Prosthet Dent* 45:186-198, 1981.

64. Mongini F: *The stomatognathic system,* Chicago, 1984, Quintessence.

65. Morris MR, Clark SK, Porter BA, Delbecq RJ: Chondrosarcoma of the temporomandibular joint: case report, *Head Neck Surg* 10:113-117, 1987.

66. Moss ML: The functional matrix concept and its relationship to temporomandibular joint dysfunction and treatment, *Dent Clin North Am* 7:445-455, 1983.

67. Musgrave MT, Westesson PL, Tallents RH et al: Improved magnetic resonance imaging of the temporomandibular joint by oblique scanning planes, *Oral Surg Oral Med Oral Pathol* 71:525-528, 1991.

68. Nortjé CJ, Farman AG, Grotepass FW et al: Chondrosarcoma of the mandibular condyle: report of a case with special reference to radiographic features, *Br J Oral Surg* 14:101-111, 1976.

69. Nwoku ALN, Koch H: The temporomandibular joint: a rare localization for bone tumors, *J Maxillofac Surg* 2:113-119, 1974.

70. Ogus HD, Toller PA: *Common disorders of the temporomandibular joint, dental practitioner handbook,* Bristol, 1981, John Wright.

71. Olson L, Eckerdal O, Hallonsten AL et al. Craniomandibular function in juvenile chronic arthritis: a clinical and radiographic study, *Swed Dent J* 15:71-83, 1991.

72. Petersson A, Nanthaviroj S: Radiography of the temporomandibular joint utilizing the transmaxillary projection, *Dentomaxillofac Radiol* 4:76-83, 1975.

73. Pettigrew J, Roberts D, Riddle R et al: Identification of an anteriorly displaced meniscus in vitro by means of three-dimensional image reconstructions, *Oral Surg* 59:535-542, 1985.

74. Pressman BD, Shellock FG: Static and kinematic MR imaging, *CDA J* 16:32-37, 1988.

75. Price C: Method of quantifying disc movement on magnetic resonance images of the temporomandibular joint: 2, application of the method to normal and deranged joints, *Dentomaxillofac Radiol* 19:63-66, 1990.

76. Pullinger A, Hollender L: Assessment of mandibular condyle position: a comparison of transcranial radiographs and linear tomograms, *Oral Surg* 60:329-334, 1985.

77. Pullinger AG, Baldioceda F, Bibb CA: Relationship of TMJ articular soft tissue to underlying bone in young adult condyles, *J Dent Res* 69:1512-1518, 1990.

78. Pullinger AG, Hollender L, Solberg WK, Petersson A: A tomographic study of mandibular condyle position in an asymptomatic population, *J Prosthet Dent* 53:706-713, 1985.

79. Rao VM, Farole A, Karasick D: Temporomandibular joint dysfunction: correlation of MR imaging, arthrography, and arthroscopy, *Radiology* 174:663-667, 1990.

80. Raustia AM, Pyhtinen J, Oikarinen KS, Altonen M: Conventional radiographic and computed tomographic findings in cases of fracture of the mandibular condylar process, *J Oral Maxillofac Surg* 48:1258-1264, 1990.

81. Richter KJ, Freeman NS, Quiek CA: Chondrosarcoma of the temporomandibular joint: report of a case, *J Oral Surg* 32:777-781, 1974.

82. Roberts D, Pettigrew J, Ram C, Joseph PM: Radiologic techniques used to evaluate the temporomandibular joint: II, computed tomography, three-dimensional imaging and nuclear magnetic resonance, *Anesth Prog* 31:241-256, 1984.

83. Roberts D, Pettigrew J, Udupa J, Ram C: Three-dimensional imaging and display of the temporomandibular joint, *Oral Surg* 58:461-474, 1984.

84. Ronquillo HI, Guay J, Tallents RH et al: Tomographic analysis of mandibular condyle position as compared to arthrographic findings of the temporomandibular joint, *J Cranio Dis Fac and Oral Pain* 2:59-64, 1988.

85. Ross JB: Diagnostic criteria and nomenclature for TMJ arthrography in sagittal section: part I, derangements, *J Cranio Disord* 1:185-201, 1987.

86. Rowe NL: Ankylosis of the temporomandibular joint, *J R Coll Surg Edinb* 27:67-79, 1982.

87. Rowe NL, Killey HC: *Fractures of the facial skeleton,* ed 2, Edinburgh, 1970, Churchill Livingstone.

88. Rugh JD, Solberg WK: Oral health status in the United States: temporomandibular disorders, *J Dent Educ* 49:398-405, 1985.

89. Sahm G, Witt E: Long-term results after childhood condylar fractures: a computer-tomographic study, *Eur J Orthod* 11:154-160, 1989.

90. Sanchez-Woodworth RE, Katzberg RW, Tallents RH, Guay JA: Radiographic assessment of temporomandibular joint pain and dysfunction in the pediatric age-group, *J Dent Child* 55:278-281, 1988.

91. Schellhas KP: Temporomandibular joint injuries, *Radiology* 173:211-216, 1989.

92. Schwaighofer BW, Tanaka TT, Klein MV et al: MR imaging of the temporomandibular joint: a cadaver study of the value of coronal images, *Am J Radiol* 154:1245-1249, 1990.

93. Simon G: *Principles of bone x-ray diagnosis,* ed 2, London, 1965, Butterworth.

94. Simon G, Kendrick R, Whitlock R: Osteochondroma of the mandibular condyle: case report and its management, *Oral Surg* 43:18-24, 1977.

95. Smith SR, Matteson SR, Phillips C, Tyndall DA: Quantitative and subjective analysis of temporomandibular joint radiographs, *J Prosthet Dent* 62:456-463, 1989.

96. Stabrun AE, Larheim TA, Hoyeraal HM, Rosler M: Reduced mandibular dimensions and asymmetry in juvenile rheumatoid arthritis: pathogenetic factors, *Arthritis Rheum* 31:602-611, 1988.

97. Syrjanen SM: The temporomandibular joint in rheumatoid arthritis, *Acta Radiol Diagn* 26:235-243, 1985.

98. Taylor RC, Ware WH, Fowler D, Kobayashi J: A study of temporomandibular joint morphology and its relationship to the dentition, *Oral Surg* 33:1002-1013, 1972.

99. Teittmen M, Josmsa T: The impact of juvenile rheumatoid arthritis on the growth of the mandible, *Proc Finn Dent Soc* 80:182-185, 1984.

100. Ten Cate AR: *Oral histology: development, structure and function,* ed 2, St Louis, 1985, Mosby.

101. Thoma KH: Tumors of the condyle and temporomandibular joint, *Oral Surg* 7:1091-1107, 1954.

102. Thoma KH: Tumors of the temporomandibular joint, *J Oral Surg* 22:157-163, 1964.

103. Toller PA: Osteoarthrosis of the mandibular condyle, *Br Dent J* 134:223-231, 1973.

104. Tyndall DA, Matteson SR: Radiographic appearance and population distribution of the pneumatized articular eminence of the temporal bone, *J Oral Maxillofac Surg* 43:493-497, 1985.

105. Van der Kuijl B, Vencken LM, de Bont LG, Boering G: Temporomandibular joint computed tomography: development of a direct sagittal technique, *J Prosthet Dent* 64:709-715, 1990.

106. Wasenko JJ, Rosenbloom SA: Temporomandibular joint chondrosarcoma: CT demonstration, *J Comput Assist Tomogr* 14:1002-1003, 1990.

107. Weinberg LA, Chastain JK: New TMJ clinical data and the implication on diagnosis and treatment, *Am Dent Assoc J* 120:305-311, 1990.

108. Weinmann JP, Sicher H: *Bone and bones,* St Louis, 1947, Mosby.

109. Wenneberg B: Inflammatory involvement of the temporomandibular joint: diagnostic and therapeutic aspects and a study of individuals with ankylosing spondylitis, *Swed Dent J Suppl* 20:1-54, 1983.

110. Wenneberg B, Hollender L, Kopp S: Radiographic changes in the temporomandibular joint in ankylosing spondylitis, *Dentomaxillofac Radiol* 12:25-30, 1983.

111. Westesson P-L: Double-contrast arthrotomography of the temporomandibular joint: introduction of an arthrographic technique for visualization of the disc and articular surfaces, *J Oral Maxillofac Surg* 41:163-172, 1983.

112. Westesson P-L: Structural hard-tissue changes in temporomandibular joints with internal derangement, *Oral Surg* 59:220-224, 1985.

113. Westesson P-L, Bronstein SL: Temporomandibular joint: comparison of single- and double-contrast arthrography, *Radiology* 164:65-70, 1987.

114. Westesson P-L, Bronstein SL, Liedberg J: Internal derangement of the temporomandibular joints: morphologic description with correlation to joint function, *Oral Surg Oral Med Oral Pathol* 59:323-331, 1985.

115. Westesson P-L, Cohen JM, Tallents RH: Magnetic resonance imaging of temporomandibular joint after surgical treatment of internal derangement, *Oral Surg Oral Med Oral Pathol* 71:407-411, 1991.

116. Westesson P-L, Eriksson L, Kurita K: Reliability of a negative clinical temporomandibular joint examination: prevalence of disk displacement in asymptomatic temporomandibular joints, *Oral Surg Oral Med Oral Pathol* 68:551-554, 1989.

117. Westesson P-L, Kurita K, Eriksson L, Katzberg RW: Cryosectional observations of functional anatomy of the temporomandibular joint, *Oral Surg Oral Med Oral Pathol* 68:247-251, 1989.

118. Wilkes CH: Internal derangements of the temporomandibular joint: pathological variations, *Arch Otolaryngol Head Neck Surg* 115:469-477, 1989.

119. Wood RE, Harris AMP, Nortjé CJ, Grotepass FW: The radiologic features of true ankylosis of the temporomandibular joint: an analysis of 25 cases, *Dentomaxillofac Radiol* 17:121-127, 1988.

120. Worman HG, Waldron CW, Radusch DF: Osteoma of the mandibular condyle, with deviation prognathic deformity, *J Oral Surg* 4:27-32, 1946.

121. Worth HM: The role of the radiologist interpretation in disease of the temporomandibular joint, *Oral Sci Rev* 6:3-51, 1974.

122. Yale SH, Allison BD, Hauptfuehrer JD: An epidemiological assessment of mandibular condylar morphology, *Oral Surg* 21:169-177, 1966.

26

Paranasal Sinuses

Many of the conditions a dental diagnostician evaluates involve not only dental structures but also the soft tissues and skeleton of the oral cavity, face, nose, nasopharynx, and even the eyes. Consequently, to perform a more thorough examination, the dentist must frequently supplement periapical films with extraoral radiographs that include the paranasal sinuses. It is important to recognize the diseases that involve the paranasal sinuses, especially the maxillary sinus, because they may refer pain to the dental structures.

The paranasal sinuses develop as evaginations from the nasal fossae. The first to develop is the *maxillary sinus,* which becomes apparent by day 17 in utero.[25] It begins just above the inferior turbinate and grows laterally. At birth it is about the size of a small bean. Initially the sinus lies medial to the orbit, but as it grows it develops laterally under the orbit. It reaches the infraorbital canal during the second year, and laterally the zygomatic bone by the ninth year. By approximately this time its inferior growth has extended to the level of the floor of the nasal fossa. Lateral growth ceases by the fifteenth year.[71] The average volume of the adult maxillary sinus is about 15 ml.[71] Hypoplasia of the maxillary sinus occurs unilaterally in about 1.7% of patients and bilaterally in 7.2%.[31] In patients with hypoplasia of the maxillary sinus, the affected sinus is more opaque than normal because of the relatively large amount of remaining maxillary bone. The configuration of the walls of the maxillary sinus frequently helps in distinguishing between a hypoplastic sinus and one that is pathologically opaque. On the Waters projection, the walls of the hypoplastic sinus bow inward, resulting in a small air cavity that appears to be opacified.

The *ethmoid sinuses* start developing as outgrowths of the nasal fossa during the fifth fetal month. These air cells continue to expand in the ethmoid bone until the end of puberty, when there are 13 to 15 paired cells.[58] The ethmoid air cells often extend into the lacrimal bone.

The development of the *frontal sinuses* does not usually begin until the fifth or sixth year.[25] They may develop either from the nasal fossa or from an anterior ethmoid air cell. A right and left frontal sinus cavity develops separately during adolescence. As these cavities expand, they approach each other in the midline where a thin bony septum separates them. This intrasinus septum may be absent in some individuals.[25] In about 4% of people, the frontal sinuses fail to develop. In the adult, the frontal sinuses are usually seen as two asymmetric cavities above the level of the supraorbital ridges and the nasion.[12] These sinuses drain directly into the nasal fossa via their frontonasal ducts (about half the cases) or into the anterior ethmoid cells, then into the nasal fossa through the infundibulum.[71]

The *sphenoid sinuses* begin growth from the nasal cavity in the fourth fetal month. The invaginations for the sphenoid sinuses are from the sphenoethmoid recess of the nasal cavity. They are present at birth as minute cavities in the sphenoid, deep within the skull. The main development takes place after puberty. The right and left sphenoid sinus, separated by a bony septum, are usually asymmetric in size. Also, the size of the sinus cavities is quite variable. They have easy access to the nasal cavity through ostia, 2 to 3 mm in diameter, which probably explains why, like the maxillary sinus, bone-destroying cysts are uncommon in the sphenoid sinuses (see the section on mucoceles later in this chapter). The mucosa of the sinuses is similar to that of the nasal cavity but with slightly fewer mucous glands. The epithelial cilia move mucus toward their respective communications with the nasal fossa.[15,25]

Clinicians have debated the function of the paranasal sinuses over the years. Various functions have been ascribed to these sinuses, including air conditioning (heating and humidification), air reservoir, ventilation, aid in olfaction, reduction in weight of the cranium, addition of resonance to voice, protection and insulation of cerebrum and orbits, participation in formation of the cranium, or evolutionary unwanted space.[74] It is clear that olfaction was the primary nasal function in early developing mammals, but the evolution of humans, with decreased emphasis on olfaction in favor of vision and thought, has led to the development of new functions for these air spaces. Some believe that as mammals progressed toward primates and humans, the function of the sinuses evolved from olfaction to assisting in respiration while adapting to changes in the cranium. Accordingly, the maxillary and ethmoid sinuses may assist in respiration, with the maxillary sinus also adjusting to the changing size of the maxillofacial area. The frontal sinus participates in the growth and development of the cerebral cranium, and the sphenoid sinus allows for adjustments of the buckling in the cranial base.[74]

PROJECTIONS

Conventional radiographic examination of the sinuses requires use of a series of skull projections (see Chapter 11). The *Caldwell posteroanterior* projection provides good visualization of the frontal sinus and the ethmoid air cells. In addition, the nasal cavity and superior portions of the maxillary antra may be examined with this view. The *Waters* projection is optimal for visualization of the maxillary sinuses, although with this view the alveolar bone and the posterior dentition obscure the posteroinferior part of the sinus.[13,81] When the mouth is open, the sphenoid sinus may also be visualized. The *lateral skull* view allows examination of the sphenoid and maxillary sinuses and the frontal and ethmoid sinuses. The *submentovertex* projection helps define the extent of the sphenoid sinus. Tomographic projections of the maxillary sinus are valuable for viewing solid masses such as an osteoma or antrolith.[34] When examining the sinuses on these projections, it is useful to remember that sinus disease is often unilateral; thus, comparison of the two sides may assist in demonstrating the abnormality.

In recent years, CT and MRI have become increasingly important for evaluation of sinus disease. These modalities are most appropriate to determine the extent of sinus disease prior to surgical treatment. High-resolution axial and coronal CT

and MRI examinations are the most revealing noninvasive techniques for the paranasal sinuses and adjacent structures and areas. CT examination is appropriate to determine the extent of disease in patients who have chronic or recurrent sinusitis, particularly when surgery is contemplated. It provides superior imaging of the anterior ethmoid air cells and the upper two thirds of the nasal cavity. CT is also best for demonstrating the bone reaction to sinus disease. MR provides superior imaging of soft tissue, especially the extension of infiltrating neoplasms into surrounding soft tissues.[40,84] Such preoperative assessment of tumors is best made with gadolinium-enhanced magnetic resonance.

The utility of *ultrasound* has been considered for examining the maxillary sinus. Sinus fluid may be detected with ultrasonography. The sensitivity of detection is proportional to the amount of fluid present. However, mucosal swelling, polyps, and cysts are poorly demonstrated by ultrasonography.[28] This technique may be most useful for follow-up treatment.

Sinuscopy is the use of short Fiberglas endoscopes for inspection of the nasal cavities. This technique provides excellent visualization of the upper nasal fossa and turbinates and sinus ostia. When the maxillary ostia are large enough, it may be used for direct inspection of the maxillary sinus.[33]

INFLAMMATORY CHANGES

Whether of infectious or allergic origin or caused by chemical irritation, introduction of a foreign body, or facial trauma, insults to the paranasal sinuses cause changes and disorders that are detectable by radiographic examination. Such changes include thickened mucosa, sinusitis, fluid levels in the sinus, polyps, empyema, or mucous retention cysts. However, viral infections may not cause a radiographic change in a sinus.[59]

Thickened mucosa

The lining membrane of the paranasal sinuses is a respiratory mucosa (or mucoperiosteum) that is normally about 1 mm thick. Normal sinus mucosa is not usually apparent in a radiograph, and the bony walls appear distinct and clear.[13] However, when the lining mucosa becomes inflamed from either an infectious or allergic process, it may increase in thickness 10 to 15 times.[34] Mucous membrane thickening greater than 3 mm is most likely pathologic.[13] The image of the thickened mucosa is readily detectable in the radiograph as a band

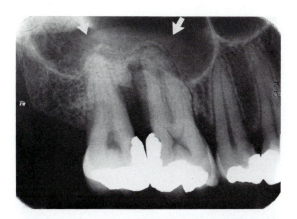

FIG. 26-1. Thickened mucoperiosteum seen as a radiopaque band on the floor of the maxillary antrum. It developed in response to a localized area of periodontal disease.

noticeably more radiopaque than the air-filled sinus and paralleling the bony wall of the sinus (Fig. 26-1).

Most of the inflammatory or allergic episodes that result in thickening of the sinus lining are unrecognized by the patient and are discovered only incidentally on a radiograph. Also, the depth of a thickened mucosa in an asymptomatic individual may vary considerably over a relatively short time. Consequently, the discovery of a thickened mucosa in an individual who is otherwise without symptoms does not necessarily imply that treatment is required. Usually when there is an identifiable cause for the mucosal thickening, such thickening will disappear following removal of the cause. If the thickening results from a periapical infection, it usually clears up in days or weeks after successful treatment of the dental infection.

Sinusitis

Sinusitis is a condition involving inflammation of the paranasal sinus mucosa. The term is usually restricted to conditions that are primarily inflammatory, cause subjective symptoms, and persist longer than 7 days, the duration of a typical viral upper respiratory tract infection. Sinusitis is usually caused by blockage of drainage from the ostiomeatal complex, the region of the ostium of the maxillary sinus and the ethmoidal ostium. This leads to ciliary dysfunction and retention of the mucosal secretions, followed by bacteria invasion and overgrowth.[55] Perhaps 10% of inflammatory episodes of the maxillary sinuses are extensions of dental infections.[34] Chronic sinusitis refers to con-

ditions lasting more than 3 months. Subacute sinusitis refers to conditions lasting from 1 to 3 months. The term *pansinusitis* describes sinusitis affecting all the paranasal sinuses. Pansinusitis in children suggests the possibility of cystic fibrosis.[59]

Clinical features. *Acute maxillary sinusitis* is often a complication of a nose cold. It is often accompanied by purulent nasal discharge or pharyngeal drainage.[68] After a few days, the stuffiness and nasal discharge increase, and the patient may complain of pain and tenderness to pressure or swelling over the involved sinus. The pain, however, may be referred to the premolar and molar teeth on the affected side, and these teeth may also be sensitive to percussion. This finding requires that these teeth be ruled out as a possible source of the pain or infection. However, the key signs and symptoms are those of sepsis: fever, chills, malaise, and an elevated leukocyte count.[49] Acute sinusitis is the most common of the sinus conditions that cause pain.

Chronic maxillary sinusitis is typically a sequela of an acute infection that fails to resolve by 3 months. In general, there are no external signs except during periods of acute exacerbations when increased pain and discomfort are apparent. Chronic sinusitis is often associated with anatomic derangements that inhibit the outflow of mucus.[55] These include deviation of the nasal septum, presence of a concha bullosa (pneumatization of the middle turbinate), or the presence of nasal polyps. Chronic sinusitis is also often associated with allergic rhinitis, asthma, cystic fibrosis, and dental infections.[18]

Radiographic features. The thickening of the mucosa and the accumulation of secretions that accompany sinusitis reduce the air content of the sinus and cause it to become increasingly radiopaque (Fig. 26-2). There may be an air-fluid level. The most common radiopaque patterns are (1) localized thickening at the base of the sinus, (2) generalized thickening of the mucoperiosteum around the entire wall of the sinus, (3) complete filling of the sinus except about the ostium on the medial wall, and (4) complete filling of the sinus.[52] Such changes are best seen in the maxillary sinus, but the frontal and sphenoid sinuses may be similarly affected.

The image of the thickened mucosa on the radiograph may be uniform or polypoid. In the case of an allergic reaction, and if the antral cavity is apparent, the mucosa tends to be more lobulated (Fig. 26-3). In contrast, in cases of infection, the

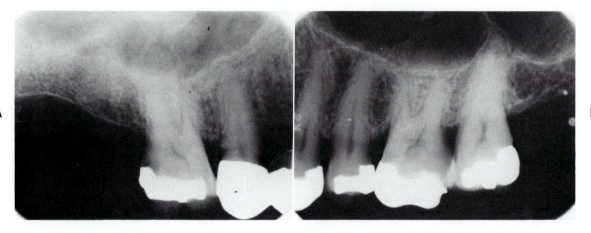

FIG. 26-2. Sinusitis seen as a thickening of the mucoperiosteum. Compare the opacified maxillary sinus, **A,** with the normal sinus, **B.**

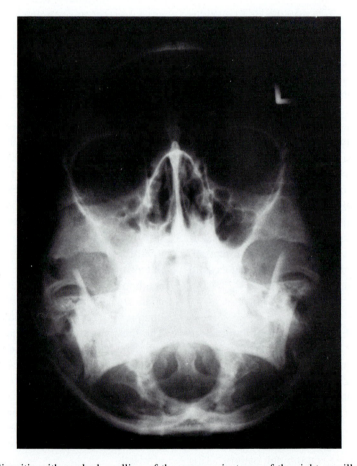

FIG. 26-3. Sinusitis with marked swelling of the mucoperiosteum of the right maxillary sinus that has nearly filled the antrum. Note the partial filling of the antrum *(left).*

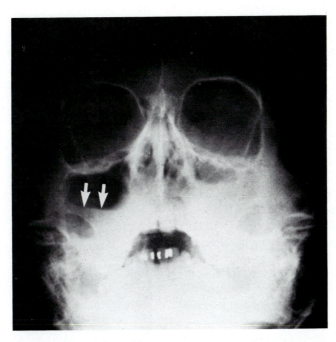

FIG. 26-4. An air-fluid level in the right maxillary antrum *(arrows)*. Note the markedly thickened mucoperiosteum in the left sinus.

mucosal outline tends to be straighter, paralleling the sinus wall.[63]

The resolution of acute sinusitis will become apparent on the radiograph as a gradual increase in the translucency of the sinus. This can first be recognized when a small clear area appears in the interior of the sinus; the thickened mucosa gradually shrinks so that it parallels the outline of the bony wall. In time, the mucosa again becomes radiographically invisible, and the sinus appears normal. Chronic sinusitis may result in persistent opacification of the sinus and sclerosis or thickening of the surrounding bone. Bony erosion is unusual.[84]

Management. The goals of treatment of sinusitis are to control the infection, promote drainage, and relieve pain. Acute sinusitis is usually treated medically with topical decongestants to reduce swelling of the mucous membranes and with antibiotics against bacteria.[27] Chronic sinusitis is primarily a disease of obstruction of the ostia; thus the goal is ventilation and drainage. This is often accomplished through endoscopic surgery to enlarge obstructed ostia.[33] When periapical or periodontal disease is the cause of sinusitis, then these dental conditions should be treated promptly.

Fluid levels

Because the radiographic densities of transudates, exudates, blood, and pathologically altered mucosa appear similar, the primary features of a questionable sinus shadow that can aid in its identification are form and distribution.[10] The presence of fluid in a sinus is indicated when the translucency of a portion of a sinus is reduced, and the line of demarcation between the more translucent and the more opaque portions is horizontal and straight (Fig. 26-4). The most common causes of fluid in a sinus are pus caused by infection and blood resulting from trauma. It is possible to confirm that one is viewing an air-fluid level boundary by tilting the head and making another radiograph.[34] This will cause a new level to form, which will eliminate any doubt as to its nature. However, when attempting to verify that such a shadow is an air-fluid level, allow sufficient time between the time the head was tilted and the second radiograph is made. If the fluid in question is a thick mucus, some minutes may be required before it attains its new level.[63] To demonstrate an air-fluid level, the patient must be upright and the x-ray beam must be horizontal at the level of the air-fluid interface.

Empyema

If a sinus ostium remains blocked by thickened, inflamed mucosa or other pathologic conditions, an empyema (a cavity filled with pus) is a possible sequela, especially in the maxillary sinus. Radiographically the sinus appears completely opaque. This condition can be distinguished from a simple mucosal thickening by the decalcification of surrounding bony wall and haziness of the trabecular bone next to the sinus wall. The bone destruction is best observed about the frontal sinus. The infection may extend into the adjacent bone with the development of an osteomyelitis.

Polyps

The thickened mucosa of a chronically inflamed sinus frequently forms into irregular folds. Polypoid hypertrophy of the mucosa may develop in an isolated area or a number of areas throughout the sinus. In differentiating a polyp from a mucosal retention cyst on a radiograph, the polyp usually occurs with a thickened mucosal lining (Fig. 26-5), because the polypoid mass is no more than an accentuation of the thickening that is affecting the entire sinus lining.[51] In most cases, however, the adjacent mucosal lining around a mucosal retention cyst is not apparent.

Polyps may cause bone displacement or destruction. Polyps in the maxillary sinus can displace or destroy the medial or lateral wall. In the ethmoid sinus, they may cause destruction of the medial wall of the orbit with subsequent unilateral proptosis. The radiographic image of the bone destruction associated with polyps frequently mimics that of a benign or malignant tumor. Because many of the sinus tumors are silent, examination of a paranasal sinus that reveals bone destruction associated with opacification is an indication for biopsy, undelayed by initial conservative treatment.[51]

Mucosal retention cysts

Another common sequela of an inflamed or hyperplastic mucosal lining of the sinus is the development of a mucosal retention cyst (also called *benign mucous cyst* or *mucous retention cyst*).[53] Mucosal retention cysts are of two general types: so-called benign retention cyst and destructive retention cyst. There are two benign varieties, one described as a mucous secretory retention cyst and the other a serous nonsecretory retention cyst. They probably have different origins.[69] The destructive mucosal retention cysts are called *mucoceles.*

The *mucous secretory retention cyst* results from an obstruction of ducts of the seromucinous glands in the lamina propria of the sinus lining. The obstruction is secondary to local inflammation, usually caused by either infection or allergy.[13] A cyst forms as the occluded glands accumulate secretion. The cyst is lined with either respiratory epithelium or, as a result of intracyst pressure, a dysplastic,

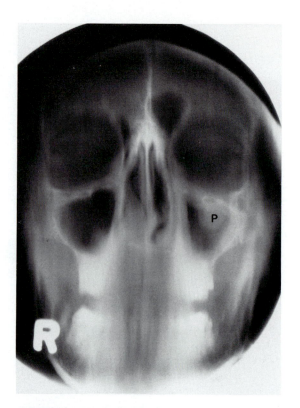

FIG. 26-5. A frontal tomogram at the level of the maxillary sinuses shows thickened mucosa of all borders of the left maxillary sinus and a polyp *(P)* suspended from the superior border of the sinus. (Courtesy Drs. A. G. Farman, C. J. Nortjé, and R. E. Wood.)

flattened, cuboidal, or squamous epithelium.[7] The cyst fluid is thick, tenacious, white or translucent, and sterile.[79]

The *serous nonsecretory retention cyst* arises as a result of cystic degeneration within an inflamed, thickened sinus lining or in a mucosal polyp. Spaces or splits develop in the lamina propria and become distended with edema fluid. The enlarging spaces merge and form a cystic lumen within the connective tissue fibers that become the cyst lining.[64] This pathogenesis precludes the development of an epithelial lining.[50] The fluid in this entity is not actively secreted but is a transudate from capillaries damaged by the inflammation. The cystic fluid is similar to plasma, is sterile, and coagulates after removal.[34]

As either type of mucosal retention cyst enlarges and fills the sinus cavity, it frequently ruptures as the result of abrupt pressure changes caused by sneezing or blowing the nose. (The cyst may be present on radiographic examination of the maxillary sinus, perhaps absent only a few days later, only to reappear on subsequent examinations.) If this does not happen, the expanding cyst usually herniates through the ostium into the nasal cavity, where it subsequently ruptures.

The maxillary sinus is the most common site of antral mucosal retention cysts, although they are occasionally found in the frontal or sphenoid sinuses.[50,85] Antral mucosal retention cysts have not been observed to be related to extractions or associated with periapical disease.[39]

Clinical features. Mucosal retention cysts in the maxillary sinus are found in all age groups,[67] but the highest incidence is observed during the third decade and twice as often in males.[1] The incidence has been reported to vary from 1.4% to 13%,[1,21,64] and the serous cyst is considerably more common.[15,85] Although the antral cysts are encountered more frequently than polyps, the differential diagnosis may be difficult.[12]

Retention cysts are usually asymptomatic, but when symptoms do occur they are generally nonspecific.[78,83] Probably fewer than 10% of individuals with retention cysts in the maxillary sinus experience pain and tenderness in the teeth and face over the sinus. Some patients report stuffiness, fullness, postnasal drip, headache,* cold symptoms, or sometimes numbness of the upper lip.[20,57] The condition of the dentition does not appear to be a factor in the development of these lesions.[48] No particular symptoms are associated with either serous or mucous cysts of the antrum.

Radiographic features. Partial images of mucosal cysts of the maxillary antrum may show on maxillary, posterior, or periapical projections, but panoramic radiographs demonstrate them best.[47,57] Although these cysts may occur bilaterally, usually only a single cyst develops. Occasionally more than one cyst may form in a sinus.[22] Both varieties of the benign cysts usually appear as a smooth, dome-shaped, homogeneous mass that is more radiopaque than the surrounding sinus cavity (Fig. 26-6). The radiopacity of the lesion is such that normal landmarks may often be seen through its image. The border of the lesion is the same density as the body of the mass. These cysts usually project from the floor of the sinus, although some may form on the lateral walls. The base of the lesions may be narrow or broad;[36] some contend that the mucous cysts are more likely to have a broad base, whereas the se-

rous are more pedunculated.[12] The remainder of the sinus appears normal if a concomitant allergic or infectious sinusitis is not present.

The images of the mucosal cysts vary in size, from that of a finger tip to completely filling the sinus and making it opaque. Mucous cysts tend to be smaller than serous cysts.[12] The condition of the mucosa lining the remainder of the sinus also helps to distinguish between the mucous and serous varieties. The mucous variety is usually associated with a thickened mucosa, whereas in the serous cyst the lining appears normal.[12] If the cyst fills the antrum, it produces a uniform cloudiness, giving no radiographic clue as to its cystic nature and appearing rather as a mild sinusitis. When the cyst completely fills the maxillary sinus cavity, it may prolapse (extrude) through the ostium and cause nasal obstruction and postnasal discharge.[46] This may be the only clinical evidence of the cyst's presence. In such case, the shadow of the antronasal polyp may also be apparent in the nasal fossa, and posteroanterior tomography of the sinuses can be extremely helpful.

Differential diagnosis. It is important to distinguish the mucosal retention cyst from odontogenic cysts (for example, radicular, dentigerous, or odontogenic keratocysts), antral polyps, or any rounded tumor mass. This can usually be done radiographically and by the patient's history.

The mucous retention cyst is dome shaped, uniformly opaque, and well defined, and it does not have the thin marginal radiopaque line representing the hyperostotic border characteristic of the odontogenic cyst. The odontogenic cyst is also more rounded or tear shaped, and most are not as homogeneous as a mucous retention cyst in the sinus. The lamina dura of the tooth or teeth associated with the odontogenic cyst is not intact in the apical area; it may be continuous with the hyperostotic outline of the odontogenic cyst. In contrast, the roots of healthy teeth projecting into or over an area of an antral cavity occupied by a mucosal retention cyst usually have the lamina dura apparent.

Antral polyps of infective or allergic origin may be distinguished radiographically from a mucous retention cyst in that they usually appear a little more opaque and more heterogeneous, are more often multiple, and are commonly associated with a thickened mucosa,[79] all of which are less frequently observed with mucosal retention cysts.

Management. Mucosal retention cysts in the maxillary sinus usually require no treatment be-

---

*Frontal headache is often referred from antral disease but only rarely caused by infection of the frontal sinus.[41]

cause they customarily resolve spontaneously without any residual effect on the antral mucosa. Surgical intervention should be considered only when there is evidence of persistent pain, headache, or expansion.[30] These signs are not characteristic of mucosal retention cysts, and their presence suggests the possibility of other conditions.

MUCOCELE

A mucocele is an expanding, destructive lesion that begins with the development of a mucous retention cyst in a sinus with a blocked ostium. The blockage may result from an infundibulum that is too long and tortuous or occluded by intra-antral or intranasal inflammation, polyps, or bony tumors.[29,87] As the cystic lesion continues to accumulate mucus after it has filled the sinus cavity, the pressure increases and the lesion becomes destructive, thinning and expanding and, in some cases, destroying the sinus walls. About 90% of these bone-destroying lesions occur in the ethmoidal and frontal sinuses;[60] they are rare in the maxillary and sphenoid sinuses.[12,59] This predilection

for the ethmoid and frontal sinuses is probably best explained by the relative difficulty a cyst has in protruding through the longer and narrower nasofrontal duct and infundibulum to the nasal cavity, in contrast to the shorter and larger ostia (the avenue of release) in the case of the maxillary and sphenoid sinuses. Such herniation into the nasal cavity reduces the destructive potential of the cyst by releasing the intracystic pressure. If a mucocele becomes infected, it is called a *pyocele* or a *mucopyocele*.

Clinical features. A mucocele in the maxillary sinus may exert pressure on the superior alveolar nerves in the resorbing sinus walls and cause radiating pain. The patient may first complain of a sensation of fullness in the cheek, and there may be swelling over the area. This swelling may first become apparent over the anteroinferior aspect of the antrum, the area where the wall is thinnest and the area in which the bony wall may first be destroyed. If the cyst expands inferiorly, it may cause loosening of the posterior teeth in the area. If it expands the medial wall of the sinus, the lateral

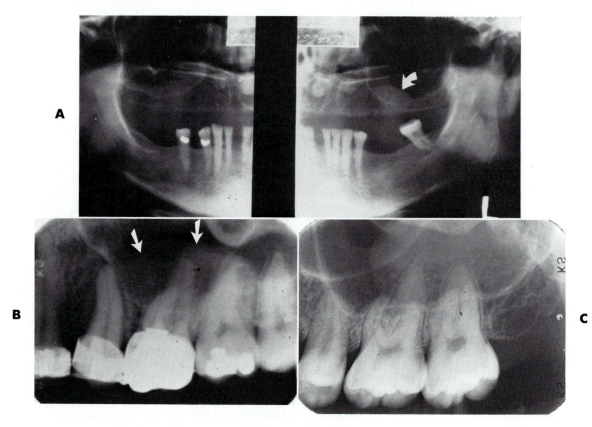

FIG. 26-6. Mucous retention cyst in the maxillary antrum *(arrows)* seen as a soft tissue opacity on panoramic **(A)**, periapical **(B** and **C)**, and Waters **(D)** projections.

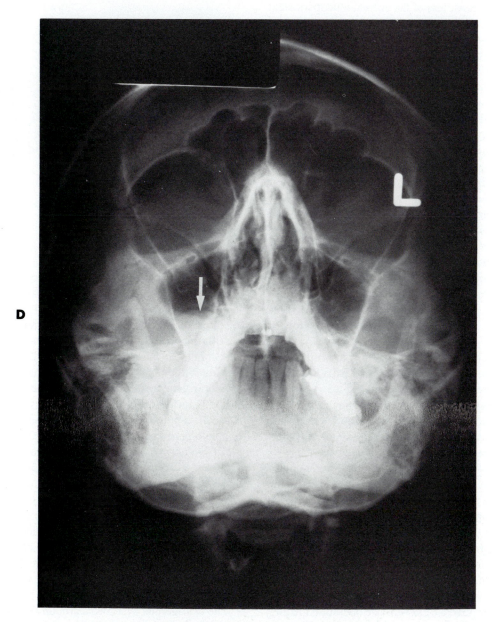

FIG. 26-6, cont'd. For legend see opposite page.

wall of the nasal cavity is deformed and the nasal airway may be obstructed. Should it expand into the orbit, it may cause diplopia (double vision) and proptosis (protrusion of the globe of the eye).

Radiographic features. Radiographically, a mucocele in the *maxillary sinus* causes opacification of the sinus, loss of the normal mucoperiosteal line, and bony expansion. Eventually, the septa and the bony walls may erode.[2]

The earliest sign of a mucocele in the *frontal sinus,* where 65% occur, is clouding that frequently subsequently seems to fade as the characteristic bony changes become apparent. The usual scalloped border of the sinus is smoothed by erosion of the septa (the intersinus septum may be displaced), the borders of the expanding sinus become sclerotic, and bone at the supramedial border of the orbit is destroyed or displaced.[2,51,71] In their later states, such lesions may be difficult to distinguish from a sinus carcinoma, which destroys the bony sinus walls.

Ethmoid mucoceles are relatively difficult to recognize radiographically because they may occur in only one of the 13 to 15 air cells, and these may obscure its presence. It may appear as a radiodensity or primarily as an expansion of the lamina papyracea. The CT scan is the examination of choice.[51,72]

Mucoceles in the *sphenoid sinus* are rare. They produce an opaque sinus and may expand superiorly, suggesting a pituitary tumor.[71]

Differential diagnosis. Although it may not be possible to distinguish between a mucocele in the maxillary antrum and a malignant tumor, any suggestion that the lesion is associated with an occluded ostium should strengthen the impression of a mucocele. Blockage of the ostium is usually the result of a previous surgical procedure, although a deviated nasal septum or polyps may be a factor. Should any of these become apparent in the patient's history, it should strengthen the diagnostician's impression that the disease is a mucocele of the antrum.

Management. Treatment of the mucocele is usually surgical, a Caldwell-Luc operation to allow excision of the lesion. The prognosis is excellent.[2]

DENTAL CYSTS

The most common group of extrinsic cysts that invade the maxillary sinus are of odontogenic origin. They comprise almost half of the lesions of the maxillary sinus.[78] Most are the radicular type, followed by dentigerous and odontogenic keratocysts.[34]

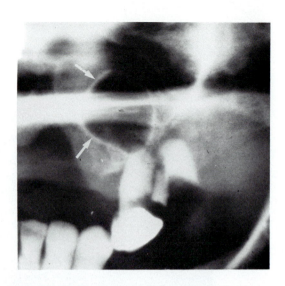

FIG. 26-7. Radicular cyst with hyperostotic borders extending into the maxillary antrum *(arrows)* on a portion of this panoramic radiograph. (Courtesy Dr. L. Hollender, Seattle.)

Radicular cyst

The radicular cyst is one of the most common periapical lesions. It is usually painless, although it may cause expansion of the cortical plates over the area of the cyst. Those that develop in the maxilla may extend and erode into the maxillary sinus (Fig. 26-7). When they approach or involve the sinus, they are likely to be responsible for an oroantral fistula after extraction of the associated tooth. Radicular cysts or granulomas may also cause elevation of the floor of the sinus, resulting in a halo appearance (Fig. 26-8). This appearance returns to normal after resolution of the lesion. On occasion, a large cyst may obliterate the sinus and make differentiation of this lesion from sinusitis difficult. Evaluation of such conditions is aided by noting that the wall of the cyst is often thicker and more uniform than that of a sinus. In addition, the normal vascular markings on the wall of the maxillary sinus are not present on the walls of a cyst.[52]

Dentigerous cyst

The dentigerous cyst forms around the crown of an unerupted or developing tooth. Although such cysts are not nearly as common in the maxilla as in the mandible, when they do occur in the upper jaw, it is most often in association with impacted third molars. Consequently, this cyst is usually associated with a tooth missing from the arch. When the cyst expands into the sinus, the radiograph usually shows a radiolucency elevating an intact wall or floor of a maxillary sinus (Fig. 26-9).

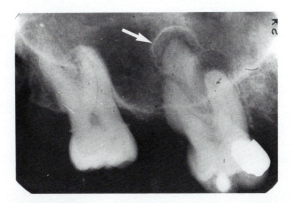

FIG. 26-8. Elevation of the floor of the maxillary sinus *(arrow)* resulting in a halo appearance around the roots of the first molar.

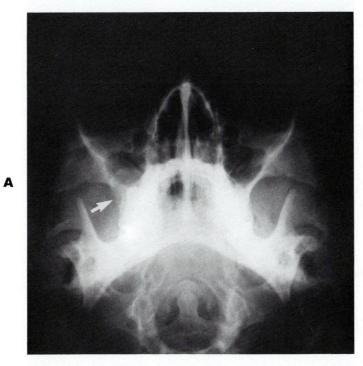

FIG. 26-9. Dentigerous cyst *(arrow)* in the maxillary antrum. **A,** Lateral expansion of the cyst wall.

Continued.

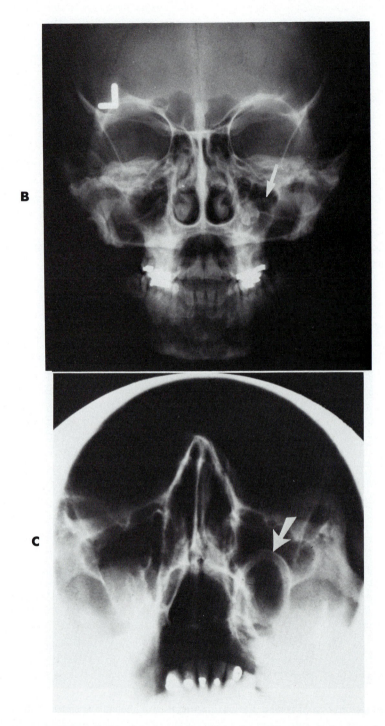

FIG. 26-9, cont'd. B and **C,** The left sinus has a thickening of its mucoperiosteum *(arrow).* (**B** and **C** courtesy Dr. L. Hollender, Seattle.)

Odontogenic keratocysts

Other cysts, such as the odontogenic keratocyst, may encroach on the maxillary sinus. These cysts are usually unilocular in the maxilla. They may act aggressively and fill the sinus, cause resorption of cortical plates, and involve adjacent soft tissue.[43]

TUMORS

Benign tumors of the paranasal sinuses other than inflammatory polyps are rare. The radiographic images of such benign tumors are nonspecific. Usually the involved portion of the sinus appears opaque because of the presence of a mass, and bone expansion may result from pressure erosion. Malignant tumors of the paranasal sinuses are usually squamous cell carcinomas and, to a lesser extent, malignant salivary gland tumors.[19] Of these carcinomas, 75% originate in the maxillary sinus.[73] Although opacification is a feature of both the usual inflammatory conditions and tumors, the tendency of the tumors is for bone destruction.

Epithelial papilloma

The epithelial papilloma is a rare tumor of respiratory epithelium that occurs in the nasal cavity and paranasal sinuses. It occurs predominantly in men and usually in the ethmoidal or maxillary sinus. Clinically, there may be unilateral nasal obstruction, nasal discharge, pain, and epistaxis. The patient may have complained of recurring sinusitis for years and a subsequent nasal obstruction on the same side as the sinusitis. The epithelial papilloma is important because, although benign and relatively rare, it has a 10% incidence of associated carcinoma.[60]

The radiographic findings are nonspecific but may suggest a soft tissue mass that may or may not fill the nasal passage or maxillary sinus. It may also appear as an isolated polyp in the nose or sinus. If bone destruction is apparent, it is the result of pressure erosion. The diagnosis can be made only by histologic examination of the tissue.

Osteoma

The osteoma is the most common of the mesenchymal tumors in the paranasal sinuses. It is usually asymptomatic and thus usually detected as an incidental finding in an examination made for another purpose. Although osteomas occasionally develop in the maxillary sinus, they more often occur in the frontal and ethmoidal sinuses. The incidence in the maxillary antrum varies between 4% and 9%, and it is almost twice as common in

males in the second, third, and fourth decades.[34,65] An osteoma in a sinus is usually slow growing and often asymptomatic. If large, it can be obstructive and expansive. When symptoms do occur, they are the result of obstruction of the sinus ostium or infundibulum or are secondary to erosion or deformity, orbital involvement, or intracranial extension. Those growing in the maxillary sinus may extend into the nose and cause nasal obstruction or a swelling of the side of the nose. They may expand the sinus and produce swelling of the cheek or hard palate. Osteomas of the maxillary sinus have been described following Caldwell-Luc operations.[14]

The radiographic appearance of the ivory osteoma is that of a lobulated or rounded homogeneous, sharply defined mass of high density (Fig. 21-33). The differential diagnosis includes antrolith, mycolith, teeth, or odontogenic tumors, including odontoma.[56] It is unusual for an osteoma to recur after removal.

Ameloblastoma

The ameloblastoma (see Chapter 21) is a benign odontogenic, epithelial tumor that is comparatively rare, although it is the most common extrinsic benign tumor affecting the maxillary sinus.[23] It occurs in the 20- to 50-year age group, about equally in both sexes, and without racial predilection. An ameloblastoma in the maxilla is relatively rare; 19% occur in the maxilla and 81% in the mandible.[70] In the maxilla, it usually arises in the cancellous bone in the premolar-molar region and invades the sinus cavity at an early stage. It is a destructive, aggressive tumor that grows slowly and may cause loosening of the teeth, nasal obstruction, and painless facial deformity. It may cause death by direct invasion. The tendency for local recurrence is strong. Although extremely rare, metastatic spread has been documented.[3,26] When an ameloblastoma occurs in the maxilla, especially posterior to the canines (where about 85% occur), it is so close to the maxillary sinus that there is a high probability that it will invade the sinus. There are no bony barriers, and the relatively good blood supply is probably also responsible for efficient local spread.[76] Because it is characteristic that the ameloblastoma is painless, slow growing, and either unilocular or multilocular, it should have a high priority in the differential diagnosis of any such lesion.

When an ameloblastoma involves the maxillary sinus, radiographs may show that the tumor expands the antral cavity and fills it with a soft tissue mass (Fig. 26-10). The bony walls are thin and eroded, and adjacent structures may also be invaded. A tooth or part of a tooth may be embedded in the tumor. Although treatment of the ameloblastoma in the mandible is generally successful, the prognosis for this entity in the maxillary sinus is less favorable. It lies in close proximity to the nasal cavity, the other paranasal sinuses, orbit, pharyngeal tissues, and base of the skull, and invasion of any of these structures complicates its excision, the most accepted mode of treatment.[54]

Squamous cell carcinoma

Malignant neoplasms of the paranasal sinuses are rare, accounting for less than 1% of all malignancies in the body.[73] Squamous cell carcinoma is by far the most common primary tumor of the paranasal sinuses, comprising 80% to 90% of the cancers in this site.[4,86] Most carcinomas occur in the maxillary sinus in males, but involvement of the frontal and sphenoid sinuses is also comparatively common.[11,77] Although maxillary sinus carcinoma has been associated with certain carcinogens and with chronic sinusitis, convincing evidence of its cause has not yet been described.[61] The early primary lesions are radiographically detectable as soft tissue masses in the sinus before they cause bone destruction, but more are extensive, involving the entire sinus, with radiographic evidence of bone destruction before clinical symptoms lead to their discovery. This situation has led to the often repeated warning that *any unexplained opacity in the maxillary sinus of an individual older than 40 years of age should be biopsied.*

Clinical features. The most common symptoms of cancer in the maxillary sinus are facial pain or swelling, nasal obstruction, and a lesion in the oral cavity. The mean age of the patient is 60 years (range 25 to 89 years); twice as many men are affected; lymph nodes are involved in about 10% of cases; and the symptoms are present for about 5 months before diagnosis.[73] The symptoms produced by neoplasms in the maxillary sinus depend on which wall(s) of the sinus is involved. The medial wall is usually the first to become eroded, leading to such nasal symptoms as obstruction, discharge, bleeding, and pain. These symptoms may appear trivial, and their significance may not be appreciated. Those lesions that arise on the floor of the sinus may first produce dental symptoms, including expansion of the alveolus, unexplained pain and numbness of the teeth, loose teeth, and

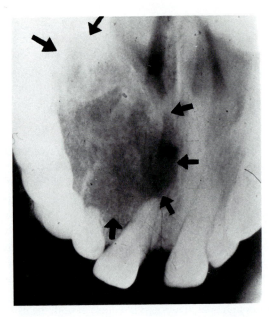

FIG. 26-10. Ameloblastoma obscuring the maxillary antrum *(arrows)*. (Courtesy Dr. L. Hollender, Seattle.)

swelling of the palate or alveolar ridge and malfitting dentures.[37] The tumor may erode the floor and penetrate into the oral cavity. Such oral manifestations appear in 25% to 35% of patients with cancer in the maxillary sinus.[5] When the lesion penetrates the lateral wall, facial and vestibular swelling become apparent and the patient may complain of pain and hyperesthesia of the maxillary teeth. Involvement of the sinus roof and the floor of the orbit cause symptoms related to the eye: diplopia, proptosis, pain, and hyperesthesia or anesthesia and pain over the cheek and upper teeth. Invasion and penetration of the posterior wall lead to invasion of the muscles of mastication causing painful trismus, obstruction of the eustachian tube causing a stuffy ear, and referred pain and hyperesthesia over the distribution of the second and third divisions of the fifth nerve.[8,9]

Radiographic features. The radiographic findings in malignant disease of the paranasal sinuses are not specific. It is not possible to differentiate the early manifestations of carcinoma in radiographs of the maxillary sinus from the clouding of the sinus that develops in sinusitis and polyp formation.[45] However, as the lesion expands, it becomes destructive, altering the outline of the sinus, destroying bone, and in general causing irregular bony radiolucencies.[45,83] The most frequent findings are erosion of the medial wall and opacifica-

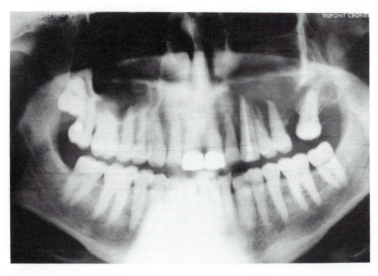

FIG. 26-11. Squamous cell carcinoma of the left maxillary sinus. Note the clouding of the sinus and the destruction of its antral walls. Compare these with the density and outline of the right maxillary sinus. (Courtesy Dr. C. Bohnfolk, Dallas.)

tion of the sinus, although any wall may show erosion.[9,37] Although the medial wall is one of the most difficult to demonstrate radiographically,[62] it is best seen on the Caldwell and Waters projections of conventional radiographs. However, as a result of the projection geometry, destruction of this wall does not appear as a frank hole; rather it seems thinner and less distinct than the contralateral wall.[51] If careful examination of a conventional radiograph of any opacified sinus reveals the slightest suggestion of bone destruction, advanced imaging is imperative (Fig. 26-11).[51] Although tomograms usually confirm or contradict the presence of destruction, it is well to note that in one study 30% of cases of medial wall involvement were not apparent even on the tomograms.[9] In addition to this radiographic evidence, the suspicion of malignancy is strengthened by a concomitant unilateral obstruction of the nasal cavity. On CT, the most characteristic sign of malignancy is disruption of the facial planes beyond the sinus walls.[24] Consequently CT is useful in revealing the extent of paranasal sinus tumors,[42] especially when there is extension into the orbit, infratemporal fossa, or cranial cavity,[16,80] areas inaccessible by conventional radiographic examination. It is also useful in staging malignant tumors of the paranasal sinuses.[24] MRI examinations are excellent for revealing the extent of soft tissue penetration into adjacent structures (Fig. 26-12).

Differential diagnosis. The differential diag-

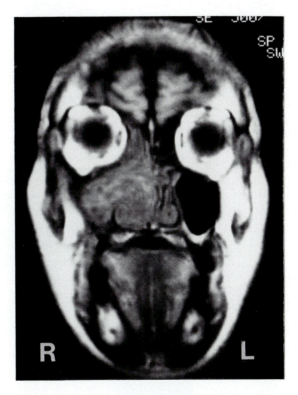

FIG. 26-12. Frontal MRI at the level of the maxillary sinuses. Note squamous cell carcinoma filling entire maxillary sinus and eroding its medial wall to fill right half of nasal fossa and superior portion of left nasal cavity as well as right ethmoid sinuses. Compare gray image of the carcinoma on right side to the normal black air-filled maxillary and ethmoid sinuses on left. (Courtesy Drs. A. G. Farman, C. J. Nortjé, and R. E. Wood.)

nosis includes all the conditions that may cause opacity of the antrum. Also, the bone destruction produced by *fibrous dysplasia* may simulate a malignant tumor. However, it is important to note that differentiation between malignant and benign disease of the sinuses on the basis of bone destruction can lead to erroneous conclusions: Bone destruction occurs in infectious and benign as well as malignant conditions.[59] Neoplasia should be suspected in any older patient in whom chronic sinusitis develops for the first time without obvious cause.[41]

Management. Treatment of squamous cell carcinoma in the paranasal sinuses generally combines surgery and radiation therapy.[73] Although there is as yet no consensus as to the merits of the various modes and sequences of treatment that have been advocated for the treatment of cancer in the maxillary sinus, it can in general be concluded that (1) the effectiveness of radiation is inversely related to tumor size, (2) almost half of tumors treated by irradiation and then surgery have viable tumor in the excised tissue, and (3) radical surgery is contraindicated in those patients with palpable lymph nodes; when the tumor has extended into the nasopharynx, sphenoid sinus, cribriform plate, and pterygopalatine fossa; and when there are distant metastases.[11] Malignant neoplasms in the paranasal sinuses usually have a poor prognosis because they are usually well advanced by the time of diagnosis.

Other factors contributing to the poor prognosis include frequently inaccurate preoperative staging and the complex anatomy of the region.[73]

FIBROUS DYSPLASIA

Fibrous dysplasia (see Chapter 23) may extend in or near one of the paranasal sinuses. Monostotic fibrous dysplasia may arise in the maxillary, sphenoid, frontal, ethmoid, and temporal bones. The involvement of the facial skeleton can result in facial asymmetry, nasal obstruction, proptosis, pituitary gland compression, impingement on cranial nerves, or sinus obliteration. The sinus obliteration results when dysplastic bone develops within the paranasal sinus or when the expanding lesion encroaches on it. The lesion may displace the roots of teeth and cause them to separate or migrate, but it usually does not cause root resorption.[44,75,82] Fibrous dysplasia is more common in children and young adults, and the lesion tends to stop growing when skeletal growth ceases.

Radiographically an expanding mass of variable opacity in the maxilla may fill the antrum, extending beyond the bony sinus walls and even elevating the orbital floor. The radiodensity of the lesion depends on its stage of development and on the relative amounts of bone present. Usually the radiopaque areas have the characteristic ground-glass appearance (Fig. 26-13). Such a painless, solitary enlargement in the jawbone of a relatively young

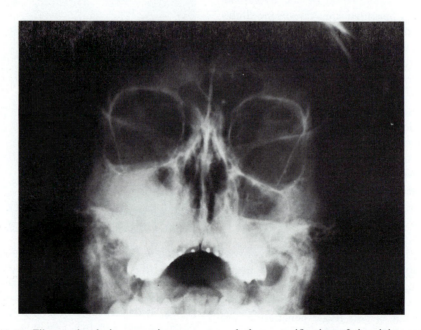

FIG. 26-13. Fibrous dysplasia, occurring as a ground-glass opacification of the right maxillary antrum. (Courtesy Dr. L. Hollender, Seattle.)

person is difficult to confuse with other radiopaque entities. Paget's disease does not usually obliterate the sinus, as does fibrous dysplasia. A complex odontoma (Fig. 26-14) usually shows unerupted teeth and a limiting border. An ossifying fibroma may also have a uniform opaque appearance (Fig. 26-15).

TRAUMATIC INJURIES TO THE PARANASAL SINUSES
Fractured roots

Extraction of teeth occasionally leads to the inadvertent fracture of the apex of the tooth. In a maxillary posterior tooth, it is possible that the fractured root tip may be forced into the maxillary sinus, either during the extraction or while efforts are made to remove the root tip. If the root tip remains in its socket, it may superimpose radiographically over the maxillary sinus but show the presence of a lamina dura, indicating its true position. If the root tip is in the maxillary sinus, no lamina dura is around it. A root tip in the sinus that is trapped under the mucoperiosteum is fixed in location. If it has penetrated through the mucoperiosteum, it may show movement in the sinus when the patient changes the orientation of the

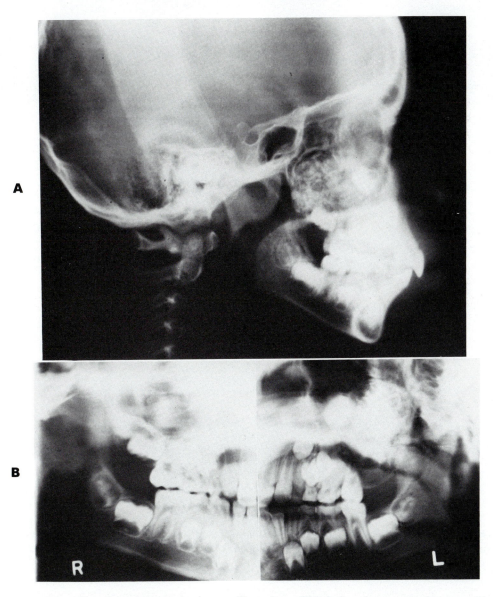

FIG. 26-14. Complex odontoma in the maxillary sinus. This lesion shows amorphous opacities surrounding and partially obscuring unerupted teeth. **A,** Lateral view; **B,** panoramic view.

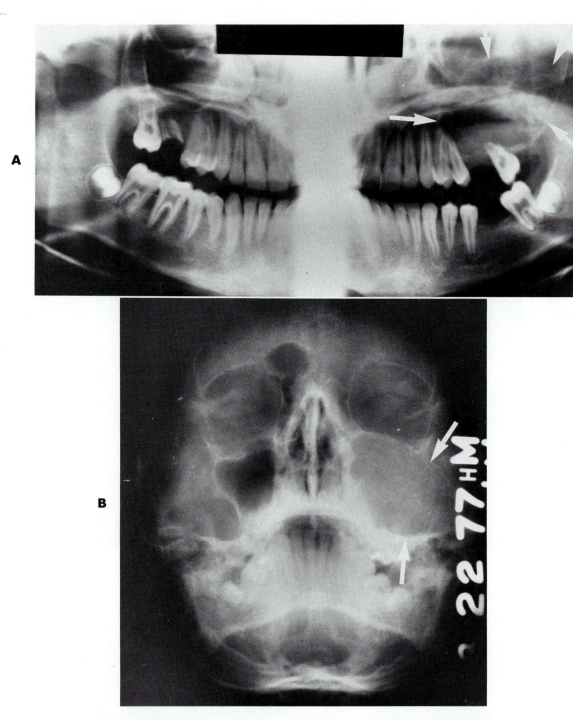

FIG. 26-15. Ossifying fibroma. **A,** A large lesion in the left maxilla with well-defined borders, displaced teeth, resorbed roots, and calcification *(arrows)*. **B,** Opacified maxillary sinus with expanded borders *(arrows)* on this Waters view.

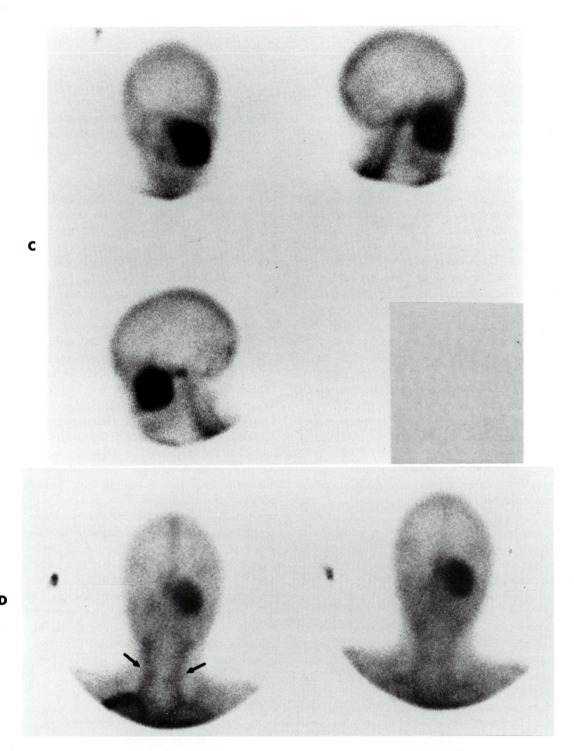

FIG. 26-15, cont'd. C, A positive radioactive bone scan shows that bone is being either destroyed or formed by the lesion. **D,** A nuclear perfusion study shows that the lesion is quite vascular (*arrows* point to the great vessels).

head. However, in spite of the convincing circumstances of the extraction, it is important to consider that the lost tooth or root tip may not be in the sinus. It may be forced into the infratemporal space or other tissue planes, for example, between the alveolar process and the periosteum or into the buccal soft tissue. There is also the possibility that it may have been displaced into a cyst that was preoperatively mistaken for a lobe of the sinus cavity.[38] Lateral maxillary occlusal views are useful for examining root tips in the maxillary sinus.[52]

Sinus contusion

Occasionally a blow to the face produces damage to the lining of the paranasal sinuses without fracturing the facial bones.[77] The term used to describe this condition is "contusion of the sinus." The traumatic force is apparently transmitted through the bony wall and absorbed by the mucosal lining, which suffers the damage. The traumatic force may cause a greenstick fracture of the sinus, with a resulting tearing injury to the mucosal lining. Deformity of the relatively elastic anterolateral wall may result in concomitant laceration of the sinus mucosa. Also, an undetected microfracture may have occurred with tearing of the blood vessels in the sinus mucosa.

The *radiographic appearance* of a sinus contusion depends on the amount of injury inflicted by the blow. One may observe a hazy sinus produced by edema of the mucosa, a soft tissue mass that mimics a retention cyst and is the result of an intramucosal hematoma, an opaque sinus, or a fluid level resulting from the hemorrhage of a mucosal tear. It is possible that the haziness resulting from edema may obscure a hematoma, which may in turn become apparent when the edema resolves. Also, the blood-filled sinus may become infected by nasal microorganisms, with the resulting complication of a sinusitis.

Differentiating between sinus contusion and sinusitis may be difficult. The diagnosis of sinus contusion is strengthened by a bloody nasal discharge, extreme tenderness of the involved sinus on pressure, rapid resolution of the soft tissue changes, absence of clinical and radiographic evidence of inflammatory changes in the other paranasal sinuses, and the absence of spontaneous pain.

Blow-out fracture

A blow-out fracture of the orbit results from a sudden increase in the intraorbital pressure, such as might result from a blow to the eye. The pressure is exerted against all the orbital walls, and because the floor of the orbit is thinnest, this is the area that is usually depressed. The pressure of the blow forces the inferior periorbital contents (fat and muscle) through the fracture, where they become entrapped. The infraorbital rim usually remains intact. There are two important clinical signs of such a fracture: diplopia, especially when the victim looks upward (caused by entrapment of the inferior rectus); and enophthalmos (depressed orbit) following reduction of the edema and fat atrophy[6] and lowering of the globe.

The *radiographic changes* produced by a blow-out fracture are opacification of the maxillary sinus with or without a fluid level, soft tissue mass in the upper portion of the sinus, and the image of depressed bone fragments (orbital floor) in the sinus (Fig. 26-16). The soft tissue mass in the superior portion of the antrum is the result of herniation of periorbital soft tissue through the floor of the orbit. The depression of the orbital floor is indicated by an increased distance between the (palpable) rim and the floor of the orbit. (On the Waters projection, the palpable margin of the orbit is the superior radiopaque line, and the orbital floor is a similar opaque line just below it.[51]) The depression fracture of the orbit is often accompanied by a fracture of the anterior wall of the maxillary sinus. This complication may go undetected on the Waters projection but is revealed on a lateral tomogram of the area. In the Waters projection fractures of the thin walls are imaged as "bright lines" (white) superimposed on the sinus. They are caused by the fragment's rotation, which results in a more tangential path of the beam through the thin bone.[51] A blow-out fracture of the floor of the orbit with downward herniation of orbital soft tissue may simulate a mucous cyst of the antral roof.[85] Although the opaque sinus may cause the blow-out fracture to be confused with sinusitis, when accompanied by a history of trauma to the eye, it can be presumptive evidence of a depressed fracture of the orbital floor.

Isolated fractures

Isolated fractures of the paranasal sinuses involve only a single wall. On radiographs, they display a fracture line (possibly a "bright line") and clouding of the involved sinus. The anterolateral wall of the maxillary sinus is the most common site for an isolated fracture. These fractures may extend to the orbital rim. Another type of isolated fracture involves the floor of the maxillary sinus

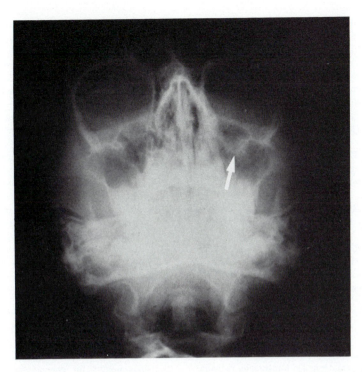

FIG. 26-16. A blowout fracture has depressed the orbital contents through the roof of the maxillary sinus *(arrow).*

into which the roots of posterior teeth are projecting. These fractures are usually iatrogenic and occur during tooth extraction.[77] A less common type involves the inferior orbital rim only.

Complex injuries of the paranasal sinuses

Zygomatic complex. A forceful blow to the zygomatic bone usually separates it from the facial skeleton. This separation ordinarily results in separation of the sutures between the zygomatic bone and the frontal and sphenoid bones, and fractures of the zygomatic arch (zygoma), the floor of the orbit (roof of the maxillary sinus), and the thin bone comprising the lateral wall of the antrum. Examination of the zygomatic arch should always be complemented by a Waters projection, the only routine view that demonstrates the complex. If there is a depression (fracture) of the arch, the smooth curve, that is, the normal image on the Waters view, will be interrupted and will not correspond to that on the contralateral side. In this case, a special zygomatic arch projection, directed to demonstrate the area where the fracture is presumed to be, is in order. The fracture involving the maxillary sinus is usually accompanied by tearing of the lining membrane and subsequent bleed-

ing into the antrum. As a result, the antrum may appear cloudy or show a fluid level. The fluid level will be apparent for only a few days before the space drains through the ipsilateral ostium and nares. Although postconvalescent radiographs of the sinus may show the mucosal changes of chronic antral infection for long periods, most patients are free of symptoms.[17,35]

Multiple sinus fractures. At least one third of patients with fractures of the facial bones sustain multiple sinus fractures (see Chapter 28). The extent of radiographic changes in the sinus depends on which facial bones are damaged. Typically, there is clouding of both maxillary sinuses, with the frontal and ethmoidal sinuses also involved.

REFERENCES

1. Allard RHB, Van der Kwast WAM, Van der Wall JI: Mucosal antral cysts: review of the literature and report of a radiographic survey, *Oral Surg* 51:2-9, 1981.
2. Atherino C, Atherino T: Maxillary sinus mucopyoceles, *Arch Otolaryngol* 110:200-202, 1984.
3. Azumi T, Nakajima T, Shigekazu T et al: Malignant ameloblastoma with metastasis to the skull: report of a case, *J Oral Surg* 39:690-696, 1981.
4. Batsakis JG: *Tumors of the head and neck,* ed 2, Baltimore, 1979, Williams & Wilkins.

5. Batsakis JG, Rice DH, Solomon AR: The pathology of head and neck tumors: squamous and mucous-gland carcinomas of the nasal cavity, paranasal sinuses and larynx: part 6, *Head Neck Surg* 2:497-508, 1980.

6. Bertz J: Maxillofacial injuries, *Clin Symp* 33:2-32, 1981.

7. Blaugrund S, Parisier SC: Benign tumors of the nasal sinuses, *Otolaryngol Clin North Am* 40:143-157, 1971.

8. Boles R: Paranasal sinuses and facial pain. In Ailing CC, Mahan PE, editors: *Facial pain,* ed 2, Philadelphia, 1977, Lea & Febiger.

9. Boone MLM, Harle TS: Malignant tumors of the paranasal sinuses, *Semin Roentgenol* 3:202-213, 1968.

10. Bret-Day RC: Secretory cysts of the maxillary antrum, *Br Dent J* 109:268-270, 1960.

11. Bridger M, Beale F, Bryce D: Carcinoma of the paranasal sinuses: a review of 158 cases, *J Otolaryngol* 7:379-88, 1978.

12. Dodd GD, Jing BS: *Radiology of the nose, paranasal sinus and nasopharynx,* Baltimore, 1977, Williams & Wilkins.

13. Dolan K, Smoker W: Paranasal sinus radiology: part 4A, maxillary sinuses, *Head Neck Surg* 5:345-362, 1983.

14. Dolan K, Smoker W: Paranasal sinus radiology: part 4B, maxillary sinuses, *Head Neck Surg* 5:428-446, 1983.

15. DuBrul EL: *Sicher's oral anatomy,* ed 7, St Louis, 1980, Mosby.

16. Eddleston B, Johnson R: A comparison of conventional radiographic imaging and computed tomography in malignant disease of the paranasal sinuses and the post-nasal space, *Clin Radiol* 56:161-172, 1983.

17. Edgerton MT: Emergency care of maxillofacial injuries. In Zuidema GD, Rutherford RB, Ballinger WF II, editors: *The management of trauma,* ed 3, Philadelphia, 1979, WB Saunders.

18. Fireman P: Diagnosis of sinusitis in children: emphasis on the history and physical examination, *J Allergy Clin Immunol* 90:433-436, 1992.

19. Goepfert H, Luna M, Lindberg R, and White A: Malignant salivary gland tumors of the paranasal sinuses and nasal cavity, *Arch Otolaryngol* 109:662-668, 1983.

20. Gothberg K, Little J, King D, and Bean L: A clinical study of cysts arising from mucosa of the maxillary sinus, *Oral Surg* 41:52-58, 1976.

21. Grossman J, Waltz HD: Nonsecreting cysts of the maxillary sinus, *Am J Roentgenol* 52:136-144, 1944.

22. Halstead CL: Mucosal cysts of the maxillary sinus: report of 75 cases, *J Am Dent Assoc* 87:1435-1441, 1973.

23. Hames RS, Rakoff SJ: Diseases of the maxillary sinus, *J Oral Med* 27:90-95, 1972.

24. Haso A: CT of tumors and tumor-like conditions of the paranasal sinuses, *Radiol Clin North Am* 22:119-130, 1984.

25. Hengerer AS: Embryonic development of the sinuses, *Ear, Nose, Throat J* 63:134-136, 1984.

26. Ikenura K, Tashior H, Hirashi F: Metastatic ameloblastoma of the mandible, *Cancer* 29:930-940, 1972.

27. Incaudo G, Gershwin ME, Nagy SM: The pathophysiology and treatment of sinusitis, *Allergol Immunopathol (Madr)* 14:423-434, 1986.

28. Jensen C, von Sydow C: Radiography and ultrasonography in paranasal sinusitis, *Acta Radiol* 28:31-34, 1987.

29. Jones JL, Kaufman PW: Mucopyocele of the maxillary sinus, *J Oral Surg* 39:948-950, 1981.

30. Kaffe I, Littner MM, Moskona D: Mucosal-antral cysts: radiographic appearance and differential diagnosis, *Clin Prev Dent* 10:3-6, 1988.

31. Karmody CS, Carter B, Vincent ME: Developmental anomalies of the maxillary sinus, *Trans Am Acad Opthalmol Otolaryngol* 84:723-728, 1977.

32. Kennedy DW: Overview, *Otolaryngol Head Neck Surg* 103:847-854, 1990.

33. Kennedy DW: Surgical update, *Otolaryngol Head Neck Surg* 103:884-886, 1990.

34. Killey HC, Kay LA: *The maxillary sinus and its dental implications,* Bristol, 1975, John Wright.

35. Knight JS, North JF: The classification of malar fractures: an analysis of displacement as a guide to treatment, *Br J Plast Surg* 13:325-339, 1961.

36. Kwapis BW, Whitten JB: Mucosal cysts of the maxillary sinus, *J Oral Surg* 29:561-566, 1971.

37. Larheim T, Kolbenstvdt A, Lien H: Carcinoma of maxillary sinus, palate and maxillary gingiva, occurrence of jaw destruction, *Scand J Dent Res* 92:235-240, 1984.

38. Lee FMS: Management of the displaced root in the maxillary sinus, *Int J Oral Surg* 7:374-379, 1978.

39. Lilly GE, Cutcher JL, Steiner M: Spherical shadows within the maxillary antrum, *J Oral Med* 23:19-21, 1968.

40. Lloyd GA: Diagnostic imaging of the nose and paranasal sinuses, *J Laryngol Otol* 103:453-460, 1989.

41. Ludman H: Paranasal sinus disease, *Br Med J* 282:1054-1057, 1981.

42. Lund V, Howard D, Lloyd G: CT evaluation of paranasal sinus tumors for cranio-facial resection, *Br J Radiol* 56:439-446, 1983.

43. MacDonald-Jankowski DS: The involvement of the maxillary antrum by odontogenic keratocysts, *Clin Radiol* 45:31-33, 1992.

44. Malcolmson KG: Ossifying fibroma of the sphenoid, *J Laryngol* 81:87-92, 1967.

45. Mancuso A, Hanafee W, Winter J, and Ward P: Extensions of paranasal sinus tumors and inflammatory disease: an evaluation by CT and pluri-directional tomography, *Neuroradiology* 16:449-453, 1978.

46. Mills CP: Secretory cysts of the maxillary antrum and their relationship to the development of antrochoanal polypi, *J Laryngol Otol* 73:324-334, 1959.

47. Ohba T, Katayama H: Comparison of panoramic radiography and Waters' projection of the diagnosis of maxillary sinus disease, *Oral Surg* 42:534-538, 1976.

48. Ohba T, Manson-Hing L: Radiologic study of cyst-like lesions in the maxillary sinus, *Dentomaxillofac Radiol* 4:100-103, 1975.

49. Palaceos E, Valvassori G: Computed axial tomography in otorhinolaryngology, *Adv Otorhinolaryngol* 24:1-8, 1978.

50. Paparella MM: Mucosal cyst of the maxillary sinus, *Arch Otorhinolaryngol* 77:650-657, 1963.

51. Potter GD: Inflammatory disease of the paranasal sinuses. In Valvassori GE, Potter GD, Hanefee WN, editors: *Radiology of the ear, nose and throat,* Philadelphia, 1982, WB Saunders.

52. Poyton H: Maxillary sinuses and the oral radiologist, *Dent Radiol Photogr* 45:43-59, 1972.

53. Poyton HG, Stoneman DW: Benign cysts of the maxillary antrum, *Can Dent Assoc J* 27:289-293, 1961.

54. Reanue C, Wesley RK, Jung B et al: Ameloblastoma of the maxillary sinus, *J Oral Surg* 38:520-521, 1980.

55. Reilly JS: The sinusitis cycle, *Otolaryngol Head Neck Surg* 103:856-862, 1990.

56. Reuben B: Odontoma of the maxillary sinus, a case report, *Quint Int* 14:287-290, 1983.

57. Rhodus NL: A comparison of periapical and panoramic radiographic surveys in the diagnosis of maxillary sinus mucous retention cysts, *Compendium* 10:275-277, 280-281, 1989.

58. Ritter FN: *The paranasal sinuses: anatomy and surgical technique,* St Louis, 1973, Mosby.

59. Robinson K: Roentgenographic manifestations of benign paranasal sinus disease, *Ear Nose Throat J* 63:144-149, 1984.

60. Rogers JH, Fredrickson JM, Noyek AM: Management of cysts, benign tumors, and bony dysplasia of the maxillary sinus, *Otolaryngol Clin North Am* 9:233-247, 1976.

61. Roush GC: Epidemiology of cancer of the nose and paranasal sinuses: current concepts, *Head Neck Surg* 2:3-11, 1979.

62. Samuel E: The opaque maxillary sinus, *Br J Radiol* 26:465-478, 1953.

63. Samuel E: Inflammatory diseases of the nose and paranasal sinuses, *Semin Roentgenol* 3:148-159, 1968.

64. Samuel E, Lloyd GAS: *Clinical radiology of the ear, nose and throat,* ed 3, Philadephia, 1978, WB Saunders.

65. Samy LL, Mostofa H: Oseoma of the nose and paranasal sinuses with a report of twenty-one caess, *J Laryngol Otol* 85:449-469, 1971.

66. Schaeffer JP: *The embryology, development and anatomy of the nose, paranasal sinuses, naso-lacrimal passageways and olfactory organ in man,* Philadelphia, 1920, P Blakiston's Son.

67. Shafer WG, Hine MK, Levy BM: *A textbook of oral pathology,* ed 4, Philadelphia, 1983, WB Saunders.

68. Shapiro GG, Rachelefsky GS: Introduction and definition of sinusitis, *J Allergy Clin Immunol* 90:417-418, 1992.

69. Shear M: *Cysts of the oral regions,* dental practitioner's handbook 3, Bristol, 1976, John Wright.

70. Small IA, Waldron CA: Ameloblastoma of the jaws, *Oral Surg* 8:281-297, 1955.

71. Som PM: The paranasal sinuses. In Bergeron RT, Osborn AG, Som PM, editors: *Head and neck imaging: excluding the brain,* St Louis, 1984, Mosby.

72. Som PM, Shogar JMA: The CT classification of ethmoid mucoceles, *J Comput Assist Tomogr* 4:199-203, 1980.

73. St-Pierre S, Baker S: Squamous cell carcinoma of the maxillary sinus: analysis of 66 cases, *Head Neck Surg* 5:508-513, 1983.

74. Takahashi R: The formation of the human paranasal sinuses, *Acta Otolaryngol Suppl (Stockh)* 408:1-28, 1984.

75. Thomas GK, Kasper KA: Ossifying fibroma of the frontal bone, *Arch Otolaryngol* 83:43-46, 1966.

76. Tsaknis PJ, Nelson JF: The maxillary ameloblastoma: an analysis of 24 cases, *J Oral Surg* 38:336-342, 1980.

77. Valvassori GE, Hord GE: Traumatic sinus disease, *Semin Roentgenol* 3:160-171, 1968.

78. Van Alyea OE: *Nasal sinuses,* Baltimore, 1951, Williams & Wilkins.

79. Van Norstrand AWP, Goodman WS: Pathologic aspects of mucosal lesions of the maxillary sinus, *Otolaryngol Clin North Am* 9:21-34, 1976.

80. Webeer A, Tadmor R, Davis R, and Roberson G: Malignant tumors of the sinuses: radiologic evaluation, including CT scanning, with clinical and pathologic correlation, *Neuroradiology* 16:443-448, 1978.

81. Williams JW Jr, Roberts L Jr, Distell B, and Simel DL: Diagnosing sinusitis by x-ray: is a single Waters view adequate? *J Gen Intern Med* 7:481-485, 566, 1992.

82. Wong A, Vaughan CW, Strong MS: Fibrous dysplasia of temporal bone, *Arch Otolaryngol* 81:131-133, 1965.

83. Wright RW: Round shadows in the maxillary sinuses, *Laryngoscope* 56:455-489, 1946.

84. Zinreich SJ: Imaging of chronic sinusitis in adults: x-ray, computed tomography, and magnetic resonance imaging, *J Allergy Clin Immunol* 90:445-451, 1992.

85. Zizmore J, Noyek AM: Cysts and benign tumors of the paranasal sinuses, *Semin Roentgenol* 3:172-201, 1968.

86. Zizmore J, Noyek AM: Cysts, benign tumors and malignant tumors of the paranasal sinuses, *Otolaryngol Clin North Am* 6:487-508, 1973.

87. Zizmore JK, Noyek AM: The radiologic diagnosis of maxillary sinus disease, *Otolaryngol Clin North Am* 9:93-115, 1976.

27

Soft Tissue Calcifications

Pathologic mineralization of soft tissues may develop in a wide variety of unrelated disorders and degenerative processes. It may occur associated with certain cutaneous tumors, scars, or inflammatory conditions. The deposited minerals are primarily calcium phosphate, but when it is amorphous and not organized, the process is referred to as *calcification*. Pathologic calcification that forms in degenerating and dead tissue is classified as *dystrophic calcification* and depends on changes in the tissues. When the minerals precipitate into normal tissue as a result of higher than normal levels of the ions in the insinuating fluids, the process is called *metastatic calcification*.[34] A third term used to characterize the development of calcarious concretions in the subcutaneous and deep connective tissues is *calcinosis*. It results from intrinsic changes in the connective tissues, such as those that occur in scleroderma.[1] In contrast, when the mineral phase is deposited as organized, well-formed bone, it is termed *heterotrophic ossification*. The bone may either be circumscribed compact bone or show some trabeculae and fatty marrow. The deposits may range from 1 mm to several centimeters in diameter, and they may be single or multiple. Sites of calcification or heterotrophic ossification typically do not cause subjective symptoms and are usually detected as incidental findings during radiographic examination. Such opacities are fairly common, being present on about 4% of panoramic radiographs.[29] In most cases, the clinician's only concern is to identify the calcification correctly, because they do not require treatment. A notable exception is the sialolith, or salivary duct stone.

LYMPH NODES

Calcification of lymph nodes is one of the more common soft tissue calcifications. A calcified lymph node indicates prior chronic infection involving the node. This condition frequently indicates a history of successfully treated tuberculosis.

Clinical features. The calcified lymph node is usually asymptomatic and first discovered as an incidental finding on a panoramic radiograph. The lesion may be single or multiple, or in some cases there may be a chain of calcified submaxillary or cervical nodes. Those that can be palpated are hard round or oblong masses.

Radiographic features. The radiographic appearance of the opaque, calcified lymph node usually suggests involvement of the entire node (Fig. 27-1). Although the border of the mass is well defined, it is more diffuse if the infection was not well contained within the node. Also, the radiodensity of the calcified mass is usually variable, showing both opaque and radiolucent areas. Occasionally, the calcified node has a laminated appearance. When dense, punctate calcifications are found on a radiograph in an area where lymph nodes usually occur, they are presumed to be lymph nodes. Because the lymph nodes in the oral region that usually calcify are in the area of the mandibular ramus or angle, they are usually considered incidental findings projected over the ramus, posterior body, or angle of the mandible or just below the angle of the mandible. This radiopaque image can usually be shifted away from the mandible with another projection. Most are unilateral.

Differential diagnosis. A radiographic diagnosis of calcified lymph nodes may only be presumed in the oral region because other types of calcification may also have similar appearance. A *sialolith* located in the hilar portion of the submandibular gland may mimic a calcified lymph node (see Chapter 30). The calcified lymph node is usually asymptomatic, in contrast to the painful sialoadenitis that frequently accompanies a sialolith. Sialography may be necessary to distinguish between the two lesions. It is usually possible to distinguish a *phlebolith* from a small calcified lymph node because the phlebolith is smaller and frequently has concentric radiopaque and radiolucent rings.

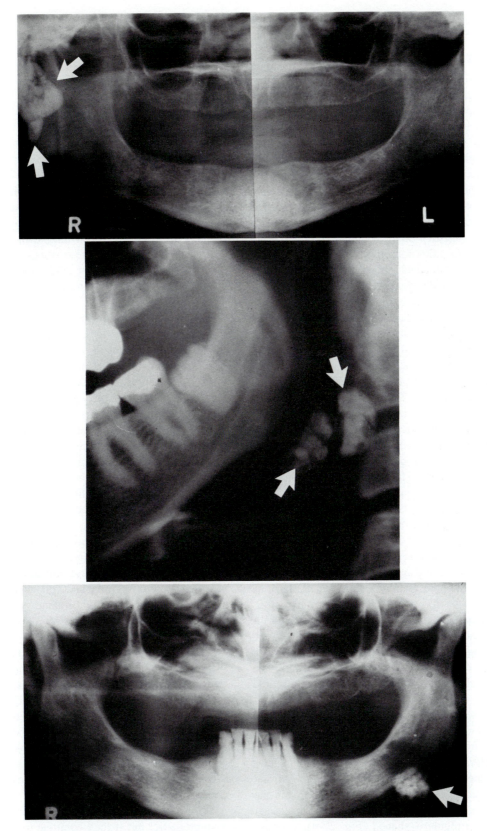

FIG. 27-1. Calcified lymph nodes appear as radiopaque masses, usually located just posterior to the ramus or inferior to the angle of the mandible.

Management. Calcified lymph nodes do not require treatment.

SIALOLITH

Sialoliths are stones within the major and minor salivary glands or in the ducts of these glands (see also Chapter 30). They are among the most common calcifications found in the soft tissues of the orofacial region. They may occur in any of the salivary gland ducts but are most common in Wharton's duct and the submandibular gland.[25] The initiation and growth of stones depend on the mechanical conditions contributing to slow flow rate (duct length and arrangement) and the physiochemical characteristics of the gland secretion.[28] Both contribute to nidus formation and to the precipitation of calcium and phosphate salts. The submandibular gland is more frequently involved (83% to 94%) than are the parotid (4% to 10%) or sublingual (1% to 7%) glands, probably because of its more viscous saliva, longer duct, and higher mineral content in the saliva.[3,26] About half the submandibular stones lie in the anterior portion of Wharton's duct, 20% in the posterior portion, and 30% in the gland.[26] The incidence at autopsy is about 1%. Sialoliths of the minor salivary glands have also been reported.[19,22]

Clinical features. Sialoliths are most common in the submandibular glands of men[32] in their middle and later years. They are usually single (70% to 80%) but may be multiple. Patients with salivary stones may be pain-free but usually have a history of pain and swelling in the floor of the mouth and in the involved gland. This discomfort may intensify at mealtimes, when salivary flow is stimulated. Because the stone usually does not block the flow of saliva, the pain gradually subsides. Perhaps as many as 9% of patients have recurrent sialolithiasis, and about 10% of patients with sialolithiasis also suffer nephrolithiasis.[26]

Radiographic features. Sialoliths located in the duct of the submandibular gland usually are cylindrical. Often they show evidence of multiple layers of calcification. The best view for visualizing these stones is a standard mandibular occlusal view, which displays the floor of the mouth without overlap from the mandible (Fig. 27-2). Occasionally, salivary stones are seen on periapical views superimposed over the mandibular premolar and molar apices (Fig. 27-3). Stones that form in the hilus of a submandibular gland tend to be larger and more irregularly shaped (Fig. 27-4). Because of their more posterior location, they are best visualized on lateral oblique radiographs. To demonstrate stones in the parotid gland duct, place a periapical film in the buccal vestibule and orient the x-ray beam through the cheek. Alternatively, stones in the parotid duct may also be demonstrated if the patient "blows out" the cheek as AP and open-mouth lateral projections are made. It is usually desirable to reduce the exposure time on radiographs made to detect sialoliths to about half the normal exposure. This helps to detect those that are lightly calcified.

About 20% or less of sialoliths in the submandibular gland and 40% of those in the parotid gland are radiolucent because of the low mineral content of their secretions.[25] When this is suspected, use sialography to visualize these stones (see Chapter 30). In the injected duct or gland, the radiolucent stone appears as a nonfilling defect.

Differential diagnosis. It is important to distinguish sialoliths from other soft tissue calcifications. Usually sialoliths are associated with pain or swelling involving a salivary gland, whereas calcifications in the lymph nodes are asymptomatic. The location of sialoliths is usually characteristic. In addition, the radiolucent stones must not be confused with a gas bubble introduced during sialography. A gas bubble in a duct is more easily moved and more circular than a sialolith, and it may not be apparent on previous or subsequent radiographs.

Management. A sialolith, whether within the duct or within the capsule of the gland, should be removed. Removal may be accomplished by manual manipulation of the stone within the duct, by simple incision of the gland or duct, or in some cases by excision of the gland. Recently, lithotripsy has been used to fragment sialoliths which are then excreted through the salivary gland ducts.[20,21]

ANTROLITHS

Antroliths are calcified masses found in the maxillary sinuses. Usually these result from calcification of masses of stagnant mucus in sites of previous inflammation, root fragments and bone chips, or foreign objects. Inasmuch as they are generally symptomless, it is not unusual to find them unexpectedly on radiographs exposed for other purposes. When antroliths are symptomatic, they may cause blood-stained nasal discharge, nasal obstruction, or facial pain.

Clinical features. The smaller antroliths are asymptomatic, but if they continue to grow, there may be an associated sinusitis.[4]

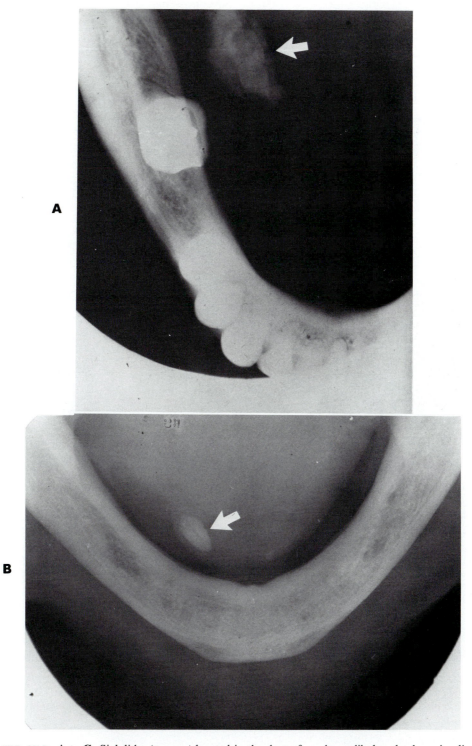

FIG. 27-2. A to **C,** Sialoliths *(arrows)* located in the duct of a submandibular gland as visualized on standard occlusal projections. Note that the exposure times are reduced to better demonstrate these concretions, which are less calcified than the mandible. **D,** Sialoliths may also be visualized on a panoramic radiograph, especially in the absence of teeth.   *Continued.*

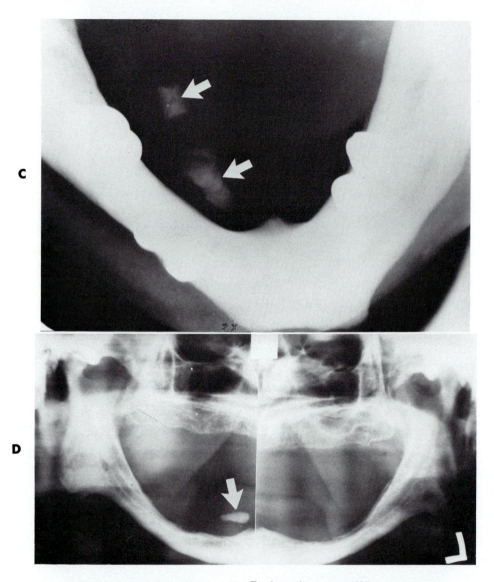

FIG. 27-2, cont'd. For legend see page 627.

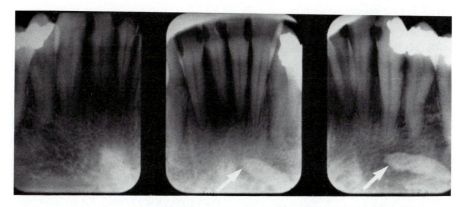

FIG. 27-3. A sialolith *(arrow)* superimposed on trabecular bone (periapical radiographs). (Courtesy Dr. L. Hollender, Seattle.)

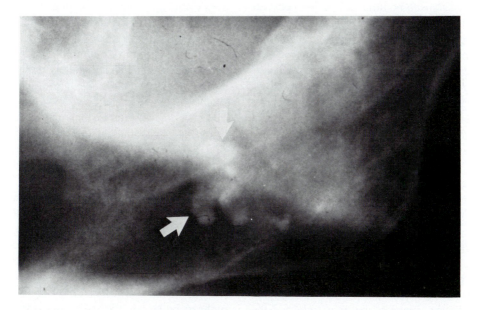

FIG. 27-4. Sialolith in the hilus of a submandibular gland *(arrow)*. Note its larger and more diffuse appearance on this portion of a panoramic radiograph.

Radiographic features. The images of antroliths vary in size, density, and outline. They may have a homogeneous or heterogeneous density, sometimes showing alternating laminations of radiolucent and radiopaque material. The outline may be rugged or smooth, and the shape may be round, oval, or irregular. They may be only slightly calcified so that only a lightly opaque mass is just visible, through which superimposed structures are easily discerned. Because these calcifications are usually attached to the wall of the sinus, their apparent position does not change when radiography is performed using different head positions.

Differential diagnosis. Antroliths may be distinguished from *root fragments* in the sinus by inspection of the mass for the usual root anatomy, such as the presence of a pulp canal. A displaced root fragment in the sinus is likely to move when radiography is performed with the head in different positions, unless it is lodged between the bone and the sinus lining. Rhinoliths are calcifications found in the nasal fossa that are comparable to antroliths.

Management. Patients who demonstrate strong presumptive evidence of antroliths should be referred to an otolaryngologist for treatment, usually removal of the concretion.

STYLOHYOID CHAIN OSSIFICATION

Ossification of the stylohyoid ligament occurs fairly commonly as an incidental feature on panoramic radiographs.[10,23] The ossification usually extends downward from the base of the skull, usually bilaterally. However, on rare occasions, ossification begins at the lesser horn of the hyoid and even more rarely in a central area of the ligament.[39]

Clinical features. Even when extensive ossification of one or both stylohyoid ligaments is seen, more than 50% of the individuals are clinically asymptomatic.[17] In one study, approximately 18% of a population examined showed more than 30 mm of the stylohyoid ligament ossified.[10] The mineralized ligament can usually be detected as a hard, pointed structure by palpation over the tonsil.[38] Although there seems to be little correlation between the extent to which the ligament has ossified and the intensity of the accompanying symptoms, in those with discomfort the anomaly is associated with vague pain on swallowing, turning the head, or opening the mouth. When this entity is associated with discomfort and there is a recent history of neck trauma (for example, tonsillectomy), it is called *Eagle's syndrome*.[6,11] The patient may describe earache, headache, dizziness, or transient syncope. The elongated styloid process probably causes these symptoms by impinging on the glossopharyngeal nerve. Similar clinical findings without a history of neck trauma are called *stylohyoid syndrome*. These individuals are usually over 40. This condition is more prevalent than Eagle's syndrome.

Radiographic features. The styloid process appears as a long, tapering, thin, radiopaque process between the ramus of the mandible and the mastoid process. The ligament shows at least some calcification in individuals of any age. It is thicker at its base and projects downward and forward (Fig. 27-5). It normally varies from about 0.5 to 2.5 cm in length. As increasing lengths of the stylohyoid ligament become ossified, the radiopaque image of the styloid process appears to extend toward the hyoid bone, roughly parallel to or superimposed on the posterior border of the mandibular ramus. The farther the radiopaque ossified ligament extends toward the hyoid bone, the more likely it is that it will be interrupted by radiolucent jointlike junctions.[12]

Differential diagnosis. Although the symptoms that complement stylohyoid and Eagle's syndrome are generally vague, when they occur with the distinctive radiographic evidence of ligament ossification, there is little chance that the complaint will be confused with another entity.

Management. The recommended treatment for Eagle's syndrome, when palpation over the tonsil is positive and the radiographic examination indicates that the stylohyoid ligament has ossified, is amputation of the stylohyoid process. For the more common stylohyoid syndrome, however, a more conservative approach of reassurance and steroid injections is recommended first.[6]

OSTEOMA CUTIS

Osteoma cutis is a rare soft tissue ossification in the skin that represents sites of normal bone formation in an abnormal location (heterotopic). It may occur anywhere, including the orofacial region. The face is the most common site, and the overlying skin and mucosa are usually normal.[30] The tongue is the most common intraoral site (osteoma mucosae).[24] Histologically these lesions are areas of dense viable bone in the dermis or subcutaneous tissue.[13] Their size may range from 0.1 mm to 5 cm, and the lesions may occur as single or multiple osteomas of the skin. They are occasionally found in diffuse scleroderma, replacing the altered collagen (in the dermis and subcutaneous septa).[1]

Clinical features. Osteoma cutis does not cause any visible change in the skin other than an occasional color change. The lesions are frequently secondary to acne of long duration, so they may develop in a scar or chronic inflammatory dermatosis. The color over the area may be normal or yellowish white. If the lesion is of reasonable size, pinhead or larger, the individual osteoma can be easily palpated. A needle inserted into one of the papules is met with stonelike resistance.[14]

Radiographic features. The osteoma cutis appears as a smoothly outlined, radiopaque, washer-shaped image, the radiolucent center of which is a cavity containing fatty marrow. Trabeculae occasionally develop in the marrow cavity of the larger entities. A larger example superimposed over the root or periapical area of a tooth may suggest an area of bone sclerosis. An AP radiograph made with the beam directed parallel to the surface of the face and the cheek blown outward demonstrates the relationship of the osteomas with the surface of the skin.

Differential diagnosis. The differential diagnosis should include *myositis ossificans, calcinosis*

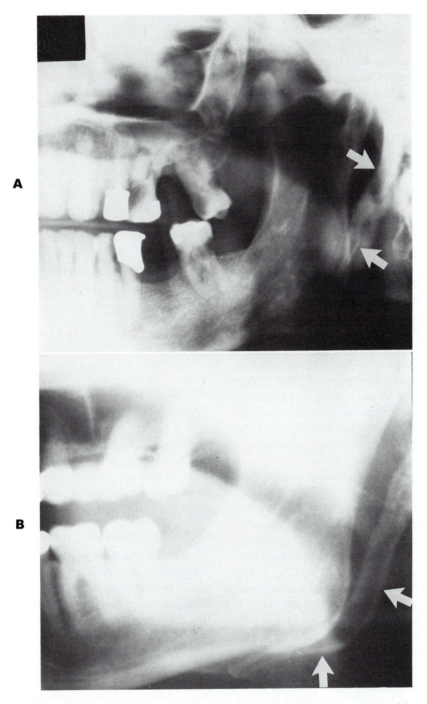

FIG. 27-5. A calcified stylohyoid ligament may be quite prominent, even in persons without symptoms.

cutis, and *osteoma mucosae.* If the "blown-out cheek" technique is used, the lesions of osteoma cutis appear as much more superficial than the mucosal lesions. Myositis ossificans is of greater proportions, in some cases causing noticeable deformity of the facial contour.

Management. Most individuals who seek attention for osteoma cutis want the lesions removed for cosmetic reasons. Although the osteoma cutis is usually quite small, it cannot be removed with a needle and must be excised.

CALCIFIED BLOOD VESSEL

Arterial walls may calcify in all forms of arteriosclerosis. Such changes may also represent sequelae of inflammatory processes affecting the vessel walls.[15] Such calcifications occasionally form in the facial arteries, as well as in the iliac, femoral, and popliteal arteries and in the abdominal aorta in occlusal arterial disease.[18] Although images of calcified arteries of the cheek and oral cavity may appear on oral radiographs of persons with arteriosclerosis obliterans, their presence does not necessarily indicate occlusive arterial disease.[2] Patients with Sturge-Weber syndrome also develop arterial wall calcification. This syndrome includes in its symptom complex capillary hemangiomas of the face, oral mucosa, and cranium. The cranial hemangiomas often show marked calcification, whereas the capillary hemangiomas found in the skin and mucosa do not. The radiopacity of the artery is the result of deposition of calcium salts within the medial coat of the vessel.

Clinical features. There are few, if any, clinical manifestations to suggest the dystrophic calcification of the facial arteries.

Radiographic features. The calcific deposits in the wall of the artery outline the image of the artery. From the side, the calcified vessel appears as a pair of thin, opaque lines. In a vessel cross-section, the calcified wall appears as a radiopaque circle. The opaque medial wall traces the vessel's tortuous path through the cheek.

Differential diagnosis. Other calcific deposits, *phleboliths* (Fig. 27-6), *miliary osteomas,* and *sialoliths* may be projected over the cheek and must be distinguished from the calcified artery. Usually the linear nature of the calcified arterial wall indicates the nature of this condition.

Management. Although the calcified vessel in the cheek does not require definitive treatment, the examiner should be alert to the possibility of other lesions in remote locations.

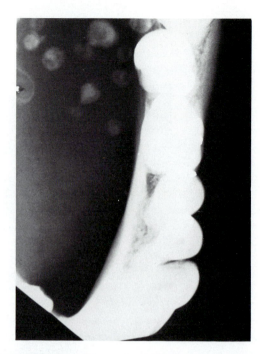

FIG. 27-6. Phleboliths are dystrophic calcifications found in veins. They are occasionally associated with hemangiomas, as seen lingual to the molars on this occlusal view.

MYOSITIS OSSIFICANS

Myositis ossificans is a condition in which ossifying interstitial connective tissue replaces muscle. Despite its name, there is little to suggest that this is an inflammatory disease in the ordinary sense.[9] There are two principal forms: *progressive* myositis ossificans and *localized* myositis ossificans.

Localized (traumatic) myositis ossificans

Localized myositis ossificans results from acute or chronic trauma or heavy muscular strain occasioned by certain occupations and sports. The injury leads to considerable hemorrhage into the muscle. The hemorrhage organizes and undergoes progressive scarring. During this healing process, cartilage may or may not form in the area, which may subsequently become calcified, but ultimately the damaged area is ossified.[34] The condition is not a myositis, and there is no actual ossification of the muscles, the calcific deposition being in the connective tissue about the muscles.[33] The mass of forming bone replaces adjacent muscle fibers. These bony lesions frequently develop in the capsules of old hematomas.

Clinical features. This lesion can develop at any age in either sex, but it occurs most often in young men who engage in vigorous activity. The most commonly involved muscles of the head and neck are the masseter and sternocleidomastoid.[37] The site of the precipitating trauma remains swollen, tender, and painful much longer than expected. The overlying skin may be red and inflamed; when this lesion involves a muscle of mastication, it may be difficult to open the jaws.[7] After about 2 or 3 weeks, the area of ossification becomes apparent in the tissues; a firm intramuscular mass can be palpated. The localized lesion may slowly enlarge, but eventually the bony mass appears to become incapable of further growth. Although this mass of heterotopic bone is not contiguous with the adjacent bone and does not arise from the periosteum, it may bind tightly to it with fibrous connective tissue and not be freely movable when examined. However, this is neither a consistent finding nor one on which a diagnosis should turn, because the lesion may not be firmly attached to the adjacent bone.

Radiographic features. Within the third or fourth week after the injury, the radiographic appearance of localized myositis ossificans is a faintly homogeneous opacity.[31] This probably represents the beginning deposition of calcium in the hemorrhage. Within another month, a delicate lacy or feathery internal structure of increased radiodensity develops, indicating that bone is being formed, sometimes with a circumscribed cortical periphery. In other cases, the mass is of uniform density. Gradually the image becomes denser and better defined. The shadow of the ossification is outside the adjacent normal bone and usually lies in the long axis of the muscle (Fig. 27-7). The internal structure of myositis ossificans does not radiographically simulate normal bony trabeculation. In contrast, there are linear streaks (pseudotrabeculae) running in the same direction as the normal muscle fibers.[33] These pseudotrabeculae are characteristic of myositis ossificans and strongly imply a diagnosis.

Differential diagnosis. The differential diagnosis of localized myositis ossificans would include *ossification of the stylohyoid ligament, dystrophic calcification* in areas of necrosis, *pathologic calcifications* in salivary glands and ducts and facial and cervical calcified lymph nodes, *phleboliths,* and *bone tumors.* There would rarely be any difficulty in distinguishing these pathologic mineralizations from myositis ossificans on the basis of their round, glandular, or lobular shapes, in contrast to the linear calcified streaks or sheets that characterize myositis ossificans. An exception may be some possible confusion with some type of ossifying bone tumors. However, in the case of myositis ossificans, the "tumor mass" has a smooth, round contour, and there is no destruction of the adjacent bone or any perpendicular striations of periosteal new bone producing the sunburst effect, as in osteosarcoma.

Management. Rest and limitation of use are recommended to diminish the extent of the calcific deposit. Early surgical removal of the lesion usually stimulates rapid (within 1 month) and extensive recurrence (from origin to insertion of the affected muscle). Recurrence is not likely, however, if the removal of the involved area of muscle is postponed until the process has become stationary.

Progressive myositis ossificans

Progressive myositis ossificans is a rare disease of unknown cause that usually affects children before 6 years of age, occasionally as early as infancy. Individuals with this condition form bone in tendons and fascia with the subsequent replacement of the adjacent muscle by the expanding bony mass. Affected individuals also frequently have congenital shortness of the first metatarsal and metacarpal bones, shortness of the little finger, and congenital hallux valgus (angulation of the great toe toward the other toes; the great toe may ride over or under the other toes). Inasmuch as fewer than 10% of the patients have a family history of the disease,[27] these associations have prompted the speculation that progressive myositis ossificans is generally a spontaneous mutation affecting the mesenchyme.[33]

Clinical features. In most cases, the heterotopic ossification starts in the muscles of the neck and upper back and moves to the extremities. The condition, which is more frequent in males,[33] starts with soft tissue swelling that is tender and painful and may show redness and heat. The acute symptoms subside, and a firm mass remains in the tissues. This condition may affect any of the striated muscles, including the heart and diaphragm.[34] In some cases, the spread of ossification is limited; in others, it becomes extensive, affecting almost all the large muscles of the body. There is a gradual increase in the stiffness and limitation of motion of the neck, chest, back, and extremities, especially the shoulder.[33] Advanced stages of the disease result in the "petrified man" condition. During

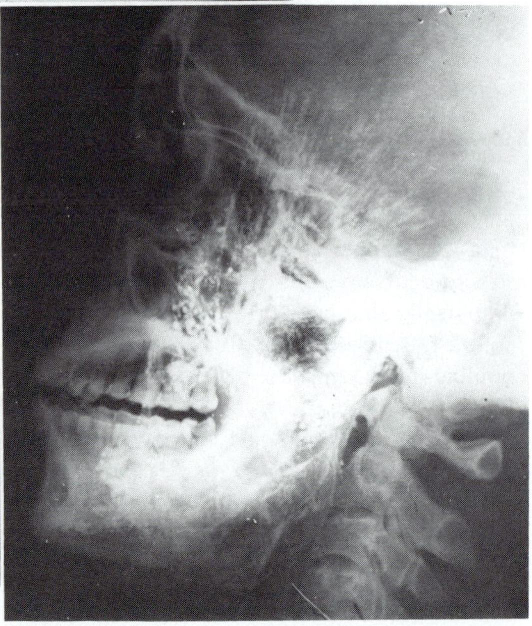

FIG. 27-7. A, Myositis ossificans, seen as bilateral linear calcifications of the sternohyoid muscle.
B and **C,** Extensive calcification of the masseter and temporalis muscles may also be seen. (**A,**
Courtesy of Dr. H. Worth, Vancouver; **B** and **C** from Shawkat AH: *Oral Surg* 23:751-754, 1967.)

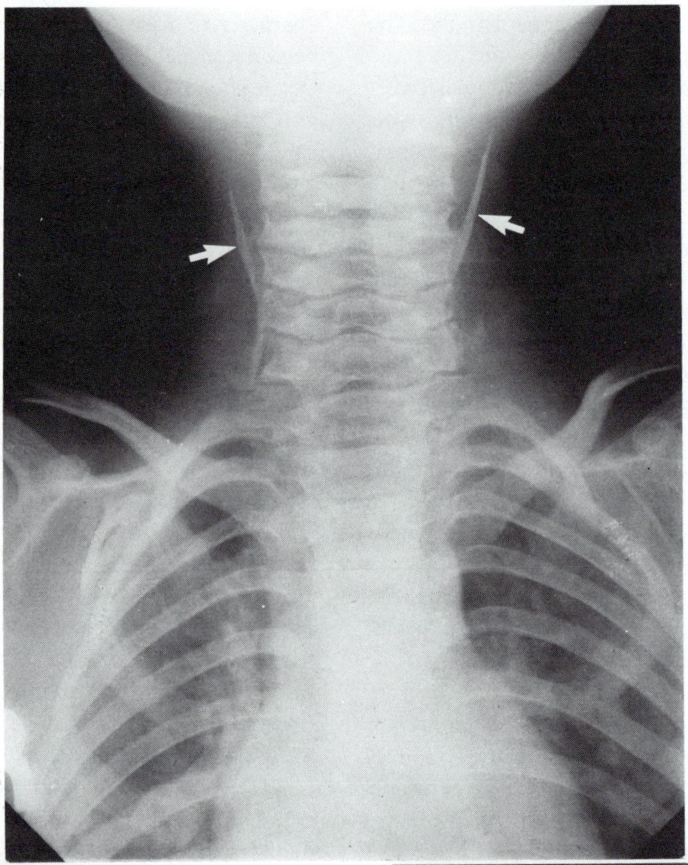

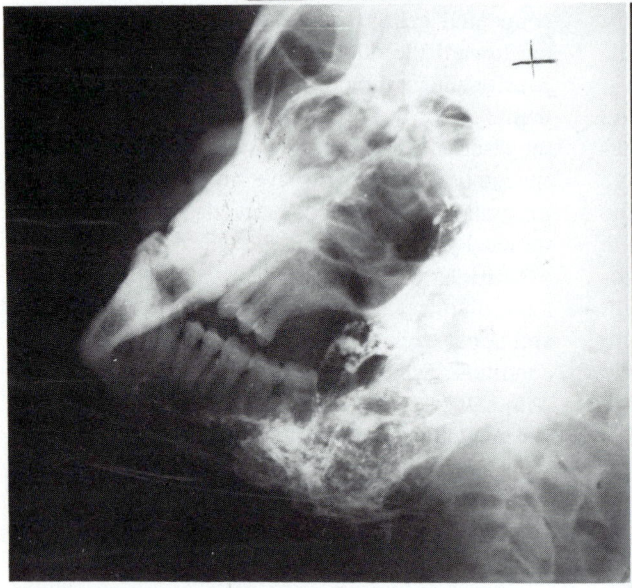

the third decade, there is usually spontaneous arrest of the process; however, most patients die during the third or fourth decade. Premature death usually results from respiratory embarrassment[5] or from inanition through the involvement of the muscles of mastication.[27]

Radiographic features. The image of the extraskeletal bone extends in the long axis of the affected muscles. The density of the heterotopic bone varies widely, and the definition of its borders is equally variable. Usually in the early stages of the disease, the calcific deposits are granular and fragmentary, and their images are distinct from those of the skeleton.[33] The skeleton becomes osteoporotic because of lack of function as muscles atrophy and joints become ankylosed.

Differential diagnosis. In the initial stages of the disease, it may be difficult to distinguish between progressive myositis ossificans and *rheumatoid arthritis*. However, the usual coexistent anomalies suggest the diagnosis. In the case of *calcinosis,* the deposits of amorphous calcium salts frequently resorb, but in progressive myositis ossificans the bone never disappears.

Management. There is no effective treatment for progressive myositis ossificans. Nodules that are traumatized and frequently ulcerate should be excised. Patients who have interference with respiration or respiratory infection in the later stages of the disease require supportive therapy.

DYSTROPHIC CALCIFICATION

When calcium salts precipitate into primary sites of chronic inflammation, dead and dying tissue, it is called *dystrophic calcification*. It is usually associated with a high local concentration of phosphatase enzymes, as in normal bone calcification,[16] and the anoxic condition within the devitalized tissue. Dystrophic calcification occurs, although the serum levels of calcium are normal and without any alteration in calcium metabolism. (In contrast, the deposition of calcium salts in vital healthy tissue is called *metastatic calcification,* but it is usually associated with some malfunctioning of the calcium metabolism that is responsible for a hypercalcemia.)

Clinical features. If the dystrophic calcification has taken place in oral tissues, the overlying tissue is frequently enlarged and ulcerated, and a solid mass of calcium salts can probably be palpated.

Radiographic features. Such dystrophic calcification is usually sparse and diffuse, rendering

detection difficult. Lesions may be single or multiple and rarely exceed 0.5 cm in diameter. The outline of the calcified area is usually irregular or indistinct, and the calcification may be homogeneous or contain punctate areas.

CYSTICERCOSIS

When eggs or gravid proglottids from *Taenia solium* (pork tapeworm) are ingested by humans, their covering is digested in the stomach and the larval form *(Cysticercus cellulosae)* is hatched. The larvae penetrate the mucosa, enter the blood vessels and lymphatics, and are distributed in the tissues all over the body, including the oral and perioral tissues, especially the muscles of mastication.[35] In body tissues other than the intestinal mucosa, the larvae die and are treated like a foreign body. After death, the larval spaces are replaced with fibrous connective tissue that may become calcified after about 3 months.[36] These areas in the tissues are referred to as *cysticerci.*

Clinical features. Mild cases of cysticercosis are completely asymptomatic. More severe cases are manifested by symptoms that range from mild to severe gastrointestinal upsets with epigastric pain and severe nausea and vomiting. Invasion of the brain may result in convulsions, irritability, and loss of consciousness.[8] Examination of the head and neck may disclose palpable firm masses up to 1 cm in diameter. Multiple small nodules may be felt in the region of the masseter and suprahyoid muscles and in the buccal mucosa and lip.

Radiographic features. Relatively radiodense elongated images of the calcified cysticerci may appear on almost any radiograph of the soft tissues of the body, including the muscles of mastication and facial expression, suprahyoid muscle, and postcervical musculature. Those that localize in muscle or subcutaneous tissue and have become calcified most often are elliptical or ovoid.[15]

Differential diagnosis. As a result of the similarity between cysticercus and a *salivary stone* in size, form, density, and occasionally location, their differentiation may be initially in doubt, especially for the cysticerci that occur in, or whose images are projected into, areas where salivary lithiasis may be expected.[15] However, in contrast to salivary stones, the calcified nodules of cysticerci are very likely to be multiple, suggesting their identity.

Management. Although prevention is the best treatment (proper preparation of pork and keeping fecal contamination to a minimum), the symptoms that accompany the initial infestation are best treated by a physician. Also, those larvae that localize in vital organs and tissues may precipitate severe symptoms and must be treated by a physician. Once the larvae have settled and calcified in the oral tissues, however, they are harmless.

REFERENCES

1. Allen AC: Skin. In Kissane JM, editor: *Anderson's pathology,* ed 8, vol 2, St Louis, 1985, Mosby.
2. Allen EV, Baker NW, Hines EA Jr: *Peripheral vascular disease,* ed 3, Philadelphia, 1962, WB Saunders.
3. Banks P: Nonneoplastic parotid swellings: a review, *Oral Surg* 25:732-745, 1968.
4. Blaschke D, Brady F: The maxillary antrolith, *Oral Surg* 48:182-189, 1979.
5. Buhain WJ, Rammohan G, Berger HW: Pulmonary function in myositis ossificans progressiva, *Am Rev Respir Dis* 110:333-337, 1974.
6. Camarda AJ, Deschamps C, Forest D: I. Stylohyoid chain ossification: a discussion of etiology, *Oral Surg* 67:508-514, 1989.
7. Cameron JR, Stetzer JJ: Myositis ossificans of the right masseter muscle: report of a case, *J Oral Surg* 3:170-173, 1945.
8. Cheraskin E, Langley LL: *Dynamics of oral diagnosis,* Chicago, 1956, Mosby.
9. Collins DH: *Pathology of bone,* London, 1966, Butterworth.
10. Correll R and others: Mineralization of the stylohyoid-stylomandibular ligament complex, *Oral Surg* 48:286-291, 1979.
11. Eagle W: Elongated styloid process, symptoms and treatment, *Arch Otolaryngol* 67:172-176, 1958.
12. Ettinger RL, Hanson JG: The styloid or "Eagle" syndrome: an unexpected consequence, *Oral Surg* 40:336-340, 1975.
13. Farhood V, Steed D, Krolls S: Osteoma cutis: cutaneous ossification with oral manifestations, *Oral Surg* 45:98-103, 1978.
14. Gasner WG: Primary osteoma cutis: report of a case, *AMA Arch Dermatol Syph* 69:101-103, 1954.
15. Gibilesco J, Turlington EG: *Oral roentgenographic diagnosis,* ed 5, Philadelphia, 1985, WB Saunders.
16. Goldstein B, Damsker J, Brady L: Dystrophic calcification in the tongue: a late sequel to radiation therapy, *Oral Surg* 46:12-17, 1978.
17. Grossman JR, Tarsitano JJ: The styloid-stylohyoid syndrome, *J Oral Surg* 35:555-560, 1977.
18. Hayes JB, Gibilisco JA, Juergens JL: Calcification of vessels in cheek of patient with medial atherosclerosis, *Oral Surg* 21:299-302, 1966.
19. Ho V, Curre WJ, Walker A: Sialolithiasis of minor salivary glands, *Br J Oral Maxillofac Surg* 30:273-275, 1992.
20. Iro H, Schneider HT, Födra C et al: Shockwave lithotripsy of salivary duct stones, *Lancet* 339:1333-1336, 1992.
21. Iro H and others: Extracorporeal piezoelectric shock-wave lithotripsy of salivary gland stones, *Laryngoscope* 102:492-494, 1992.
22. Jensen J, Howell F, Rich G, and Correll R: Minor salivary gland calculi: a clinicopathologic study of forty-seven new cases, *Oral Surg* 47:44-50, 1979.
23. Kaufman SM, Elzay RP, Irish EF: Styloid process variation: radiographic and clinical study, *Arch Otolaryngol* 91:460-463, 1970.
24. Krolls SO, Jacoway JR, Alexander WN: Osseous choristomas of intraoral soft tissue, *Oral Surg* 32:588-595, 1971.
25. Lowman RM, Cheng GK: Diagnostic radiology. In Rankow RM, Polayer IM, editors: *Diseases of the salivary glands,* Philadelphia, 1976, WB Saunders.
26. Lustmann J, Regev E, Melamed Y: Sialolithiasis: a survey on 245 patients and a review of the literature, *Int J Oral Maxillofac Surg* 19:135-138, 1990.
27. Lutwak L: Myositis ossificans progressiva: mineral metabolic and radioactive calcium studies of the effects of hormones, *Am J Med* 37:269-293, 1964.
28. Mandel ID, Thompson RH Jr: The chemistry of parotid and submaxillary saliva in heavy calculus formers and nonformers, *J Periodontol* 38:310-315, 1967.
29. Monsour PA, Romaniuk K, Hutchings RD: Soft tissue calcifications in the differential diagnosis of opacities superimposed over the mandible by dental panoramic radiography, *Aust Dent J* 36:94-101, 1991.
30. Peterson WC Jr, Mandel SL: Primary osteomas of the skin, *Arch Dermatol* 87:626-632, 1963.
31. Pugh DG: *Roentgenologic diagnosis of diseases of bones,* New York, 1951, Thomas Nelson.
32. Rauch S, Gorlin RJ: Diseases of the salivary glands. In Gorlin RJ, Goldman HM, editors: *Thoma's oral pathology,* ed 6, vol 2, St Louis, 1970, Mosby.
33. Ritvo M: *Bone and joint x-ray diagnosis,* Philadelphia, 1955, Lea & Febiger.
34. Robbins SL: *Pathologic basis of disease,* Philadelphia, 1974, WB Saunders.
35. Rosencrans M, Barack J: Parasitic infection of the mouth: a case report of *Cysticercus cellulosea, NY State Dent J* 35:371-373, 1963.
36. Shear M: *Cysts of the oral regions,* Bristol, England, 1976, John Wright.
37. Standish SM: Diseases of the muscles of the face and oral regions. In Tiecke RW, editor: *Oral pathology,* New York, 1965, McGraw-Hill.
38. Winkler S, Sammatino FJ Sr, Sammatino FJ Jr, and Monari JH: Styloid syndrome: report of a case, *Oral Surg* 51:215-217, 1981.
39. Worth HM: *Principles and practice of oral radiologic interpretation,* Chicago, 1963, Mosby.

28

Trauma to Teeth and Facial Structures

Radiography of the orofacial region often plays a critical role in evaluating the effects of a traumatic injury. Radiographs serve to identify the location and orientation of fractures and indicate the degree of separation or displacement of fracture margins. They may also serve to locate a foreign object associated with the trauma. Multiple projections, especially right-angle views, are often most useful and may be essential for establishing the precise location of an injury. Often patients who have suffered recent trauma are difficult to work with because of discomfort, medication, or wound dressings. Achieving a satisfactory examination may require patience and ingenuity. When radiographs are obtained, study them systematically for evidence of abnormality. It is often valuable to confirm suspected abnormalities with additional films that provide alternate views of the region. However, despite the significant manner in which radiographs can contribute to the description of an injury, they are only supplementary to a careful history and clinical examination. Follow-up radiographs are useful in evaluating the extent of healing in the interval following an injury and the development of long-term changes resulting from the trauma.

TRAUMATIC INJURIES OF THE TEETH
Concussion

The term *concussion* describes those circumstances where the traumatic event caused some injury to the supporting structures but without abnormal loosening or displacement of the tooth.[16] There is some crushing injury to the vascular structures at the apex and to the periodontal ligament, with resulting inflammatory edema. This frequently tends to elevate the tooth to a degree that may cause some masticatory interference.

Clinical features. The patient usually complains that the traumatized tooth is sore. On examination, the tooth is markedly sensitive to both horizontal and vertical percussion. It may also be sensitive to biting forces, but patients usually modify their bite to remove occlusal stress for the short period that the periodontal ligament is inflamed.

Radiographic features. The radiographic appearance of a dental concussion is widening of the periodontal ligament space.[27] This widening usually occurs only in the apical portion of the periodontal ligament space because the raising of the tooth results in an essentially parallel movement of the coronal two thirds of the root surface with the lamina dura (Fig. 28-1). Reduction in the size of the pulp chamber and pulp canals may develop in the months and years following such traumatic

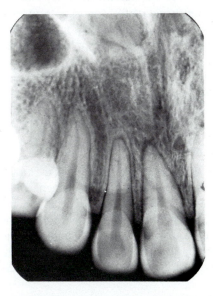

FIG. 28-1. Dental concussion has resulted in widening of the periodontal ligament space of the lateral and central incisors.

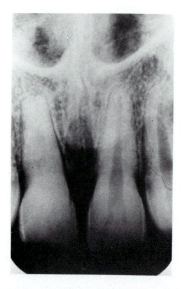

FIG. 28-2. Dental concussion has led to obliteration of the pulp chamber and external resorption of the root following an injury.

injury (Fig. 28-2). This reduction in the size of the pulp may be accompanied by pupal necrosis and development of a periapical lesion. Occasionally, there is lack of the usual reduction of pulp size in developing teeth, which also indicates pulpal necrosis.

Management. Because there is no apparent displacement of the tooth (teeth), the appropriate treatment for permanent teeth is conservative: slight adjustment of the opposing teeth, if necessary, and repeated vitality tests during a postinjury period of clinical and radiographic examination. If the patient is seen shortly after the trauma, digital pressure applied to the incisal edge will assure that the tooth is not extruded. Deciduous teeth that have sustained a concussion require only subsequent clinical and radiographic observation.

Luxation

Luxation of teeth is dislocation of the articulation (represented by the periodontal attachment) of the tooth. Such teeth are both abnormally mobile and displaced. Subluxation of the tooth corresponds to a sprain in that it denotes an injury to the tooth's supporting structures that has resulted in abnormal loosening of the tooth, but without frank dislocation.

Traumatic forces, depending on their nature and orientation, can cause intrusive luxation (displacement of teeth into the alveolar bone), extrusive

luxation (partial displacement of teeth out of the socket), or lateral displacement (movement of teeth other than axial displacement). In intrusive and lateral luxation, comminution (crushing) or fracture of the supporting alveolar bone accompanies dislocation of the tooth.

The movement of the apex and the disruption of the circulation to the traumatized tooth that accompanies luxation usually induce temporary or permanent pulpal changes, which may conclude in complete or partial pulpal necrosis. If the pulp survives, the rate of hard tissue formation by the pulp accelerates and continues until it obliterates the pulp chamber and canal. This may take place in permanent and deciduous teeth.

The teeth most frequently subjected to luxation are the maxillary incisors in both the deciduous and permanent dentitions. The mandibular teeth are seldom involved.[4] The type of luxation varies with age, possibly as an expression of change in the physical nature of the bone. Intrusions and extrusions are the primary dislocations found in the deciduous teeth. In the permanent dentition, the intrusive type of luxation is seen less frequently, and those that do occur are seen in the younger individuals in this group.[2] When teeth are luxated, in either dentition, usually two or more are involved, and seldom just a single tooth.[65]

Clinical features. It is important to obtain an adequate history before beginning the clinical examination because it is basic to the examination. It is especially helpful in identifying the condition affecting a malpositioned tender tooth and in prompting the appropriate therapy.

Teeth that have been subluxated are in their normal location but abnormally mobile. There may be some bleeding from the gingival crevice, indicating periodontal ligament damage. Subluxated teeth are extremely sensitive to percussion and masticatory forces. When evaluating the mobility of a luxated tooth, test both the horizontal and vertical mobility.

The clinical crowns of intruded teeth may appear shortened. Maxillary incisors may even be driven so deeply into the alveolar ridge that they appear completely avulsed (lost). Although this is especially true of deciduous teeth, deep intrusive luxations of permanent teeth also occur. Depending on the orientation and magnitude of the force and the shape of the root, the root may be pushed through the buccal alveolar plate, where it can be seen or palpated. The root might also be dislocated lingually. In this case, it might cause some damage to adjacent developing teeth, including its succe-

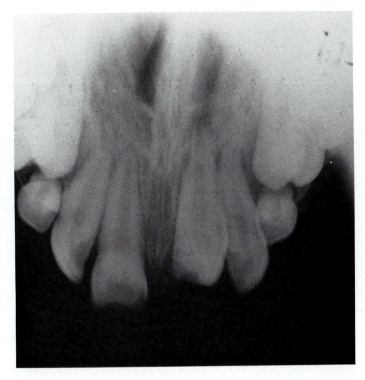

FIG. 28-3. Intruded maxillary central incisor following trauma. Note the obliteration of the apical lamina dura and the fractured incisal edges of both centrals.

daneous tooth. On repeated vitality testing, the sensitivity of a luxated tooth may be temporarily decreased or nondetectable, especially shortly after the accident. Vitality may return, however, after weeks or even several months.

Radiographic features. Radiographic examinations of luxated teeth may demonstrate the extent of the injury to the root, periodontal ligament, and alveolar bone and the stage of tooth formation when appropriate. Further, a radiograph made at the time of injury will serve as a valuable reference point for comparison with subsequent radiographs. Make radiographs of the traumatized tooth and nearby teeth in both jaws. It is usually appropriate to use the bisecting-angle technique for the intraoral radiographs to reduce pressure on the injured teeth. Any error in the extent of displacement it imposes will be minimal.

As with dental concussion, the minor damage associated with subluxation may be only an apparent elevation of the traumatized tooth. The sole radiographic finding may be a widening of the apical portion of the periodontal ligament space. However, the increase in this space may be so slight and the geometric variables so difficult to control that recognizable radiographic change is not ap-

parent. In this case, it is necessary to make the diagnosis on the clinical finding of abnormal mobility.

Dislocation of teeth is easily diagnosed if the radiographic examination is properly executed. Its demonstration is often dependent on the angle of the central beam. Make a second radiograph at an altered angle of projection before concluding that the tooth is not luxated.

The depressed position of the crown of an intruded tooth is often apparent on the radiograph (Fig. 28-3). It may also cause partial or total obliteration of the periodontal ligament space. A lateral projection of the dislocated tooth shows its direction of displacement and its relationship to vestibular bone and developing permanent teeth (if the intruded tooth is deciduous). A minimally or moderately intruded tooth may be difficult to demonstrate radiographically. Extrusively luxated teeth result in increased width of the periodontal ligament space. The widening may be accentuated in the apical region, whereas in a more severely extruded tooth the space about the profile of the entire root may be increased. A laterally luxated tooth usually demonstrates a widened periodontal ligament space about the root. The increase in width

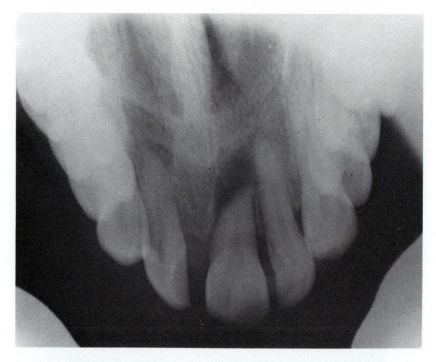

FIG. 28-4. This central incisor has been extruded following trauma. Note the periapical radiolucency caused by the revealed socket and the secondary inflammatory destruction of bone.

is greater on the side of impact (Fig. 28-4). Often these teeth are somewhat extruded.

Management. A subluxated permanent tooth that is causing discomfort as a result of extruding from the alveolus may be restored to its normal position by digital pressure shortly after the accident. If swelling precludes repositioning, minimal reduction of antagonists to relieve discomfort may be necessary. Periodically examine a subluxated primary tooth after the injury. If it causes some discomfort as the result of extrusion, it can be removed without undue concern for occlusal problems.

Reposition extruded and laterally luxated permanent teeth by digital manipulation. Stabilize them by splinting to prevent further damage to the pulp and periodontal ligament. However, remove the dislocated tooth if its apex is near its succedaneous tooth. If the alveolar bone over the root of a luxated tooth has been fragmented and displaced, reposition the fragments by digital pressure. Finally, expect fragments of radiopaque material in the soft tissues if crown fractures are clinically apparent.

Avulsion

Avulsion (or exarticulation) is the term used to describe the complete displacement of a tooth from

its alveolus. Teeth may be avulsed by direct trauma when the force is applied directly to the tooth or by indirect trauma, for example, when the force causes the jaws to strike together and the force is indirectly applied to the teeth.[62] Avusion occurs in about 15% of traumatic injuries to the teeth.[2] Fights are responsible for the avulsion of most permanent teeth, whereas accidental falls account for the traumatic loss of most deciduous teeth.[4] The maxillary central incisors are most often avulsed from both dentitions.[13]

Clinical features. When a tooth has been avulsed, it will also be missing from the arch. The appearance of the alveolus depends on the time between its loss and the clinical examination. Typically, this injury occurs in a relatively young age group, when the permenent central incisors are just erupting[44] and the periodontal ligament is immature. Most often only a single tooth is lost, and fractures of the alveolar wall and lip injuries are frequently seen.[2]

Radiographic features. The radiographic examination of an avulsed tooth shows a dental socket without the corresponding tooth. The displaced tooth may be in adjacent soft tissue, and its image may occasionally project on radiographs near the empty alveolus. In the case of a deciduous tooth, the radiograph may show that a tooth presumed to

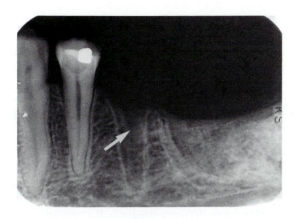

FIG. 28-5. Bone formation in a healing socket develops from the lateral walls and may leave a central radiolucent line *(arrow)* that is suggestive of a pulp canal in a retained root fragment.

be avulsed has in reality suffered intrusive luxation or was fractured with retention of a root tip.

In a recent wound, the lamina dura probably is apparent because it usually persists for several months after the loss of function.[76] The replacement of the socket site with new bone requires months and, in some cases, years. As new bone forms and the opposite walls of the healing socket approach each other, the vertical radiolucent shadow between the constricting walls resembles a pulp canal on the radiograph. The sclerosing socket may resemble a retained ankylosed root (complete with an apparent pulp canal but without a periodontal ligament space) for some time (Fig. 28-5).

Management. Reimplanting permanent teeth after avulsion often restores function. If the tooth is intact and without extensive caries or periodontal disease, and the extraoral period has not been extensive, the chances for success are enhanced. Successful reimplantation depends largely on the viability of the residual periodontal ligament fibers. The shorter the extraoral period, the better the prognosis.[37] Reimplanting avulsed deciduous teeth carries the danger of interfering with the developing succedaneous teeth. If the apical foramen is open, endodontic therapy may not be required. It can be delayed until the first signs of apical resorption are radiographically detected (usually 2 or 3 weeks after replantation). If the apical foramen is closed, endodontic treatment will be required, but should be delayed 1 or 2 weeks. External root resorption may occur in the months and years following replantation, and the resorption may progress to virtually complete destruction of the root.

Fractures of the teeth

Dental crown fractures. Fracture of the dental crowns most frequently involves anterior teeth. They represent about 25% of the traumatic injuries to the permanent teeth and 40% to the deciduous teeth.[5] The most common event responsible for the fracture of permanent teeth is a fall, followed by accidents involving vehicles (e.g., bicycles, autos) and blows from foreign bodies striking the teeth.[2] Fractures involving only the crown normally fall into three categories: (1) fractures that involve only the enamel without the loss of enamel substance (infraction of the crown or crack); (2) fractures involving enamel or enamel and dentin with loss of tooth substance but without pulpal involvement (uncomplicated fracture); and (3) fractures that pass through enamel, dentin, and pulp with loss of tooth substance (complicated fracture).

Clinical features. Infractions or cracks in the enamel are quite common but frequently overlooked because they are not readily detectable in the usual direct illumination used for dental examination. Illuminating crowns with indirect light (directing the beam in the long axis of the tooth) causes cracks to appear distinctly in the enamel. Direct impact to the enamel causes these cracks. Histologic studies show that they pass through the enamel but not into the dentin.[66] The pattern and distribution of these cracks are unpredictable and apparently relate to the trauma. The recognition of infraction lines should suggest the possibility that other traumatic injuries may be present and require attention.

The uncomplicated crown fracture that does not involve the dentin usually occurs at the mesial or distal corner of the maxillary central incisor.[28] Loss of the central portion of the incisal edge is also fairly common. Fractures that involve both the enamel and dentin but are not complicated by pulpal exposure are more frequent in the permanent dentition than are the complicated cases.[31] In contrast, the incidence of complicated and uncomplicated fractures is about equal in the deciduous teeth. Fractures that involve dentin can be readily recognized clinically because a segment of the crown is missing, and the dentin is identifiable by the contrast in color between it and the peripheral layer of enamel. The exposed dentin is usually sensitive to chemical, thermal, and mechanical stimulation. In deep fractures, the pink image of the pulp may shine through the thin remaining dentinal wall.

The complicated crown fractures are usually distinguishable by the missing part(s) and by frank

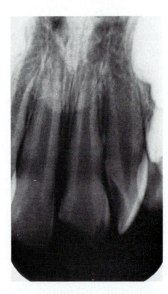

FIG. 28-6. Fracture of this maxillary central incisor has resulted in a loss of enamel and dentin but left the pulp intact.

bleeding from the exposed pulp or by droplets of blood forming from pinpoint exposures. The pulp is likewise visible. If treatment has been delayed for weeks, there may be proliferation of the pulpal tissue from the open pulp chamber. The exposed pulp is sensitive to most forms of stimulation.

Radiographic features. The radiograph of a fractured tooth shows the size and position of the pulp chamber, another perspective of the location and extent of the exposure, and the stage of root development (Fig. 28-6). Such information complements the clinical findings and aids in the identification of such complications as root fracture, apical involvement, or luxation, all of which play a role in treatment planning.

Management. Although crown infractions do not require treatment, the implication of trauma does suggest that the vitality of the tooth should be questioned and determined. Because an uncomplicated fracture limited to the enamel results in only a small defect in the profile of the tooth, it can be corrected by grinding, especially if the sharp edges of enamel are causing some discomfort. When a fracture is so extensive that it cannot be aesthetically corrected by grinding alone, restoration is in order. Delay this procedure for a number of weeks until the pulp has recovered from its initial shock and is starting to lay down secondary dentin. The prognosis for teeth with fractures limited to the enamel is quite good, and pulpal necrosis de-

velops in fewer than 2% of such cases.[59] When a fracture involves both dentin and enamel, the frequency of pulpal necrosis is about 3%.[60] Oblique fractures have a worse prognosis than horizontal fractures because a greater amount of dentin is exposed. The frequency of pulpal necrosis increases greatly if there is also concussion and mobility of the tooth.

Treatment of complicated crown fractures of permanent teeth may involve pulp capping, pulpotomy, or pulpectomy, depending on the stage of root formation. When a coronal fracture of a deciduous tooth involves the pulp, it is usually best treated by extraction.

Dental root fractures. Fractures of tooth roots limited to the dentin and pulp are uncommon.[32] They account for 7% or fewer of the traumatic injuries to permanent teeth and for about half that many in deciduous teeth.[25] This difference probably results from the fact that the deciduous teeth are less firmly anchored in the alveolus.

Clinical features. Most root fractures occur in maxillary central incisors.[37] The coronal fragments are usually displaced lingually and slightly extruded.[5] The degree of mobility of the crown relates to the level of the fracture: The closer the fracture to the apex, the more stable the tooth. When testing the mobility of a traumatized tooth, place a finger over the alveolar bone. If only movement of the crown can be detected, root fracture is likely. Fractures of the root may occur with fracture of the alveolar bone. This is most often observed in the anterior region of the mandible, where root fractures are infrequent.[28] It is probable that many bony fractures in one alveolar wall are overlooked. Although root fracture is usually associated with temporary loss of sensitivity (by all usual criteria), the sensitivity of most teeth returns to normal within about 6 months.[46]

Radiographic features. Fractures of the dental root may occur at any level and involve one or all the roots of multirooted teeth (Fig. 28-7). When the orientation of the x-ray beam is parallel with the plane of a root fracture, the fracture appears as a sharp radiolucent line between the fragments. If, however, the orientation of the beam is not directly through the fracture but some of the tooth structure is superimposed over the fracture, the image of the fracture appears as a more poorly defined gray shadow. Most nondisplaced root fractures are usually difficult to demonstrate radiographically, and several views may be necessary.

Most of the fractures confined to the root occur

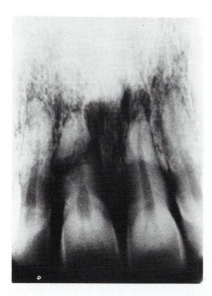

FIG. 28-7. Transverse root fracture of the central incisor.

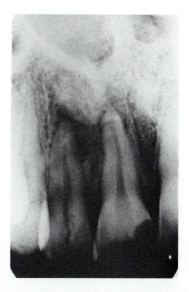

FIG. 28-8. An oblique fracture of the central incisor root mimics a comminuted fracture. There is also a longitudinal fracture of the lateral incisor. On this radiograph, note how the soft tissue outline of the nose simulates a fracture of the central incisor root tip.

in the middle third of the root.[6] They are usually transverse and oblique, casting an ellipsoid image of the single fracture, which may result in the images of the buccal and lingual margins mimicking a multiple (comminuted) fracture (Fig. 28-8). Longitudinal root fractures are relatively uncommon but are most likely in teeth with posts that have been subjected to trauma. Root fractures tend to open with time, probably as a result of hemorrhage, edema, or granulation tissue displacing the fragments, and some early resorption of the fractured surfaces. This may result in the subsequent identification of a root fracture that was initially overlooked. Over the long term, calcification and obliteration of the pulp chamber and canal may be seen.[10]

Differential diagnosis. The superimposition of soft tissue structures such as the lip, ala of the nose, and the nasolabial fold with the image of a root may suggest a root fracture with the fragment in place (Fig. 28-8). Avoid this diagnostic error by noting that the soft tissue image (of the "lip line") usually extends beyond the tooth margins. Bony fractures may also suggest fractures of tooth roots.

Management. When there are permanent teeth with fractures in the middle or apical third of the root, manually restore the teeth to their proper position and immobilize them. There is a generally favorable prognosis; the incidence of pulpal necrosis is about 20% to 24%.[10] The more apical the fracture, the better the prognosis. Perform endodontic therapy only when there is evidence of

pulpal necrosis. If a radiolucency does develop, it is usually at the site of the fracture rather than at the apex.[34] When the fracture occurs in the coronal third of the root, the prognosis is poor and extraction is indicated unless the root fragment can be extruded orthodontically and restored. The roots of fractured deciduous teeth that are not badly dislocated may be retained with the expectation that they will be normally shed. If they are dislocated, they should be removed because the pulp is likely to become necrotic. Apical fragments of fractured primary teeth that remain after removal of the coronal portion are likely to be resorbed. Any effort to remove them may result in damage to the developing succedaneous tooth.[5]

Crown-root fractures. Crown-root fractures involve both the crown and root(s).[11] Such fractures are likely to be intra-alveolar and extra-alveolar. Although uncomplicated fractures may occur, they usually involve the pulp.[55] About twice as many affect the permanent as the deciduous teeth.[2] Most crown-root fractures of the anterior teeth are the result of direct trauma. Many posterior teeth are predisposed to such fractures by large restorations or extensive caries.

Clinical features. The typical crown-root fracture of an anterior tooth has a labial margin in the gingival third of the crown and courses obliquely to exit below the gingival attachment on the lingual surface. Displacement of the fragments is usually minimal. Crown-root fractures in completely erupted teeth frequently involve the pulp, whereas teeth in the process of erupting usually sustain uncomplicated crown-root fractures. The patient with a crown-root fracture usually complains of pain during mastication. The teeth are sensitive to occlusal forces, which cause separation of the fragments.

Radiographic features. The fact that the course of the most common crown-root fracture of anterior teeth is perpendicular to the direction of the beam generally used to radiograph these teeth precludes its easy recognition on the radiograph. In addition, the fragments are usually maintained in close contact by the periodontal ligament fibers. This also minimizes visualization of the fracture margins. However, because the labial margin of the fracture is usually apparent, radiographic detection is not of primary importance. The vertical fractures of crown and root that are mainly tangential to the direction of the radiographic beam are readily apparent on the radiograph. Unfortunately, this is not common.

Management. For adequate evaluation of the injury, examine the fractured surfaces directly by removal of the coronal fragment. If the coronal fragment includes as much as 3 to 4 mm of clinical root, successful restoration of the tooth is doubtful and removal of the residual root is recommended.[42] Also, if the crown-root fracture is vertical, prognosis is poor regardless of treatment. If the pulp is not exposed and the fracture does not extend more than 3 to 4 mm below the epithelial attachment, conservative treatment is likely to be successful.

Uncomplicated crown-root fractures are frequently encountered in posterior teeth, and with the appropriate crown-lengthening procedures (gingivectomy and ostectomy), the tooth is likely to be amenable to successful restoration.[51] If only a small amount of root is lost with the coronal fragment but the pulp has been compromised, it is likely that the tooth can be restored after endodontic treatment with a crown over a post and core.[20]

Vertical root fractures. Vertical root fractures (cracked tooth syndrome) run lengthwise from the crown toward the apex of the tooth. They usually occur in the posterior teeth in adults, especially in mandibular molars. These fractures are usually iatrogenic following insertion of retention screws or pins into vital or nonvital teeth.[9] Uncrowned posterior teeth that have been treated endodontically

are most at risk. This results from weakening of the tooth caused by dehydration and loss of tooth structure during root canal therapy. Traumatic occlusion is another source of vertical root fracture, particularly in restored teeth. Usually both sides of a root are involved.[73] The crack is usually oriented in the facial lingual plane in both anterior and posterior teeth.[56,73]

Clinical features. Patients with vertical root fractures complain of persistent dull pain, often of long duration. It may be elicited by applying pressure to the involved tooth. The pain may vary from nonexistent to mild. A BB shot held in tape has been used to localize sensitive fractured teeth with great accuracy.[47] The patient may have a periodontal lesion resembling a chronic abscess[45] or a history of repeated failed endodontic therapy.[36] Occasionally, definitive diagnosis can be made only by inspection after surgical exposure.[56]

Radiographic features. If the central ray of the x-ray beam lies in the plane of the fracture, the fracture may be visible as a radiolucent line on the radiograph. Usually, however, radiographs are not useful in identifying vertical root fractures in their early stages. Later, after there has been bacterial invasion of the pulp through the fracture, radiographs usually show thickening of the periodontal ligament or a diffuse radiolucent lesion. This radiolucency may be quite different from that usually seen, because it may extend quite far coronally along the side of a tooth toward the crestal bone.[56] Lesions may also extend apically from the alveolar crest and resemble periodontal lesions.

Management. Single rooted teeth with vertical root fractures must be extracted.[9,56] Multirooted teeth may be hemisected and the intact remaining half of the tooth restored with endodontic therapy and a crown.[4,47,56]

TRAUMATIC INJURIES TO FACIAL BONES

Injury to the facial bones may occur in one bone or involve multiple bones. Faical fractures most frequently occur in the zygoma or mandible and, to a lesser extent, in the maxilla.[14] Radiography plays a critical role in the management of traumatic injuries to the facial bones. It is important that a complete clinical and radiographic examination of each traumatized tooth be conducted, including appropriate skull films with right-angle views, which will enable the radiologist to identify the location of fractures and the amount of separation of bony fragments and recognize soft tissue reactions such as sinus opacification. Determine the integrity of the remaining dentition because it may be used for fixation of the fracture(s). Recognize, however, that the fragments of some fractures are not displaced and are oriented oblique to the direction of the x-ray beam and thus will not be detected radiographically. Accordingly, appreciate that radiographs and the clinical examination are complementary, and neither should be solely used to exclude the possibility of a fracture.

Mandibular fractures

The most common mandibular fracture sites are the condyle, body, and angle, followed less frequently by the symphysis, ramus, coronoid process, and alveolus.[1,26,54] The most common cause of mandibular fractures is assault, followed by automobile accidents, falls, and sports injuries.[1,15,26,75] About half of all mandibular fractures occur in individuals between 16 and 35 years of age,[1,26,75] and fractures are more likely on Fridays and Saturdays than on other days of the week.[1] Males are affected about three times as frequently as females.[26,54] Trauma to the mandible is often associated with other injuries, most commonly concussion (loss of consciousness) and other fractures, usually of the maxilla, zygoma, and skull.[1,7]

Mandibular body. The mandible is the most commonly fractured facial bone. Although it may fracture in any region, the most common locations are in the body or condylar process. It is important to realize that a fracture of the mandibular body on one side is frequently accompanied by a fracture of the condylar process on the opposite side. Trauma to the anterior mandible that does not fracture this region may still result in a unilateral or bilateral fracture of the condylar processes. When a heavy force strikes a small area laterally, fracture of the angle, ramus, or even the coronoid process may result. In children, fractures of the mandibular body usually occur in the anterior region.

Mandibular fractures are classified as favorable or unfavorable depending on their orientation. Unfavorable fractures are those where the action of muscles attached to the mandible are likely to displace the fracture margins. If a fracture site in the body of the mandible slants posteriorly and inferiorly such that the masseter and internal pterygoid muscles pull the ramus segment away from the body of the mandible, the fracture is unfavorable. In favorable fractures, muscle action tends to reduce the fracture. The assessment of fractures as favorable or unfavorable is important in the planning of treatment.

Clinical features. There is usually a history of injury, substantiated by some evidence of the trauma that caused the fracture, such as contusions or wounds in the skin. There is frequently swelling and a deformity that is accentuated when the patient opens the mouth. There is often a discrepancy in the occlusal plane, and manipulation may produce crepitus or abnormal mobility.[70] Intraoral examination may reveal ecchymosis in the floor of the mouth.[12] If there are bilateral fractures to the mandible, there is the risk that the digastric and mylohyoid muscles will pull the mandible against the pharynx and compromise the airway.[68,71]

Radiographic features. The radiographic examination of a suspected fracture of the mandibular body should include the entire mandible. Panoramic views are useful as a general survey,[14,50,52] but it is often wise to supplement them with right-angle, extraoral views.[18,61] Reverse Towne projections are excellent for examining the condylar processes, and posteroanterior skull views allow examination of the mandibular rami. A submentovertex view and occlusal projection demonstrate the body and symphyseal regions of the mandible. Frequently such supplemental views disclose fractures or displacement of fracture margins not evident on panoramic projections. CT examinations of nondisplaced fractures of the mandible, however, are less sensitive than conventional radiography.[21] This appears to result from the tomographic orientation and volume averaging.

The margins of fractures usually project as sharply defined radiolucent (dark) lines where the margins of the bone at the fracture site have separated. They are best visualized when the x-ray beam lies in the plane of the fracture. If there is displacement of the fragments, a cortical discontinuity or "step" is evident (Fig. 28-9). An irregularity in the occlusal plane is often apparent, indicating the fracture site. Occasionally, the margins of the fracture overlap each other, resulting in radiopaque lines at the fracture site.

Nondisplaced mandibular fractures may involve both buccal and lingual cortical plates or only one cortical plate. An incomplete fracture involving only one cortical plate is often called a *greenstick* fracture. Such fractures usually occur in children. An oblique fracture that extends through each of the two cortical plates may cause some diagnostic difficulties if the image of the fracture in the buccal plate does not superimpose on the fracture in the lingual plate (Fig. 28-10). In such cases, two separate fracture lines project on the film and the ra-

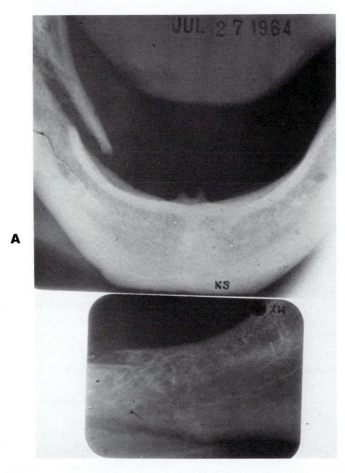

FIG. 28-9. Mandibular fractures. **A,** Of the mandibular body, showing medial and superior displacement of the posterior fragment.

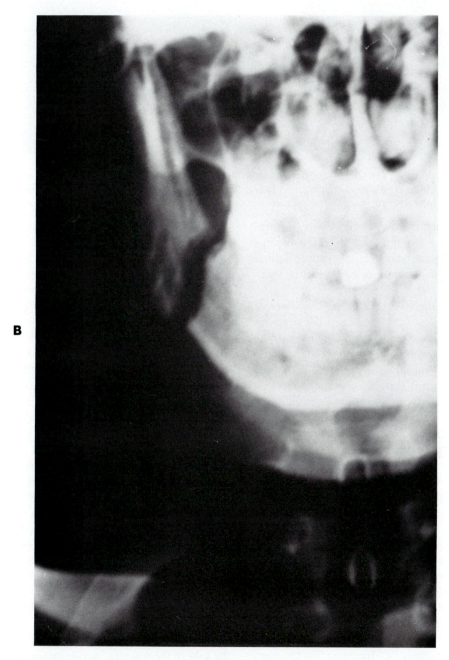

FIG. 28-9, cont'd. B, Through the angle of the mandible, with lateral displacement of the ramus. (**B** courtesy Dr. B. Sanders, Los Angeles.)

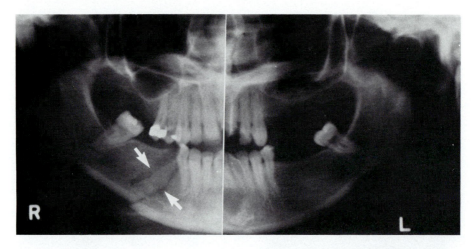

FIG. 28-10. Single fracture of the mandibular body, with separation of the fracture lines on the buccal and lingual plates simulating two fractures *(arrows)*. Note how the fracture lines meet at the inferior cortex.

diogaphic examination may suggest two fractures when there is actually only one.[53] To resolve this confusion, note that both lines of fracture join at the same point on the inferior border of the mandible.

Differential diagnosis. Error in diagnosis of jaw fractures have arisen because of the superimposition of soft tissue shadows on the image of the mandible. The combination of dense tongue tissue with the oral pharyngeal airway produces a definite line along the dorsal surface of the tongue. This air–soft tissue interface projects on the mandibular image in lateral jaw radiographs and is sometimes mistakenly interpreted as a mandibular fracture. Similar difficulties may arise from projection of the soft palate over portions of the mandibular ramus. On panoramic views, this air space between the soft palate and the dorsum of the tongue may suggest a fracture through the mandibular angle or ramus.

Management. The management of a fracture of the mandible presents a variety of surgical problems that involve the proper reduction, fixation, and immobilization of the fractured bone. Minimally displaced fractures are managed by closed reduction and intermaxillary fixation, whereas fractures with more severely displaced fragments may require open reduction.[30,75] Treatment for fractures of the body often includes antibiotic therapy because a tooth root may be in the line of the fracture. When the fracture line involves third molars, severely mobile teeth, or teeth with at least half their roots exposed in the fracture line, the involved teeth are often extracted to reduce the risk of infection and problems with fixation.[17]

Mandibular condyle. Fractures in the region of the condyle usually occur below the condylar head. When the condylar process fractures, the head usually displaces medially, inferiorly, and anteriorly (as a result of pull from the lateral pterygoid muscle). The fracture stump moves laterally. Fractures of the condylar head itself inside the articular capsule are relatively infrequent. Severe trauma may displace the condylar head into the skull or sinuses. Consequently, an apparently missing condyle should be sought by broad radiologic examination. Almost half of patients with condylar fractures also have fractures in the mandibular body.[64] In most cases, masticatory function is restored following healing of the fractures.[67]

Clinical features. The clinical symptoms of a fractured condylar process are not always clear, so the preauricular area and the region around the external meatus of the ear must be carefully examined and palpated. Movement of the jaw may cause crepitus. The patient may have pain on opening or closing the mouth, but there may be so much swelling and trismus that the patient is unable to move the jaw. There is usually an anterior open bite, with the last molars in contact. Also, the mandible may be displaced forward or, in case of a unilateral fracture, the mandible is deviated toward the side of the fracture. A significant feature is the patient's inability to bring the jaw forward because the external pterygoid muscle is attached to the condyle.[69] Similarly, a condylar fracture may be suspected when the clinician cannot palpate the condyle in the external ear canal when the jaw is closed.[12]

Radiographic features. Radiographic exami-

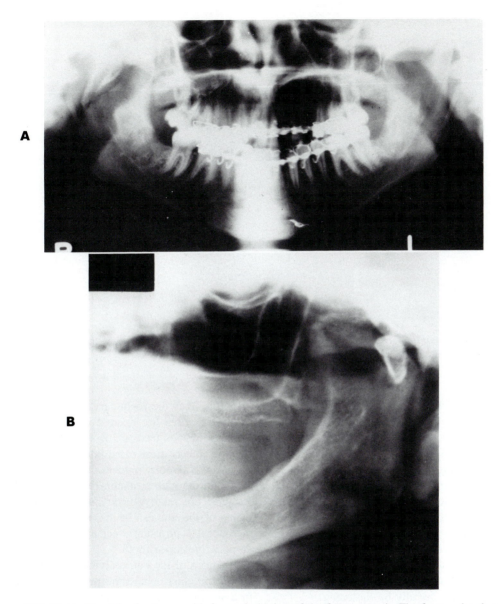

FIG. 28-11. Condylar fractures, with forward rotation of the fragments. **A,** The fracture has been stabilized by intermaxillary fixation. **B,** Fracture in an edentulous individual.

nation of the condyles for evidence of fracture should always include both condyles and lateral and anteroposterior views of each condyle. Appropriate lateral projections include panoramic (Fig. 28-11), infracranial (Fig. 28-12), or lateral oblique views of the ramus and condylar regions. Frontal views of value include occipitofrontal (reverse Towne) or transorbital projections. Nondisplaced fractures of the condylar process may be difficult to detect on lateral views and are best demonstrated on anteroposterior views. Displaced condylar fractures are usually well demonstrated on both an-

teroposterior and lateral projections. Occasionally, overriding bone edges over the fracture site may obscure condylar fractures on lateral jaw films. Anteroposterior films are most helpful in such cases. In addition, careful tracing of the anatomy of the posterior border of the ramus and of the condylar notch on the lateral projection usually reveal the presence of such apparently impacted fractures.

Studies of remodeling of fractured condyles show that young persons have much greater remodeling potential than do adults. In children younger than 12 years, most fractured condyles

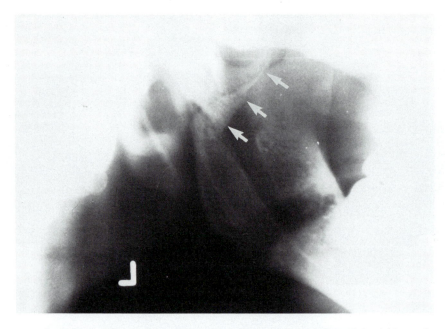

FIG. 28-12. An infracranial projection demonstrates fracture of the left condyle, with overlapping of the bony margins *(arrows)*.

showed a radiographic return to normal morphology after healing, whereas in teenagers the remodeling is less complete, and in adults only minor remodeling is observed.[23] The extent of remodeling is also greater with high condylar fractures than with low condylar fractures with luxation of the condylar head.[63] The most common deformities are medial inclination of the condyle, abnormal shape of the condyle, shortening of the neck, erosion, and flattening.[58] With increasing age, it is more likely that there is apposition of bone on the posterior aspect of the condyle. Often the mandibular fossa also remodels, usually by flattening.

Management. The technical details of treating condylar fractures vary according to whether one or both are involved, the extent of displacement, and the occurrence and severity of concomitant fractures. Direct treatment to relieve acute symptoms, restore proper anatomic relationships, and prevent bony ankylosis. If a malocclusion develops, intermaxillary fixation may be required to restore proper occlusion. Early mobilization is necessary to minimize scarring.[30]

Maxillary fractures

Alveolar ridge. These injuries to the supporting bone may involve the buccal or lingual walls of the alveolar ridge. Anterior alveolar fractures are some of the most common fractures of the maxilla.

As a rule, they are secondary to traumatic injuries to the teeth that are luxated with or without dislocation. Several teeth are usually affected, and the fracture line is most often horizontal.[2] The labial plate of the alveolar process is more prone to fracture than the palatal plate. These simple alveolar fractures are relatively rare in the posterior segments of the arches. In this location, fracture of the buccal plate usually occurs during removal of an upper posterior tooth.

Fractures of the entire alveolar process also occur in the anterior and the premolar regions, but in a somewhat older age group than the alveolar wall fractures. The line of fracture extends through the process (in contrast to the alveolar wall fracture described previously) and may be subapical or involve the tooth socket. These are also commonly associated with dental injuries, extrusive luxations with and without root fractures.[3]

Clinical features. A characteristic feature of alveolar process fracture is marked malocclusion along with displacement and mobility of the fragment. When testing the mobility of a single tooth, the extent of the injury is well illustrated when the entire fragment moves. The teeth in the fragment also has a recognizable dull sound when percussed. The detached bone may include the floor of the maxillary sinus, which may cause bleeding from the nose on the involved side. Ecchymosis of the

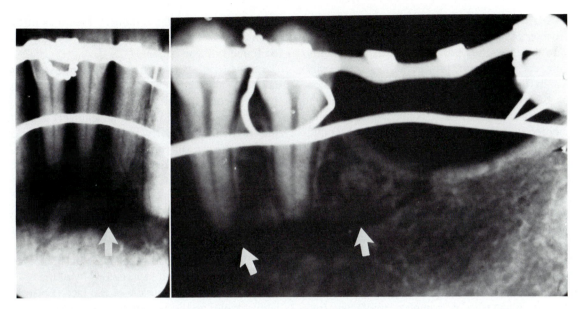

FIG. 28-13. Alveolar ridge fracture at the level of the root apices. In both these cases, metallic stabilizing splints are securing the fracture fragments. (Courtesy Dr. L. Hollender, Seattle.)

buccal vestibule is usually evident.

Radiographic features. Intraoral radiographs often do not reveal fractures of a single wall of the alveolar process, although evidence that the teeth have been luxated may be well demonstrated. However, a labial wall fracture is usually apparent on a lateral extraoral radiograph if there is some bone displacement and if the film and beam are oriented to project the bony defect at the margin of the alveolar image.

Fractures of both plates of the alveolar process (from buccal or labial to palatal plate) are usually well visualized on either an intraoral or extraoral radiograph (Fig. 28-13). The closer the fracture to the alveolar crest, the greater the possibility that root fractures will be found.[72] An alveolar fracture associated with a root mimics a root fracture, although the fracture image is usually less dark and not so well defined. Further, the bony fracture extends beyond the margin of the root. Also, after exposing a second radiograph with an altered vertical angulation, the position of the suspected fracture line on the tooth changes, but the root fracture does not.

Fractures of the posterior alveolus are best demonstrated by periapical radiographs. Assume that fractures of the posterior alveolus that demonstrate a break in the floor of the sinus have damaged the sinus mucosa. A sinus examination is indicated to determine the presence of an edematous mucosa or hemorrhage filling the sinus.

Management. Treat socket wall fractures by repositioning the displaced teeth and associated bone fragments by digital pressure. Suture gingival lacerations, if present. Splint luxated permanent teeth. If the splinted teeth are stable, intermaxillary fixation is not necessary. In the case of permanent teeth in adults, keep the splints in place for about 6 weeks. The faster healing in children permits their removal in about half that time. A soft diet for 10 to 14 days is recommended. Provide antibiotic coverage because of communication with tooth sockets. Teeth that have lost their vascular supply may eventually require endodontic treatment.

Midface fractures. Fractures of the midfacial region may be limited to the maxilla alone or may involve other bones, including the frontal, nasal, lacrimal zygoma, vomer, ethmoid, and sphenoid. Such complex fractures may be quite variable but often follow general patterns classified by Rene Le Forte: the zygomatic (complex), horizontal, pyramidal, and the craniofacial disjunction fractures.[8,43] These fractures may be evident clinically or radiographically. They are rare in children.

The radiographic examination of the midface is difficult because of the complex anatomy in this region and the multiple superimpositions of structures. An initial examination should include posteroanterior, Waters, reverse Towne, lateral skull, and submentovertex projections. It is important to view each of these projections systematically. Search for fractures in the frontal bone, the nasion, the orbital walls, the zygomatic arches, and the maxillary antrum.[33] Fractures may appear as linear radiolucencies that are usually widest at discontinuities in margins of bone, alterations of normal skeletal contour, or displacement of fragments. Also, one may see separation of bony sutures. Often it is not possible to visualize fractures known clinically to be present. This results from either minimal separation of the bony margins, orientation of the fracture at an oblique angle to the x-ray beam, or superimposition of the fracture lines over other complex anatomic structures.

Computed tomography is especially effective for the diagnosis of complex midfacial fractures.[35,39,40,49,52] It is useful both to reveal the bony fractures and for imaging changes in the soft tissues, such as herniation of orbital fat and extraoccular muscle and tissue swelling. Usually axial and coronal studies are performed with a 5-mm-thick slice and extended bone window. CT is particularly advantageous for examining comminuted facial fractures because of high bony resolution, soft tissue contrast, absence of overlapping shadows, and the ability to reformat two- and three-dimensional images.

Abnormal soft tissue densities may both help and hinder the examination of facial trauma. When the fracture tears the antral or nasal mucosa, radiographs reveal densities associated with edema and bleeding in those areas and thus help to identify regions of fracture. However, facial edema detracts from the clarity of the radiographs, and preexisting inflammatory or allergic paranasal sinus disease may be misleading.[33]

Horizontal fracture (Le Fort I). This is a relatively horizontal fracture in the body of the maxilla that results in a maxillary tooth-bearing fragment being detached from the middle face. It is the result of a traumatic force directed to the lower maxillary region.[24] The fracture line passes above the teeth, below the zygomatic process, through the maxillary sinuses and the tuberosities, to the inferior portion of the pterygoid processes (Fig. 28-14). It may be unilateral or bilateral. In the unilateral fracture, there is an auxiliary fracture in the midline of the palate. The unilateral fracture must be distinguished from a fracture of the alveolar process (as discussed previously), which

does not extend to the midline.[41] Fractures of the mandible (54%) or of the zygoma (23%) may also be found in these patients.[48]

CLINICAL FEATURES. If the fragment is not distally impacted, it can be easily moved by the teeth. If the fracture line is at a high level, the fragment includes the pterygoid muscle attachments that pull the fragment posteriorly and depress its posterior margin. As a result, the posterior maxillary teeth force the mandible open, resulting in open bite, retruded chin, and long face, an appearance indicative of this type of fracture. If the fracture is at a low level, the pterygoid muscles do not displace it, and the fracture may be overlooked. However, the evidence of trauma is not difficult to recognize. There are swelling and bruising about both eyes, pain over the nose and face, deformity of the nose, and flattening of the middle of the face. Epistaxis is inevitable, and occasionally there are double vision and varying degrees of paresthesia over the distribution of the infraorbital nerve. Manipulation may reveal a mobile maxilla and crepitation.

RADIOGRAPHIC FEATURES. This fracture is difficult to see, but it should be identifiable on the posteroanterior, lateral skull, and Waters projections. Both maxillary sinuses are cloudy and may show air-fluid levels. The lateral view may disclose a slight posterior displacement of the fragment (the inferior portion of the maxilla below the fracture line), if it has occurred, and the fracture line through the pterygoid bones. Carefully distinguish between Le Fort I fractures and the intervertebral spaces of the cervical spine. This type of fracture unites rapidly, so if there is a period of a few days between injury and the radiographic examination the fracture may not be detectable radiographically.

MANAGEMENT. If the fracture is not displaced and at a relatively low level of the maxilla, it can be treated by intermaxillary fixation. Those that are high, with the fragment displaced posteriorly or pronounced separation, require craniomaxillary fixation in addition to intermaxillary fixation. A unilateral horizontal fracture is usually immobilized by intermaxillary fixation. However, if it cannot be reduced manually, elastic traction in the required direction (across the palate or between the arches) is employed. Antibiotics are usually administered because the fracture line involves the maxillary sinuses.

Pyramidal fracture (Le Fort II). This fracture has a pyramidal appearance on the posteroanterior skull radiograph, hence the name. It results from a violent force applied to the central region of the

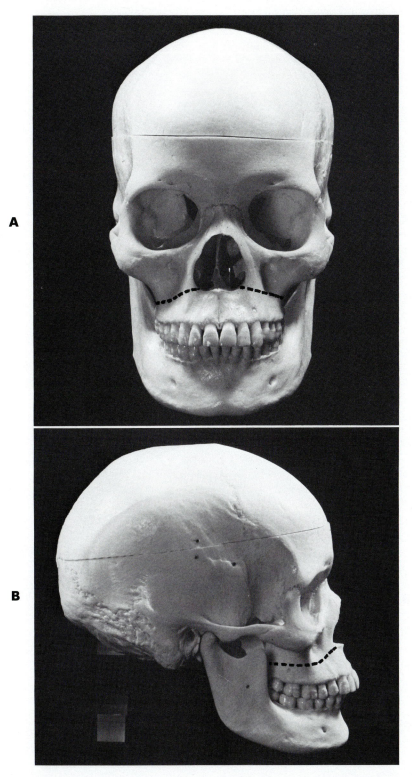

FIG. 28-14. Usual position of the Le Fort I horizontal fracture on a frontal (**A**) and a lateral (**B**) view.

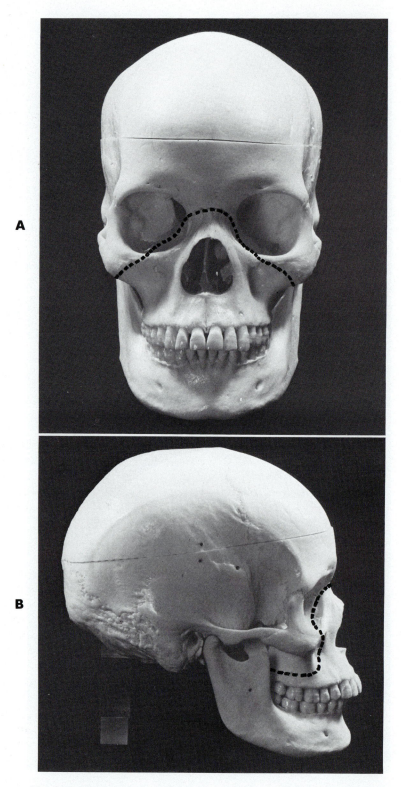

FIG. 28-15. Usual position of the Le Fort II pyramidal fracture on a frontal (**A**) and a lateral (**B**) view.

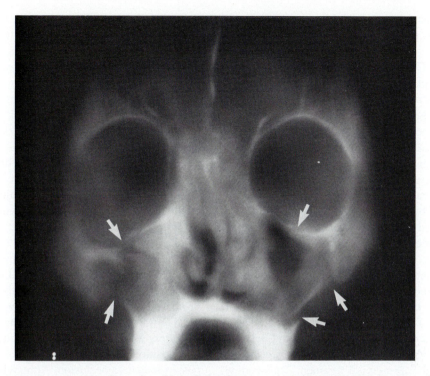

FIG. 28-16. Tomographic view of multiple facial fractures, including a Le Fort II, through the ethmoid bone, infraorbital rims *(arrows)*, and lateral wall of the maxilla *(arrows)*. (Courtesy Dr. C. Schow, Galveston.)

middle third of the facial skeleton.[62] This force separates the maxilla from the base of the skull by causing fractures of the nasal bones and frontal processes of the maxilla. The fractures extend laterally through the lacrimal bones, floors of the orbits, and inferiorly through the zygomaticomaxillary sutures (Fig. 28-15). Frequently on one side the fracture passes through the suture or through the zygoma, and the other side it passes around and beneath the base of the zygomatic process of the maxilla. From this area, it then passes posteriorly along the lateral wall of the maxilla, across the pterygomaxillary fossa and through the pterygoid plates. It usually extends through the maxillary sinuses. The frontal and ethmoid sinuses are involved in about 10% of the cases, especially with severe comminuted fractures.

CLINICAL FEATURES. In contrast to the Le Fort I (horizontal) fracture, characterized by only slight swelling about the upper lips, the Le Fort II injury results in massive edema and marked swelling of the middle third of the face. Typically, an ecchymosis around the eyes develops within minutes of the injury. Attending edema about the eyes is likely to be so severe that it is impossible to see the eyes

without prying them open. The conjunctiva over the inner quadrants of the eyes are bloodshot; if the zygomatic bones are involved, this subconjunctiva ecchymosis is also over the outer quadrant. The broken nose is displaced; because the face has fallen, the nose and face are lengthened. There is an anterior open bite (with molars in contact). Epistaxis is inevitable, and there may also be a cerebrospinal fluid rhinorrhea. Palpation reveals the discontinuity of the lower borders of the orbits. By applying pressure between the bridge of the nose and palate, the "pyramid" of bone can be moved. There are usually double vision and variable degrees of paresthesia over the distribution of the infraorbital nerve.

RADIOGRAPHIC FEATURES. The radiographic examination reveals fractures of the nasal bones and both frontal processes of the maxilla (and ethmoid and frontal sinuses, if involved), the infraorbital rims on both sides (and floor of both orbits), fractures near (in zygoma or zygomatic process of maxilla) or separation of the zygomaticomaxillary sutures on both sides, deformity and discontinuity of the lateral walls of both maxillary sinuses, thickening of the lining mucosa or clouding of the maxillary sinus and sometimes the frontal and ethmoid sinuses, and, finally, fractures through both pterygoid plates (Fig. 28-16). Tomograms, stereo views, or a CT examination may be required to supplement plane views of the skull because of multiple superimposition of structures.

Exercise special care in evaluating the floor of an orbit. In the usual sinus skull examinations, the relationship of the x-ray beam to the skull is such that two lower limits to the orbit can be projected. One is the actual floor of the orbit, which is often thin and difficult to discern. The other is the inferior rim of the orbit, which usually is of heavier bone and more easily seen. It appears above the floor of the orbit in the Waters projection. The infraorbital foramen may project into the space between the shadow of the floor of the orbit and the shadow of the lower rim of the orbit. The presence of the less distinct floor of the orbit underneath the level of the shadow of the rim of the orbit may suggest a blow-out fracture of the floor of the orbit because some wisps of apparent orbital floor project below the level of the infraorbital foramen. The shadow of herniated orbital contents through the floor of the orbit is a useful sign for the determination of fracture of the orbital floor. However, orbital floor fractures do not always have associated soft tissue herniation. Complex motion tomography in the frontal plane provides a valuable demonstration of herniated orbital contents.[52]

MANAGEMENT. The treatment of this fracture is accomplished by reduction of the downward displacement of the maxilla. It is fixed in place by intermaxillary wires or arch bars. Usually, treatment includes open reduction and interosseous wiring of the infraorbital rims. The accompanying fractures of the nose, nasal septum, orbital floor, and detached medial canthal ligaments also require repair.[30] If there is leakage of cerebrospinal fluid, a neurosurgeon should attend to its repair. Antibiotics are required because of communication of the fractures with the paranasal sinuses.[30]

Craniofacial disjunction (Le Fort III). This type of midface fracture results when the force of the traumatic incident is of sufficient magnitude (so violent) to completely separate the middle third of the facial skeleton from the cranium. The fracture line usually extends through the nasal bones and the frontal processes of the maxilla or nasofrontal and maxillofrontal sutures, across the floors of the orbits, through the ethmoid and sphenoid sinuses and the zygomaticofrontal sutures (Fig. 28-17). It passes across both pterygomaxillary fissures and

separates the pterygoid plates where they arise from the sphenoid bone (at their roots). If the maxilla is displaced and freely movable, a fracture must also have occurred in the area of the zygomaticotemporal suture. Because the zygoma or zygomatic arch is involved, these injuries are, as a rule, associated with multiple other maxillary fractures. Mandibular fractures are also observed in half the cases.[48]

CLINICAL FEATURES. Clinically, the craniofacial disjunction produces an appearance similar to pyramidal fracture. However, this injury is considerably more extensive. The soft tissue injuries are severe, with massive edema. The nose may be blocked with blood clot, or there may be blood, serum, or cerebrospinal fluid rhinorrhea. There may be bleeding into the periorbital tissues and all quadrants of the conjunctiva; a number of eye signs of neurologic importance are likely to be present. A "dish face" deformity is characteristic of these fractures, as is an anterior open bite (because of retroposition of the maxillary incisors) with the posterior teeth in occlusion. Although the mandible is wide open, the patient is unable to separate the molars. Intraoral and extraoral palpation reveals irregular contours and step deformities, and crepitation is also apparent when moving the fragments.

RADIOGRAPHIC FEATURES. The radiographic projections of Le Fort III fractures usually are hazy because of the soft tissue swelling. The main radiographic findings are separated sutures: the nasofrontal, maxillofrontal, zygomaticofrontal, and the zygomaticotemporal (Fig. 28-18). The nasal bones, frontal processes of the maxilla, both orbital floors, and pterygoid plates are likely to show radiolucent lines and discontinuity in some of these areas. The ethmoid and sphenoid sinuses are probably cloudy, indicating their fracture; the frontal sinus are also frequently opaque. Associated fractures of other facial bones that commonly accompany transverse fractures also disrupt the integrity of the maxillary sinuses, which may show a diffuse opacity.

It is important to emphasize that in spite of these precise descriptions, radiographs of the maxilla are difficult to interpret. Fractures are easier to interpret when the margins are displaced. However, so many structures are superimposed on the radiographs of this area that to establish a diagnosis it must be confirmed both clinically and radiographically. Tomographic views are useful.

MANAGEMENT. The severe trauma required to cause this fracture often causes considerable soft

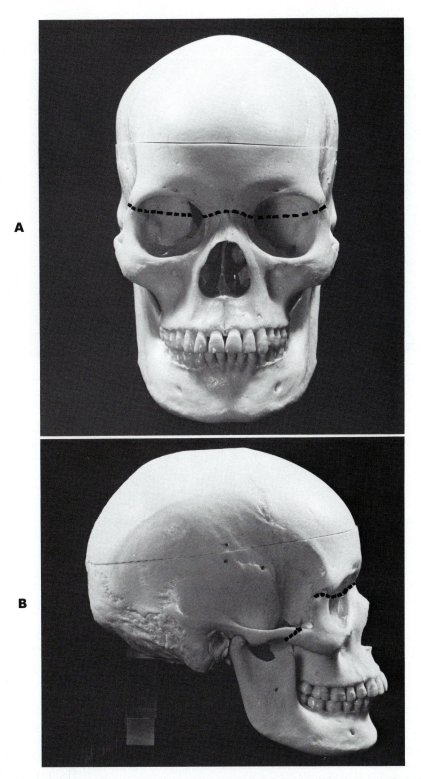

FIG. 28-17. Usual position of the Le Fort III craniofacial disjunction fracture on a frontal (**A**) and a lateral (**B**) view.

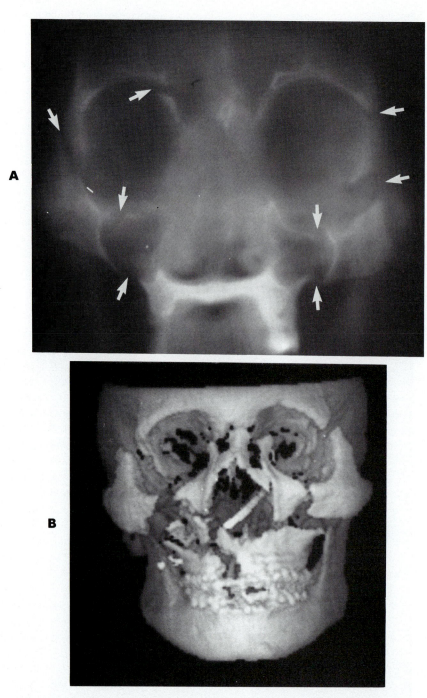

FIG. 28-18. A, Tomographic view of multiple facial fractures, including a Le Fort III, through the ethmoid bone, lateral walls of the orbits *(arrows)*, infraorbital rims *(arrows)*, and lateral walls of the maxilla *(arrows)*. **B,** Three-dimensional computed tomographic views of another patient with comparable facial fractures. Note the separation of each zygomaticofrontal suture as well as fractures of the ethmoid bone, each anterior maxilla inferior to the orbit, and the maxillary alveolar ridge from the midface. (**A** courtesy Dr. C. Schow, Galveston; **B** courtesy Dr. Marden Alder, San Antonio.)

tissue injury. Accordingly, it is often necessary to initially control hemorrhage, maintain the airway, and close lacerations. Surgery may be delayed until the edema has sufficiently resolved.[30] The treatment of transverse fractures is complicated because fixation of the loose middle third of the facial skeleton is difficult, as the zygoma and probably the zygomatic arch are fractured. The only possibilities are external immobilization or immobilization with the tissues.[8] In the former, the loose maxilla is suspended by wires through the cheeks from a metal head frame (halo) or fixed by using external pins anchored in solid bone.[19] The other possibility is immobility within the tissues by using internal wiring to the closest solid bone superior to the fracture. A number of complications may develop during or after this treatment including malunion or nonunion,[22] diplopia caused by depressed orbital floor, persistent periorbital edema, poor occlusion and facial disfigurement, poorly functioning nose and damaged sinus lining, and dimness of vision, even leading to blindness, caused by hematoma pressing on the optic nerve.[41]

Zygomatic fractures

Unilateral fractures involving the zygoma are of two types: zygomatic arch fractures in which just the arch is fractured and zygomatic complex fractures in which the zygoma is separated from its frontal, maxillary, and temporal connections. Bilateral zygomatic fractures occur in association with Le Forte II and Le Forte III fractures, described previously. The body of the zygoma itself is rarely fractured. Injuries to the zygomatic arch usually result from a forceful blow to the side of the face. Although the blow may displace the fragment medially, the arch is so well supported superiorly by the temporal muscle and inferiorly by the masseter muscle that it is rarely displaced upward or downward. The arch may fracture at its center, resulting in a V-shaped medial displacement, or near its articulation with the zygomatic process of the maxilla, resulting in medial displacement of the anterior end of the zygoma.

The body of the zygoma is at times pushed so far medially against the wall of the maxillary sinus (maxilla) that a zygomatic complex fracture is caused. Resulting hemorrhage fills the antrum and in turn drains through the ostium, causing an ipsilateral epistaxis. The medially displaced zygoma may interfere with the movement of the coronoid process of the mandible, and the patient may be unable either to open or to close the mouth, de-

pending on the position of the mandible at impact. Posterior displacement of the zygoma is important because of loss of support for the orbit and the resultant diplopia.

Clinical features. Examine the zygomatic arch along its entire length. Direct particular attention to the articulation of the arch with the zygomatic bone and with the articular eminence. Flattening of the upper cheek with tenderness and dimpling of the skin over the zygomatic arch and zygomaticofrontal suture and a fullness of the lower cheek may occur after zygomatic complex fracture. Step defects may be palpated in the zygomaticofrontal area and along the infraorbital rim. Some of the clinical characteristics of a zygomatic fracture may not be apparent much longer than an hour after the trauma.[41] Subsequently, they are masked by edema for about a week. It is almost certain that circumorbital ecchymosis and hemorrhage into the sclera (near the outer canthus) will occur. The examiner probably also finds unilateral epistaxis (for a short time after the accident), anesthesia or paresthesia of the cheek, and an altered level of the eye. The presence of diplopia suggests a significant injury to the floor of the orbit.[57] There may be limitation of mandibular movement if the displaced zygomatic bone impinges on the coronoid process.

Radiographic features. Because edema may obscure many clinical features of zygomatic fracture, the radiographic examination may provide the only means of determining the presence and extent of the injury. The occipitomental (Waters) radiograph provides an image of the whole zygoma and the maxillary sinus. The submentovertex projection provides a good view of the zygomatic arch (Fig. 28-19). The examiner can anticipate that the radiographs will have a haziness caused by the attending edema of the face. CT examinations have also proved to be of considerable value in assessing fractures of the zygoma.[29]

A variety of findings may be observed, including a separation or fracture of the frontozygomatic suture. Dislocation of the greater wing of the sphenoid from the zygomatic bone may be evident on the radiograph. The zygomatic arch may also fracture at its weakest point, about 1 cm posterior to the zygomaticotemporal suture. Displacement of the zygoma usually does not occur at the thick and sturdy zygomaticomaxillary suture but medial to this line of juncture in the thin bone comprising the lateral wall of the antrum (as described previously). In addition, as a result of bleeding into the sinus from the torn lining membrane, the antrum

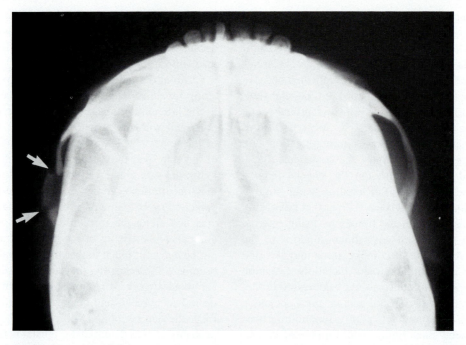

FIG. 28-19. Fractures of the zygomatic arch *(arrows)* demonstrated on this submentovertex projection with reduced exposure time.

may appear cloudy or show a fluid level. The fluid level is apparent for only a few days before the space drains through the ostium. In some cases, the zygomatic process of the maxilla can fracture from the lateral wall of the sinus and be slightly depressed without injury to the sinus mucosa. In such cases, there is no opacification of the antrum, and possibly a depressed fracture may be overlooked. Hence, careful tracing of the lateral wall of the sinus is always indicated in radiologic examinations for zygomatic fractures.

Panoramic views of the zygomatic arch often reveal the zygomaticotemporal suture as a radiolucent space, which may even have the appearance of a discontinuity in the inferior border. Take care not to confuse this normal variant with a fracture in the zygomatic arch.

Management. When there is minimal displacment of the zygoma and no cosmetic deformity or impairment of eye movement, no treatment may be required.[30,74] Otherwise, reduction is usually indicated. Fractures of the arch may be reduced through an intraoral or extraoral approach. If a fractured zygoma is treated within 5 days, the bones frequently snap into place and do not require fixation. When treatment has been delayed more than 5 days, the fragments can usually be reduced, but they will not remain in place. In such delayed treatment cases, the zygoma is fixed in place by elastic traction anchored to a headcap. Should the fracture's treatment be delayed for several months, it is almost impossible to reduce, and treatment is not generally undertaken. In this instance, the treatment is focused on the associated structures with the objective of restoring function and appearance.[41]

Facial bone fracture follow-up

Radiographic examination of the facial bones after trauma is usually necessary to measure the degree of reduction from treatment and to monitor the continued immobilization of the fracture site during repair. Ultimately, it is desirable to demonstrate remineralization of the fracture site. During normal healing, expansion of the fracture site may be expected in about 2 weeks after reduction of the fracture. This space results from the resorption of small sequestered fragments of bone that may not have been seen on the initial radiologic examination. The monitoring of fracture repair should include examination of both the alignment of the cortical plates of the involved bone and remodeling and remineralization of the fracture site. Evidence of remineralization usually occurs 5 to 6 weeks after treatment. The complete remodeling of the fracture site with obliteration of the fracture line seen on radiographic examinations may take several months. On rare occasions, fracture lines may persist for years, even when the patient has made a clinically complete recovery. A study of patients following orthognathic surgery revealed surgical complications in 10% of cases.[38] These included inadvertent fractures in the mandible or nasal septum, transection of teeth, nonunion of osteotomy fragments, and bilateral dislocation of the mandibular condyles. Other complications reported include avascular necrosis of the proximal mandibular osteotomy fragments and dislocation of graft material. The presence of blood in the sinus following maxillary osteotomies is common and should not be confused with sinusitis.

SPECIFIC REFERENCES

1. Andersson L, Hultin M, Nordenram A, Ramstrom G: Jaw fractures in the county of Stockholm (1978-1980): I, general survey, *Int J Oral Surg* 13:194-199, 1984.
2. Andreasen JO: Etiology and pathogenesis of traumatic dental injuries: a clinical study of 1298 cases, *Scand J Dent Res* 78:329-342, 1970.
3. Andreasen JO: Fractures of the alveolar process of the jaw: a clinical and radiographic follow-up study, *Scand J Dent Res* 78:263-272, 1970.
4. Andreasen JO: Luxation of permanent teeth due to trauma: a clinical and radiographic follow-up study of 189 injured teeth, *Scand J Dent Res* 78:273-286, 1970.
5. Andreasen JO: *Traumatic injuries of the teeth*, Philadelphia, 1981, WB Saunders.
6. Andreasen JO, Hjorting-Hansen E: Intraalveolar root fractures: radiographic and histologic study of 50 cases, *J Oral Surg* 25:414-426, 1967.
7. Bailey BJ, Clark WD: Management of mandibular fractures, *Ear Nose Throat J* 62:371-378, 1983.
8. Banks P: *Kiley's fractures of the middle third of the facial skeleton*, Bristol, 1981, Wright.
9. Bender IB, Freedland JB: Adult root fracture, *J Am Dent Assoc* 107:413-419, 1983.
10. Bender IB, Freedland JB: Clinical considerations in the diagnosis and treatment of intra-alveolar root fractures, *J Am Dent Assoc* 107:595-600, 1983.
11. Bennett DT: Traumatized anterior teeth, *Br Dent J* 115:309-311, 1963.
12. Bertz J: Maxillofacial injuries, *Clinical Symposia CIBA* 33:2-32, 1981.
13. Braham RL, Roberts MW, Morris ME: Management of dental trauma in children and adolescents, *J Trauma* 17:857-865, 1977.
14. Brook IW, Wood N: Aetiology and incidence of facial fractures in adults, *Int J Oral Surg* 12:293-298, 1983.
15. Carter E: The management of fractures of the facial skeleton, *Aust Dent J* 27:227-233, 1982.
16. Castaldi CR, Bass GA: *Dentistry for the adolescent*, Philadelphia, 1980, WB Saunders.
17. Chan DM: Management of mandibular fractures in unreliable patient populations, *Ann Plast Surg* 13:298-303, 1984.
18. Chayra GA, Meador LR, Laskin DM: Comparison of panoramic and standard radiographs for the diagnosis of mandibular fractures, *J Oral Maxillofac Surg* 44:677-679, 1986.
19. Close LG: Fractures of the maxilla, *Ear Nose Throat J* 62:365-370, 1983.
20. Clyde JS: Transverse-oblique fractures of the crown with extension below the epithelial attachment, *Br Dent J* 120:402-406, 1968.
21. Creasman CN, Markowitz BL, Kawamoto HK Jr et al: Computed tomography versus standard radiography in the assessment of fractures of the mandible, *Ann Plast Surg* 29:109-113, 1992.
22. Crosby JF, Woodward HW: Autogenous bone graft for repair of nonunion of maxillary fractures: report of case, *J Oral Surg* 23:441-445, 1965.
23. Dahlström L, Kahnberg KE, Lindahl L: 15 years follow-up on condylar fractures, *Int J Oral Maxillofac Surg* 18:18-23, 1989.
24. Dodd GD, Jing Boa-Shan: *Radiology of the nose, paranasal sinuses and nasopharynx*, Baltimore, 1977, Wiliams & Wilkins.
25. Down CH: The treatment of permanent incisor teeth of children following traumatic injury, *Aust Dent J* 2:9-24, 1957.
26. Ellis E, Moos KF, El-Attar A: Ten years of mandibular fractures: an analysis of 2,137 cases, *Oral Surg* 59:120-129, 1985.
27. Finn SB: *Clinical pedodontics*, Philadelphia, 1973, WB Saunders.
28. Fujii N: Classification of malar complex fractures using computed tomography, *J Oral Maxillofac Surg* 41: 562-567, 1983.
29. Gelbien S: Injured anterior teeth in children: a preliminary report, *Br Dent J* 123:331-335, 1967.
30. Gerlock AJ Jr, Sinn DP, McBride KL: *Clinical and radiographic interpretation of facial fractures*, Boston, 1981, Little, Brown.
31. Gutz DP: Fractured permanent incisors in a clinic population, *J Dent Child* 38:94-95, 1971.
32. Hardwick JL, Newman PA: Some observations on the incidence and emergency treatment of fractured permanent anterior teeth of children, *J Dent Res* 33:730, 1954.
33. Harris JH, Ray RD, Rauschkolb EN, Rappaport NJ: An approach to mid-facial fractures, CRC *Crit Rev Diagn Imaging* 21:105-132, 1984.
34. Jacobsen I: *Traumatized teeth, clinical studies of root fractures and pulp complications*, thesis, University of Oslo, 1981.
35. Johnson DH: CT of maxillofacial trauma, *Radiol Clin North Am* 22:131-144, 1984.
36. Johnson WT, Leary JM: Vertical root fractures: diagnosis and treatment, *Gen Dent* 32:425-429, 1984.
37. Josell SD, Abrams RG: Traumatic injuries to the dentition and its supporting structures, *Pediatr Clin North Am* 29:717-741, 1982.
38. Kaplan PA, Tu HK, Koment MA et al: Radiography after orthognathic surgery: part II, surgical complications, *Radiology* 167:195-198, 1988.
39. Kassel EE, Noyek AM, Cooper PW: CT in facial trauma, *J Otolaryngol* 12:2-15, 1983.
40. Kreipke D, Moss J, Franco J et al: Computed tomography and thin-sectioned tomography in facial trauma, *Am J Roentgenol* 142:1041-1045, 1984.

41. Kruger GO: *Textbook of oral and maxillofacial surgery,* ed 6, St Louis, 1984, Mosby.

42. Langdon JD: Treatment of oblique fractures of incisors involving the epithelial attachment: a case report, *Br Dent J* 125:72-74, 1968.

43. Le Forte R: Etude experimentale sure les fractures de las machoire superieire, *Rev Chir (Paris)* 23:208-360, 1901.

44. Lenstrup K, Steiller V: A follow-up study of teeth replanted after accidental loss, *Acta Odont Scand* 17:503-509, 1959.

45. Lin LM, Langeland K: Vertical root fracture, *J Endodont* 8:558-562, 1982.

46. Lindhal B: Transverse intra-alveolar root fractures: roentgen diagnosis and prognosis, *Odont Rev* 9:10-24, 1958.

47. Luebke RG: Vertical crown-root fractures in posterior teeth, *Dent Clin North Am* 28:883-894, 1984.

48. Manson P, Hoopes J, Su C: Structural pillars of the facial skeleton: an approach to the management of Le Forte fractures, *Plastic Reconstr Surg* 66:54-61, 1980.

49. Marsh JL, Vannier MW, Gado M, Stevens WG: In vivo delineation of facial fractures: the application of advanced medical imaging technology, *Ann Plast Surg* 17:364-376, 1986.

50. Matteson S, Tyndall D: Pantomographic radiology: II, pantomography of trauma and inflammation of the jaws, *Dental Radiol Photogr* 56:21-48, 1982.

51. Natkin E: Diagnosis and treatment of traumatic injuries and their sequelae. In Ingle JI, editor: *Endodontics,* Philadelphia, 1965, Lea & Febiger.

52. Noyek AM and others: Contemporary radiologic evaluation in maxillofacial trauma, *Otolaryngol Clin North Am* 16:473-508, 1983.

53. Olech E: Fracture lines in mandible, *Dent Radiol Photogr* 28:21-26, 1955.

54. Olson RA, Fonseca RJ, Zeitler DL, Osborn DB: Fractures of the mandible: a review of 580 cases, *J Oral Maxillofac Surg* 40:23-28, 1982.

55. Pindborg JJ: *Pathology of the dental hard tissues,* Philadelphia, 1970, WB Saunders.

56. Pitts DL, Natkin E: Diagnosis and treatment of vertical root fractures, *J Endodont* 9:338-346, 1983.

57. Prendergast ML, Wildes TO: Evaluation of the orbital floor in zygoma fractures, *Arch Otolaryngol Head Neck Surg* 114:446-450, 1988.

58. Raustia AM, Pyhtinen J, Oikarinen KS, Altonen M: Conventional radiographic and computed tomographic findings in cases of fracture of the mandibular condylar process, *J Oral Maxillofac Surg* 48:1258-1264, 1990.

59. Ravn JJ; Follow-up study of permanent incisors with enamel fractures as a result of acute trauma, *Scand J Dent Res* 89:213-217, 1981.

60. Ravn JJ: Follow-up study of permanent incisors with enamel-dentin fracture after acute trauma, *Scand J Dent Res* 89:355-365, 1981.

61. Reiner SA and others: Accurate radiographic evaluation of mandibular fractures, *Arch Otolaryngol Head Neck Surg* 115:1083-1085, 1989.

62. Rowe NL, Killey HC: *Fractures of the facial skeleton,* Bristol, 1965, John Wright.

63. Sahm G, Witt E: Long-term results after childhood condylar fractures: A computer-tomographic study, *Eur J Orthod* 11:154-160, 1989.

64. Silvennoinen U, Iizuka T, Lindqvist C, Oikarinen K: Different patterns of condylar fractures: an analysis of 382 patients in a 3-year period, *J Oral Maxillofac Surg* 50:1032-1037, 1992.

65. Skieller V: The prognosis for young teeth loosened after mechanical injuries, *Acta Odont Scand* 18:171-181, 1960.

66. Sutton PRN: Fissured fractures: 2,501 transverse crack lines in permanent incisors, *Aust Dent J* 6:144-150, 1969.

67. Tarlowska W, Markiewicz H, Awillo K: A clinical and radiographic long-term follow-up study of fractures of the mandibular condyle, *Dent Maxillofac Radiol Suppl* 7:156, 1985 (abstract).

68. Teichgraeber JF, Rappaport NJ, Harris JH Jr: The radiology of upper airway obstruction in maxillofacial trauma, *Ann Plast Surg* 27:103-109, 1991.

69. Thoma KH: *Oral pathology,* ed 5, St Louis, 1954, Mosby.

70. Thoma KH: *Oral surgery,* ed 5, St Louis, 1969, Mosby.

71. Trimble LD: Severe facial trauma resulting in airway obstruction, *Oral Surg Oral Med Oral Pathol* 62:476-478, 1986.

72. Valvassori GE, Hard GE: Traumatic sinus disease, *Semin Roentgenol* 3:160-171, 1968.

73. Walton RE, Michelich RJ, Smith GN: The histopathogenesis of vertical root fractures, *J Endodont* 10:48-56, 1984.

74. Winstanley RP: The management of fractures of the zygoma, *Int J Oral Surg* 10(suppl 1):235-240, 1981.

75. Winstanley RP: The management of fractures of the mandible, *Br J Oral Maxillofac Surg* 22:170-177, 1984.

76. Wood NK, Goaz PW: *Differential diagnosis of oral lesions,* ed 4, St Louis, 1991, Mosby.

29

Developmental Disturbances of the Face and Jaws

The events associated with embryogenesis and development are a complex of actions and interactions of highly integrated systems that are coordinated by poorly understood control mechanisms. These developmental mechanisms must withstand multiple genetic and environmental assaults on the embryo and fetus if defects in the phenotype are to be averted. The long process of morphogenesis is yet to be fully described, and it is difficult to determine the critical periods during which teratogenesis might occur. Consequently, the study of deviations in the phenotype (as in this chapter) has been largely limited to descriptive analysis of abnormal structures. In spite of the spectrum of abnormalities that may affect humans, the overpowering wonder is that more anatomic and functional variants do not occur, as the developmental process is dependent on so many unpredictable and uncontrollable events. This chapter considers some of the most common developmental abnormalities that affect the face and jaws.

CLEIDOCRANIAL DYSPLASIA

Cleidocranial dysplasia (previously known as *cleidocranial dysostosis*) is a developmental anomaly of the skeleton and teeth. This condition may be inherited, be transmitted as a dominant characteristic in either sex, or appear spontaneously.

Clinical Features. Cleidocranial dysplasia primarily affects the skull, clavicle, and dentition. The characteristic skull findings are brachycephaly (reduced anteroposterior dimension but increased skull width), delayed or failed closure of the fontanelles, and the presence of open skull sutures and multiple wormian bones (small, irregular bones in the sutures of the skull that are formed by secondary centers of ossification in the suture lines). The maxilla and paranasal sinuses characteristically are underdeveloped, resulting in maxillary micrognathia.

Typically the clavicles are underdeveloped to varying degrees and, in approximately 10% of cases, are completely absent. This allows excessive mobility of the shoulder girdle (Fig. 29-1). Other bones may also be affected, including long bones, the vertebral column, the pelvis, and bones of the hands and feet. The mandible is not involved.

Characteristically, patients with cleidocranial dysplasia show prolonged retention of the primary dentition and delayed eruption of the permanent dentition.[15] Extraction of primary teeth does not stimulate eruption of underlying permanent teeth. Adults with this condition usually have mixed dentition.[35] A study of teeth from patients with cleidocranial dysplasia revealed a paucity or complete absence of cellular cementum on both erupted and unerupted teeth.[23] In addition, patients with this condition frequently show a large number of unerupted supernumerary teeth. As many as 63 unerupted teeth have been described in one patient.[34] These teeth may be well formed, often having the appearance of premolars. There may be considerable crowding and disorganization of the developing permanent dentition.

Radiographic features. The radiographic findings are consistent with the clincial observations. Skull films may reveal open sutures and the presence of wormian bones. Chest films may show malformation or absence of the clavicles. Films of the jaws often show prolonged retention of the primary dentition and typically multiple unerupted supernumerary teeth (Fig. 29-2). Characteristically, the unerupted teeth develop in the anterior regions, extending as far posterior as the first molar.

Differential diagnosis. Cleidocranial dysplasia may be identified by the family history, excessive mobility of the shoulder, clinical examination of the skull, and the pathognomonic radiographic findings of prolonged retention of primary teeth

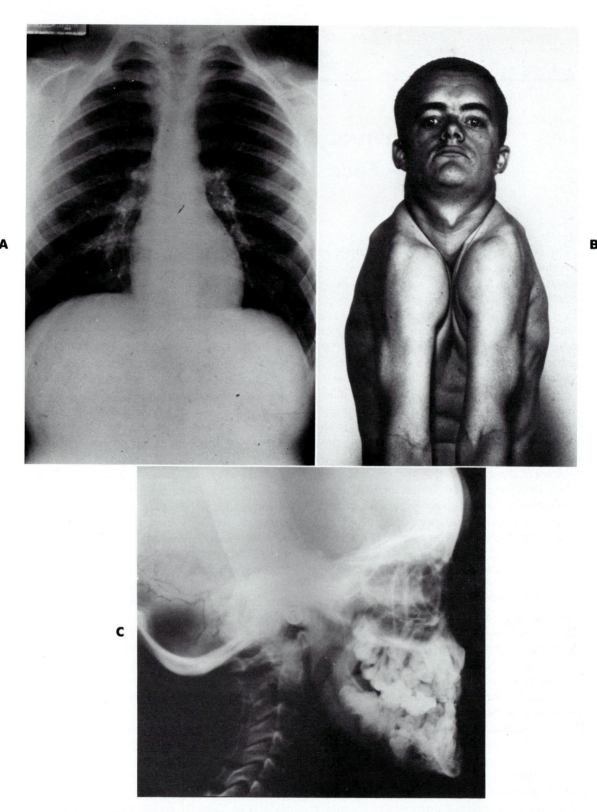

FIG. 29-1. Cleidocranial dysplasia. **A,** Chest radiograph of a patient. Note the absence of clavicles. **B,** The result is excessive mobility of the shoulders. Note also the frontal bossing and underdeveloped maxilla on this patient. **C,** On a lateral radiograph of a boy, note the wormian (sutural) bones and supernumerary teeth.

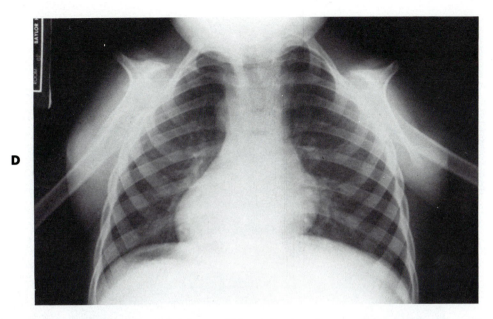

FIG. 29-1, cont'd. D, Chest of a 5-year-old boy, showing absence of the clavicles. (**D** courtesy Department of Radiology, Baylor University Hospital, Dallas.)

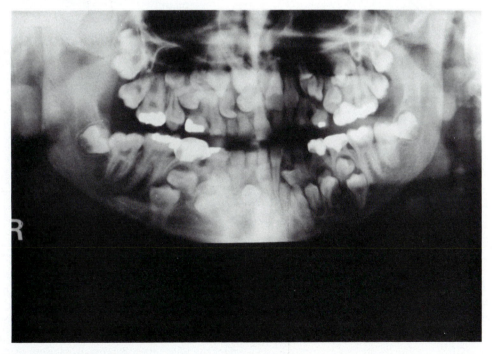

FIG. 29-2. Cleidocranial dysplasia results in prolonged retention of the primary dentition and multiple unerupted supernumerary teeth.

Continued.

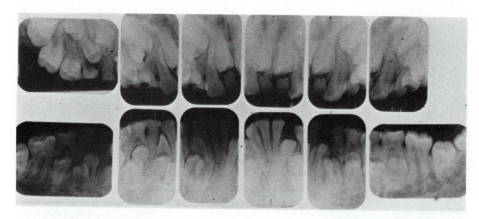

FIG. 29-2, cont'd. For legend, see page 665.

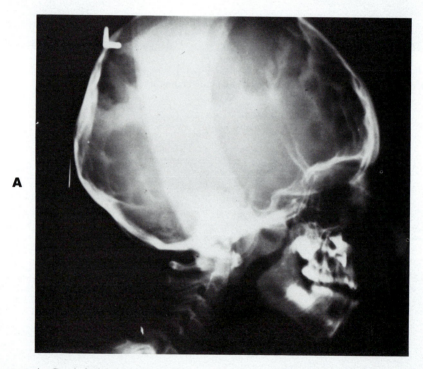

FIG. 29-3. A, Craniofacial dysplasia results in early closure of the cranial sutures and depressions on the inner surface of the calvarium (digital impressions) from growth of the brain.

with multiple unerupted supernumerary teeth.

Management. Care in cleidocranial dysostosis is directed toward retention of the erupted primary teeth.

CRANIOFACIAL DYSOSTOSIS

Craniofacial dysostosis (Crouzon's disease) is a developmental anomaly of unknown cause, although there is some evidence it may be transmitted as an autosomal dominant trait. In patients with this condition, all cranial sutures close early. This causes various skull malformations as the result of increased intracranial pressure.

Clinical features. Characteristically, patients show bulging of the frontal bone in the midline over the nose and a downward sloping of the back of the head.[35] The eyes may develop wide apart (hypertelorism) or protrude (exophthalmos). Patients may become blind as a result of early suture closure and increased intracranial pressure. A prominent and pointed nose often occurs. The maxilla is frequently narrow and underdeveloped.

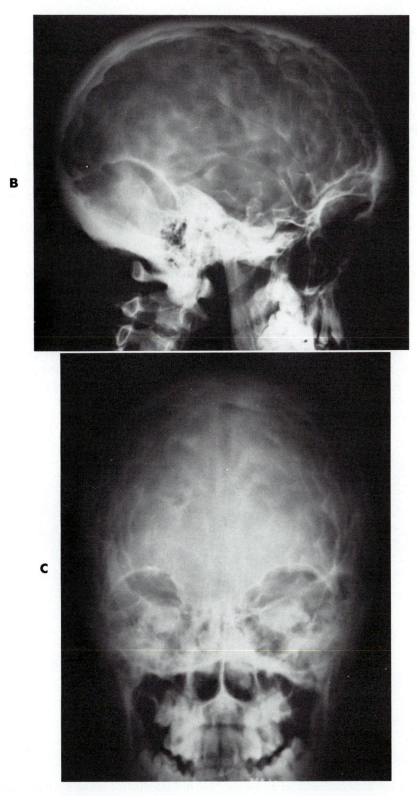

FIG. 29-3, cont'd. B and **C,** Closure of the cranial sutures in another patient. Note also the prominent digital markings. (**B** and **C** courtesy Department of Radiology, Baylor University Hospital, Dallas.)

Radiographic features. Skull examination reveals the absence of sutures. There are prominent cranial markings resulting from increased intracranial pressure from the brain. These markings may be seen as multiple radiolucencies appearing as depressions (digital impressions) covering the inner surface of the cranial vault (Fig. 29-3).

Differential diagnosis. Skull radiographs that show definite and widespread digital impressions and premature synostosis suggest craniofacial dysostosis. However, this condition must be differentiated from others also presenting with craniosynostosis.[9,12]

Management. Although many patients have progressive impairment and some have mental retardation, they have normal life spans. Consequently, maxillofacial surgery may be considered for correction of facial deformity, and neurosurgery for the progressive visual complications and to open the sutures.

MANDIBULOFACIAL DYSOSTOSIS

Mandibulofacial dysostosis (Treacher Collins syndrome) is a developmental anomaly that is often inherited as an autosomal dominant trait, but at least half of the cases arise as spontaneous mutations.

Clinical features. Individuals with mandibulofacial dysostosis often show a wide range of anomalies, depending on the severity of the condition. The most common clinical findings are relative underdevelopment of the zygomatic bones, resulting in midfacial deformity, a downward inclination of the palpebral fissures, underdevelopment of the mandible with a steep mandibular angle, macrostomia, malformation of the external ears, absence of the external auditory canal, and occasional facial clefts. The palate develops with a high arch or cleft in 30% of the cases.[3] Because of the steep mandibular angle, the patient may have an anterior open bite. Maldevelopment of the external ear and auditory canal may result in partial or complete deafness.

Radiographic features. Radiographic findings largely are consistent with the clinical observations (Fig. 29-4). A striking finding is the reduction in size of the zygomatic bones. The maxillary sinuses may also be underdeveloped or completely absent. There may also be underdevelopment of the articular eminence.[33] Radiographic examination may also reveal reduction or absence of the auditory canal. The mastoid air cells have also been reported to be reduced or absent.[3]

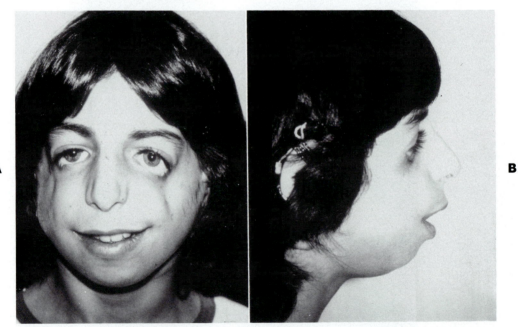

FIG. 29-4. A and **B,** Mandibulofacial dysostosis. Note the characteristic facies: downward-sloping palpebral fissures, colobomas of the outer third of the lower lids, depressed cheek bones, receding chin, little if any nasofrontal angle, and a nose that appears relatively large. **C** to **E,** Correlation of radiographic with clinical features: short mandibular rami, steep mandibular angle, and an anterior open bite. The zygomas are poorly formed.

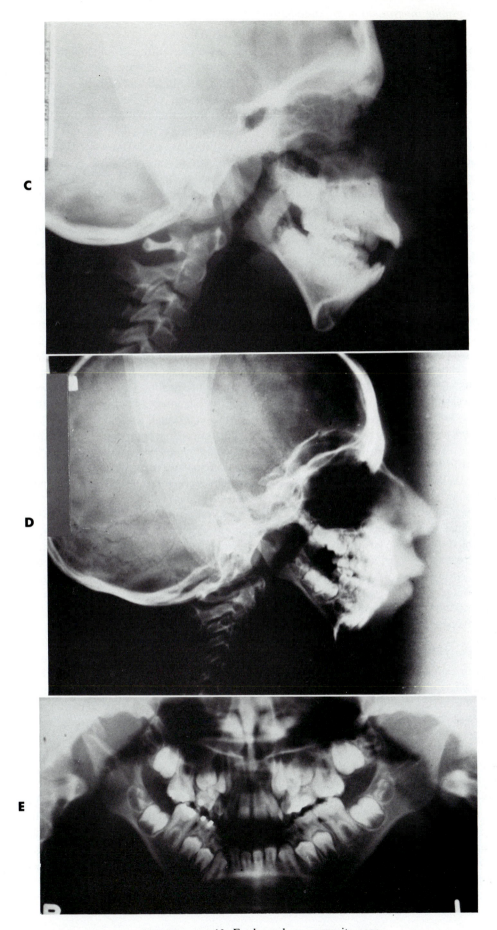

FIG. 29-4, cont'd. For legend, see opposite page.

Management. Growth of the facial bones during adolescence results in some cosmetic improvement.[27] Surgical intervention may also be used to improve the osseous and ear defects.

HEMIFACIAL HYPERTROPHY

Hemifacial hypertrophy is a condition in which half of the face and jaws, alone or in concert with other parts of the body, grow to unusual proportions. The cause of this condition is unknown, but it seems unlikely that heredity plays a part.

Clinical features. This condition begins during youth, sometimes at birth, and usually continues throughout the growing years. It often occurs wih other abnormalities, including mental deficiency, skin abnormalities, compensatory scoliosis,[20] genitourinary tract anomalies, and various neoplasms, including Wilms' tumor of the kidney, adrenocortical tumor, and hepatoblastoma.[8] Females and males are affected with approximately equal frequency.[8] The dentition of affected individuals may show enlargement of the canine, premolar, and first molar crowns and roots and accelerated development.[21] Primary teeth are usually shed prematurely. The tongue and alveolar bone enlarge on the involved side.

Radiographic features. Radiographic examination of the skulls of these patients reveals, on the affected side, enlargement of the bones, including the mandible (Fig. 29-5), maxilla, zygoma, and frontal and temporal bones.

Differential diagnosis. The differential diagnosis should consider *hemifacial hypoplasia (of the opposite side), arteriovenous aneurysms,* and *congenital lymphedema.*[35] The presence of the enlarged teeth and the rapid eruption of the dentition suggest hemifacial hypertrophy.

HEMIFACIAL HYPOPLASIA

Patients with hemifacial hypoplasia (also known as *hemifacial microsomia*) display reduced growth of half of the face. This condition may involve the whole of one side of the face or just the mandible. When the whole face is involved, there is reduction in the size of the mandible, maxilla, zygoma, external and middle ear, parotid gland, fifth and seventh cranial nerves, musculature, and other soft tissues.[5] Its cause is unknown.

Clinical features. Hemifacial hypoplasia usually begins early in life, but its onset may be delayed to any time until the cessation of facial growth. Patients with this condition have a striking appearance as a result of progressive failure of growth of the affected side, with the result that there is a reduced dimension of the involved side of the face. In addition, there is aplasia or hypoplasia of the external ear (crumpled, distorted pinna) in almost 100% of cases.[6] The ear canal is often missing.[11] In some patients the skull is reduced in size. There does not appear to be a sex predilection, and there is no evidence of a hereditary pattern. In about 90% of cases, malocclusion is present on the affected side, but the teeth are of normal size and shape.[11,22]

Radiographic features. The primary radiographic findings associated with this condition are a reduction in the size of the bones on the affected side. These changes are most clear in the mandible, which may show a reduction in the size of the condyle, coronoid process, or overall dimension of the body and ramus of the mandible (Fig. 29-6). The dentition on the affected side may show a reduction in the number or size of the teeth. CT examination shows a reduction in size of the muscles of mastication.[18] Three-dimension reformatting of CT images readily displays the extent of skeletal abnormalities.[32]

Differential diagnosis. The clinical and radiographic findings of this condition are characteristic of it. Exposure of the face of a child to radiation therapy may also cause underdevelopment of the tissues in the irradiated region.

Management. Orthodontic intervention may correct or prevent malocclusion. Also, the ear and mandibular abnormalities may be repaired by plastic surgery.[6] The hearing loss should be evaluated and may be (partially) corrected by hearing aids or possibly by surgery.[9]

HYPERPLASIA OF MAXILLARY TUBEROSITY

Hyperplasia of the maxillary tuberosity is a condition in which there is excessive enlargement of each maxillary tuberosity. Its cause is unknown.

Clinical features. This condition results in bilateral enlargement of the maxillary tuberosities, a situation easily identified on clinical examination. This condition develops in adults and may result in difficulty in wearing dentures and in normal mastication.

Radiographic features. The radiographic features of hyperplasia of the maxillary tuberosities are those of bilaterally enlarged maxillary tuberosities (Fig. 29-7). The bone is typically more opaque than normal, most probably because of its large dimension.

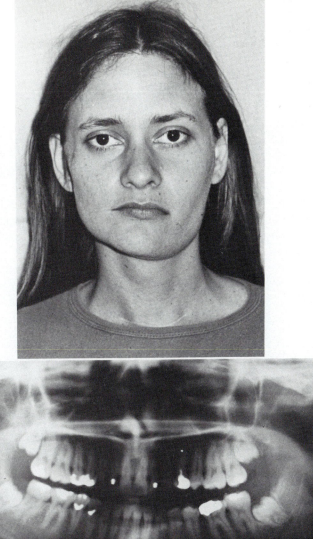

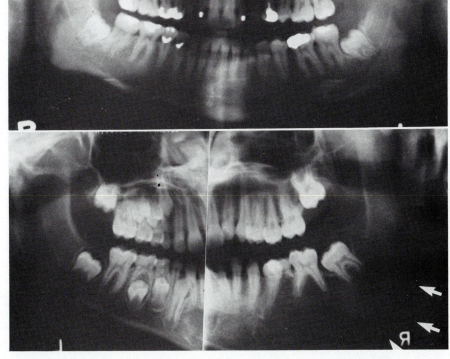

FIG. 29-5. A and **B,** Hemifacial hypertrophy, revealing enlargement of the left mandible and maxilla. **C,** Note the marked enlargement of the right maxilla and mandible and the accelerated development of the dentition on that side.

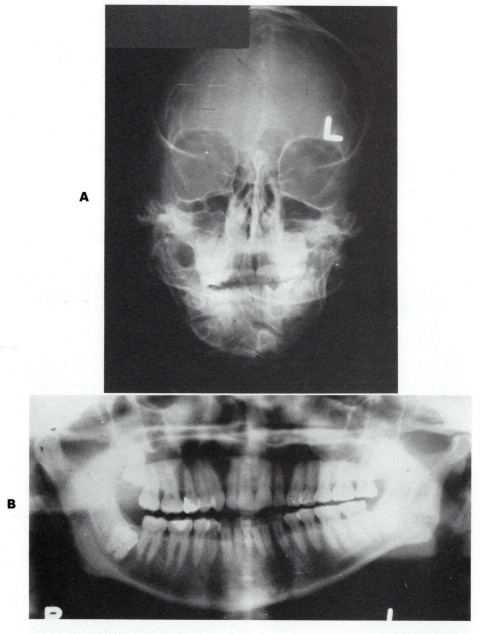

FIG. 29-6. **A** and **B,** Hemifacial hypoplasia, showing reduced size of the left maxilla and mandible.

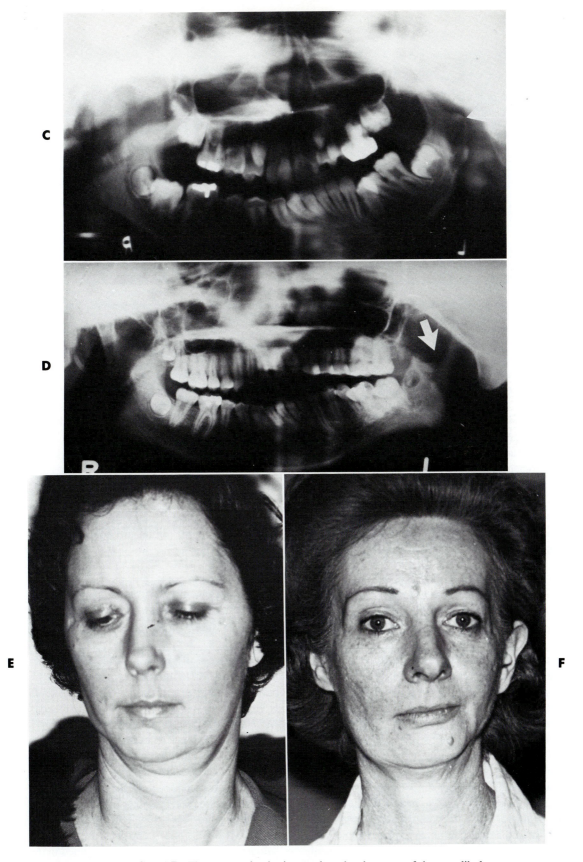

FIG. 29-6, cont'd. **C** and **D,** There may also be incomplete development of the mandibular ramus and condyle *(arrow)*. Note the delayed third molar development on the affected side in each case. **E** and **F,** Two women with hemifacial hypoplasia. (**E** and **F** courtesy Department of Oral Diagnosis, Baylor College of Dentistry, Dallas.)

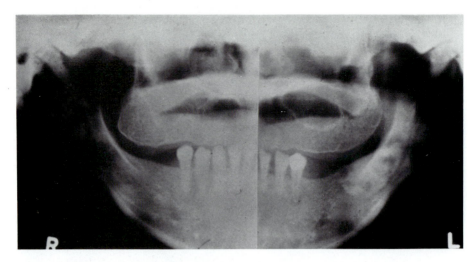

FIG. 29-7. Hyperplasia of the maxillary tuberosities, revealed as opaque bony enlargements of these regions of the maxilla.

Differential diagnosis. The clinical and radiographic appearances of the hyperplastic tuberosities are so distinctive that there is little difficulty in recognizing them.

Management. This entity is usually innocuous. In those relatively rare cases in which the enlargements reach such proportions that they interfere with mastication or the proper construction of dentures, they must be surgically reduced. Presurgical radiographs demonstrate the proximity of the sinus and the extent to which it may have expanded into the hypertrophied tuberosity.

DEVELOPMENTAL SALIVARY GLAND DEFECT

The developmental salivary gland defect of the mandible (also called *static bone cavity* or *latent bone cyst*) is a deep, well-defined depression in the lingual surface of the posterior body of the mandible. In those developmental bone defects investigated surgically, an aberrant lobe of the submandibular gland extends into the bony depression. The cause of this condition is uncertain, but it has been suggested that the mandible develops around the lobe during embryonic life. However, one report describes the development of this defect after middle age,[30] and another at the age of 11 years, requiring the next 5 years to reach its full size.[13] Similar depressions are occasionally found in the molar-premolar and canine areas of the mandibular body. These probably bear a similar relationship to the sublingual gland.

Clinical features. Developmental salivary gland defects are relatively rare, with an incidence of about 4 in every 1000 adults.[16] They are asymptomatic and next to impossible to palpate manually, so they are discovered only during radiographic examination of the area. More cases have been reported in men than in women.

Radiographic features. The image of the developmental salivary gland defect is a round or ovoid radiolucency that ranges in diameter from 1 to 3 cm (Fig. 29-8). It generally develops below the mandibular canal and above the inferior border of the mandible, just anterior to the angle of the jaw and below and just behind the third molar. The margins of the radiolucent defect are well defined by a dense radiopaque line. This is the result of the x-rays passing tangentially through the relatively thick walls of the depression. The lesion may involve the inferior border of the mandible.

Differential diagnosis. The appearance and location of the radiographic image of the developmental bone defect are so characteristic that it is readily recognized. It may be mistaken for a *radicular cyst* if it is situated more anteriorly and is projected over the apices of teeth. It may resemble a *residual cyst* if found more superiorly than its usual location and in an area from which a tooth has been extracted.

Management. The recognition of the lesion should preclude any treatment or surgical exploration. However, one should at least be aware that salivary gland neoplasms have developed in the soft tissue within the defect. Consequently, carefully examine images of these defects and palpate the area for signs of abnormal growth. Make a repeat

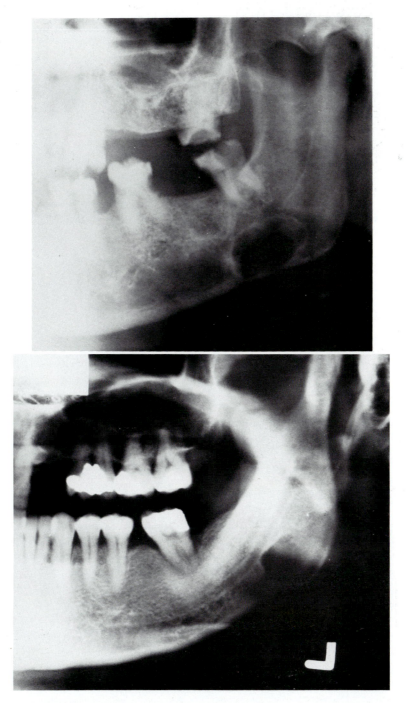

FIG. 29-8. Developmental salivary gland defects are usually seen as sharply defined radiolucencies beneath the mandibular canal in the region of the third molars. They can erode the inferior border of the mandible.

Continued.

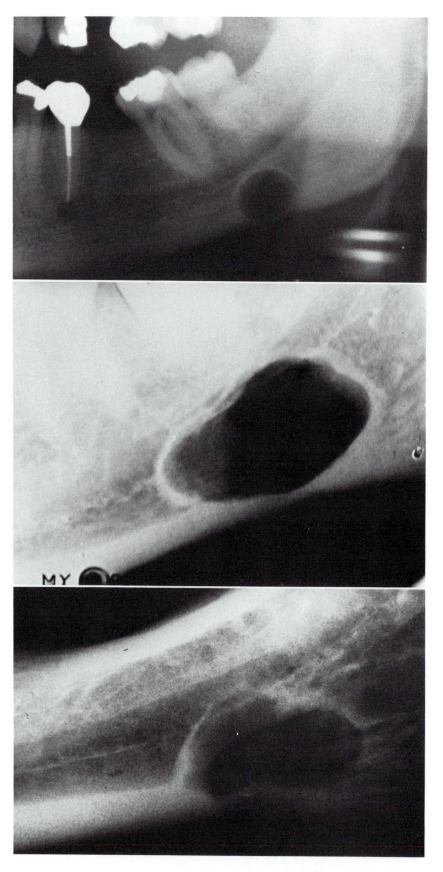

FIG. 29-8, cont'd. For legend, see page 675.

radiographic examination after 3 to 6 months to confirm that the defect is not growing.

CLEFT PALATE

A failure of fusion of the developmental processes of the face during embryonic life may result in a variety of facial clefts. The most prevalent of these conditions are cleft lip, with or without cleft palate, and isolated cleft palate. The overall incidence of cleft lip and cleft palate is about 3 per 1000 live births.[24,31] Clefts of the mandibular lip or jaw are extremely rare. The causes of facial clefts are not fully understood, but hereditary factors are considered to be most important. Other factors that have received considerable attention include nutritional disturbances, environmental teratogenic agents, stress resulting in increased secretion of hydrocortisone, defects of vascular supply to the involved region, and mechanical in-terference with the closure of the embryonic processes.

Clinical features. Clefts of the lip may be either unilateral or bilateral. There are sex differences in the frequency of occurrence, but these differences vary among races. Also, regardless of sex, the left side alone is involved in 70% of cases.[7] The cleft may extend just through the lip or may extend up into the nostril. Clefts of the palate may also vary in severity, involving only the uvula or soft palate or extending all the way through the palate and including the alveolar ridge on one or both sides. Defects in the alveolar ridge usually occur near the maxillary lateral incisor. The palatal defect may result in impaired speech.

Radiographic features. Radiographic examination may reveal a cleft of the alveolar bone as well as numerous dental anomalies (Fig. 29-9) that may include the absence of the maxillary lateral

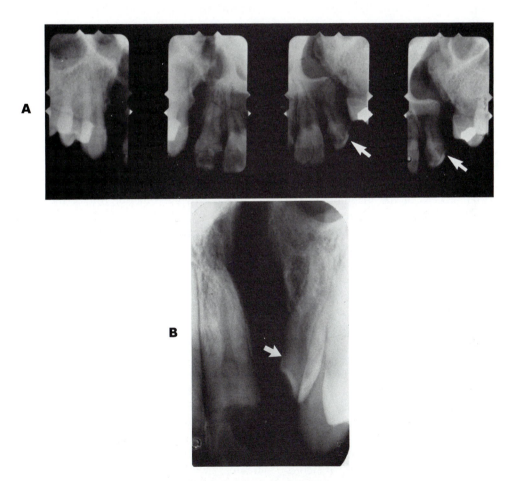

FIG. 29-9. Cleft palate results in defects in the alveolar ridge and abnormalities of the dentition. **A,** Bilateral cysts with absence of the right lateral incisor and malformation of the left lateral *(arrow)*. **B,** Cyst and a supernumerary tooth *(arrow)*.

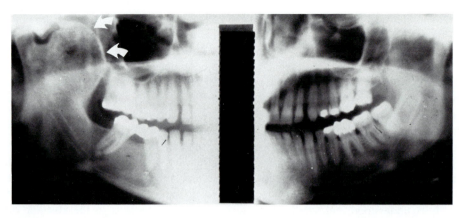

FIG. 29-10. Hyperplasia of the coronoid process of the mandible *(arrows)*. (Courtesy Dr. B. Gratt, Los Angeles.)

incisor and the presence of supernumerary teeth in this region. Often the teeth in this region are malformed and poorly positioned. In boys with unilateral clefts of the lip, alveolus, and palate, there is a mild retardation in development of maxillary and mandibular teeth.[2,14,17] Affected children of both sexes also have an increased incidence of hypodontia in both arches.

Management. Management of these defects is complex, requiring the coordinated efforts of a surgeon, orthodontist, dentist, speech therapist, and occasionally a psychologist.

HYPERPLASIA OF CORONOID PROCESS

On occasion, one may observe hypertrophy of the coronoid process of the mandible.[19] The causes of this hypertrophy are unknown. It also occurs as a component of the trismus-pseudocampylodactyly syndrome in combination with a trismus (caused by the coronoid process enlargement) and curvature of the fingers on dorsiflexion of the wrist.[29]

Clinical features. Hyperplasia of the coronoid process is usually detected in adults, although the onset is around the time of puberty.[10] Such patients have a history of limited opening and may describe pain unilaterally or bilaterally, somewhat anterior to the temporomandibular joint.

Radiographic features. Enlargement of the coronoid processes may be recognized radiographically on lateral films, such as panoramic views, or on the Waters projection (Fig. 29-10). The panoramic projection shows the position of the coronoid process in relation to the posterior wall of the zygomatic process of the maxilla. The Waters projection reveals the mediolateral position of the cor-

onoid process in relation to the zygomatic arch. Comparison of the patient's right and left sides on these projections readily demonstrates unilateral hyperplasia of the coronoid process. By making these views with the mouth open as far as possible, the coronoid process may be seen impinging anteriorly on the posterior wall of the zygomatic process of the maxilla or laterally on the medial aspect of the zygomatic arch.

Differential diagnosis. The recognition of this entity is not difficult if, when the mouth is open, the distance between the central incisors is markedly restricted, there is some pain over one or both sides of the jaws, and the radiograph shows an image of an elongated coronoid process more than 5 mm above the superior rim of the zygomatic arch.[19]

Management. Surgical removal of the coronoid process will permit the patient to open the mouth normally and without symptoms.

FOCAL OSTEOPOROTIC BONE MARROW DEFECTS

Focal osteoporotic bone marrow defects are radiolucent defects discovered in the jaws on routine radiographic examination. Histologic examination reveals areas of hematopoietic or fatty marrow. Their pathogenesis is unknown, but they have been postulated to be derived from (1) bone marrow hyperplasia secondary to a demand for blood cells, (2) persistent embryologic marrow remnants, or (3) sites of abnormal healing following extraction, trauma, or local inflammation.[1,25]

Clinical features. Focal osteoporotic bone marrow defects are usually clinically asymptomatic. They are discovered only as incidental findings on

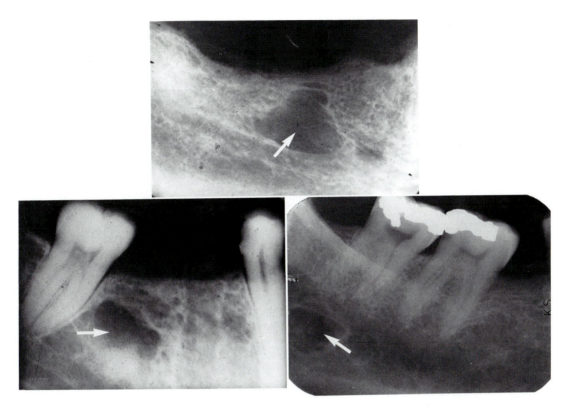

FIG. 29-11. Focal osteoporotic bone marrow defect, seen as a radiolucency *(arrow)* usually with internal trabeculation and variable margins.

radiographic examinations. Some patients have a history of pain in the region. Often these lesions develop in association with a previous extraction site, impacted teeth, periapical cemental dysplasia, or other conditions.[1] The lesions are more common in middle-aged women.[1,4,25,28] The most common site is the mandibular molar-premolar region.

Radiographic features. The radiographic appearance of focal osteoporotic bone marrow defects is quite variable. The lesion is radiolucent and usually demonstrates internal trabeculation (Fig. 29-11). The margins may be ill defined or well defined. They may be corticated or noncorticated. The lesions are most common in edentulous areas.

Differential diagnosis. The variety of subtle features that may attend these radiolucent lesions and that are usually recognized radiographically may cause the following entities to be included in the differential diagnosis: *residual dental infection, central neoplasm,* and *traumatic bone cyst.*[26]

Management. Because the radiographic appearance of focal osteoporotic bone marrow defects of the jaw is not pathognomonic and may mimic more serious entities, a biopsy is indicated. If the

diagnosis of osteoporotic bone marrow defect is established histologically, no treatment is required.[26]

REFERENCES

1. Barker B, Jensen J, Howell F: Focal osteoporotic bone marrow defects of the jaws, *Oral Surg* 38:404-413, 1974.
2. Brouwers HJ, Kuijpers-Jagtman AM: Development of permanent tooth length in patients with unilateral cleft lip and palate, *Am J Orthod Dentofacial Orthop* 99:543-549, 1991.
3. Cohen MM Jr: Dysmorphic syndromes and craniofacial manifestations. In Stewart RE, Prescott GG, editors: *Oral facial genetics,* St Louis, 1976, Mosby.
4. Crawford B, Weathers D: Osteoporotic marrow defects of the jaws, *J Oral Surg* 28:600-603, 1970.
5. Figueroa AA, Fields H: Craniovertebral malformation in hemifacial microsomia, *J Cranio Genet Dev Biol* 1(suppl):167-178, 1985.
6. Finegold M: Hemifacial microstomia. In Bergsma D, editor: *Birth defects compendium,* ed 2, New York, 1973, Alan R Liss.
7. Fraser GR, Calnan JS: Cleft lip and palate: seasonal incidence, birth weight, birth rank, sex, site associated malformations and parental age, *Arch Dis Child* 36:420-423, 1961.
8. Fraumeni JF, Geiser CF, Manning MD: Wilms' tumor and

congenital hemihypertrophy: report of five new cases and review of literature, *Pediatrics* 40:886-899, 1967.

9. Goodman RM, Gorlin RJ: *Atlas of the face in genetic disorders,* ed 2, St Louis, 1977, Mosby.

10. Gorlin RJ, Goldman HM: *Thoma's oral pathology,* ed 6, vol 1, St Louis, 1970, Mosby.

11. Gorlin RJ, Pindborg JJ: *Syndromes of the head and neck,* New York, 1964, McGraw-Hill.

12. Gorlin RJ, Cohen MM, Levin LS: *Syndromes of the head and neck,* ed 3, New York, 1990, Oxford University Press.

13. Hansson L: Development of a lingual mandibular bone cavity in an 11-year-old boy, *Oral Surg* 49:376-378, 1980.

14. Harris EF, Hullings JG: Delayed dental development in children with isolated cleft lip and palate, *Arch Oral Biol* 35:469-473, 1990.

15. Jensen BL, Kreiborg S: Development of the dentition in cleidocranial dysplasia, *J Oral Pathol Med* 19:89-93, 1990.

16. Karmiol M, Walsh R: Incidence of static bone defect of the mandible, *Oral Surg* 26:225-228, 1968.

17. Loevy HT, Aduss H: Tooth maturation in cleft lip, cleft palate, or both, *Cleft Palate J* 25:343-347, 1988.

18. Marsh JL, Baca D, Vannier MW: Facial musculoskeletal asymmetry in hemifacial microsomia, *Cleft Palate J* 26:292-302, 1989.

19. Mauer RM, Wildin RE: Hypertrophy of the coronoid process of the mandible, a case of restricted opening of the mouth, *Radiology* 83:1060-1063, 1964.

20. Ringrose RE, Jabbour FT, Keele DK: Hemihypertrophy, *Pediatrics* 36:434-448, 1965.

21. Rowe NH: Hemifacial hypertrophy: review of the literature and addition of four cases, *Oral Surg* 15:572-589, 1962.

22. Rushton MA: A case of unilateral micrognathia, aural atresia and macrostomia, *Br Dent J* 64:549-552, 1938.

23. Rushton MA: Anomaly of cementum in cleidocranial dysostosis, *Br Dent J* 100:81-83, 1956.

24. Sayetta RB, Weinrich MC, Coston GN: Incidence and prevalence of cleft lip and palate: what we think we know, *Cleft Palate J* 26:242-248, 1989.

25. Schneider LC, Mesa ML, Fraenkel D: Osteoporotic bone marrow defect: radiographic features and pathogenic factors, *Oral Surg* 65:127-129, 1988.

26. Shafer WG, Hine MK, Levy BM: *Oral pathology,* ed 4, Philadelphia, 1983, WB Saunders.

27. Smith D: *Recognizable patterns of human malformation: genetic, embryologic, and clinical aspects,* vol 7. *Major problems in clinical pediatrics,* Philadelphia, 1970, WB Saunders.

28. Standish S, Shafer W: Focal osteoporotic bone marrow defects of the jaws, *J Oral Surg* 20:123-128, 1962.

29. Ter Haar BGA, Van Hoof RF: The trismuspseudocampylodactyly syndrome, *J Med Genet* 11:41-49, 1974.

30. Tolman DE, Stafne EC: Developmental bone defects of the mandible, *Oral Surg* 24:488-490, 1967.

31. Vanderas AP: Incidence of cleft lip, palate, and cleft lip and palate among races: a review, *Cleft Palate J* 24:216-225, 1987.

32. Whyman RA, Doyle TC, Harding WJ, Ferguson MM: An unusual case of hemifacial atrophy, *Oral Surg Oral Med Oral Pathol* 73:564-569, 1992.

33. Worth HM: *Principles and practice of oral radiologic interpretation,* Chicago, 1963, Year Book.

34. Yamamoto H, Sakae T, Davies JE: Cleidocranial dysplasia: a light microscope, electron microscope, and crystallographic study, *Oral Surg Oral Med Oral Pathol* 68:195-200, 1989.

35. Zegarelli E, Kutscher A, Hyman G: *Diagnosis of diseases of the mouth and jaws,* ed 2, Philadelphia, 1978, Lea & Febiger.

30

BYRON W. BENSON

Salivary Gland Radiology

Disorders of the salivary glands fall within the dental diagnostician's area of responsibility. A familiarity with these disorders and applicable imaging techniques are essential elements of the clinician's armamentarium. The major salivary glands are symmetrically paired and located adjacent to the ramus and body of the mandible. They are the parotid, the submandibular (submaxillary), and the sublingual glands. The major glands are complemented by numerous minor salivary glands found on the buccal, palatal, and sublingual mucosal surfaces of the oral cavity.[46]

The early development of the salivary glands is similar to that of the teeth, hair follicles, and other glands or epithelially derived structures. The development of the parotid precedes the other major and minor salivary glands.[58] By 5 months in utero, the tubular components are formed and terminal clusters are differentiating into acini.[41,48] The general pattern of the ducts, starting from the secreting acini, is smaller ducts successively merging into ducts of larger caliber. The smallest ducts originating at the secretory acini are the intercalated ducts, which merge with the larger striated (or secretory) branches, which in turn join the terminal excretory duct.[48] The excretory duct of the parotid is Stensen's duct and the excretory duct of the submandibular gland is Wharton's duct. The intercalated and smaller secretory ducts are considered to be intralobular; the larger secretory and excretory ducts are considered to be interlobular in orientation.[46]

Acinar cells may be either serous or mucous.[48] The parotid acini are almost entirely serous. The sublingual acini are essentially mucous. The submandibular acini are mixed; however, the serous acini are more numerous. Lymph nodes are frequently included within the capsule of the parotid during its development. The mesenchyme adjacent to the developing submandibular and sublingual glands condenses early, which precludes the inclusion of lymphatic tissue in these glands.[48]

DIAGNOSTIC IMAGING OF THE SALIVARY GLANDS

Diagnostic imaging of salivary gland disease is undertaken to differentiate between inflammatory and neoplastic disease, distinguish between diffuse and focal suppurative disease, identify and locate salivary stones, and demonstrate ductal morphology. In addition, diagnostic imaging attempts to determine the anatomic location of a tumor, differentiate between benign and malignant disease, demonstrate the relationship between a tumor and adjacent structures, and differentiate between intrinsic and extrinsic masses.

Plain film radiography

Plain film radiography is an important part of the examination of the salivary glands and may provide sufficient information to preclude the use of more sophisticated and expensive imaging techniques. Plain film radiography has the potential to identify unrelated osseous diseases in the areas of the salivary glands that may be mistakenly identified as salivary gland disease, such as resorptive or osteoblastic changes in adjacent bone that may cause periauricular swelling, mimicking a parotid tumor. Panoramic or conventional posteroanterior (PA) radiographs (see Chapter 11) may demonstrate bony involvement, thus eliminating salivary disease from the differential diagnosis. Hypertrophy of the masseter muscle may mimic a salivary tumor, but a panoramic radiograph may demonstrate a deep antegonial notch, overdeveloped mandibular angle, and exostosis on the outer surface of the angle, which are indicative of muscle hypertrophy.[29,61]

Plain film radiographs are most useful when the

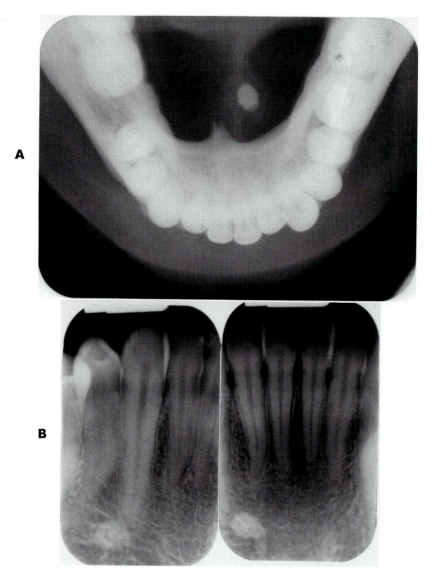

FIG. 30-1. Sialolith. **A,** Underexposed mandibular occlusal radiograph demonstrating radiopaque sialolith/calculus in Wharton's duct. Note the classical laminated appearance. **B,** Periapical radiographs of the same case. The radiopaque sialolith can be localized lingual to the teeth by applying appropriate object localization rules.

clinical impression, supported by a compatible history, suggests the presence of sialoliths (stones or calculi) or phleboliths.[10] Such an examination should include both intraoral and extraoral images to demonstrate the entire ductal system. Several sialoliths may be present at different locations. It is expedient to use about half of the usual exposure to avoid overexposure of the sialoliths. However, the usefulness of this technique is somewhat limited in that about 20% of the obstructions in the submandibular gland and 40% of those in the parotid are radiolucent.[32,49] The radiolucent variety (mucous plugs) are rarely found in the sublingual glands. If clinically suspected stones are not demonstrated by plain film radiography, sialography is indicated. The radiographic image of a sialolith superimposed over bone must be differentiated from calcified lymph nodes, phleboliths, myositis ossificans, multiple miliary osteomas of the skin, and calcified acne scars.[27]

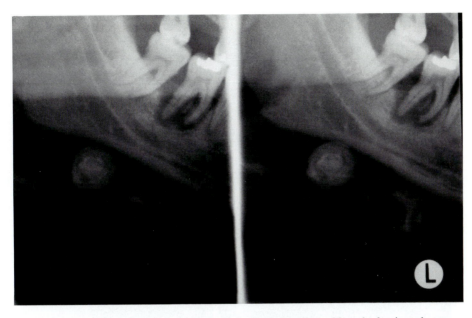

FIG. 30-2. Sialolith. Stereoscopic panoramic plain film projections. Note the laminated appearance of this sialolith in the submandibular gland. The image of the sialolith is magnified because of its relatively lingual placement in the image layer. Taken from slightly different horizontal angles, a three-dimensional appearance is presented when viewed with stereo binoculars.

Intraoral radiography

Calculi in the anterior two thirds of the submandibular duct are typically imaged with a cross-sectional mandibular occlusal projection as described in Chapter 9 (Fig. 30-1). The posterior part of the duct is demonstrated with a posterior oblique view, wherein the patient's head is tilted back and maximally inclined toward the unaffected side. The central ray is directed parallel with the mandible in the area of the submandibular fossa and into the posterior part of the floor of the mouth.

Parotid calculi are more difficult to demonstrate than the submandibular variety as a result of the tortuous course of Stensen's duct around the anterior border of the masseter and through the buccinator muscle. As a rule, only calculi in the anterior part of the duct, distal to the masseter muscle, can be imaged on an intraoral film. To demonstrate calculi in the anterior part of the duct, an intraoral film is held with a hemostat against the cheek, as high as possible in the buccal sulcus and over the parotid papilla. The central ray is directed perpendicular to the center of the film.

Extraoral radiography

A panoramic projection (see Chapter 12) frequently demonstrates calculi in the posterior (interglandular) duct in the submandibular gland if the calculus is in the image layer (Fig. 30-2). Because most calculi are superimposed over the ramus and body of the mandible, lateral oblique radiographs are of limited value. To demonstrate calculi in the submandibular gland, a lateral projection is made by opening the mouth, extending the chin, and depressing the tongue with the index finger. This will usually move the calculus inferiorly below the mandibular border, where its image will be apparent.

Calculi in the distal portion of Stensen's duct or in the parotid are difficult to demonstrate by intraoral or lateral extraoral views. However, a posteroanterior (PA) projection (see Chapter 11) with the cheeks puffed out may move the calculus free of the bone and be apparent on the image. This technique may also demonstrate calculi in the gland, which would be obscured during sialography. However, less mineralized calculi may be obscured by a heavy soft tissue shadow in the PA view.[48]

Sialography. Sialography is a radiographic technique in which a radiopaque contrast agent is infused into the ductal system of a salivary gland prior to imaging with plain films, fluoroscopy, panoramic radiography, tomography, or computed tomography.[29,48] Sialography provides a straightforward demonstration of the ductal system (Fig. 30-3). The parotid and submandibular gland are more commonly studied with this technique than the sub-

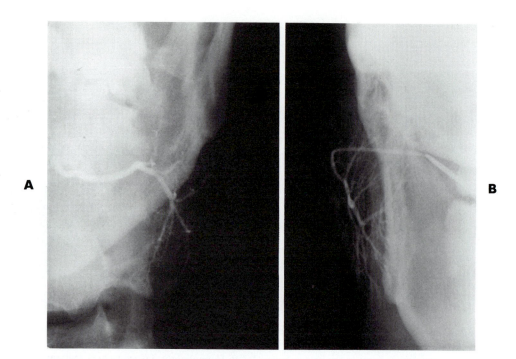

FIG. 30-3. Sialograms. **A,** PA projection of submandibular gland demonstrating prominent superior and posterior extensions of the gland. It may be appreciated that the peripheral margins of the submandibular gland lie in close proximity to inferior and anterior margins of the parotid. **B,** PA projection of parotid. Gland was filled using pressure-regulated pump for optimal parenchymal opacification. Lack of parenchyma blush suggests edema.

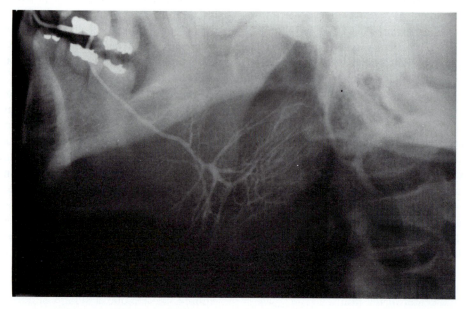

FIG. 30-4. Sialogram of normal submandibular gland. This lateral view demonstrates the ductal filling stage prior to parenchymal opacification.

lingual gland. Although the sublingual gland is difficult to infuse intentionally, it may be fortuitously opacified while infusing Wharton's duct to opacify the submandibular gland.[21]

A survey ("scout") film is usually made prior to the introduction of the contrast solution into the ductal system to aid in determining the correct exposure and patient positioning parameters. Radiopaque calculi may also be demonstrated, along with extraglandular and bone disease that may in fact be responsible for the clinical symptoms.

The closed-system sialographic technique is frequently recommended. A lacrimal probe is used to dilate the sphincter at the ductal orifice prior to passing a cannula (blunt needle or catheter) connected by extension tubing to a syringe containing contrast agent.[30,48] Lipid soluble (e.g., Ethiodol) or non-lipid soluble (e.g., Sinographin) contrast solution is slowly infused until the patient feels discomfort (usually between 0.2 and 1.5 ml, depending on the gland being studied).[1] Fluoroscopic monitoring of the filling phase is recommended by some;[37,48] otherwise, the procedure is monitored with static films. The intent is to opacify the ductal system all the way to the acini. The syringe containing the contrast agent is then taped to the patient's chest or shoulder outside of the area of interest. The image of the ductal system appears as tree limbs, with no area of the gland devoid of ducts (Fig. 30-4). With acinar filling, the "tree" comes into "bloom," which is the typical appearance of the parenchymal opacification phase[45] (Fig. 30-5). The gland is allowed to empty for 5 minutes. If imaging suggests contrast retention, a sialogogue such as lemon juice or 2% citric acid may be administered to augment the emptying phase by stimulating secretion.[21]

Sialography is indicated for the evaluation of chronic inflammatory or ductal diseases. However, it is no longer considered the study of choice for space-occupying masses. Contraindications to siography include acute infection, known sensitivity to iodine-containing compounds, and anticipated thyroid function tests.*

Computed tomography (CT). See Chapter 13 for a description of the process by which CT images are acquired. This technique is useful in evaluating structures in and adjacent to salivary glands, as CT distinguishes both soft and hard tissues, along with minute differences in soft tissue densities (Fig. 30-6). Glandular tissues are usually easily discernible

---
*References 13, 28, 35, 48, 49, 69, 79.

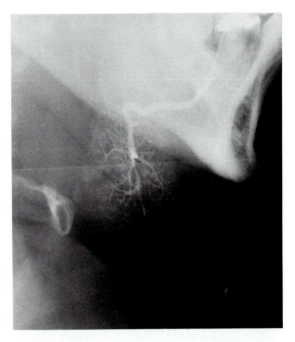

FIG. 30-5. Sialogram of normal submandibular gland. This lateral view demonstrates parenchymal filling. Normal fine branching is visible. Lack of parenchymal blush at the anteroinferior margin is caused by radiographic burnout.

from neighboring fat and muscle. The parotids are more radiodense than the surrounding fat but less dense than adjacent muscles.[10] Although the submandibular and sublingual glands are similar in density to adjacent muscles, they are readily identified on the basis of shape and location.[69] The submandibular and sublingual glands are most easily identified on contrast-enhanced coronal CT scans.[31]

CT is useful for the assessment of acute inflammatory processes and abscesses. An acutely inflamed gland is enlarged and of increased density. Abscess formation on routine CT appears as an area of decreased density within the enlarged gland. Spatial resolution of CT is inadequate to detect small irregularities in the ductal system.[73]

CT images of cysts and mucoceles demonstrate well-circumscribed margins and thin walls. The radiographic density of the lumen may vary, depending on the composition of the fluid contained therein.[6]

CT is sensitive for neoplasia and is extremely helpful in distinguishing between intrinsic and extrinsic masses. It is the method of choice for the investigation of masses in or about the salivary

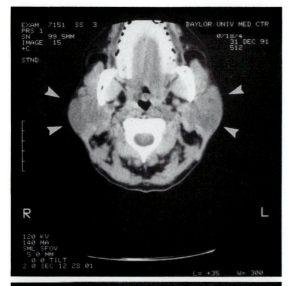

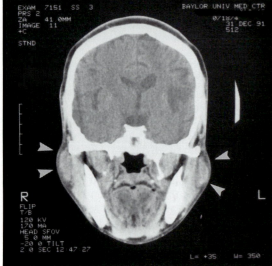

FIG. 30-6. CT images. **A,** Axial view demonstrating bilateral enlargement of the parotids *(arrows).* **B,** Coronal view of the same patient. The clinical/histopathologic diagnosis was autoimmune parotitis. (Courtesy Radiology Dept., Baylor University Medical Center, Dallas.)

glands.[6] Benign tumors within the gland are usually well defined (encapsulated), denser than adjacent normal glandular tissue, and have a homogeneous composition. However, these combinations of features are also suggestive of low-grade malignancies and benign cysts. In contrast, the borders of high-grade and recurrent malignant tumors are usually not well defined, which is indicative of an infiltrative tumor. These tumors have high density and a

heterogeneous pattern. These distinguishing characteristics are not absolute; they are only general guidelines. Exceptions are encountered so often that it is not always possible to differentiate between malignant and benign lesions on the basis of their CT presentation.[40] A combination of CT, CT-sialography, and enhanced CT may be necessary to define the submandibular gland, which is denser than the parotid and comparable with that of adjacent tissue. Plain CT usually provides sufficient delineation of extraglandular tumors adjacent to the parotid or Stensen's duct.[47] Foci of fat (lipomas and liposarcomas) are characteristic on CT images because of the distinctive low density (dark image) of lipid.[53]

Magnetic resonance imaging (MRI). See Chapter 13 for a description of the basic concepts and principles of nuclear magnetic resonance imaging. MRI provides better soft tissue images than CT and fewer problems with streak artifacts from dental amalgam that are sometimes seen in CT[69,76] (Fig. 30-7). Whereas indications for CT and MRI occasionally overlap, MRI demonstrates as well as or better than CT the margins of salivary gland masses, internal structure, and regional extension of lesions into adjacent tissues or spaces, as occurs with some lesions of the deep lobe of the parotid. MRI also discloses the major vessels identified as areas of low signal (dark) without the use of contrast medium.[34,43,55,65]

Scintigraphy (nuclear medicine). See Chapter 13 for a description of the nuclear medicine procedures used to acquire images. This technique provides a functional study of the salivary glands, taking advantage of the selective concentration of specific radiopharmaceuticals in the glands. When ^{99m}Tc-pertechnetate is injected intravenously, it is concentrated in and excreted by glandular structures including salivary, thyroid, and mammary glands. The radionuclide appears in the ducts of the salivary glands within minutes and reaches maximum concentration within 30 to 45 minutes. A sialogogue is then administered to evaluate secretory capacity. All major salivary glands can be studied at once by scintigraphy, and it is especially advantageous in the conditions where sialography is contraindicated as well as for those whose ducts cannot be cannulated. Although this technique is very sensitive, it lacks specificity and demonstrates little morphology.[8,10,76] Diffusely increased uptake is found in acute inflammation, granulomatous disease, and lymphoma. The concentration of radionuclide will be more focal in sialosis because of

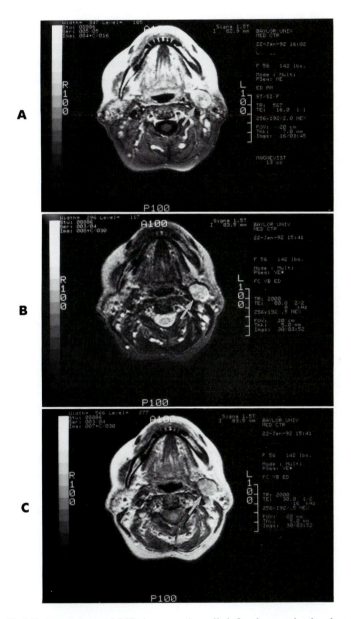

FIG. 30-7. Gadolinium-enhanced MR images. A well-defined mass in the deep lobe of the left parotid *(arrow)* as imaged with T1- **(A)**, T2- **(B)**, and proton **(C)** density–weighted formats. The appearance is typical of benign salivary tumors. Histopathologic diagnosis was pleomorphic adenoma. (Courtesy Radiology Dept., Baylor University Medical Center, Dallas.)

obstruction and in oncocytoma and Warthin's tumor (Fig. 30-8). Decreased uptake is seen in aging, viral infections. Sjögren's syndrome, and most primary and metastatic tumors. Areas of abscess formation do not concentrate radionuclide.

In chronic sialadenitis there are various degrees of tissue damage and fibrosis, and findings depend upon the amount of functional tissue remaining. There is usually decreased uptake ("cold spots") because of the atrophy and fibrosis of the glandular tissue.[24] Following the secretory phase there may be secondary retention images ("hot spots") in dilated ducts and abscess cavities. Diffuse unilateral decreased uptake is suggestive of previous radiotherapy, postsurgical parotitis, chronic recurrent sialadenitis, and trauma.

The diagnosis of salivary gland tumors from nuclear medicine scans is not completely reliable.[39,70] Current levels of resolution consistently visualize only tumors exceeding 1 to 1.5 cm. Some malignant tumors and the majority of benign tumors demonstrate "cold spots" with [99m]Tc. Exceptions that show "hot spots" include Warthin's tumor, oncocytoma, and infrequently pleomorphic adenoma.[1] Most malignant tumors show increased uptake of ^{67}Ga-labeled citrate, whereas most benign tumors show decreased uptake.[20,70] Ductal obstructions can trap the isotope, resulting in persistent activity in the gland (hot spots) following the excretory phase.[71] CT and MRI are preferred for the evaluation of salivary masses.

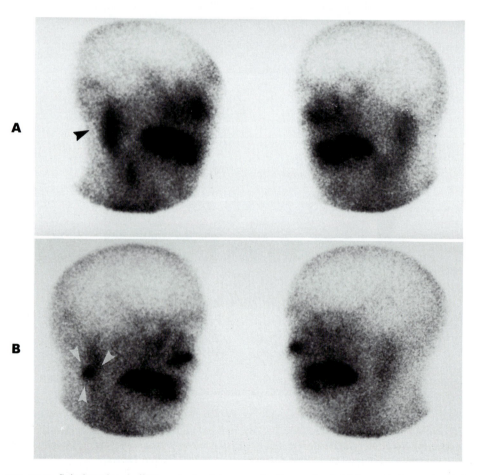

FIG. 30-8. Scintigraphy. **A,** [99m]Tc pertechnetate scan of salivary glands (right and left anterior oblique views) demonstrate increased uptake of radioisotope in right parotid *(black arrow).* **B,** Scintigram following administration of sialogogue (lemon juice) demonstrates retention of isotope in right parotid *(white arrows).* This is a typical presentation of salivary stasis, Warthin's tumor, or oncocytoma.

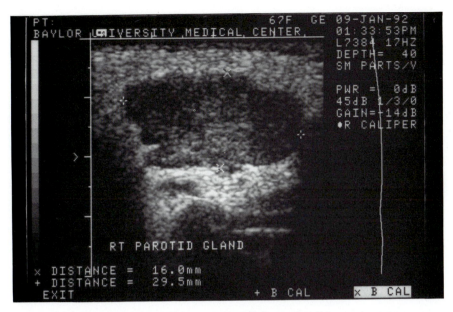

FIG. 30-9. Ultrasound image of left parotid. A well-delineated, solid mass is apparent, suggested by echo returns within the lesion. (The lesion borders are marked with *x* and + signs.) Ultrasound appearance is typical of a benign salivary tumor. (Courtesy Radiology Dept., Baylor University Medical Center, Dallas.)

Ultrasonography

For a description of ultrasonography, see Chapter 13. Compared to CT and MR, ultrasonography has the advantages of being relatively inexpensive, widely available, painless, easy to perform, and noninvasive.[11,69] The main application of ultrasonography is the differentiation between solid and cystic masses.[11,22,42,78] Solid masses are echogenic, producing internal echoes. Cystic or fluid-filled lesions are echo-free with enhancement of the deep wall. Solid tumors larger than 5 mm are usually well visualized. Benign masses are typically less echogenic than parenchyma, sharply defined, and of homogeneous echo strength and density (Fig. 30-9). Malignant masses typically have irregular, ill-defined margins, are of heterogeneous echo strength, and demonstrate a relatively reduced echo pattern.[51]

Ultrasonography has limited value in the diagnosis of inflammatory and obstructive diseases, but recent studies indicate it is fairly reliable in demonstrating calculi.[69] More than 90% of stones larger than 2 mm are detected as echo-dense spots with a characteristic acoustic shadow.[76,78] Unexpected abscesses may be detected with ultrasound in cases of chronic sialadenitis and autoimmune disorders.[53]

IMAGE INTERPRETATION OF SALIVARY GLAND DISORDERS

Disorders of the salivary glands may be generally classified as inflammatory, noninflammatory, or space-occupying masses. Inflammatory lesions are either acute or chronic, and space-occupying masses are either cystic or neoplastic.[9,57,68] The diagnosis of salivary gland diseases is based on history, clinical and laboratory examination, and biopsy. Occasionally, radiographic procedures such as conventional radiography and contrast sialography are helpful in confirming the diagnostician's clinical impression. Infrequently, one of the more sophisticated imaging techniques such as CT, MRI, scintigraphy, or ultrasound may be useful in establishing the diagnosis and formulating appropriate clinical management protocols.

Inflammatory disorders (sialadenitis)

Acute sialadenitis. The most common acute viral infection of the salivary glands is mumps (epidemic parotitis). Eighty-five percent of the cases occur in the parotid, but the submandibular gland may occasionally be enlarged. Painful swelling of either the parotid or submandibular gland may be unilateral but is typically bilateral. Most commonly

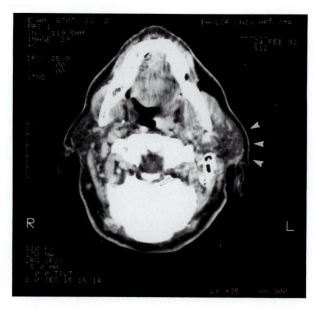

FIG. 30-10. Contrast-enhanced CT image. The left submandibular gland *(arrows)* is larger than the right with no suggestion of abscess formation. Appearance is compatible with diffuse parotitis and cellulitis. (Courtesy Radiology Dept., Baylor University Medical Center, Dallas.)

children between ages 2 and 14, constitutional symptoms are usually present. Diagnosis is based on clinical symptoms and a history of contact with an infected individual.[3,57] Infection by the mumps virus usually confers lifelong immunity, although other viruses such as the Coxsackie, parainfluenza, herpes, echo, and influenza viruses can cause an acute parotitis.[20]

Acute bacterial infections most commonly affect the parotid, but the submandibular gland may also be involved. Most cases are unilateral and may occur at any age. Commonly afflicted are elderly, postoperative, and/or debilitated patients who have poor hygiene as a result of reduced salivary secretion and retrograde infection by the oral flora (usually *Staphylococcus aureus* and *Streptococcus viridans*).[68] Reduced salivary secretion may also be drug related or secondary to occlusion of a major duct.[75] Untreated acute suppurative infections typically form abscesses.[61] Diagnosis is based on clinical observation, constitutional symptoms, and the expression of pus from the duct.

Image interpretation. Sialography is contraindicated in acute infections. Ultrasound may distinguish between diffuse inflammation (echo-free, light image) and suppuration (less echo-free, darker image) along with detection of calculi that are at least 2 mm in diameter.[10,27] Plain films may also

detect radiopaque calculi. MRI, CT, and scintigraphy are not likely to provide additional useful information unless the clinician feels there is some other disorder coincident with the acute infection[4,10,21] (Fig. 30-10).

Chronic sialadenitis. Chronic inflammation may affect any of the major salivary glands, cause extensive swelling, and culminate in fibrosis. This may be a consequence of an untreated acute sialadenitis or associated with some type of obstruction due to calculi, noncalcified organic debris, or stricture (scar or fibrosis) formation in the excretory ducts. Bacteria or viruses may not be demonstrated in the gland or saliva.[1,10] The parotid is most often involved. During periods of painful swelling, pus may be expressed from the ductal orifice, and salivary stimulation may cause pain. Episodic in nature, there are seldom signs of generalized sepsis.

Obstruction of the secretory ducts may result in chronic infections. The obstruction may be congenital or secondary to calculus (sialolithiasis), trauma, infection, or neoplasia. The symptoms are intermittent swelling, pain with eating, and superimposed infection due to stasis. Calculi may form in any of the major or minor salivary glands or their ducts, but usually only one gland is involved. The submandibular gland and Wharton's duct are

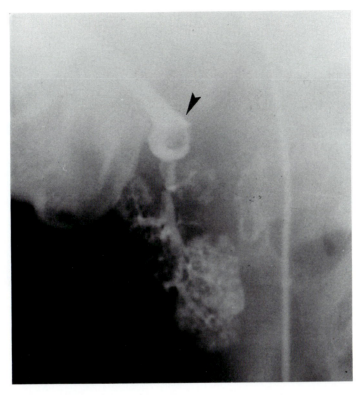

FIG. 30-11. Sialogram. Slightly oblique lateral view demonstrating parenchymal opacification of submandibular gland. Arrow points to a radiolucent obstruction within main duct. Filling of gland parenchyma is patchy, resulting from fibrosis occurring secondary to chronic obstruction.

by far the most frequently involved (83% of cases).[1,27,35] If one stone is found, there is at least a 25% chance that others are present.

Image interpretation. Plain films and ultrasound images are appropriate examinations when there is a clinical suspicion of obstructive calculi (Fig. 30-1). Specific plain film techniques have been described earlier in this chapter. Sialography is helpful in locating obstructions that were not detected with plain radiography, especially if the obstructions are radiolucent (mucous plugs).[17] The contrast agent usually flows around the calculi to fill the duct proximal to the obstruction. The ductal system is frequently dilated proximal to the obstruction. If the obstruction itself is not recognizable, its presence is inferred by the ductal dilation. The calculus is typically less radiodense than the adjacent contrast agent that has flowed around it (Fig. 30-11). Small calculi distal to the end of the cannula or those that are superimposed with contrast agent may be obscured by the technique. Radiolucent obstructions (mucous plugs) appear as filling defects (Fig. 30-12). Sialography should not

be performed if a radiopaque stone has been shown by plain radiography to be in the distal portion of the duct because the procedure may displace it proximally into the ductal system, which might complicate its subsequent removal.

Dilation of the ductal system (sialodochitis) is a prominent sialographic feature of chronic recurrent sialadenitis, most common in the submandibular gland, but seen almost as often in the affected parotid (Fig. 30-13).[1,9,48] If interstitial fibrosis develops, it is evidenced by the sausage-string appearance of the main duct and its major branches produced by alternate strictures and dilations.

CT, MRI, and scintigraphy are not typically indicated in the diagnosis of inflammatory diseases of the salivary glands. It is costly and nonspecific and probably will not provide any more useful information than ultrasonography or sialography. Scintigraphy is an appropriate alternate examination in cases where sialography is contraindicated or not technically possible[73] (Fig. 30-8).

As imaged by ultrasound, dilated ducts and duc-

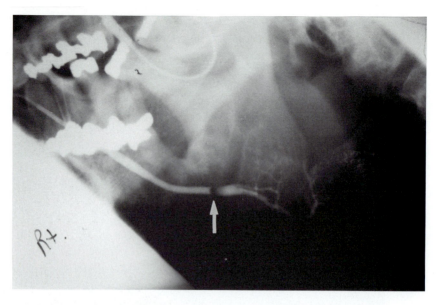

FIG. 30-12. Sialogram. Lateral view of submandibular gland demonstrating a radiolucent obstruction (mucous plug) in the main duct *(arrow)*.

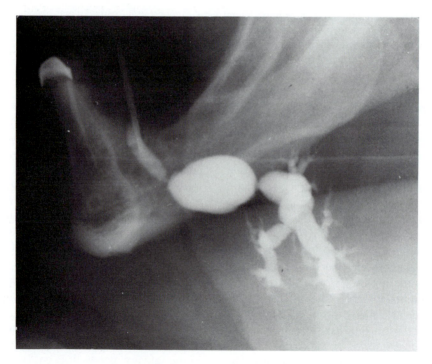

FIG. 30-13. Sialogram. Lateral view of submandibular gland shows intermittent stricture and dilation of the main ducts, referred to as *sialodochitis*.

tal cysts appear as echo-free, dark areas. However, the ultrasound appearance of chronic inflammation is not very specific. Calculi 2 mm or larger can be seen as echo-dense spots, but if they are near the orifice of Wharton's duct, they may be missed because of acoustic shadowing of the mandible.

Autoimmune sialadenitis (myoepithelial sialadenitis). Autoimmune diseases are a group of disorders that affect the salivary glands and that share an autosensitivity. The range of clinical and histopathological manifestations suggests that these disorders represent different developmental stages of the same immunologic mechanisms, differing only in extent and intensity of tissue reaction and that the different forms have a common etiology.[58] The clinical manifestations range from recurrent, painless, unilateral or bilateral swelling of the salivary glands (usually the parotid), to a stage that includes enlargement of the lacrimal glands (Mikulicz's disease). Glandular swelling may be accompanied by xerostomia and xerophthalmia (primary Sjögen's syndrome) and subsequently by a connective tissue disease such as rheumatoid arthritis, progressive systemic sclerosis, systemic lupus erythematosus, or polymyositis (secondary Sjögren's syndrome). The process may progress to benign lymphoepithelial lesions that can assume the proportions of a tumor.[44] A presumptive diagnosis can be made on the basis of any two of the three features: dry mouth, dry eyes, and/or rheumatoid arthritis.[56]

Image interpretation. Sialography is helpful in the diagnosis and staging of autoimmune disorders. Early in the disease, there is the initiation of sialectasia indicated by punctate (smaller than 1 mm) and globular (1 to 2 mm) spherical collections of contrast agent evenly distributed throughout the glands (Fig. 30-14). These collections are referred to as *sialectases*. At this stage, the ductal system typically appears normal. However, the main duct may appear to be normal, but the intraglandular ducts may be narrowed or not even evident.[15] Sialectasia remains after the administration of a sialogogue, which is an indication that contrast agent is pooled extraductally and the acini are still functional.[62,77]

As the disease progresses, the collections of contrast agent increase in size (greater than 2 mm in diameter) and are irregular in shape. These pools of contrast agent are termed *cavitary sialectases*. Cavitary sialectases are fewer in number and less uniformly distributed throughout the glands than are the punctate or globular sialectases (Fig. 30-

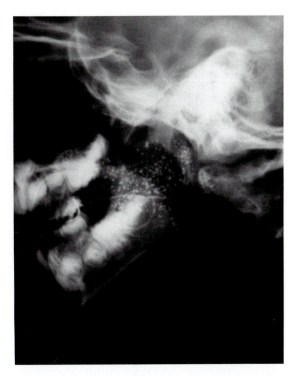

FIG. 30-14. Sialogram of left parotid. Punctate sialectases distributed throughout the gland are suggestive of early stage autoimmune disease. Clinical/histopathologic diagnosis was Sjögren's syndrome. (Courtesy Radiology Dept., Baylor University Medical Center, Dallas.)

15). Progressively larger cavities of contrast agent and dilation of the main ductal system may also be present. At the endpoint of this disorder, there is complete destruction of the gland. Cavitation and glandular fibrosis are the result of intercurrent inflammation.[62,77]

There is a consensus that scintigraphy with ^{99m}Tc pertechnetate is useful for diagnosing and monitoring the progression of Sjögren's syndrome. Impairment of the parotid and submandibular glands is demonstrated by decreased uptake of the pertechnetate as well as the delay in its stimulated excretion.[2] CT, MRI, and ultrasonography are not particularly diagnostic for autoimmune disorders of the salivary glands (see Fig. 30-6).

Noninflammatory disorders (sialadenosis, sialosis)

Metabolic and secretory disorders of the parenchyma are associated with diseases of nearly all the endocrine glands (hormonal sialedenosis), protein deficiencies,[54] malnutrition (dystrophic-

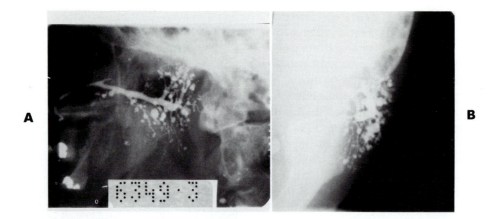

FIG. 30-15. Sialogram of left parotid. Punctate (small spherical), globular (larger spherical), and cavitary (largest nonspherical) sialectases are demonstrated and, with dilation of the main duct, suggests advanced autoimmune disease with retrograde infection in lateral (**A**) and PA (**B**) projections. Clinical/histopathologic diagnosis was Sjögren's syndrome. (Courtesy Radiology Dept., Baylor University Medical Center, Dallas.)

metabolic sialadenosis) in alcoholics,[39] in vitamin deficiencies,[52] and in neurologic disorders (neurogenic sialadenosis).[9] Affected glands are typically hypotrophic.

Image interpretation. Although sialography demonstrates atrophy of the affected glands, CT and MRI provide a more straightforward depiction of the smaller than normal glands. Diminished salivary gland size and a decrease in radioisotope uptake may be apparent upon scintigraphic examination.

Space-occupying masses

Cystic lesions. Cysts of the salivary glands are rare (less than 5% of all salivary gland masses) and most commonly occur unilaterally in the parotid. They may progress to proportions that are clinically palpable and must be distinguished from neoplasia. Salivary gland cysts may be congenital (branchial), lymphoepithelial, dermoid, or acquired, including the mucous retention cyst (obstruction from any etiology).[3,61] Cystic salivary lesions may be intraglandular or extraglandular in nature. Cystic neoplasms are discussed separately in this chapter. Mucous extravasation pseudocysts lack an epithelial lining and result from ductal rupture. Mucous retention cysts occur secondary to partial obstruction of a minor salivary gland. Ranulas are retention cysts that usually occur secondary to obstruction of the sublingual duct. Benign lymphoepithelial cysts are thought to be a sequel of cystic degeneration of salivary inclusions within lymph nodes.

HIV-associated multicentric parotid cysts have been reported. These lesions are accompanied with cervical lymphadenopathy, occur bilaterally, and are usually in the superficial portion of the parotid[59,63] (Fig. 30-16). A secondary parotitis may develop.[36]

Image interpretation. Upon sialographic examination, cystic masses are only indirectly visualized by the displacement of the ducts arching around it.[72] Cystic lesions typically appear as well-circumscribed, low-density areas when examined with CT, with CT numbers between 10 and 18 HU.[61] The scintigraphic appearance of a salivary gland cyst, like other space-occupying lesions, is that of an area of decreased radioisotope uptake ("cold spot"). As such, scintigraphy does not contribute to the development of a differential diagnosis because malignant tumors also do not take up the radioisotope.[4] When imaged with ultrasound, cysts demonstrate sharp margins and are echo-free (represented as a dark area)[25] (Fig. 30-17).

Benign tumors. Salivary gland tumors are relatively uncommon and occur in less than 0.003% of the population.[64] They account for about 3% of all tumors.[18] About 80% of the salivary tumors arise in the parotid, 5% in the submandibular, 1% in the sublingual, and 10% to 15% in the minor salivary glands.[16] The majority (70% to 80%) of these tumors occur in the superficial lobe of the parotid. Most are benign or low-grade malignancies. High-grade malignancies are uncommon.[60,66] Thus, the incidence of benign neoplasms of major

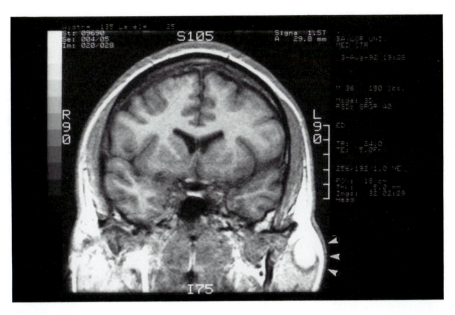

FIG. 30-16. Coronal section MR image. High signal mass *(arrows)* in left parotid diagnosed as a cyst. This patient was found to be HIV-positive. (Courtesy Radiology Dept., Baylor University Medical Center, Dallas.)

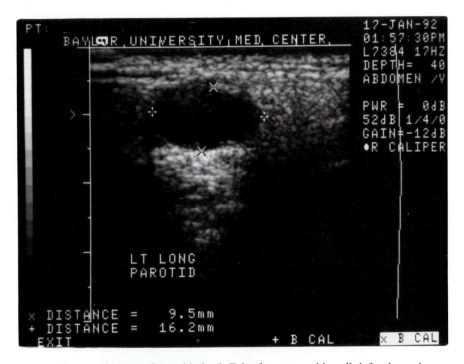

FIG. 30-17. Ultrasound image of parotid gland. Echo-free mass with well-defined margins presents a typical cystic appearance. (The lesion borders are marked with *x* and + signs.) (Courtesy Radiology Dept., Baylor University Medical Center, Dallas.)

salivary glands appears to increase with the size of the gland.[48]

Pleomorphic adenoma (benign mixed tumor). Of the salivary gland tumors, 75% are pleomorphic adenomas:[16] 80% found in the parotid, 4% in the submandibular gland, 1% in the sublingual gland, and 10% in the minor salivary glands. Those in the minor salivary glands occur most frequently in the palate, cheek, tongue, lip, and floor of the mouth, respectively.[57] This tumor most likely arises from ductal epithelium and typically occurs in the fifth decade of life as a slow-growing, unilateral, encapsulated, asymptomatic mass.[74] There is a slight female predilection.[38] The pleomorphic adenoma is characteristically sharply circumscribed and infrequently lobulated.[7] Following excision, 50% of the cases recur.

IMAGE INTERPRETATION. Benign tumors and low-grade malignancies typically have well-defined margins, which are most apparent on CT or MRI examinations. The CT image of a pleomorphic adenoma is a sharply circumscribed and essentially round lesion that is homogeneous and has a higher density than the adjacent glandular tissue. The higher density of the submandibular gland often obscures the tumor in this area and

requires intravenous contrast infusion CT procedures to enhance the diagnostic value of the image.[69] CT sialography may also be helpful in delineating the tumor. Measurement of the CT densities of tumors is not predictive except for lipid-containing or vascular tumors.[6,47]

T1-weighted MRI images show the pleomorphic adenoma as an area of relatively low signal intensity (dark) compared to adjacent glandular tissue. The tumor has a greater intensity (intermediate brightness) on proton density–weighted MRI images and appears as a homogeneous high-intensity (bright) area on T2-weighted images (see Fig. 30-7). Foci of low signal intensity (dark) usually represent areas of fibrosis or dystrophic calcifications. The presence of calcification (signal void) in a parotid neoplasm favors pleomorphic adenoma as the diagnosis.[19]

Pleomorphic adenoma does not usually concentrate [99m]Tc. Thus, the tumor appears as a cold spot when examined by scintigraphy.[14] The ultrasound appearance of the tumor is characteristically that of a hypoechoic, slightly heterogeneous, solid lesion with distinct borders. Sialography is of limited value but may suggest a space-occupying mass when the ducts are compressed or smoothly dis-

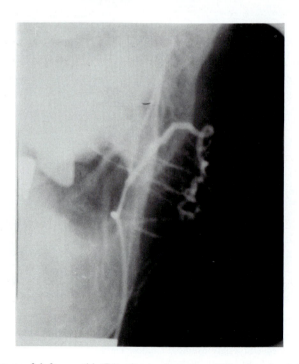

FIG. 30-18. Sialogram of left parotid (PA view). A mass within the gland is inferred by the appearance of the ducts displaced around the lesion. This is referred to as the "ball-in-hand" appearance, which is typical of a space-occupying mass. (Courtesy Radiology Dept., Baylor University Medical Center, Dallas.)

placed around the lesion (the "ball-in-hand" appearance)[27,61] (Fig. 30-18).

Warthin's tumor (papillary cystadenoma lymphomatosum). Warthin's tumor is the second most common benign neoplasm of the salivary gland, accounting for 2% to 6% of the parotid tumors. In the parotid, it is usually found in the inferior lobe of the gland. This unusual type of tumor probably arises from proliferating salivary ducts trapped in lymph nodes during embryogenesis. Slow growing and painless, it is frequently bilateral, and 30% are cystic. Warthin's tumor typically afflicts males over the age of 40.[8]

IMAGE INTERPRETATION. CT, MRI, and scintigraphy are the preferred techniques for imaging Warthin's tumor. The CT and MRI appearance of this tumor is not specific and is typical of benign salivary tumors as described for pleomorphic adenoma.[64,66] In general, the detection of this lesion with MRI is as good as or better than with CT.[55]

Warthin's tumors are characteristically intensely "hot" on ^{99m}Tc scans. Oncocytomas (oxyphil adenoma) may also accumulate the ^{99m}Tc, but they are less common (less than 1% of all salivary gland tumors) and less likely to be bilateral[50] (see Fig. 30-8). The ultrasound presentation is that of a solid mass (hypoechoic)[25] (see Fig. 30-9).

Hemangioma. Hemangioma is the most frequent nonepithelial salivary neoplasm, accounting for 50% of the cases;[12] 85% arise in the parotid. It is the most common salivary gland tumor during infancy and childhood. The average age at diagnosis is 10 years, with 65% occurring in the first two decades of life. They are frequently unilateral and asymptomatic. There is a 2:1 female predilection.[23] Treatment is by local excision and is sometimes delayed, as some hemangiomas undergo spontaneous remission.

IMAGE INTERPRETATION. Phleboliths are common in this tumor and are well demonstrated on plain films. They appear as calculi with a radiolucent center. Displaced ducts curving about the mass may also be apparent on sialography.[61] Hemangiomas image as cold spots with scinigraphy.[14] The CT presentation of hemangioma is a soft tissue mass that is well distinguished from surrounding tissue, especially when IV contrast enhancement is used.

Although the ultrasound image of this tumor usually demonstrates well-defined margins, ill-defined margins also occur. Strongly hypoechoic, hemangiomas may have a complex ultrasonographic appearance due to the multiple interfaces in the lesion.[25] Phleboliths appear as multiple hyperechoic areas within the body of the gland itself.[10]

Lipoma. Although lipoma is the most common mesenchymal tumor, it is rare in the salivary glands.[5,13] Occurring predominantly in females, the clinical presentation is typical of benign salivary tumors. Most are found in the parotid as round or ovoid, moderately firm nodules that are usually painless and mobile. The treatment of choice is local excision, and the prognosis is good.[12]

IMAGE INTERPRETATION. CT is particularly helpful in imaging lipomas because of the high lipid content of the tumor, which has a very low CT number (-80 HU). T2-weighted MRI examinations demonstrate lipomas as dark masses, which differ from the bright T2 appearance of most salivary tumors.[48] The sialographic, ultrasound, and scintigraphic appearances of the lipoma are typical of those previously described for benign salivary tumors.

Malignant tumors. About 20% of tumors in the parotid are malignant as compared with 50% to 60% of the submandibular tumors, 90% of the sublingual tumors, and 60% to 75% of minor salivary tumors. Thus, the incidence of malignant tumors appears to decrease with increasing size of the gland.[48]

Mucoepidermoid carcinoma. The mucoepidermoid carcinoma is the most common salivary gland malignancy (35%).[1,27] Just over half occur in the major salivary glands; the rest are found in the minor glands, where the palate is the most frequent location. The aggressiveness of the lesion is variable. Although the highest prevalence is in the fifth decade of life, mucoepidermoid carcinoma is the most common malignant salivary gland tumor in children.[23,67] There is a slight predilection for females. The low-grade variety rarely metastasizes. Clinically, this tumor appears as a movable, slow-growing, painless nodule not unlike a pleomorphic adenoma. It is usually only 1 to 4 cm in diameter. The prognosis is good, with more than 95% of the patients surviving 5 years.[26]

In contrast to the low-grade variety of this tumor, high-grade mucoepidermoid carcinoma often causes facial pain and paralysis, has ill-defined margins, and is relatively immobile. Metastasis by blood and lymph are common, with recurrence in half of the patients following excision. The prognosis is poor, with only a 25% 5-year survival rate.[26]

IMAGE INTERPRETATION (LOW-GRADE TUMOR). Low-grade mucoepidermoid carcinomas are not

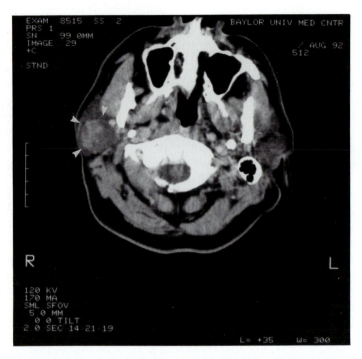

FIG. 30-19. Contrast-enhanced CT images. Mass in right parotid *(arrows)* demonstrates a poorly defined, heterogeneous, slightly lobulated appearance. Poorly defined margins suggest a low-grade malignancy rather than a benign tumor, even though the CT appearance of both is similar. Histopathologic diagnosis was low-grade mucoepidermoid carcinoma. (Courtesy Radiology Dept., Baylor University Medical Center, Dallas.)

apparent on plain films unless destructive changes to adjacent osseous structures have occurred. The sialographic, CT, MRI, ultrasonographic, and scintigraphic presentations of this tumor are similar to those previously described for benign salivary tumors. However, low-grade mucoepidermoid carcinoma may present a lobulated or irregular sharply circumscribed appearance on CT or MRI scans[20,33] (Fig. 30-19).

IMAGE INTERPRETATION (HIGH-GRADE TUMOR). The radiographic diagnosis of high-grade mucoepidermoid carcinoma typically rests on the appearance of irregular margins and/or ill-defined form when the mass is examined with CT or MRI. The CT section shows the tumor as an irregular homogeneous mass, not much denser than the parenchyma. A CT-sialogram shows the tumor as a sharply defined homogeneous mass that is considerably denser than on the conventional CT. CT is also a reliable technique for the detection of bony invasion.[31,47]

In contrast to the low-grade malignancies and benign neoplasms, high-grade mucoepidermoid carcinomas, like most high-grade malignancies,

have low signal intensity on T1-weighted and T2-weighted MRI images.[7,60] The T1-weighted images have lower intensity (dark) than the surrounding structures and are relatively homogeneous. T2-weighted images of the tumor are more intense (brighter) than T1-weighted images, just slightly lower than the surrounding tissues and more heterogeneous than on the T1-weighted images. It follows then that, regardless of clinical presentation and margins, low signal intensity is suggestive of a high-grade malignancy.[60]

Cavitary sialectasia and ductal displacement may be noted on sialographic images. Like most malignant tumors, the ultrasonographic presentation of high-grade mucoepidermoid carcinoma is a homogeneous echo pattern with low to medium reflectivity (due to the densely packed cells) and attenuation. Diffuse or poorly defined margins are also apparent on ultrasound. Although benign tumors and low-grade malignancies usually have well-defined margins and high-grade malignancies usually have poorly defined margins, an inflammatory response in a benign neoplasm may mimic the appearance of a high-grade malignancy.[3,60]

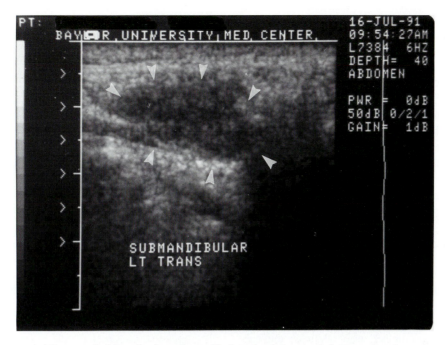

FIG. 30-20. Ultrasound. Mass in the submandibular gland *(arrows)* demonstrates heterogeneous hypoechoic pattern compared to adjacent tissue. The histopathologic diagnosis was adenoid cystic carcinoma. (Courtesy Radiology Dept., Baylor University Medical Center, Dallas.)

Malignant mixed tumor. Comprising about 15% of malignant salivary neoplasms, the term *malignant mixed tumor* actually applies to three histopathologic variations. The first is that of a pleomorphic adenoma that inexplicably metastasizes. The second variation contains malignant epithelial or mesenchymal components (carcinosarcoma). The third is a pleomorphic adenoma in which the epithelial component is malignant (carcinoma ex pleomorphic adenoma).[12] The latter is the most common of the three. The tumor typically begins as a slowly growing mass that suddenly undergoes rapid proliferation often accompanied by pain and facial paralysis. Metastasis is early, and the prognosis is unfavorable.

IMAGE INTERPRETATION. The image of this tumor is similar to that of the high-grade mucoepidermoid carcinoma previously described.

Adenoid cystic carcinoma. Of all malignant salivary gland tumors, 23% are adenoid cystic carcinomas. It is the most common malignant neoplasm to develop in the minor salivary glands (70%), usually occurring on the palate. The balance of those in the major salivary glands occur in the parotid. Occurring most often between the ages of 40 and 60 years, there is no gender predilection. Although this slow-growing tumor appears histologically benign, it does metastasize by the blood (usually to the liver) and recurs locally. Only 30% of patients are free of tumor 5 years after removal. Spreading of the tumor along nerve sheaths often causes burning and stinging pain, hypoesthesia, and paralysis in the distribution of a cranial nerve.[33] Paralysis may develop before the tumor is clinically evident.[3]

IMAGE INTERPRETATION. The appearance of this tumor is nonspecific and similar to that of high-grade mucoepidermoid carcinoma, previously described. Ultrasonography may demonstrate echo-free cystic areas (Fig. 30-20).

Adenocarcinoma. The adenocarcinoma accounts for 6.4% of all salivary gland tuimors. Typically occurring in older individuals (40 to 79 years), adenocarcinoma has a slight female gender predilection; 50% occur in the parotid, 15% in the submandibular, 12% in the sublingual, and 15% in the minor salivary glands. The mass is usually about 2 to 3 cm in diameter when first diagnosed. Some are reported to be as large as 2.5 cm in diameter. Of the affected individuals, 25% experience pain or paresthesia. The tumor spreads to adjacent tissues by direct invasion in approximately 25% of the cases. The prognosis for parotid adenocarcinomas is much more favorable than for those of the submandibular gland.[26,76]

IMAGE INTERPRETATION. The image of this tumor is nonspecific and similar to that previously described for mucoepidermoid carcinoma.

Acinic cell carcinoma. The vast majority (96%) of acinic cell carcinomas occur in the parotid. This tumor has a slight female predilection, and peak incidence is 30 to 49 years of age. It is typically low grade and less than 3 cm in size upon diagnosis. Pain and paresthesia may be present in high-grade cases. Interestingly, the pain associated with acinic cell carcinoma is not considered to be as grave a sign as in other malignant salivary tumors.[12,26]

IMAGE INTERPRETATION. The appearance of this tumor is nonspecific and similar to that previously described for mucoepidermoid carcinoma.

Lymphoma. Although primary lymphoma of the salivary glands is rare, metastatic lymphomas are relatively common. The typical site is the parotid, but this tumor can also occur in the submandibular gland. Peak incidence is 50 to 70 years of age. There is a 2:1 female gender predilection. Most malignant lymphomas are low- or intermediate-grade tumors.[12,26] Malignant lymphoma has an incidence 40 times greater in patients with Sjögren's syndrome than in the general population.[57]

IMAGE INTERPRETATION. The image of this tumor is nonspecific and similar to that previously described for mucoepidermoid carcinoma.

Squamous cell carcinoma. About 2% of salivary gland neoplasms and 8% of malignancies are squamous cell carcinomas. The clinical presentation is similar to that described for low- and high-grade mucoepidermoid carcinomas.[26]

IMAGE INTERPRETATION. The appearance of this tumor is nonspecific and similar to that previously described for mucoepidermoid carcinoma.

Metastatic tumors. Metastasis of tumors to the salivary glands may occur. Metastatic lesions in the parotid are more common than to the other salivary glands because of the parotid's extensive lymphatic and circulatory components. Most metastatic lesions of the parotid are via the lymphatic system and include squamous cell carcinoma, lymphoma, and melanoma. Although considerably fewer lesions are the result of hematogenous dissemination, metastasis from the lung, breast, kidney, and gastrointestinal tract has been reported.[26,66]

IMAGE INTERPRETATION. The variable and nonspecific interpretive appearance of metastatic tumors of the salivary glands is similar to that previously described for mucoepidermoid carcinoma.

REFERENCES

1. Adams GL: Disorders of the salivary glands. In Adams GL, Boies LR, Hilger PA, editors: *Boies fundamentals of otolaryngology,* Philadelphia, 1989, WB Saunders.
2. Arrago JP and others: Scintigraphy of the salivary glands in Sjögren's syndrome, *J Clin Path* 40:1463-1467, 1987.
3. Batsakis JG: *Tumors of the head and neck: clinical and pathological considerations,* Baltimore, 1979, Williams & Wilkins.
4. Bocchini T and others: Bilateral Warthin's tumor, *Clin Nucl Med* 13:892-895, 1988.
5. Boering G: *Diseases of the oral cavity and salivary glands,* Baltimore, 1971, Williams & Wilkins.
6. Bryan RN, Miller RH, Ferreyro RI, Sessions RB: Computed tomography of the major salivary glands, *AJR* 139:547-554, 1982.
7. Byrne MN, Spector G, Garvin CF, and Gado MH: Preoperative assessment of parotid masses: a comparative evaluation of radiographic techniques to histologic diagnosis, *Laryngoscope* 99:284-292, 1989.
8. Chaudhuri TK, Stadalnik RC: Salivary gland imaging, *Sem Nucl Med* 10:400-401, 1980.
9. Chilla R: Sialadenosis of the salivary glands of the head, *Acta Otorhinolaryngolgica* 26:1-38, 1981.
10. Curtin HD: Assessment of salivary gland pathology, *Otolaryngol Clin North Am* 21:547-573, 1988.
11. Da-Xi S, Hai-Xiong S, Qiang Y: The diagnostic value of transonography and sialography in salivary gland masses, *Dentomaxillofac Radiol* 16:37-45, 1987.
12. Del Balso AM and others: Diagnostic imaging of the salivary glands and periglandular regions. In Del Balso AM, editor: *Maxillofacial imaging,* Philadelphia, 1990, WB Saunders.
13. Del Balso AM, Williams E, Tane TT: Parotid masses: current modes of diagnostic imaging, *Oral Surg* 54:360-364, 1982.
14. De Rossi G, Salvatori M, Valenza Y: Radioisotope studies under pathologic conditions. In De Rossi G: *Radioisotope study of salivary glands,* Boca Raton, 1987, CRC.
15. Dijkstra PF: Classification and differential diagnosis of sialographic characteristics in Sjögren syndrome, *Semin Arthritis Rheum* 190:10-187, 1980.
16. Eneroth C-M: Salivary gland tumors in the parotid gland and the palate region, *Cancer* 27:1415-1418, 1971.
17. Epivatianos A, Harrison JD, Dimitriou T: Ultrastructural and histochemical observations on microcalculi in chronic submandibular sialadenitis, *J Oral Path* 16:514-517, 1987.
18. Evans RW, Cruickshank AH: Epithelial tumors of the salivary glands. In Bennington JL, editor: *Major problems in pathology,* vol 1, Philadelphia, 1970, WB Saunders.
19. Freling JJM, Graamans K: Magnetic resonance imaging of the parotid gland. In Graamans K, Van Den Akker HP, editors: *Diagnosis of salivary gland disorders,* Boston, 1991, Kluwer.
20. Garcia RR: Differential diagnosis of tumors of the salivary glands with radioactive isotopes, *Int J Oral Surg* 3:330-334, 1974.
21. Gates GA: Sialography and scanning of the salivary glands, *Otolaryngol Clin North Am* 10:379-390, 1977.
22. Gooding GAW: Gray scale ultrasound of the parotid gland, *AJR* 134:469-472, 1980.
23. Greer RO, Mierau GW: *Tumors of the oral mucosa and jaws in infants and children,* Denver, 1980, University of Colorado Medical Center.

24. Greyson ND, Nikko AM: Radionuclide salivary scanning, *J Otolaryngol* 11:3-47, 1982.

25. Gritzman G: Sonography of the salivary glands, *AJR* 153:161-166, 1989.

26. King JJ, Fletcher GH: Malignant tumors of the major salivary glands, *Radiology* 100:381-384, 1971.

27. Langlais RP, Benson BW, Barnett DA: Salivary gland dysfunction: infections, sialoliths, and tumors, *Ear Nose Throat J* 68:758-770, 1989.

28. Langlais RP, Kasle MJ: Sialolithiasis: the radiolucent stones, *Oral Surg Oral Med Oral Pathol* 40:686-690, 1975.

29. Langland OE, Langlais RP, McDavid WD, DelBalso AM: *Panoramic radiology*, ed 2, Philadelphia, 1989, Lea & Febiger.

30. Langland OE, Sippy FH, Langlais RP: *Textbook of dental radiology*, Springfield, 1984, Charles C Thomas.

31. Lloyd RE, Ho KH: Combined CT scanning and sialography in the management of parotid tumors, *Oral Surg Oral Med Oral Pathol* 65:142-144, 1988.

32. Lowman RM, Cheng GK: Diagnostic radiology. In Rankow RM, Polayes IM, editors: *Diseases of the salivary glands*, Philadelphia, 1976, WB Saunders.

33. Lufkin RB, Hanafee WN: *MRI of the head and neck*, New York, 1992, Raven.

34. Mafee MF: Oral cavity, oropharynx, upper neck and salivary glands. In Valvassori GE, Buckingham RA, Carter BL, et al, editors: *Head and neck imaging*, New York, 1988, Thieme.

35. Manashil GB: *Clinical sialography*, Springfield, Ill, 1978, Charles C Thomas.

36. Marcusen AC, Sooy CD: Otolaryngologic and head and neck manifestations of acquired immunodeficiency syndrome (AIDS), *Laryngoscope* 95:401-405, 1985.

37. McGahan JP, Walter JP, Bernstein L: Evaluation of the parotid gland: comparison of sialography, non-contrast computed tomography, and CT sialography, *Radiology* 152:453-458, 1984.

38. Mirich DR, McArdle CB, Kulkarni MV: Benign pleomorphic adenomas of the salivary glands: surface coil MR imaging versus CT, *J Comp Assist Tomogr* 11:620-623, 1987.

39. Mishkin FS: Radionuclide salivary gland imaging, *Sem Nucl Med* 11:258-265, 1981.

40. Mooyaart EL, Panders AK, Vermeij A: CT scanning of tumors in or near the parotid or submandibular glands, *Diagn Imaging Clin Med* 53:177-181, 1984.

41. Moss-Salentijn L, Moss ML: Developmental and functional anatomy. In Rankow RM, Polayes IM, editors: *Diseases of the salivary glands*, Philadelphia, 1976, WB Saunders.

42. Neiman HL, Phillips JF, Jaques DA, Brown, TL: Ultrasound of the parotid gland, *J Clin Ultrasound* 4:11-13, 1975.

43. New PFJ, Rosen BR, Brady TJ, et al: Potential hazards and artifacts of ferromagnetic and nonferromagnetic surgical and dental materials and devices in nuclear magnetic resonance imaging, *Radiology* 147:139-148, 1983.

44. Oestberg Y: The clinical picture of benign lymphoepithelial lesions, *Clin Otolaryngol* 8:381-390, 1983.

45. Ollerenshaw R, Ross SS: Radiological diagnosis of salivary gland disease, *Br J Radiol* 24:538-548, 1951.

46. Provenza DV: *Fundamentals of oral histology and embryology*, Philadelphia, 1972, JB Lippincott.

47. Rabinov K, Kell T, Gordon PH: CT of the salivary glands, *Radiol Clin North Am* 22:145-159, 1984.

48. Rabinov K, Weber AL: *Radiology of the salivary glands*, Boston, 1985, GK Hall.

49. Rankow RM, Polayes IM: *Diseases of the salivary glands*, Philadelphia, 1976, WB Saunders.

50. Reede DL, Bergeron RT, Osborn AG: CT of the soft tissues of the neck. In Bergeron RT, Osborn AG, Som PM, editors: *Head and neck imaging excluding the brain*, St Louis, 1984, Mosby.

51. Rothberg R, Noyek AM, Goldfinger M, Kassel EE: Diagnostic ultrasound imaging of parotid disease: a contemporary clinical perspective, *J Otolaryngol* 13:232-240, 1984.

52. Salomon T: Enlarged parotids and pellagra, *J Trop Med Hyg* 61:253-259, 1958.

53. Saluk PH, Swartz JD, Korsvik H, Marlowe FI: High resolution computed tomography of the major salivary glands: current status, *J Comput Assist Tomogr* 9:39-50, 1985.

54. Sandstead HR, Koehn CJ, Sessions SM: Enlargement of the parotid gland in malnutrition, *Am J Clin Nutr* 3:198-214, 1955.

55. Schaefer SD, Maravilla KR, Close LG, et al: Evaluation of NMR versus CT for parotid masses: a preliminary report, *Laryngoscope* 95:945-950, 1985.

56. Scully C: Sjögren's syndrome: clinical and laboratory features, immunopathogenesis, and management, *Oral Surg* 62:510-523, 1986.

57. Seifert G, Miehlke A, et al: *Diseases of the salivary glands*, Stuttgart, 1986, George Thieme Verlag.

58. Shafer WG, Hine MK, Levy BM: *A textbook of oral pathology*, ed 4, Philadelphia, 1983, WB Saunders.

59. Shugar JMA, Som PM, Jacobson AL, et al: Multicentric parotid cysts and cervical adenopathy in AIDS patients, a newly recognized entity: CT and MR manifestations, *Laryngoscope* 98:772-775, 1988.

60. Som PM, Biller HF: High-grade malignancies of the parotid gland identification with MR imaging, *Radiology* 173:823-826, 1989.

61. Som PM, Sanders RE: The salivary glands. In Bergeron RT, Osborne AG, Som PM, editors: *Head and neck imaging excluding the brain*, St Louis, 1984, Mosby.

62. Som PM, Shugar JM, Train JS, Biller HF: Manifestations of parotid gland enlargement: radiographic, pathologic, and clinical correlation, part 1, the autoimmune pseudosialectasias, *Radiology* 141:415-419, 1981.

63. Sooy CD: The impact of AIDS on otolaryngology—head and neck surgery. In EN Meyeres, editor: *Advances in otolaryngology—head and neck surgery,* vol 1, Chicago, 1987, Year Book.

64. Swartz JD and others: MR imaging of parotid mass lesions: attempts at histopathologic differentiation, *J Comput Assist Tomogr* 13:789-796, 1989.

65. Tabor EK, Curtin HD: MR of the salivary glands, *Radiol Clin North Am* 27:379-392, 1989.

66. Thawley SE, Panbje WR: *Comprehensive management of head and neck tumors*, Philadelphia, 1987, WB Saunders.

67. Tran L, Sadeghi A, Hanson D, et al: Major salivary gland tumors: treatment results and prognostic factors, *Laryngoscope* 96:1139-1144, 1986.

68. Travis LW, Hecht DW: Acute and chronic inflammatory diseases of the salivary glands: diagnosis and management, *Otolaryngol Clin North Am* 10:329-338, 1977.

69. Van den Akker HP: Diagnostic imaging in salivary gland disease, *Oral Surg* 66:625-637, 1988.

70. Van den Akker HP, Busemann-Sokole E: Absolute indications for salivary gland scintigraphy with ^{99m}Tc-pertechnetate, *Oral Surg* 60:440-447, 1985.

71. Van den Akker HP, Busemann-Sokole E: Salivary gland scintigraphy with 99m Tc-pertechnetate. In Graamans K, Van den Akker HP, editors: *Diagnosis of salivary gland disorders,* Boston, 1991, Kluwer.

72. Van den Akker HP, Dijkstra PF: Plain radiography and sialography. In Graamans K, Van den Akker HP, editors: *Diagnosis of salivary gland disorders,* Boston, 1991, Kluwer.

73. Van den Akker HP, Graamans K: Concluding remarks and recommendations. In Graamans K, Van den Akker HP, editors: *Diagnosis of salivary gland disorders,* Boston, 1991, Kluwer.

74. Vermey A, Oldhoff J, Panders AK, et al: Benign epithelial parotid tumors: results of treatment, *J Clin Oncol* 5:389, 1979.

75. Warpeha RL: Masses in the neck. In Wood NK, Goaz PW, editors: *Differential diagnosis of oral lesions,* ed 4, St Louis, 1991, Mosby.

76. Watson MG: Investigation of salivary gland disease, *Ear Nose Throat J* 68:84-93, 1989.

77. Whaley K and others: Sialographic abnormalities in Sjögren's syndrome, rheumatoid arthritis, and other arthridities and connective tissue diseases: a clinical and radiological investigation using hydro-static sialography, *Clin Radiol* 23:474-482, 1972.

78. Wittich GR, Scheible WF, Hajek PC: Ultrasonography of the salivary glands, *Radiol Clin North Am* 23:29-37, 1985.

79. Yune HY, Klatte EC: Current status of sialography, *Am J Roent Rad Therapy Nuc Med* 115:420-428, 1972.

31

BARTON M. GRATT and VIVEK SHETTY

Implant Radiology

PURPOSE AND DEFINITION OF A DENTAL IMPLANT

Dental implants are devices made of biocompatible materials, such as titanium root-forms, that are used to restore form and function to the oral cavity. Implants aid in the replacement of missing teeth and missing bone, and provide a preferable alternative to standard fixed and removable dental appliances. Successful implants depend on close physical contact between the implant fixture and the supporting bone. Such intimate fixture-to-bone integration may be best observed with light microscopy.[5] Dental implants work as part of a system combining metal fixtures integrated with bone, abutments screwed to fixtures, and a variety of dental appliances attached to abutments. In the clinical practice of implant therapy, (1) treatment planning, (2) the assessment of implant integration, and (3) ongoing implant function are all assisted by radiography.

TYPES OF IMPLANTS

Dentistry uses a wide variety of implants that integrate with bone and are readily identified on radiographs. The most common types of dental implants are manufactured in the form of a root (Fig. 31-1). These are called *endosteal* implants as they are placed in bone. Additional types of endosteal dental implants are formed as metal blades (Fig. 31-2). Subperiosteal implants are custom-made to the shape of the alveolar ridge, where they are secured in place with screws (Fig. 31-3). They are often used to support complete dentures. Fractured mandibles are commonly repaired using bone plates, another type of implant system (Fig. 31-4). Bone tray implants are used to support bone marrow or bone fragments to induce new bone formation (Fig. 31-5). Other implant systems are also used to replace condyles, articular eminences, mental tubercles, or missing bone (Fig. 31-6). This chapter focuses on the use of radiographs for treatment planning and follow-up of patients receiving endosteal dental implants.

CLINICAL ASSESSMENT OF PATIENTS FOR DENTAL IMPLANTS

To determine if a patient will benefit from dental implant therapy, it is necessary to conduct a careful clinical assessment of the patient's overall health. Specific medical conditions that increase risk of

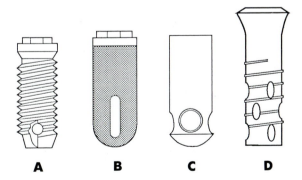

FIG. 31-1. Four varieties of root-form implant fixtures designed for bone integration: **A,** Brånemark; **B,** IMZ; **C,** Integral; **D,** ITI.

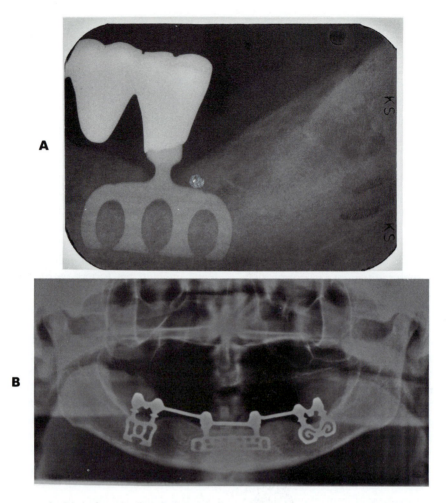

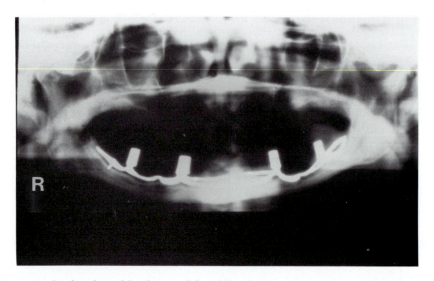

FIG. 31-2. A, Blade-form implant integrated with bone to support a fixed bridge (periapical radiograph of the mandibular molar region). **B,** Three blade implants integrated with bone using common abutments to support a mandibular denture (panoramic radiograph). (**A** courtesy Dr. Krishan Kapur, Los Angeles.)

FIG. 31-3. A subperiosteal implant used for aiding denture support (panoramic radiograph).

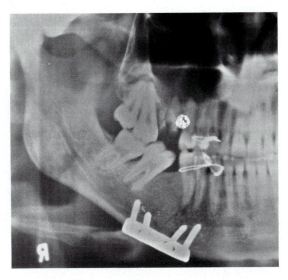

FIG. 31-4. A bone plate (with screws) used to aid the healing of a fractured mandible (panoramic radiograph).

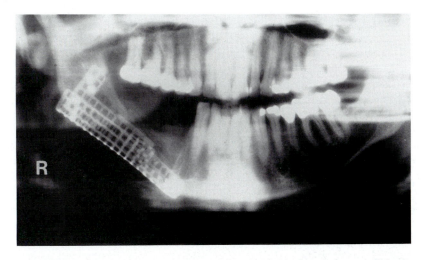

FIG. 31-5. A bone tray used to reconstruct a defect in the body of the mandible (panoramic radiograph).

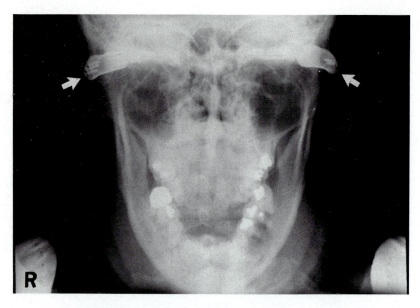

FIG. 31-6. Two bone replacement implants substituting for the surgically altered right and left articular eminences (reverse Towne [skull] projection).

TABLE 31-1. Commonly used radiographic procedures with time intervals for treatment planning and assessment of dental implants.

	Time (months)	Radiographic procedures
Treatment planning	−1	Periapical, panoramic, cross-sectional tomography, CT, cephalometry
Surgery (fixture placement)	0	Films only for corrections of problems
Healing	0–3	Films only for correction of problems
Remodeling	4–12	Periapical, panoramic (assess loading of fixture)
Maintenance (without problems)	13+	Periapical, panoramic (follow-up every 3 years)
Problem present (any time)		Periapical, panoramic, cross-sectional tomography, stereoscopy

implant failure include uncontrolled diabetes, alcoholism, blood dyscrasia, and immunosuppression from drug therapy[10] or other diseases. In addition, it is necessary to evaluate the implant site clinically and radiographically. The clinician must rule out the presence of periapical or periodontal diseases that could adversely affect implantation as well as the physical adequacy of the site.

RADIOLOGIC ASSESSMENT OF DENTAL IMPLANT SITES (TREATMENT PLANNING)
Overview of implant imaging procedures

Common radiographic procedures used for treatment planning and the ongoing evaluations of den-

tal implants are shown in Table 31-1. The selection and timing of each phase of implant therapy vary according to individual patient needs. The variety of radiographic techniques available to assist the clinician include periapical radiography, panoramic radiography, cross-sectional tomography, computer-aided tomography (CT), lateral skull or cephalometric radiography, and stereoscopic (paired) x-ray imaging. Each of these imaging modalities offers the clinician unique diagnostic information in the assessment of dental implants.

Treatment planning

Radiography offers the sole method of noninvasive analysis of the bone required for implant

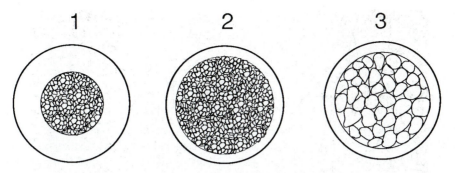

FIG. 31-7. Wide variations in bone quality present in potential implant therapy patients: *1*, greatest thickness of cortical bone, most desirable for supporting an implant; *2*, less cortical bone; *3*, least favorable for implants, having similar cortical bone to no. 2 but with thinner cancellous bone and larger trabecular spaces; this type offers the least support for an implant. These differences in bone quality reflect function. (Adapted from Brånemark P-I, Zarb GA, Albrektsson T: *Tissue integrated prostheses*, Chicago, 1985, Quintessence.)

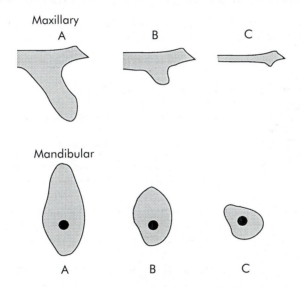

FIG. 31-8. Wide variations in morphology of the anterior maxilla and posterior mandible in potential implant therapy patients. In the maxilla note the anterior nasal spine (to the *right* in each drawing) and the floor of the nasal fossa *(top)*. **A,** No resorption of the alveolar bone. **B,** Effect of progressive resorption or loss of alveolar bone. **C,** Virtually complete resorption. In the mandible **A** shows complete alveolar bone and **C** extreme resorption of the alveolar bone. (Adapted from Brånemark P-I, Zarb GA, Albrektsson T: *Tissue integrated prostheses*, Chicago, 1985, Quintessence.)

therapy.[19] Bone assessment includes an analysis of the quantity and quality of the bone that is available by location. It is important that the bone has the necessary dimensions and quality to provide support for the implant fixture. Cortical bone is best suited to withstand the functional loading forces placed on dental implants. A greater thickness of cortical bone increases the likelihood of successful implantation with osseous integration. Similarly, the larger the vertical height of the available bone,

the longer the implant that can be placed (Fig. 31-7). The chances of successful implantation are increased as more bone is available for anchorage and over which the masticatory forces will be distributed. Figure 31-8 is a diagram of a classification system for assessing maxillary and mandibular residual ridges. It is important to evaluate the potential implant site carefully for any evidence of abnormality. Potential problems such as impacted teeth, root tips, osteomyelitis or other pathologic bone changes must be corrected before or during implant surgery.

Dental implants vary from approximately 5 to 15 mm in length. Accurate bone measurements help to determine the optimal length of the proposed implant. Radiographic images may be magnified, with the magnification factor varying with the radiographic technique used. This magnification factor must be taken into account when calculating the dimensions of bone at the implant site. The dimensions obtained from the radiographs (usually in millimeters) are divided by the magnification factor (usually 1.0 to 1.8) to obtain the actual dimensions of the available bone. Particular attention should be given to adjoining anatomic structures including the mental foramen, inferior alveolar canal, incisal canals, existing teeth, and the borders of the maxillary sinus and nasal fossa, all of which may limit the placement of longer implants. Each radiographic technique has a different magnification factor; some are variable (panoramic, periapical), others are fixed (tomography), and still others may be corrected to life size by computer (reformatted CT scan). Following a successful clinical assessment, the minimum radiological assessment for initiating implant therapy employs periapical radiography and, when necessary, panoramic radiography.

Periapical radiographs

Periapical radiographs are commonly used in implant therapy treatment planning.[14] Maxillary and mandibular periapical radiographs may be used to evaluate remaining teeth and remaining alveolar bone in the mesial-to-distal dimension. They may also be used to assess the alveolar bone for vertical height, architecture (or shape), and quality (bone density, amount of cortical bone, and amount of trabecular bone). Some clinicians have advocated special repositioning devices to aid realignment of the film with the implant fixture and the x-ray beam over time.

Panoramic radiographs

In treatment planning, panoramic radiographs are useful to evaluate the alveolar bone, all remaining teeth, and the location of critical anatomic structures and to rule out the presence of bone disease. Panoramics have broader anatomic coverage as compared to periapical radiographs. This is useful for estimating crestal alveolar bone and cortical boundaries of the inferior alveolar nerve, maxillary sinus, and nasal fossa. However, it must

be emphasized that panoramics have variable magnification that may vary on an individual panoramic radiograph from 10% to 30% (see Chapter 12). Also, structures on panoramic radiographs are not localized in the facial-lingual dimension.

Cross-sectional tomographs

Alveolar bone height and width and the location of critical anatomic structures in the proposed surgical field can be best determined with cross-sectional tomographs.[2,6,8,17,18] Cross-sectional tomography employs a coordinated movement of the x-ray beam and the film allowing for a selected image plane (see Chapter 13). For cross-sectional implant tomography, the x-ray beam is directed perpendicular to the bone in the region of the proposed implant. This orientation is critical for accurate imaging. Cross-sectional radiographs are generally made on multidirectional tomographic equipment (such as Scanora, Tomax, Polytome, Stratomatic). Magnification on cross-sectional tomographic x-ray units varies from machine to machine, but the magnification for any individual unit is fixed, uniform, and known. The magnification factor must be considered when making bone measurements from the tomograms. Uniform magnification with cross-sectional tomography allows for accurate bone height and bone width measurements in a facial-to-lingual and vertical dimension (Fig. 31-9, *A* and *B*).

Panoramic radiographs may also be used with dental splints (stents) containing metal markers (ball bearings) as an aid to cross-sectional tomography. The metal markers are placed in a hole(s) drilled in the splint over the area of the potential implant site. The splint is placed in the mouth before making the radiograph. These markers are radiographic guides for selecting the sites for the cross-sectional tomographs. The panoramic radiograph shows the markers in the mesial-to-distal dimension, whereas the cross-sectional tomographs image the marker and all bony structures in the facial-to-lingual and vertical dimension (Fig. 31-9, *C*).

Computer-aided tomography (CT scan)

Computer-aided tomography (CT scan) is a computer-generated tomographic image (see Chapter 13) commonly used for implant treatment planning, especially for edentulous patients requiring a large number of implants.[4] Typically during treatment planning, a patient receives a tomographic or CT examination, but not both. The patient is placed in

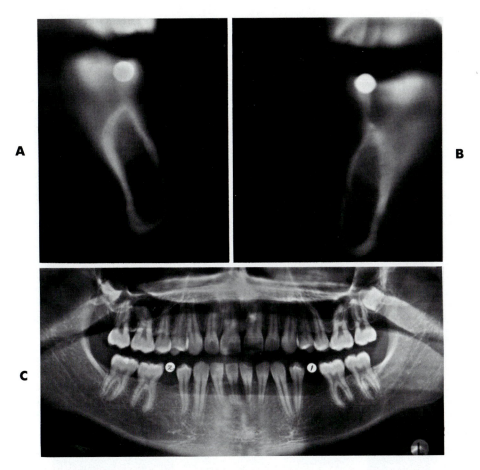

FIG. 31-9. A and **B,** Examples of a cross-sectional tomogram of the mandible. Note the use of metal markers for confirming the location of the tomographic section (or slice). **C,** Panoramic radiograph taken with the splint in place (containing metal guide markers) used in treatment planning for implant therapy.

a supine position in the CT scanner, and multiple scans are made in the axial plane. The patient's head must be still during scanning. Restrain the patient's head in a head holder to limit movement if necessary. When imaging the maxillary arch, position the hard palate perpendicular to the floor (or CT table). For imaging the mandibular arch, align the alveolar ridge of the mandible perpendicular to the floor.[12,13] To verify proper head alignment view the lateral or "scout" radiograph of the selected jaw and make alignment corrections as needed. Each axial CT image is 1.5 mm thick. The mandible usually requires 30 to 35 axial CT sections, the maxilla 20 to 30.[6,9,12,13]

After axial CT images are acquired, they undergo computer manipulation termed *multiplanar reformatting* (or MPR).[3,15,16,21] Typically three ba-

sic images are produced: axial images with a superimposed curve, cross-sectional images, and panoramic images. This advanced computer technique allows the formation of two-dimensional images in multiple-image planes. Using a reformatting dynamic mode and bone algorithm, it is possible to produce cross-sectional images from axial CT scans that are either perpendicular or parallel to an individually selected dental arch. One of the axial scans that demonstrates the full contour of the mandible (or maxilla) and is at the level of the dental roots is used for reformatting. Using the computer, a series of sequential dots is placed on the selected scan and an arch (or curve) is generated by the computer connecting these dots (Fig. 31-10). This arch is unique for each jaw. The computer then generates a series of lines perpendicular to the

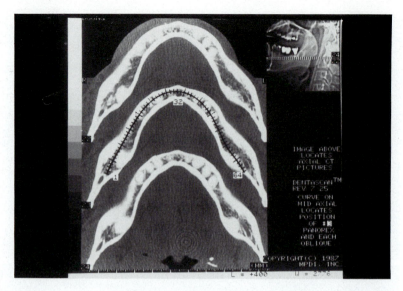

FIG. 31-10. Three axial CT scans of the mandible with an operator-drawn arch and computer-generated 2 mm spaced cross-hatches *(middle image)*. Each crosshatch relates to a numbered reformatted cross-sectional projection of the mandible (or maxilla). The scout orientation image *(upper right corner)* indicates the orientation of the mandible during scanning.

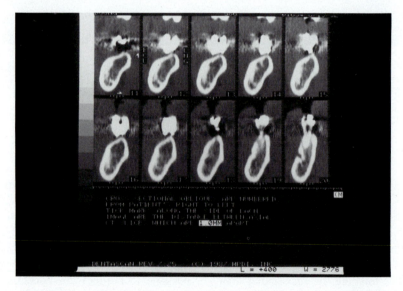

FIG. 31-11. CT data reconstructed using a special (bone-shaping) program to enhance visibility of bone trabeculae. Axial cross-sectional data are reformatted into frontal and lateral planes of view using a selected software reformatting program (CT/MPR). Oblique planes of view are reformatted perpendicular to the curved line *(arch)* demarcating the curvature of the alveolar ridge (Fig. 31-10). These oblique images represent true cross-sections of the mandible. The CT cross-sectional images contain a measuring scale that allows accurate measurements to be made from the radiographic images.

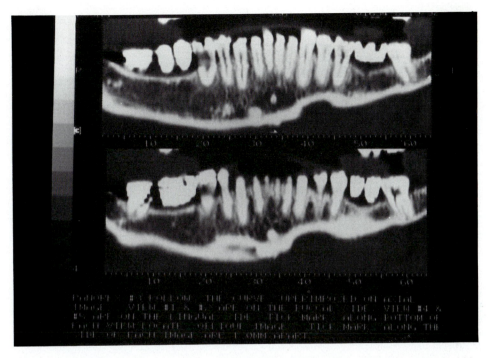

FIG. 31-12. Same CT data reformatted parallel with the curved line *(arch)* of the alveolar ridge (Fig. 31-10). These images are similar in orientation to panoramic radiographs. The reformatted images contain a measuring scale that allows for accurate anatomic measurement.

previously drawn arch. These lines are numbered sequentially and can be varied from 1 to 10 mm apart, usually at 2-mm intervals. These marks indicate the position of each axial slice and the corresponding cross-sectional image (Fig. 31-11). In addition, the computer displays a ruler next to the image to allow measurements of the cross-sectional images. Finally, the computer may draw additional arches paralleling the original hand-drawn arch. It then makes panoramic-type reformations along the planes indicated by the lines (Fig. 31-12). Dental splints with opaque markers are sometimes used during the scanning procedure.[7] The splints are used to correlate position and inclination of proposed fixture placement.[13]

In contrast to cross-sectional tomography, CT-reformatted implant studies usually display life-size images. Like tomographic examinations, reformatted CT implant studies provide information regarding the continuity of cortical plates of bone and vertical bone height measurements of the mandible and the maxilla. Unlike tomograms, reformatted CT implant studies can provide radiographic density values of cortical plates and medullary bone. In addition, the dimensions and contour of

soft tissue may also be evaluated.[9] The presence of any metallic restorations, however, may cause considerable image artifact. In addition, a CT examination subjects a patient to greater radiation exposure than cross-sectional tomography. CT examinations are typically more expensive than tomographic examinations.

Lateral cephalometric radiography (lateral skull radiography)

Lateral cephalometric radiography (or lateral skull projection) (see Chapter 11) is occasionally used for implant treatment planning. The lateral skull projection may be taken with or without the patient wearing a splint containing metal markers. The projection provides an overview of the jaws giving information regarding inclinations of existing teeth, potential inclinations of implants, and an overview of the relationships of the anterior dentoalveolar structures. It also provides an especially good view of the maxillary sinuses. In addition, it is a useful cross-sectional type of projection for evaluation of the middle structures of the lower and middle face, including the alveolar bone in the maxillary and mandibular midline (Fig. 31-13).

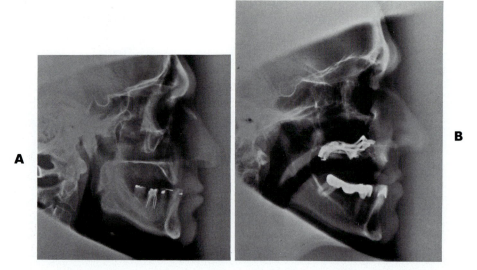

FIG. 31-13. Lateral cephalometric radiographs used to develop treatment plan and evaluate dental implants. **A,** Radiograph for assessing the midline alveolar bone of the mandible and the maxilla. **B,** Radiograph for evaluating a subperiosteal implant positioned over the maxilla. In addition to imaging the midline alveolar bone, this projection demonstrates the maxillary sinus region.

SURGICAL IMPLANTATION

Upon completion of treatment planning, the next phase of implant therapy is surgical insertion of the implant. It is important to prepare the implant site for insertion of the fixture with great care. Injury to the bone around the implant fixture by excessive thermal or mechanical trauma during surgery may reduce the probability of successful osseous integration.

Usually there is no indication for radiography at the time of surgery. If some surgical complication arises (e.g., unplanned perforation of cortical bone), individually selected radiographs may be useful (e.g., periapical radiographs, panoramic radiographs, cross-sectional tomographs). Some clinicians have advocated the application of electronic digital imaging systems (e.g., RVG System, Visualix System, Flashdent System, Sens-A-Ray System, see Chapter 13). All of these electronic systems are useful for rapid bone imaging during surgery. Rapidly obtained electronic images may be useful for determining the depth of a hole created in bone and for evaluating implant positioning relative to other anatomic structures (e.g., the mandibular canal).

FOLLOW-UP ASSESSMENT

It is common to use periapical radiographs in the ongoing assessment of dental implants.[14] Mesial and distal marginal bone height is measured utiliz-

ing predetermined fixture threads as a reference point. This is compared to the bone level in previous radiographs. The presence of distinct bone margins indicates successful osseous integration. Resorptive changes, if present, are evidenced by the apical migration of the alveolar bone or the development of indistinct margins (Fig. 31-14). These adverse changes are progressive and should be differentiated from the initial resorptive changes (bone loss) around the cervical area induced by surgery. Studies indicate that the rate of marginal bone loss after successful implantation is 1.2 mm in the first year and subsequently tapers off to about 0.1 mm in the succeeding years.[19] Sometimes areas of marginal bone gain may also be noted.

A clinically stable fixture is invariably associated with the radiographic appearance of normal bone in intimate contact with the implant surface.[19] The development of a thin radiolucent area that closely follows the outline of the implant usually correlates with implant mobility and is an important indicator of failed osseous integration (Fig. 31-15). In addition, changes in the periodontal ligament space of the nearest tooth (natural abutment) are useful in demonstrating functional competence of the prostheses-implant system. Any widening of the periodontal ligament space, as compared to preoperative radiographs, indicates poor stress distribution and forecasts implant failure.

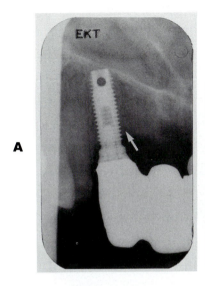

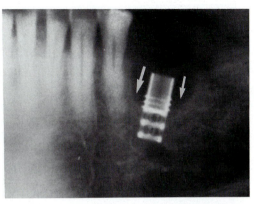

FIG. 31-14. **A,** Marginal bone loss ("saucerization" type) around the cervical region of a root-form dental implant (periapical radiograph). **B,** Marginal bone loss around the cervical region of a root-form dental implant (panoramic radiograph). (**A** courtesy Dr. Michael Hamada, Los Angeles.)

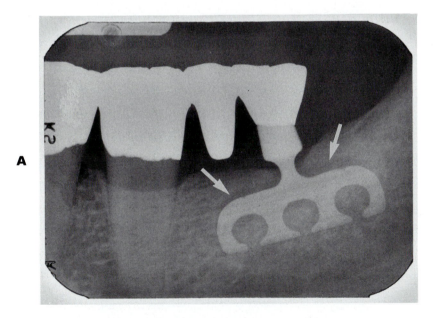

FIG. 31-15. **A,** Perifixtural bone loss around a blade-type dental implant, indicating failed osseous integration (periapical radiograph). *Continued.*

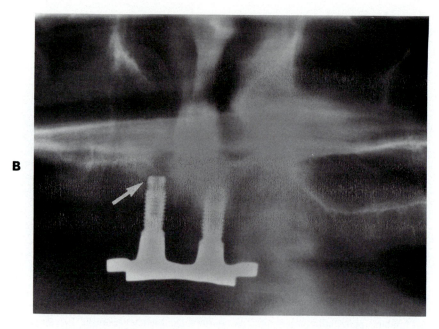

FIG. 31-15, cont'd. B, Perifixtural bone loss around a root-form dental implant, indicating failed osseous integration (panoramic radiograph). (**A** courtesy Dr. Krishan Kapur, Los Angeles.)

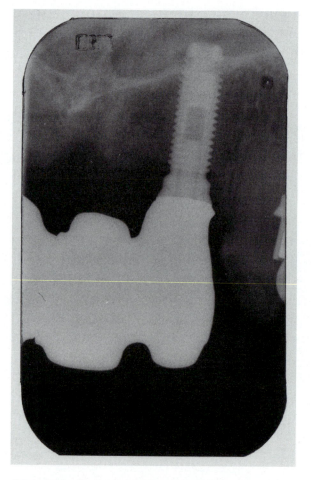

FIG. 31-16. Successful dental implant, in place for more than 5 years (periapical radiograph). It is supporting a fixed bridge. (Courtesy Dr. Michael Hamada, Los Angeles.)

Periapical radiographs are made at the time of abutment attachment in order to verify correct seating of the abutment on the implant. After these radiographs have been made, and in the apparent absence of any problems, periapical radiographs should be made at approximately 3-year intervals to assess the ongoing success of the dental implant (Fig. 31-16). Panoramic radiographs also assist in the ongoing evaluation of implant systems. Like periapical radiographs, they may be used to evaluate the alveolar bone around the implant for integration, to check the adaptation of the abutment to the fixture, to assess the implant system for fracture, and, finally, to assess the surrounding bone and teeth for viability and the absence of disease.

PROBLEM ASSESSMENT

Problems may arise at any time following the placement of dental implants. When the problem is limited to a specific region, a periapical radiograph may be sufficient for bone and implant evaluation. Panoramic radiographs may be appropriate to examine a broader region. In cases where alveolar bone height cannot be readily determined from a single periapical or panoramic radiograph (due to superimposition of anatomic structures, for example), stereoscopic paired radiographs are useful.[4,19] To observe these paired images, use specially designed stereoviewing glasses. The three-dimensional images allow the observer to localize the alveolar bone margin and are also helpful in detecting infrabony pockets or a soft tissue layer between the implant fixture and the bone. This finding indicates failed bony integration. Stereoscopic images are also useful for inspecting the fixture for fracture and assessing the functional relations of the mechanical parts of the dental implant.[19]

GENERAL REFERENCES

Brånemark P-I, Zarb GA, Albrektsson T: *Tissue integrated prostheses,* Chicago, 1985, Quintessence, p 350.

Worthington P, Brånemark P-I: *Advanced osseointegration surgery: applications in the maxillofacial region,* Chicago, 1992, Quintessence, p 403.

SPECIFIC REFERENCES

1. Abrahams JJ: CT assessment of dental implant planning, *Oral Maxillofacial Surg Clin North Am* 4:1-18, 1992.
2. Fernandes RJ, Azarbal M, Ismail YH, Curtin HD: A cephalometric tomographic technique to visualize the buccolingual and vertical dimensions of the mandible, *J Prosthet Dent* 58:466-470, 1987.
3. Golec TS: CAD-CAM multiplanar diagnostic imaging for subperiosteal implants, *Dent Clin North Am* 30:85-95, 1986.
4. Hollender L, Rockler B: Radiographic evaluation of osseointegrated implants of the jaws, *Dentomaxillafac Radiol* 9:91-95, 1980.
5. Jeffcoat MK: Digital radiology for implant treatment planning and evaluation, *J Dentomaxillofac Radiol* 21:203-207, 1992.
6. Klinge B, Petersson A, Maly P: Location of the mandibular canal: comparison of macroscopic findings, conventional radiography, and computed tomography, *Int J Oral Maxillofac Implants* 4:327-331, 1989.
7. Kopp CD: Stent-assisted CT in three phases of osseointegration, *Academy Osseointegration* 1:1-6, 1985.
8. Lindh C, Petersson AR: Radiologic examination of the mandibular canal: a comparison between panoramic radiography and conventional tomography, *Int J Oral Maxillofac Implants* 4:249-253, 1989.
9. McGivney GP, Haughton V, Stradt JA, et al: A comparison of computer-assisted tomography and data-gathering modalities in prosthodontics, *Int J Oral Maxillofac Implants* 1:55-59, 1986.
10. Schnitman P: Implant success through patient education, *Dentistry Today* 11:38-41, 1992.
11. Schwarz MS, Rothman SLG, Rhodes L, et al: Computed tomography: part I, preoperative assessment of the mandible for endosseous implant surgery, *Int J Oral Maxillofac Implants* 2:137-142, 1987.
12. Schwarz MS, Rothman SLG, Rhodes L, et al: Computed tomography: part II, preoperative assessment of the maxilla for endosseous implant surgery, *Int J Oral Maxillofac Implants* 2:143-148, 1987.
13. Schwarz MS, Rothman SLG, Chafetz N, et al: Computed tomography in dental implantation surgery: osseointegration, *Dent Clin North Am* 33:555-597, 1989.
14. Sewerin I: Identification of dental implants on radiographs, *Quintessence Int* 23:611-618, 1992.
15. Shimura M, Babbush CA, Majima H, et al: Presurgical evaluation for dental implants using a reformatting program of computed tomography: maxilla/mandible shape pattern analysis (MSPA), *Int J Oral Maxillofac Implants* 5:175-180, 1990.
16. Smith RA: New developments and advances in dental implantology, *Oral Maxillofac Surg Infections* 2:42-54, 1992.
17. Stella JP, Tharanon W: A precise radiographic method to determine the location of the inferior alveolar canal in the posterior edentulous mandible: implications for dental implants. Part 1, technique, *Int J Oral Maxillofac Implants* 5:15-22, 1990.
18. Stella JP, Tharanon W: A precise radiographic method to determine the location of the inferior alveolar canal in the posterior edentulous mandible: implications for dental implants. Part 2, clinical application, *Int J Oral Maxillofac Implants* 5:23-28, 1990.
19. Strid K-G: Radiographic results. In Brånemark P-I, Zarb GA, Albrektsson T, editors: *Tissue integrated prostheses,* Chicago, 1985, Quintessence.
20. Strid K-G: Radiographic procedures. In Brånemark P-I, Zarb GA, Albrektsson T: *Tissue integrated prostheses,* Chicago, 1985, Quintessence.
21. Wishan MS, Bahat O, Krane M: Computed tomography as an adjunct in dental implant surgery, *Int J Oral Maxillofac Implants* 8:31-47, 1988.

Index

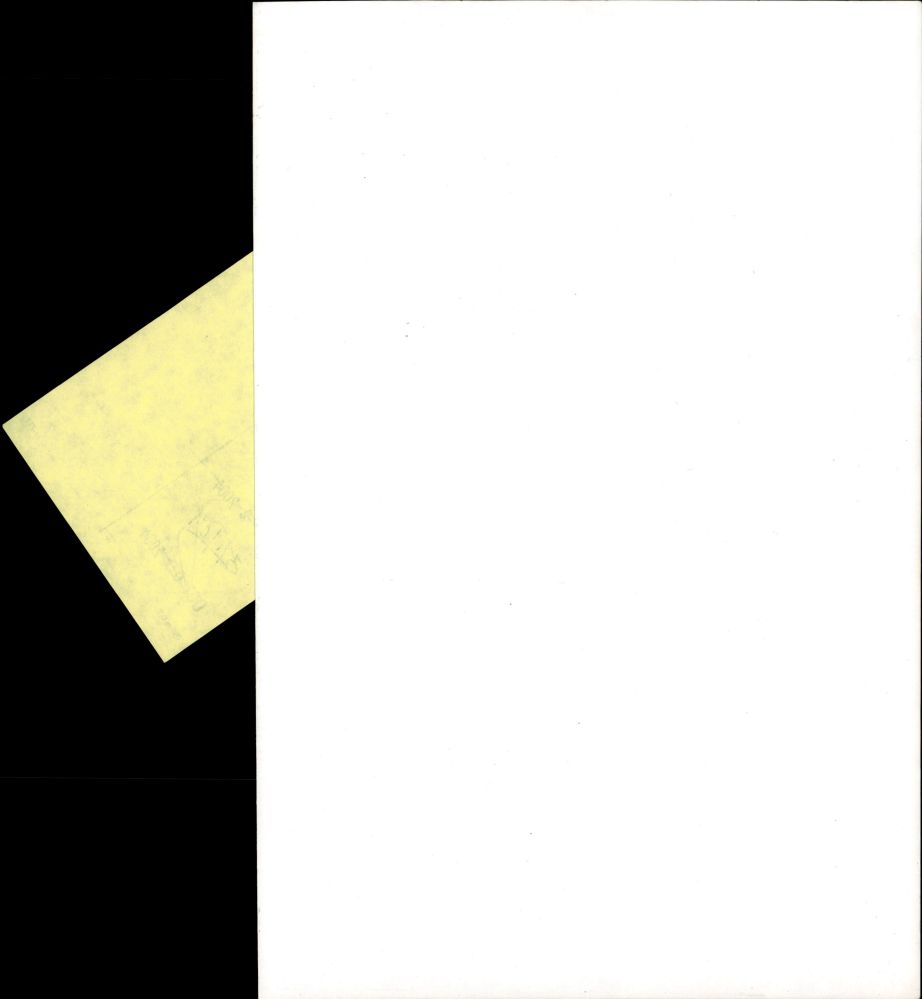

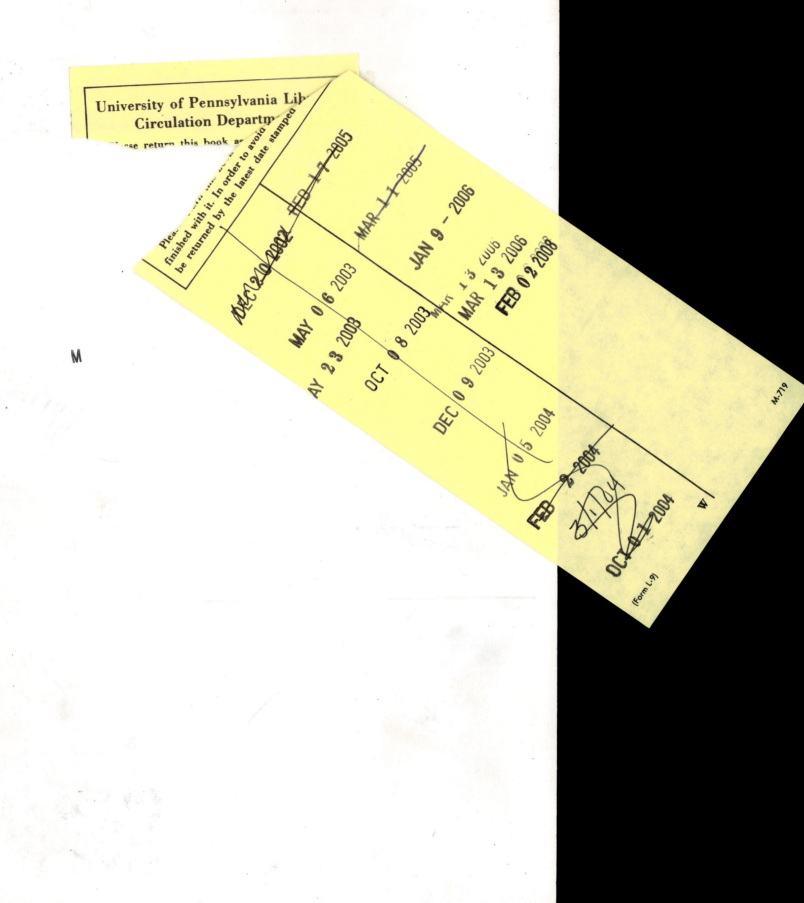